ACSM's
Exercise Testing and Prescription

ACSM's Exercise Testing and Prescription

EDITORS

Madeline Paternostro Bayles, PhD, FACSM, ACSM-CEP, ACSM-PD

Department of Kinesiology, Health, and Sport Science
Indiana University of Pennsylvania
Indiana, Pennsylvania

Ann M. Swank, PhD, FACSM, ACSM-CEP, ACSM-PD

Human Performance Lab
University of Louisville
Louisville, Kentucky

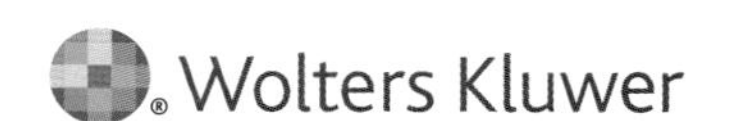

Philadelphia • Baltimore • New York • London
Buenos Aires • Hong Kong • Sydney • Tokyo

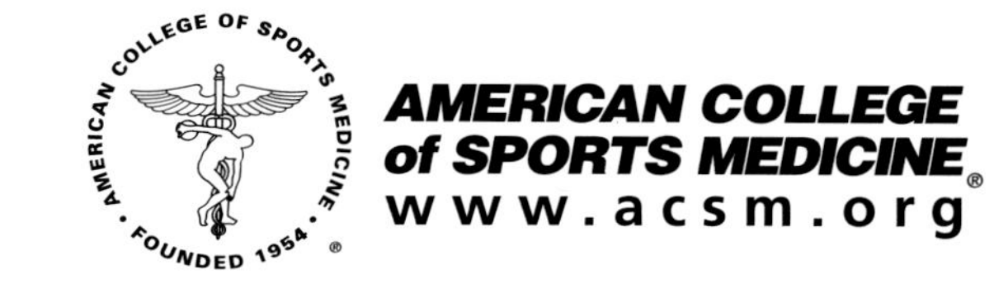

Executive Editor: Michael Nobel
Senior Product Development Editor: Amy Millholen
Editorial Coordinator: Lindsay Ries
Marketing Manager: Shauna Kelley
Production Project Manager: Barton Dudlick
Design Coordinator: Stephen Druding
Manufacturing Coordinator: Margie Orzech
Compositor: Absolute Service, Inc.
ACSM Publications Committee Chair: Jeffrey Potteiger, PhD, FACSM
ACSM Chief Content Officer: Katie Feltman
ACSM Development Editor: Angela Chastain

First Edition

9 8 7 6 5 4 3 2 1

Printed in China

Library of Congress Cataloging-in-Publication Data

Names: Bayles, Madeline P., editor. | Swank, Ann Marie, editor. | American College of Sports Medicine, issuing body.
Title: ACSM's exercise testing and prescription / editors, Madeline P. Bayles, Ann M. Swank.
Other titles: American College of Sports Medicine's exercise testing and prescription | Exercise testing and prescription
Description: First edition. | Philadelphia : Wolters Kluwer, [2018] | Includes bibliographical references and index.
Identifiers: LCCN 2017046016 | ISBN 9781496338792
Subjects: | MESH: Exercise Test | Exercise Tolerance | Exercise Therapy
Classification: LCC RM701.6 | NLM WG 141.5.F9 | DDC 615.8/2076--dc23 LC record available at https://lccn.loc.gov/2017046016

To purchase additional copies of this book, call our customer service department at (800) 638-3030 or fax orders to (301) 223-2320. International customers should call (301) 223-2300.

For more information concerning the American College of Sports Medicine certification and suggested preparatory materials, call (800) 486-5643 or visit the American College of Sports Medicine Website at www.acsm.org.

Foreword

ACSM's Resource Manual for Guidelines for Exercise Testing and Prescription, first published in 1988, was developed to be a comprehensive, explanatory companion text to *ACSM's Guidelines for Exercise Testing and Prescription*. After much consideration and research, ACSM's Publications Committee, with the support of ACSM's Committee on Certification and Registry Board (CCRB), determined that there was a need to reenvision the *Resource Manual* to meet the evolving needs of the field. Out of this strategic planning, two resources that could be paired with *Guidelines* in a classroom setting were developed: this book — *ACSM's Exercise Testing and Prescription* — and another book (*ACSM's Clinical Exercise Physiology*).

We couldn't have selected better editors than the two individuals who led this project. Madeline Paternostro Bayles and Ann M. Swank brought together leading experts in the field to present the most accurate and up-to-date information. You'll find they have provided the latest scientific information in accordance with the standard set forth by *ACSM's Guidelines for Exercise Testing and Prescription*.

We hope you will be as pleased as we are with their work and find *ACSM's Exercise Testing and Prescription*, first edition, to be an asset to your toolbox.

Jeffrey A. Potteiger, PhD, FACSM
Chair, ACSM's Publications Committee
Dean, The Graduate School
Authorizing Institutional Official
Research Integrity Officer
Grand Valley State University
Grand Rapids, Michigan

Preface

This first edition of *ACSM's Exercise Testing and Prescription* is geared toward undergraduate students studying exercise physiology as well as those seeking ACSM certifications. This book will be a useful resource for those wishing to translate the knowledge of exercise into practice. *ACSM's Exercise Testing and Prescription* is based on the most up-to-date information provided in *ACSM's Guidelines for Exercise Testing and Prescription*, 10th edition.

Organization

This book is divided into four separate parts to assist the reader in navigating the deeper knowledge base within each area. **Part I: Physical Activity and Health** covers the description, the recommended amounts, and the benefits of physical activity as well as the detrimental impact of inactivity. **Part II: Preparticipation Screening, Fitness Assessment, and Interpretation** provides the latest of the preparticipation health screening recommendations and health-related components of fitness (cardiorespiratory fitness, muscular fitness, body composition, and functional and flexibility assessments). **Part III: Exercise Prescription** covers the general principles of exercise prescription and provides guidelines for three stages that occur across the lifespan (pregnancy, children and youth, and older adults. **Part IV: Exercise Testing and Prescription for Special Populations** refines the exercise testing, prescription, and progression information for a variety of special populations beyond the content presented in *ACSM's Guidelines for Exercise Testing and Prescription*, 10th edition.

Features

Parts I–III emphasize educating the reader regarding a variety of topics important to the health and fitness practitioner from physical activity to screening to prescription. Chapters 9–23 include frequency, intensity, time, and type (FITT) **tables**, which expand on the FITT principle presented in *ACSM's Guidelines for Exercise Testing and Prescription*, 10th edition. Each chapter within Part IV presents a real-world **case study** selected specifically for the special population to bridge the gap between science and practice and also provide contextual framework for practitioners in working with each of these special populations. **Case study questions** are integrated throughout these chapters to guide the reader through assessment and prescription.

Additional Resources

ACSM's Exercise Testing and Prescription includes additional resources for students and instructors that are available on the book's companion Web site at http://thepoint.lww.com.

Students can access:

- Online Case Studies

Approved adopting instructors will be given access to the following resources:

- PowerPoint lecture outlines
- Test Generator
- Image Bank, including all figures and tables from the text

See inside the front cover of this text for more details, including the passcode you will need to gain access to the Web site.

Updates for the book can be found at http://certification.acsm.org/updates.

Acknowledgments

The authors wish to thank members of the ACSM's Committee on Certification and Registry Board (CCRB) for the original concept of this book as well as the ACSM's Publications Committee, Greg Dwyer, Jeffrey A. Potteiger, and, in particular, Dierdra Bycura, for the effort they took to get this diverse publication reviewed. The hardworking individuals from both these committees are tireless in their efforts to produce excellent work that represents the ACSM. Thank you to Deb Riebe and coauthors of *ACSM's Guidelines for Exercise Testing and Prescription*, 10th edition (*GETP10*) for always accepting my calls and for producing a book of such high standards and quality which served as a guide in the development of this publication. Finally, thank you to the individual chapter authors. Thank you for the high-quality work that we asked you to create and the attention you paid to making sure that this book is a useful tool for all students and exercise professionals.

Additionally, this publication could not have come to a completion without the patience (lots of it) and guidance of Katie Feltman, ACSM Chief Content Officer, and Michael Nobel, WK Executive Editor. Additional gratitude and thanks to Amy Millholen, WK Senior Product Development Editor; Robin Bushing, Developmental Editor; and Angela Chastain, ACSM Editorial Assistant; for their enormous display of patience and hard work in working with Ann and I through this process.

From Madeline Paternostro Bayles: On a personal note, I want to thank my family, son, and daughter for their support and especially my husband, Bob, to whom I promised not to say yes to writing anything else. Also, my IUP colleagues who put up with me during this process. Also, this book is dedicated to the memory of an extraordinary person and member of the CCRB, Dr. Teresa Connelly Fitts, FACSM — gone too soon, but an inspiration to all who knew her.

From Ann M. Swank: On a personal note, I would like to thank my family (every one of them) and my colleagues for helping me through this very worthwhile project. I am very happy to have this textbook as my last professional activity before retiring. I would also like to thank the entire staff of ACSM and WK for their patience and strong work ethics and professionalism in completing this project. It has been worthwhile.

Madeline Paternostro Bayles, PhD, FACSM, ACSM-CEP, ACSM-PD
Ann M. Swank, PhD, FACSM, ACSM-CEP, ACSM-PD

Contributors

Robert S. Axtell III, PhD, FACSM, ACSM-ETT
Southern Connecticut State University
New Haven, Connecticut
Chapters 5 and 9

Frank J. Bosso, PhD
Youngstown State University
Youngstown, Ohio
Chapter 6

Richard Casaburi, MD, PhD
Los Angeles Biomedical Research Center
Torrance, California
Chapter 16

Scott Cheatham, DPT, PhD
California State University Dominguez Hills
Carson, California
Chapter 19

Dawn Podulka Coe, PhD, FACSM, ACSM-CEP
University of Tennessee
Knoxville, Tennessee
Chapter 9

Sheri R. Colberg-Ochs, PhD, FACSM
Old Dominion University (Emerita)
Norfolk, Virginia
Chapter 14

Donald M. Cummings, PhD
East Stroudsburg University
East Stroudsburg, Pennsylvania
Chapter 8

Jay Dawes, PhD, ACSM-EPC
University of Colorado, Colorado Springs
Colorado Springs, Colorado
Chapter 7

Gregory B. Dwyer, PhD, FACSM, ACSM-CEP, ACSM-RCEP, ACSM-PD, ACSM-ETT, ACSM-EIM3
East Stroudsburg University
East Stroudsburg, Pennsylvania
Chapter 8

Yvonne L. Eaglehouse, MPH, PhD, ACSM-EPC, ACSM-EIM2
John P. Murtha Cancer Center
Walter Reed National Military Medical Center
Bethesda, Maryland
Chapter 20

Nicholas H. Evans, MHS, ACSM-CEP
Beyond Therapy and The Pulse Spinal Cord Injury Laboratory
Shepherd Center
Atlanta, Georgia
Chapter 23

Chris Garvey, MSN, MPA, FNP
University of California, San Francisco
San Francisco, California
Chapter 16

Patrick S. Hagerman, PhD
Scotlea Enterprises, Inc.
Waunakee, Wisconsin
Chapter 7

Aaron W. Harding, MS, ACSM-CEP, ACSM-RCEP
Oregon Heart & Vascular Institute
Springfield, Oregon
Chapter 13

Julie M. Hughes, PhD
U.S. Army Research Institute of Environmental Medicine (USARIEM)
Natick, Massachusetts
Chapter 21

Kristi King, PhD
University of Louisville
Louisville, Kentucky
Chapter 1

Morey J. Kolber, PT, PhD
Nova Southeastern University
Fort Lauderdale, Florida
Chapter 19

Trina M. Limberg, BS, RRT, FAARC, MAACVPR
UC San Diego Health
San Diego, California
Chapter 17

David G. Lorenzi, PhD, CHES
Indiana University of Pennsylvania
Indiana, Pennsylvania
Chapter 23

Mark A. Patterson, MEd, ACSM-RCEP
Kaiser Permanente Colorado Franklin Medical Offices
Denver, Colorado
Chapter 13

Janette T. Poppenberg, ACSM-EPC, ACSM/ACS-CET
Cancer Exercise Trainer
Pittsburgh, Pennsylvania
Chapter 20

Joseph A. Quatrochi, PhD, ACSM-EPC
Metropolitan State University of Denver
Denver, Colorado
Chapter 6

Amy D. Rickman, RD, PhD, LDN, FACSM
Slippery Rock University of Pennsylvania
Slippery Rock, Pennsylvania
Chapter 18

Marc I. Robertson, PhD
Southern Connecticut State University
New Haven, Connecticut
Chapter 9

Bonny Rockette-Wagner, PhD
University of Pittsburgh
Pittsburgh, Pennsylvania
Chapter 2

Peter J. Ronai, MS, FACSM, ACSM-CEP, ACSM-RCEP, ACSM-PD, ACSM-EPC, ACSM-ETT, ACSM-EIM3
Sacred Heart University
Fairfield, Connecticut
Chapter 19

Patrick D. Savage, MS
University of Vermont College of Medicine
Burlington, Vermont
Chapter 10

Lesley M. Scibora, DC, PhD
University of St. Thomas
St. Paul, Minnesota
Chapter 21

Ray W. Squires, PhD, FACSM, ACSM-CEP, ACSM-PD
Mayo Clinic
Rochester, Minnesota
Chapter 11

Ann M. Swank, PhD, FACSM, ACSM-CEP, ACSM-PD
University of Louisville
Louisville, Kentucky
Chapter 12

Beth A. Taylor, PhD, FACSM
University of Connecticut
Storrs, Connecticut
Chapter 15

Benjamin C. Thompson, PhD, FACSM, ACSM-EPC, ACSM-EIM2
Metropolitan State University of Denver
Denver, Colorado
Chapters 3 and 4

Steven D. Verba, PhD
Slippery Rock University of Pennsylvania
Slippery Rock, Pennsylvania
Chapter 18

Kathryn E. Wilson, PhD
University of Nebraska Medical Center
Omaha, Nebraska
Chapter 22

Amanda Zaleski, MS
Hartford Hospital
Hartford, Connecticut
Chapter 15

Reviewers

Sarah E. Baker, PhD
Mayo Clinic
Rochester, Minnesota

James Christopher Baldi, PhD, FACSM
University of Otago
Dunedin, New Zealand

Christopher G. Berger, PhD, ACSM-EPC
Arizona State University
Phoenix, Arizona

Robert J. Buresh, PhD, ACSM-EPC
Kennesaw State University
Kennesaw, Georgia

Dierdra Bycura, EdD, ACSM-EPC, ACSM-CPT
Northern Arizona University
Flagstaff, Arizona

Shawn M. Drake, PT, PhD, ACSM-CEP, ACSM-PD, ACSM-EIM3
Arkansas State University
Jonesboro, Arkansas

Tiffany A. Esmat, PhD, ACSM-EPC, ACSM/NCHPAD-CIFT
Kennesaw State University
Kennesaw, Georgia

Michael A. Figueroa, EdD
William Paterson University
Wayne, New Jersey

Kenneth D. Fitch, MD, FACSM
University of Western Australia
Crawley, Western Australia, Australia

Beau K. Greer, PhD
Sacred Heart University
Fairfield, Connecticut

Garrett M. Hester, PhD, ACSM-CPT
Kennesaw State University
Kennesaw, Georgia

Simon D. Holzapfel, MS, ACSM-EPC
Arizona State University
Tempe, Arizona

Benjamin D. Levine, MD, FACSM
Texas Health Presbyterian Hospital
Dallas, Texas

Kate Lyden, PhD
University of Massachusetts
Amherst, Massachusetts

Christopher P. Repka, PhD
Northern Arizona University
Flagstaff, Arizona

Kelly Rice, PhD
Eastern Oregon University
La Grande, Oregon

John M. Schuna Jr, PhD
Oregon State University
Corvallis, Oregon

Eric Scibek, MS
Sacred Heart University
Fairfield, Connecticut

Lauren M. Smith, PhD
La Plata Integrated Healthcare, Axis Health System
Durango, Colorado

Alicja B. Stannard, PhD
Sacred Heart University
Fairfield, Connecticut

Trisha A. VanDusseldorp, PhD
Kennesaw State University
Kennesaw, Georgia

Valerie A. Wherley, PhD, ACSM-CPT, ACSM-EPC
Sacred Heart University
Fairfield, Connecticut

Contents

PART I

Physical Activity and Health

CHAPTER 1

The Health Benefits of Physical Activity

INTRODUCTION

Exercise science, public health, and medical experts recommend that everyone engage in regular physical activity throughout their lifespans (86–88). Engaging in regular physical activity is a behavior that serves as a modifiable risk factor for preventing premature mortality as well as preventing or managing chronic diseases. Considering that physical inactivity is the fourth leading cause of death worldwide (99), that half of the adults in the United States have a chronic disease such as heart disease, cancer, or diabetes (94), and that these diseases contribute to disability and premature death (56,101), it is imperative that physical activity, along with eating a healthy diet (85) and avoiding tobacco use (90), be promoted as part of a healthy lifestyle so that people can decrease their risk of chronic disease and/or manage their conditions. The purposes of this chapter are to describe physical activity and the recommended amounts as well as provide several examples of the benefits of physical activity.

The terms *physical activity*, *exercise*, and *physical fitness* are often used in research studies and are worthy of clearly defining. **Physical activity** is defined as "any bodily movement produced by skeletal muscles that results in energy expenditure. The energy expenditure can be measured in kilocalories" (19). The total amount of caloric expenditure associated with physical activity is determined by the amount of muscle mass producing bodily movements and the **intensity**, duration, and **frequency** of muscular contractions (83). Examples of physical activity include walking, gardening, or riding a bicycle.

Physical activity should not be confused with **exercise**, which is a subset of physical activity performed for the purpose of improving or maintaining physical fitness (19). **Physical fitness** is an attained set of attributes (*e.g.*, **muscular strength**, **muscular endurance**, cardiorespiratory endurance, **flexibility**, and **body composition**) that relates to the ability to perform physical activity (3). Typically, exercise is planned, structured, and repetitive as in jogging or swimming. Although physical activity and physical fitness both show a strong dose-response relationship with healthy outcomes, the relationship is more pronounced for physical fitness and healthy outcomes (3,13,96). In fact, the terms *physical activity* and *exercise* are sometimes used interchangeably. As some experts noted, "The intent is to recognize that many **types** of physical movement may have a positive effect on physical fitness, morbidity, and mortality" (22).

Given that the majority of Americans and many others throughout the world are not engaging in adequate health-maintaining and disease-preventing physical activity, promoting physical activity may be more conducive to engaging sedentary populations prior to recommending exercise or physical fitness. Although exercise or physical fitness may have more health benefits, engaging in physical activity as opposed to exercise may be a healthy first step for most physically inactive people.

Physical activity and exercise are behaviors, whereas physical fitness is an outcome of behaviors. It can often be confusing to determine which term to use. Each term represents a variable that can be measured. For example, cardiorespiratory endurance (a component of physical fitness and an outcome of exercise behavior) can be measured by conducting the exercise and testing protocol as outlined in the *ACSM's Guidelines for Exercise Testing and Prescription, 9th edition* (67). Although **cardiorespiratory fitness** testing is reliable and valid and can be conducted accurately by exercise professionals, it can also be time-consuming and labor-intensive. Physical activity can be assessed through large-scale surveys or by using objective monitoring devices (*e.g.*, pedometers, accelerometers); however, the accuracy or precision of the physical activity assessment may not compare favorably with the accuracy or precision of physical fitness. For large-scale, population-based studies, such as epidemiological or public health studies, physical activity may be the most feasible, cost-effective, and practical behavior to measure. For purposes of this chapter, literature review searches using the terms *physical activity*, *exercise*, and *physical fitness* were used when determining relationships to chronic diseases.

There has been substantial research regarding decreasing sedentary behavior in addition to engaging in adequate physical activity (11). **Sedentary behavior** can be defined as sitting or reclined while engaging in minimal energy expenditure (≤1.5 **metabolic equivalents** [**METs**]) (75,81). **Physical inactivity** can be defined as not meeting the recommended 30 minutes of moderate-intensity physical activity on at least 5 days every week, 20 minutes of vigorous-intensity physical activity on at least 3 days every week, or an equivalent combination achieving 600 MET-minutes per week (30). One MET represents 3.5 $mL \cdot kg^{-1} \cdot min^{-1}$ of oxygen consumption and is a method for estimating energy expenditure during physical activity (1,2). Light-intensity physical activity (*e.g.*, walking) can be defined as requiring <3.0 METs, moderate-intensity physical activity (*e.g.*, jogging) as 3.0–5.9 METs, and vigorous-intensity physical activity (*e.g.*, running) as ≥6 METs (31,78). A variety of physical activity and their ancillary METs can be found at https://sites.google.com/site/compendiumofphysicalactivities/. It is recommended that individuals who are less fit begin with lesser intense physical activity prior to engaging in more intense activity (31). Regarding obesity and weight loss, further guidelines recommend from 45 to 90 minutes of moderate- to vigorous-intensity physical activity (74,84).

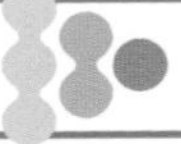

Domains of Physical Activity

Physical activity is a behavior that represents the interaction of the person and his or her social and physical environments and can be categorized in numerous ways (19,71). Typically, four **physical activity domains** include recreation, transport, occupation, and household. *Active living* incorporates exercise, recreational activities, household and occupational activities, and active transportation (72). Likewise, physical inactivity, or the lack of meeting the recommended amount of physical activity, may include categorizations such as sedentary behavior, walking, and sitting (see Chapter 2 for a more detailed discussion of physical inactivity and sedentary behavior).

Addressing physical activity behavior in an ecological model framework helps exercise scientists, public health, and medical experts plan, develop, implement, and evaluate physical activity interventions and policies (71,73,78). Physical activity behavior is influenced by intrapersonal (biological, psychological), interpersonal/cultural, organizational, physical environment (built, natural), and policy (laws, rules, regulations, codes) (54). Physical activity interventions and policies are most effective when they operate on multiple levels (40).

Physical Activity Recommendations

The current guidelines for physical activity are published in the *2008 Physical Activity Guidelines for Americans*, also known as the current federal physical activity guidelines (86). The guidelines are the following:

> All adults should avoid inactivity. Some physical activity is better than none, and adults who participate in any amount of physical activity gain some health benefits.
>
> For substantial health benefits, adults should do at least 150 minutes (2 hours and 30 minutes) a week of moderate-intensity, or 75 minutes (1 hour and 15 minutes) a week of vigorous-intensity aerobic physical activity, or an equivalent combination of moderate- and vigorous-intensity aerobic activity. Aerobic activity should be performed in episodes of at least 10 minutes, and preferably, it should be spread throughout the week.
>
> For additional and more extensive health benefits, adults should increase their aerobic physical activity to 300 minutes (5 hours) a week of moderate-intensity, or 150 minutes a week of vigorous-intensity aerobic physical activity, or an equivalent combination of moderate- and vigorous-intensity activity. Additional health benefits are gained by engaging in physical activity beyond this amount.
>
> Adults should also do muscle-strengthening activities that are moderate or high intensity and involve all major muscle groups on 2 or more days a week, as these activities provide additional health benefits.

Furthermore, *Healthy People 2020* (32), the nation's health agenda, set a goal to improve health, fitness, and quality of life through daily physical activity and delineated 36 objectives related to the promotion of physical activity across the lifespan (Box 1.1).

Box 1.1 Healthy People 2020 Physical Activity Objectives

Healthy People 2020 Physical Activity Objectives	For Adults and/or Children
PA-1 Reduce the proportion of adults who engage in no leisure-time physical activity	Adults
PA-2 Increase the proportion of adults who meet current Federal physical activity guidelines for aerobic physical activity and for muscle-strengthening activity	Adults
PA-2.1 Increase the proportion of adults who engage in aerobic physical activity of at least moderate intensity for at least 150 minutes/week, or 75 minutes/week of vigorous intensity, or an equivalent combination	Adults
PA-2.2 Increase the proportion of adults who engage in aerobic physical activity of at least moderate intensity for more than 300 minutes/week, or more than 150 minutes/week of vigorous intensity, or an equivalent combination	Adults
PA-2.3 Increase the proportion of adults who perform muscle-strengthening activities on 2 or more days of the week	Adults
PA-2.4 Increase the proportion of adults who meet the objectives for aerobic physical activity and for muscle-strengthening activity	Adults
PA-3 Increase the proportion of adolescents who meet current Federal physical activity guidelines for aerobic physical activity and for muscle-strengthening activity	Children
PA-3.1 Increase the proportion of adolescents who meet current Federal physical activity guidelines for aerobic physical activity — Revised	Children
PA-3.2 Increase the proportion of adolescents who meet current Federal physical activity guidelines for muscle-strengthening activity	Children
PA-3.3 Increase the proportion of adolescents who meet current Federal physical activity guidelines for aerobic physical activity and muscle-strengthening activity	Children
PA-4 Increase the proportion of the Nation's public and private schools that require daily physical education for all students	Children
PA-4.1 Increase the proportion of the Nation's public and private elementary schools that require daily physical education for all students	Children
PA-4.2 Increase the proportion of the Nation's public and private middle and junior high schools that require daily physical education for all students	Children
PA-4.3 Increase the proportion of the Nation's public and private senior high schools that require daily physical education for all students	Children
PA-5 Increase the proportion of adolescents who participate in daily school physical education	Children
PA-6 Increase regularly scheduled elementary school recess in the United States	Children
PA-6.1 Increase the number of States that require regularly scheduled elementary school recess	Children
PA-6.2 Increase the proportion of school districts that require regularly scheduled elementary school recess	Children

(continued)

Box 1.1 Healthy People 2020 Physical Activity Objectives (*continued*)

Healthy People 2020 Physical Activity Objectives	For Adults and/or Children
PA-7 Increase the proportion of school districts that require or recommend elementary school recess for an appropriate period of time	Children
PA-8 Increase the proportion of children and adolescents who do not exceed recommended limits for screen time	Children
PA-8.1 Increase the proportion of children aged 0 to 2 years who view no television or videos on an average weekday	Children
PA-8.2 Increase the proportion of children and adolescents aged 2 years through 12th grade who view television, videos, or play video games for no more than 2 hours a day	Children
PA-8.2.1 Increase the proportion of children aged 2 to 5 years who view television, videos, or play video games for no more than 2 hours a day	Children
PA-8.2.2 Increase the proportion of children and adolescents aged 6 to 14 years who view television, videos, or play video games for no more than 2 hours a day	Children
PA-8.2.3 Increase the proportion of adolescents in grades 9 through 12 who view television, videos, or play video games for no more than 2 hours a day	Children
PA-8.3 Increase the proportion of children and adolescents aged 2 years to 12th grade who use a computer or play computer games outside of school (for nonschool work) for no more than 2 hours a day	Children
PA-8.3.1 Increase the proportion of children aged 2 to 5 years who use a computer or play computer games outside of school (for nonschool work) for no more than 2 hours a day	Children
PA-8.3.2 Increase the proportion of children and adolescents aged 6 to 14 years who use a computer or play computer games outside of school (for nonschool work) for no more than 2 hours a day	Children
PA-8.3.3 Increase the proportion of adolescents in grades 9 through 12 who use a computer or play computer games outside of school (for nonschool work) for no more than 2 hours a day	Children
PA-9 Increase the number of States with licensing regulations for physical activity provided in child care	Children
PA-9.1 Increase the number of States with licensing regulations for physical activity in child care that require activity programs providing large muscle or gross motor activity, development, and/or equipment	Children
PA-9.2 Increase the number of States with licensing regulations for physical activity in child care that require children to engage in vigorous or moderate physical activity	Children
PA-9.3 Increase the number of States with licensing regulations for physical activity in child care that require a number of minutes of physical activity per day or by length of time in care	Children

Healthy People 2020 Physical Activity Objectives		For Adults and/or Children
PA-10	Increase the proportion of the Nation's public and private schools that provide access to their physical activity spaces and facilities for all persons outside of normal school hours (that is, before and after the school day, on weekends, and during summer and other vacations)	Adults
PA-11	Increase the proportion of physician office visits that include counseling or education related to physical activity	Adults Children
PA-11.1	Increase the proportion of office visits made by patients with a diagnosis of cardiovascular disease, diabetes, or hyperlipidemia that include counseling or education related to exercise	Adults Children
PA-11.2	Increase the proportion of physician visits made by all child and adult patients that include counseling about exercise	Adults Children
PA-12	(Developmental) Increase the proportion of employed adults who have access to and participate in employer-based exercise facilities and exercise programs	Adults
PA-13	Increase the proportion of trips made by walking	Adults Children
PA-13.1	Increase the proportion of trips of 1 mile or less made by walking by adults aged 18 years and older — Revised	Adults
PA-13.2	Increase the proportion of trips of 1 mile or less made to school by walking by children and adolescents aged 5 to 15 years — Revised	Children
PA-14	Increase the proportion of trips made by bicycling	Adults Children
PA 14.1	Increase the proportion of trips of 5 miles or less made by bicycling by adults aged 18 years and older	Adults
PA-14.2	(Developmental) Increase the proportion of trips of 2 miles or less made to school by bicycling by children and adolescents aged 5 to 15 years	Children
PA-15	(Developmental) Increase legislative policies for the built environment that enhance access to and availability of physical activity opportunities	Adults Children
PA-15.1	(Developmental) Increase community-scale policies for the built environment that enhance access to and availability of physical activity opportunities	Adults Children
PA-15.2	(Developmental) Increase street-scale policies for the built environment that enhance access to and availability of physical activity opportunities	Adults Children
PA-15.3	(Developmental) Increase transportation and travel policies for the built environment that enhance access to and availability of physical activity opportunities	Adults Children

HealthyPeople.gov. *Physical Activity* [Internet]. Washington (DC): Office of Disease Prevention and Health Promotion; [cited 2017 Oct 2]. Available from: https://www.healthypeople.gov/2020/topics-objectives/topic/physical-activity/objectives

Healthy People 2020's objectives were derived from seminal research and meta-analyses in exercise physiology, public health, and medicine to reach all Americans in achieving optimal quality and quantity of life. For example, Objective PA-2, "Increase the proportion of adults who meet current Federal physical activity guidelines for aerobic physical activity and for muscle-strengthening activity," is derived from the Centers for Disease Control and Prevention (CDC) and American College of Sports Medicine's (ACSM) issuance of a public health recommendation on the types and amounts of physical activity for health promotion and disease prevention across the lifespan. The special communication article, published in the *Journal of the American Medical Association*, concluded that "every US adult should accumulate 30 minutes or more of moderate-intensity physical activity on most, preferably all, days of the week" (66).

Later, the American Heart Association (AHA) and ACSM's expert panel of scientists, physicians, epidemiologists, exercise scientists, and public health specialists convened to update and clarify the recommendations. These updates published in *Medicine & Science in Sports & Exercise®* (31), as well as in *Circulation* (2007), included the following:

> To promote and maintain health, all healthy adults aged 18 to 65 yr need moderate-intensity aerobic (endurance) physical activity for a minimum of 30 min on five days each week or vigorous-intensity aerobic physical activity for a minimum of 20 min on three days each week.
> I (A). Combinations of moderate- and vigorous-intensity activity can be performed to meet this recommendation.
> IIa (B). For example, a person can meet the recommendation by walking briskly for 30 min twice during the week and then jogging for 20 min on two other days. Moderate-intensity aerobic activity, which is generally equivalent to a brisk walk and noticeably accelerates the heart rate, can be accumulated toward the 30-min minimum by performing bouts each lasting 10 or more minutes.
> I (B). Vigorous-intensity activity is exemplified by jogging, and causes rapid breathing and a substantial increase in heart rate. In addition, every adult should perform activities that maintain or increase muscular strength and endurance a minimum of two days each week.
> IIa (A). Because of the dose-response relation between physical activity and health, persons who wish to further improve their personal fitness, reduce their risk for chronic diseases and disabilities or prevent unhealthy weight gain may benefit by exceeding the minimum recommended amounts of physical activity.

The aforementioned physical activity recommendations describe minimal frequency, intensity, and **time** amounts in order to achieve or maintain health. The recommendations also suggest that accumulating more than the recommended amounts is better. Furthermore, other health behaviors, such as healthy eating, may be considered when trying to achieve energy balance or weight loss (31,35).

Prevalence of Physical Activity

Considering that 1 in 4 adults (20% of men and 27% of women) worldwide are insufficiently physically active, physical inactivity has been listed as a global pandemic (42,100). In the United States, approximately one-half of the proportion of adults and about one quarter of high school students meet the guidelines for **aerobic** physical activity (12,37,38). Typically, reports refer to the aerobic recommendations, although there are muscle-strengthening and flexibility recommendations as well. The latest self-report data indicate that 47% of adults in the United States meet neither the aerobic nor muscle-strengthening guideline, 3% meet the muscle-strengthening guideline only, 29% meet the aerobic guideline only, and 21% meet the full guidelines for both aerobic and muscle-strengthening activity based on their participation in leisure-time physical activity (12).

Health Equity and Health Disparities

The prevalence of those meeting physical activity recommendations is not equitable among demographic sectors. Health equity is achieved when every individual has the opportunity to "attain his or her full health potential," and no one is "disadvantaged from achieving this potential because of social position or other socially determined circumstances" (20). Differences in sex, race/ethnicity, age, educational attainment, family income, family type, country of birth, disability status, geographic location, health insurance status, sexual orientation, and marital status in national physical activity data reveal that disparities exist.

An example of a health disparity is the difference in physical activity behaviors between men and women. In 2008, self-report survey results indicated that 47.4% of men met the recommendation, and the number steadily increased to 54.1% in 2013. For women, the gains were not as noteworthy. In 2008, 43.6% of women met the physical activity recommendation, and the proportion increased to 46.1% in 2013. Furthermore, men were more likely than women to have met the aerobic and muscle-strengthening physical activity recommendations (12).

Recent data indicate that non-Hispanic White adults (23%) are more likely to meet the full guidelines for both aerobic and muscle-strengthening activity based on their participation in leisure-time physical activity than Hispanic adults (16%) or non-Hispanic African American adults (17%) (12). Also, younger adults are more active than **older adults**, and as age increases, physical activity decreases.

Social and environmental circumstances, or social determinants of health, can have an impact on a person's ability to be physically active. For example, not having access to safe recreational facilities or sidewalks for families to walk to school or work may negatively affect engagement in physical activity. Research results indicate that as poverty levels decrease, the percentage of adults who are physically active increases (12). See Box 1.2 for other examples of disparities in physical activity among certain demographic characteristics.

Box 1.2 Prevalence of Disparities for Meeting Physical Activity Recommendations

- More men (54.1%) met the recommendations than women (46.1%).
- More Native Hawaiian or other Pacific Islander (64.5%) met the recommendation than White, non-Hispanic (53.4%), two or more races (50.7%), Asian (49.8%), American Indian or Alaska Native (46.6%), Hispanic or Latino (42.7%), and non-Hispanic African American adults (41.3%).
- More younger adults, aged 18–24 years (61.5%), met the recommendations than adults aged 25–44 years (55.1%), 45–54 years (48.4%), 55–64 years (44.1%), 65–74 years (41.8%), 75–84 years (31.2%), and 85 years and older (18.3%).
- For adults aged 25 years and older, those with higher educational attainment reported a higher rate of meeting the recommendation than those with lower educational attainment (*e.g.*, advanced degree, 64.7%; 4-yr college degree, 59.4%; associate degree, 50.3%; some college education, 49.1%; high school graduate, 39.7%; and less than high school education, 30.5%).
- Those who lived in a family with a higher income met the recommendations more than those who live with families with lower income (*e.g.*, >600% over the poverty threshold, 65.8%; 400%–599%, 57.2%; 200%–399%; 48.3%; 100%–199%, 38.6%; and <100%, 35.6%).
- Adults who had a spouse or partner were more active (55.3%) than single (52.6%), two-parent family with child or children (52.8%), single parent with child or children (41.5%), or other (43.0%).
- Adults who were born in the United States (51.6%) met the recommendations more than adults who were not born in the United States (43.6%).
- Those individuals without activity limitations (53.9%) met the guidelines for physical activity more than individuals with activity limitations (30.5%).

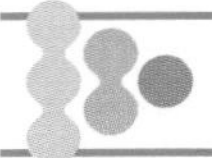

Benefits of Physical Activity and Chronic Disease

Participation in regular physical activity can attenuate the prevalence, morbidity, or mortality of many of the leading causes of death (28,100). In addition to preventing all-cause mortality, a plethora of physiological and psychological benefits are attributed to regular physical activity.

Physical Activity and All-Cause Mortality

Not engaging in sufficient physical activity has been identified as the fourth leading risk factor for mortality and is attributed to 3.2 million deaths globally (100). Numerous studies, meta-analyses, and reviews underscore the relationship between physical activity and all-cause mortality (23,41,47,49,52,98). For example, as part of the longitudinal Harvard Alumni Health Study, results from physical activity behaviors survey data (*i.e.*, walking, stair climbing, sports/recreation) and mortality rates (*i.e.*, death certificates) from 13,485 Harvard alumni indicated that men who engaged in moderate- (4–<6 METs) and vigorous-intensity (≥6 METs) physical activity lived longer than those who engaged in light-intensity (<4 METs) physical activity (47). These findings support the public health recommendation of engaging in moderate-intensity physical activity for overall general health purposes; however, they also support that greater health benefits may be achieved for those who are able to engage in vigorous-intensity physical activity without contraindications.

Physical Activity and Chronic Diseases

In addition to all-cause mortality, a synopsis of the benefits of physical activity in the treatment or maintenance of chronic diseases is presented throughout this section. Chronic diseases (also called *noncommunicable diseases*) develop over time and are not infectious (also called *communicable*) or transferred from person to person. Worldwide, the four most prevalent types of chronic diseases are cardiovascular diseases, cancers, chronic respiratory diseases, and diabetes (101). The *Global Recommendations on Physical Activity for Health* developed by the World Health Organization promote physical activity for the improvement or maintenance of cardiovascular health, cancer, metabolic health (diabetes and obesity), musculoskeletal health (bone health, osteoporosis), functional health and prevention of falls, and depression (99).

In the United States, the 10 most prevalent leading causes of death are cardiovascular diseases, cancers, chronic lower respiratory diseases, stroke, unintentional injuries, Alzheimer disease, diabetes mellitus, pneumonia and influenza, kidney disease, and suicide (59). Seven of these 10 leading causes of death are chronic diseases, two of which (heart disease and cancer) account for approximately half of all deaths each year and are among the most common, costly, and preventable of all health problems in the United States (12).

Physical Activity and Cardiovascular Disease

Cardiovascular disease, also called *heart disease*, is an overarching term for a variety of diseases of the heart and blood vessels. These diseases or conditions can include coronary heart disease, stroke, hypertension, and heart failure. Ischemic heart disease is the leading cause of death worldwide with 7.4 million deaths in 2012 (101). Heart disease is the leading cause of death in the United States (614,348 deaths in 2014) (59).

The positive relationship between physical activity and cardiovascular health has been well established in research studies (47,48,55,63,64,76,93). Physical activity improves cardiorespiratory fitness and reduces risk of cardiovascular disease. Cardiorespiratory fitness has a direct dose-response relationship between frequency, intensity, time, and volume. Achieving the minimal recommended guidelines for physical activity is suggested to reduce risks and improve cardiorespiratory health and additional health benefits (86). Furthermore, experts suggest that engaging in more physical activity than recommended in the guidelines may be needed for greater reduction in risks for heart disease (76) and heart failure (64). Even among overweight and obese women, there is an inverse relationship between the risk of heart disease and increased physical activity (95).

Physical Activity and Stroke

Worldwide, stroke accounted for 6.7 million deaths and is the second leading cause of death (101). A stroke occurs when blood flow (*e.g.*, oxygen and glucose) to an area of the brain is blocked due to a clot or a hemorrhage of a blood vessel. In the United States, stroke was the fifth leading cause of death among 133,103 deaths in 2014 (37,59). Hypertension and heart disease are among the primary risk factors for stroke. In a meta-analysis of 13 studies determining the relationship between physical activity level and stroke outcomes, researchers concluded that the higher the intensity of physical activity, the greater the reduction in risk of stroke and related outcomes (25). For men and women, moderate-intensity physical activity was associated with an 11% reduction in risk of stroke outcomes when compared with low-intensity physical activity, whereas higher intensity physical activity was associated with a 19% reduction in risk. When examining men and women separately, men showed a 12% reduction in risk associated with moderate-intensity physical activity, whereas women did not show a significant reduction in risk. Furthermore, men and women who engaged in high-intensity physical activity showed an even greater risk reduction for stroke outcome than when engaging in moderate-intensity physical activity (men = 19% and women = 24%). The results of the meta-analysis indicated that for women, higher intensity physical activity may be required to reduce risks compared with men.

Physical Activity and Cancer

Worldwide, cancer ranks as one of the leading causes of morbidity and mortality. Approximately 14 million new cases and 8.2 million cancer-related deaths occurred in 2012 (101). The most common causes of cancer death are lung (1.6 million deaths, the fifth leading cause of death worldwide), liver (745,000 deaths), stomach (723,000 deaths), colorectal (694,000 deaths), breast (521,000 deaths), and esophageal cancer (400,000 deaths). Lung, prostate, colorectal, stomach, and liver cancer are the most prevalent cancers among men, and breast, colorectal, lung, cervix, and stomach cancers are the most prevalent cancers among women. In the United States, cancer is the second leading cause of death (591,699 deaths) (37,59) and is projected to surpass cardiovascular disease as the primary leading cause of death.

A variety of behavioral as well as genetic and environmental factors can contribute to cancer. Globally, physical inactivity, lower fruit and vegetable consumption, tobacco use, alcohol use, and overweight or obesity have been listed as the primary behaviors that contribute to one-third of cancer deaths (7). Research studies linking an association between physical activity and the prevention and/or maintenance of certain cancers are well documented (16,17,26,29,39,45,65,79,80,82,97).

In the United States, tobacco smoking is responsible for approximately 1 in 5 (480,000) deaths annually (90). Interestingly, physical activity has been shown to play a role in having inverse relationship with lung cancer risk (17,79,82). In a **systematic review and meta-analysis** of 28 studies, individuals who engaged in higher amounts of physical activity had a reduced risk of lung cancer (16). The authors noted, however, that results should be interpreted with caution because the number of studies in the analysis that focused on determining the physical activity and lung cancer association among those individuals who had never smoked was small — only four studies.

296,395 participants and 10,815 incident cases, indicate that moderate- and vigorous-intensity physical activity are associated with decreased incidence of Type 2 diabetes. The authors note, however, that higher intensity physical activity is more beneficial in decreasing the incidence of Type 2 diabetes than moderate-intensity physical activity (33). Although physical activity is beneficial, the American Diabetes Association (ADA) and ACSM published a position statement indicating that the majority of U.S. adults with diabetes or prediabetes are not sufficiently active (22).

It is crucial to consider health disparities when addressing diabetes. For example, the majority of older U.S. adults with diabetes are less likely to engage in recommended levels of physical activity than their peers without the condition (102). Furthermore, physical activity levels typically decline with age, and women are typically less active than men. In a study of older U.S. adults with diabetes, less than half of older adults with diabetes were physically active at baseline, and over a 6-year period, the probability of engaging in physical activity declined by more than 30% with no significant variation by gender. Considering that women were less active than men at baseline and experienced a decrease in their physical activity accumulation over the 6 years, the odds of men engaging in physical activity were 85% higher than for women (53). Although men and women experienced similar declines in physical activity, the physical activity trajectory for women started and remained less favorable than for men. Interestingly, the fact that older women were less likely to engage in physical activity than older men is consistent with published findings for those with and without diabetes (102). In fact, in the population-based study of 99,172 adults, 18,370 of whom had diabetes mellitus, 25% and 42% of older adults with diabetes mellitus met recommendations for total physical activity based on the 2007 ADA (6) and the *2008 Physical Activity Guidelines for Americans* (86), respectively. Adults with Type 2 diabetes were 31%–34% less likely to engage in physical activity at recommended levels and 13%–19% less likely to be physically active at insufficient levels than those without Type 2 diabetes (102).

Physical Activity and Obesity

More than two-thirds of adults (68.5%; 78 million) in the United States were either overweight or obese, 34.9% were obese, and 6.4% were extremely obese (grade 3 obesity) in 2011–2012 (62). Overweight is defined as a **body mass index (BMI)** of 25–29.9 kg $\cdot$ m^{-2} and obesity as a BMI of ≥30 kg $\cdot$ m^{-2} with further levels — grade 1 (BMI 30–34 kg $\cdot$ m^{-2}), grade 2 (BMI 35–39 kg $\cdot$ m^{-2}), and grade 3 (BMI ≥40 kg $\cdot$ m^{-2}) (60,61). The prevalence of obesity rose to 36.5% during 2011–2014 (61), which is higher than the Healthy People 2020 goal of 30.5% (32). Fewer younger adults (aged 20–39 yr, 32.3%) were obese than middle-aged (aged 40–59 yr, 40.2%) and older adults (aged 60 yr and older, 37.0%) (61). Furthermore, other health disparities were exhibited by gender and race. More women (38.3%) were obese than men (34.3%), and the highest prevalence of obesity was among non-Hispanic African American (48.1%), followed by Hispanic (42.5%), non-Hispanic White (34.5%), and non-Hispanic Asian adults (11.7%) (61). Obesity rates remained level at approximately 17% for youth (61). Obesity has health risks such as risk of morbidity from hypertension, dyslipidemia, Type 2 diabetes, cardiovascular disease, stroke, gallbladder disease, osteoarthritis, sleep apnea and respiratory problems, and some cancers (35,61,92). Furthermore,

Given that lung cancer can still occur for individuals who have never smoked, more research is needed to investigate the relationship (80).

Results of two meta-analyses show beneficial relationships between physical activity and breast cancer risks and outcomes (29,44). A systematic review and meta-analysis of 22 studies, including 123,574 participants, indicated there were significant associations between lifetime and recent prediagnosis physical activity and risk of breast cancer-related death. Furthermore, for those individuals who were physically active after being diagnosed with cancer, there were also significant reductions in the risk of breast cancer–related death. The authors warned readers, however, that results should be interpreted with caution due to the limitations (*e.g.*, heterogeneity) when conducting a meta-analysis with differing outcomes (44).

Results of the other meta-analysis indicated that physical activity is associated with reductions in postmenopausal breast cancer (evidence is not consistent in premenopausal women) (29).

Physical activity can serve as a protective factor and has been related to reductions in colon cancer (65). Results of a meta-analysis of 56 studies show an inverse relationship between physical activity and colon cancer (97). There are growing numbers of studies connecting the positive associations between physical activity and the reduction in risks or deaths from other cancer sites (45), including pancreatic (an 11% risk reduction in pancreatic cancer risk for those who engaged in physical activity) (26) and endometrial (97) cancers.

Physical Activity and Diabetes

Diabetes is the seventh leading cause of death worldwide with 1.5 million (2.7%) deaths in 2012, an increase from 1.0 million (2.0%) deaths in 2000 (101). In the United States, diabetes is the seventh leading cause of death (76,488 deaths in 2014) (37,59); however, the number of individuals living with diabetes was almost 24 million, with an estimate that 2.6 million individuals do not have their diabetes under control (37). Although there are different types of diabetes, the disease has become a widespread epidemic primarily because of the increasing prevalence and incidence of Type 2 diabetes mellitus, which accounts for 90%–95% of cases (5).

Type 2 diabetes is a condition in which a person's body becomes insulin-resistant. It is also estimated that almost 60 million people have prediabetes, a condition in which blood glucose levels are above normal, thus greatly increasing their risk for Type 2 diabetes. Diabetes is a significant cause of premature mortality and is associated with examples of morbidity caused from cardiovascular disease, blindness, kidney and nerve disease, and amputation.

The rate of developing diabetes is increasing. Some experts estimated that 1 out of 3 adults in the United States are projected to have diabetes (14), a 198% increase from 16.2 million in 2005 to 48.3 million in 2050 (57). Among certain demographic characteristics such as age, sex, country of birth, and ethnicity, it is estimated that 1 out of 2 adults will develop diabetes (58). For example, it is projected that men will see an increase from 7.59 million in 2005 to 20.81 million in 2050 (174% increase), whereas women will experience a 220% increase from 8.59 million to 27.47 million. Older adults will experience higher rates of diabetes than younger people. Disparities regarding the prevalence of diabetes will exist among race/ethnicities as well. Increases in the number of those with diabetes will be largest for minority groups; between 2005 and 2050, the number is projected to increase 481% among Hispanics, 208% among African Americans, and 113% among Whites. The race/ethnicity and age group with the largest increase will be for African Americans and 75 years of age or older (increased 606%) (57).

Regular physical activity promotes glycemic control and enhances insulin action (22), thus improving blood glucose, lipid, blood pressure control abnormalities, and weight loss and/or maintenance (7). Medications and/or insulin may be recommended as well in addition to healthy behaviors (7). Research findings conclude that regular physical activity may prevent or delay diabetes and its complications (33,51,53,102). For example, results from a meta-analysis of eight studies, including

Physical Activity and Disabilities, Aging, Functional Independence, and Activities of Daily Living

Approximately 57 million people in the United States (11.6%) of all ages have a hearing, vision, mobility, or cognition disability or have emotional or behavioral disorders (15), and although disability prevalence increases with age, most adults with disabilities are between 18 and 64 years of age (8,21). Furthermore, 7 million adults reported not being able to accomplish **activities of daily living (ADL)** due to depression or anxiety (15). Disability-associated health care expenditures have been estimated at nearly $400 billion (8). Furthermore, being obese adds additional health care expenditures for people with disabilities (9).

Adults with disabilities are more likely to be physically inactive (47.1%) than adults without disabilities (26.1%) (18). Furthermore, those adults with disabilities who are inactive (50.0%; 10.1 million) are more likely to have one or more chronic diseases than those with disabilities who are physically active. Physical activity is recommended to all persons, including those with disabilities and may be adapted according to ability (32,91).

Cognitive function refers to those mental processes that are crucial for the conduct of the ADL. In the United States, Alzheimer disease is the sixth leading cause of death (93,451 deaths in 2014) (59) and actually may be higher due to the underreporting of dementia in death certificates (34). However, as the older population has grown, the proportion and number of deaths from Alzheimer disease has increased slowly and steadily. In 2011, Alzheimer disease–attributed deaths accounted for 84,974 deaths, or 3.4% of total deaths. A systematic review (247 studies) and meta-analysis (31 studies) of modifiable factors (*e.g.*, smoking, alcohol, caffeine, nutrition, physical activity) and cognitive function was conducted resulting in were retrieved for systematic review. Physical activity was among the strongest predictors of risk reduction for Alzheimer disease (10). In a systematic review of 13 randomized controlled trials with 896 older adults with dementia, authors reported that older people with dementia can be successfully engaged in activity and will regularly attend sessions, and undertaking exercise shows some physical benefits (68). Although physical activity is recommended, in a meta-analysis of 19 studies of older adults in long-term residential facilities, physical rehabilitation appears to have a small effect on ADL (24).

Lastly, suicide is the 10th leading cause of death in the United States (42,733 deaths in 2014) (59). Although a variety of factors are associated with suicide such as adverse **child** events, depression is one factor that may be modifiable with physical activity. The research supporting the inverse association of physical activity and depression is expansive (88). For example, physical activity is associated with lower rates and severity of depression among older adults (69). Physical activity is being considered as a treatment for those experiencing posttraumatic stress disorder, although the research to support the claim is still underway (70). Additionally, individuals who are severely obese who participated in physical activity lifestyle interventions have reported improvements in their quality of life (36).

campaign to increase physical activity, thus reducing obesity among children (50). A multisector approach engaging stakeholders at individual, social, organizational, community, and policy levels is encouraged (71), outlined in the National Physical Activity Plan, and promoted by the AHA (43).

It is important to address health disparities and to focus on delivering a variety of interventions within an ecological framework, thus improving social support and environmental conditions promoting physical activity for individuals with diabetes (43).

Consider what social determinants of health may have a positive or negative impact on your patient's ability to engage in physical activity. Consider your patient's age, income, whether children are living at home, and disability status when designing an **exercise prescription**. Also, consider physical characteristics such as neighborhood safety and access to sidewalks and parks during exercise prescription.

REFERENCES

1. Ainsworth BE, Haskell WL, Herrmann SD, et al. 2011 Compendium of Physical Activities: a second update of codes and MET values. *Med Sci Sports Exerc.* 2011;43(8):1575–81.
2. Ainsworth BE, Haskell WL, Whitt MC, et al. Compendium of Physical Activities: an update of activity codes and MET intensities. *Med Sci Sports Exerc.* 2000;32(9 suppl):S498–504.
3. American College of Sports Medicine. *ACSM's Resource Manual for Guidelines for Exercise Testing and Prescription.* 7th ed. Baltimore (MD): Lippincott Williams & Wilkins; 2014. 896 p.
4. American College of Sports Medicine. *What is Exercise is Medicine®* [Internet]. Indianapolis (IN): American College of Sports Medicine; [cited 2016 Jun 10]. Available from: http://www.exerciseismedicine.org/support_page.php/about/
5. American Diabetes Association. Diagnosis and classification of diabetes mellitus. *Diabetes Care.* 2010;33(suppl 1):S62–9.
6. American Diabetes Association. Standards of medical care in diabetes — 2007. *Diabetes Care.* 2007;30(suppl 1):S4–41.
7. American Diabetes Association. *Type 2* [Internet]. Arlington (VA): American Diabetes Association; [cited 2016 May 23]. Available from: http://www.diabetes.org/diabetes-basics/type-2/
8. Anderson WL, Armour BS, Finkelstein EA, Wiener JM. Estimates of state-level health-care expenditures associated with disability. *Public Health Rep.* 2010;125(1):44–51.
9. Anderson WL, Wiener JM, Khatutsky G, Armour BS. Obesity and people with disabilities: the implications for health care expenditures. *Obesity (Silver Spring).* 2013;21(12):E798–804.
10. Beydoun MA, Beydoun HA, Gamaldo AA, Teel A, Zonderman AB, Wang Y. Epidemiologic studies of modifiable factors associated with cognition and dementia: systematic review and meta-analysis. *BMC Public Health.* 2014;14:643.
11. Biswas A, Oh PI, Faulkner GE, et al. Sedentary time and its association with risk for disease incidence, mortality, and hospitalization in adults: a systematic review and meta-analysis. *Ann Intern Med.* 2015;162(2):123–32.
12. Blackwell DL, Lucas JW, Clarke TC. Summary health statistics for U.S. adults: National Health Interview Survey, 2012. *Vital Health Stat.* 2014;10(260):1–161.
13. Blair SN, Jackson AS. Physical fitness and activity as separate heart disease risk factors: a meta-analysis. *Med Sci Sports Exerc.* 2001;33(5):762–4.
14. Boyle JP, Thompson TJ, Gregg EW, Barker LE, Williamson DF. Projection of the year 2050 burden of diabetes in the US adult population: dynamic modeling of incidence, mortality, and prediabetes prevalence. *Popul Health Metr.* 2010;8:29.
15. Brault MW. *Americans With Disabilities: 2010. Current Population Reports No. 70-131.* Washington (DC): United States Census Bureau; 2012. 23 p.
16. Brenner DR, Yannitsos DH, Farris MS, Johansson M, Friedenreich CM. Leisure-time physical activity and lung cancer risk: a systematic review and meta-analysis. *Lung Cancer.* 2016;95:17–27.
17. Buffart LM, Singh AS, van Loon EC, Vermeulen HI, Brug J, Chinapaw MJ. Physical activity and the risk of developing lung cancer among smokers: a meta-analysis. *J Sci Med Sport.* 2014;17(1):67–71.
18. Carroll DD, Courtney-Long EA, Stevens AC, et al. Vital signs: disability and physical activity — United States, 2009-2012. *MMWR Morb Mortal Wkly Rep.* 2014;63(18):407–13.
19. Caspersen CJ, Powell KE, Christenson GM. Physical activity, exercise, and physical fitness: definitions and distinctions for health-related research. *Public Health Rep.* 1985;100(2):126–31.
20. Centers for Disease Control and Prevention. CDC grand rounds: public health practices to include persons with disabilities. *MMWR Morb Mortal Wkly Rep.* 2013;62(34):697–701.

21. Centers for Disease Control and Prevention. *Health Equity* [Internet]. Atlanta (GA): Centers for Disease Control and Prevention; [cited 2017 Oct 2]. Available from: http://www.cdc.gov/chronicdisease/healthequity/index.htm
22. Colberg SR, Albright AL, Blissmer BJ, et al. Exercise and type 2 diabetes: American College of Sports Medicine and the American Diabetes Association: joint position statement. Exercise and type 2 diabetes. *Med Sci Sports Exerc.* 2010;42(12):2282–303.
23. Cooper R, Kuh D, Hardy R. Objectively measured physical capability levels and mortality: systematic review and meta-analysis. *BMJ.* 2010;341:c4467.
24. Crocker T, Young J, Forster A, Brown L, Ozer S, Greenwood DC. The effect of physical rehabilitation on activities of daily living in older residents of long-term care facilities: systematic review with meta-analysis. *Age Ageing.* 2013;42(6):682–8.
25. Diep L, Kwagyan J, Kurantsin-Mills J, Weir R, Jayam-Trouth A. Association of physical activity level and stroke outcomes in men and women: a meta-analysis. *J Womens Health (Larchmt).* 2010;19(10):1815–22.
26. Farris MS, Mosli MH, McFadden AA, Friedenreich CM, Brenner DR. The association between leisure time physical activity and pancreatic cancer risk in adults: a systematic review and meta-analysis. *Cancer Epidemiol Biomarkers Prev.* 2015;24(10):1462–73.
27. Finkelstein EA, Trogdon JG, Cohen JW, Dietz WA. Annual medical spending attributable to obesity: payer- and service-specific estimates. *Health Aff (Millwood).* 2009;28(5):w822–31.
28. Ford ES, Ajani UA, Croft JB, et al. Explaining the decrease in U.S. deaths from coronary disease, 1980-2000. *N Engl J Med.* 2007;356(23):2388–98.
29. Gonçalves AK, Dantas Florêncio GL, de Atayde Silva MJ, Cobucci RN, Giraldo PC, Cote NM. Effects of physical activity on breast cancer prevention: a systematic review. *J Phys Act Health.* 2014;11(2):445–54.
30. Hallal PC, Andersen LB, Bull FC, Guthold R, Haskell W, Ekelund U. Global physical activity levels: surveillance progress, pitfalls, and prospects. *Lancet.* 2012;380(9838):247–57.
31. Haskell WL, Lee I-M, Pate RR, et al. Physical activity and public health: updated recommendation for adults from the American College of Sports Medicine and the American Heart Association. *Med Sci Sports Exerc.* 2007;39(8):1423–34.
32. HealthyPeople.gov. *Physical Activity* [Internet]. Washington (DC): Office of Disease Prevention and Health Promotion; [cited 2017 Oct 2]. Available from: http://www.healthypeople.gov/2020/topicsobjectives2020/overview.aspx?topicId=33
33. Huai P, Han H, Reilly KH, Guo X, Zhang J, Xu A. Leisure-time physical activity and risk of type 2 diabetes: a meta-analysis of prospective cohort studies. *Endocrine.* 2016;52(2):226–30.
34. James BD, Leurgans SE, Hebert LE, Scherr PA, Yaffe K, Bennett DA. Contribution of Alzheimer disease to mortality in the United States. *Neurology.* 2014;82(12):1045–50.
35. Jensen MD, Ryan DH, Apovian CM, et al. 2013 AHA/ACC/TOS guideline for the management of overweight and obesity in adults: a report of the American College of Cardiology/American Heart Association Task Force on Practice Guidelines and the Obesity Society. *J Am Coll Cardiol.* 2014;63(25 pt B):2985–3023.
36. Jepsen R, Aadland E, Robertson L, Kolotkin RL, Andersen JR, Natvig GK. Physical activity and quality of life in severely obese adults during a two-year lifestyle intervention programme. *J Obes.* 2015;2015:314194.
37. Johnson NB, Hayes LD, Brown K, Hoo EC, Ethier KA. CDC National Health Report: leading causes of morbidity and mortality and associated behavioral risk and protective factors — United States, 2005-2013. *MMWR Suppl.* 2014;63:3–27.
38. Kann L, Kinchen S, Shanklin SL, et al. Youth Risk Behavior Surveillance — United States, 2013. *MMWR Suppl.* 2014;63(4):1–168.
39. Keum N, Ju W, Lee DH, et al. Leisure-time physical activity and endometrial cancer risk: dose–response meta-analysis of epidemiological studies. *Int J Cancer.* 2014;135(3):682–94.
40. King AC, Stokols D, Talen E, Brassington GS, Killingsworth R. Theoretical approaches to the promotion of physical activity: forging a transdisciplinary paradigm. *Am J Prev Med.* 2002;23(2 suppl):15–25.
41. Kodama S, Saito K, Tanaka S, et al. Cardiorespiratory fitness as a quantitative predictor of all-cause mortality and cardiovascular events in healthy men and women: a meta-analysis. *JAMA.* 2009;301(19):2024–35.
42. Kohl HW III, Craig CL, Lambert EV, et al. The pandemic of physical inactivity: global action for public health. *Lancet.* 2012;380(9838):294–305.
43. Kraus WE, Bittner V, Appel L, et al. The National Physical Activity Plan: a call to action from the American Heart Association: a science advisory from the American Heart Association. *Circulation.* 2015;131(21):1932–40.
44. Lahart IM, Metsios GS, Nevill AM, Carmichael AR. Physical activity, risk of death and recurrence in breast cancer survivors: a systematic review and meta-analysis of epidemiological studies. *Acta Oncol.* 2015;54(5):635–54.
45. Lee I-M. Physical activity and cancer prevention — data from epidemiologic studies. *Med Sci Sports Exerc.* 2003;35(11):1823–7.
46. Lee I-M, Djoussé L, Sesso HD, Wang L, Buring JE. Physical activity and weight gain prevention. *JAMA.* 2010;303(12):1173–9.
47. Lee I-M, Paffenbarger RS Jr. Associations of light, moderate, and vigorous intensity physical activity with longevity. The Harvard Alumni Health Study. *Am J Epidemiol.* 2000;151(3):293–9.
48. Lee I-M, Paffenbarger RS Jr. Change in body weight and longevity. *JAMA.* 1992;268(15):2045–9.
49. Lee I-M, Shiroma EJ, Lobelo F, Puska P, Blair SN, Katzmarzyk PT. Effect of physical inactivity on major non-communicable diseases worldwide: an analysis of burden of disease and life expectancy. *Lancet.* 2012;380(9838):219–29.
50. Let's Move! *Eat Healthy* [Internet]. Washington (DC); Let's Move!; [cited 2017 Oct 2]. Available from: https://letsmove.obamawhitehouse.archives.gov/eat-healthy
51. Liubaoerjijin Y, Terada T, Fletcher K, Boulé NG. Effect of aerobic exercise intensity on glycemic control in type 2 diabetes: a meta-analysis of head-to-head randomized trials. *Acta Diabetol.* 2016;53(5):769–81.

52. Löllgen H, Böckenhoff A, Knapp G. Physical activity and all-cause mortality: an updated meta-analysis with different intensity categories. *Int J Sports Med.* 2009;30(3):213–24.
53. McLaughlin SJ, Connell CM, Janevic MR. Gender differences in trajectories of physical activity among older Americans with diabetes. *J Aging Health.* 2016;28(3):460–80.
54. McLeroy KR, Bibeau D, Steckler A, Glanz K. An ecological perspective on health promotion programs. *Health Educ Q.* 1988;15(4):351–77.
55. Morris JN, Heady JA, Raffle PA, Roberts CG, Parks JW. Coronary heart-disease and physical activity of work. *Lancet.* 1953;265(6795):1053–7.
56. Murray CJ, Abraham K, Ali MK, et al. The state of US health, 1990-2010: burden of diseases, injuries, and risk factors. *JAMA.* 2013;310(6):591–608.
57. Narayan KMV, Boyle JP, Geiss LS, Saaddine JB, Thompson TJ. Impact of recent increase in incidence on future diabetes burden: U.S., 2005–2050. *Diabetes Care.* 2006;29(9):2114–6.
58. Narayan KMV, Boyle JP, Thompson TJ, Sorensen SW, Williamson DF. Lifetime risk for diabetes mellitus in the United States. *JAMA.* 2003;290(14):1884–90.
59. National Center for Health Statistics. *Health, United States, 2015: With Special Feature on Racial and Ethnic Health Disparities.* Hyattsville (MD): National Center for Health Statistics; 2016. 461 p.
60. National Institutes of Health. Clinical guidelines on the identification, evaluation, and treatment of overweight and obesity in adults — the evidence report. *Obes Res.* 1998;6(suppl 2):51S–209S.
61. Ogden CL, Carroll MD, Fryar CD, Flegal KM. Prevalence of obesity among adults and youth: United States, 2011–2014. *NCHS Data Brief.* 2015;(219):1–8.
62. Ogden CL, Carroll MD, Kit BK, Flegal KM. Prevalence of childhood and adult obesity in the United States, 2011-2012. *JAMA.* 2014;311(8):806–14.
63. Paffenbarger RS Jr, Lee IM. A natural history of athleticism, health and longevity. *J Sports Sci.* 1998;16(suppl):S31–45.
64. Pandey A, Garg S, Khunger M, et al. Dose-response relationship between physical activity and risk of heart failure: a meta-analysis. *Circulation.* 2015;132(19):1786–94.
65. Parent M-É, Rousseau M-C, El-Zein M, Latreille B, Désy M, Siemiatycki J. Occupational and recreational physical activity during adult life and the risk of cancer among men. *Cancer Epidemiol.* 2011;35(2):151–9.
66. Pate RR, Pratt M, Blair SN, et al. Physical activity and public health. A recommendation for the Centers for Disease Control and Prevention and the American College of Sports Medicine. *JAMA.* 1995;273:402–7.
67. Pescatello LS. *ACSM's Guidelines for Exercise Testing and Prescription.* 9th ed. Philadelphia (PA): Wolters Kluwer; 2014. 456 p.
68. Potter R, Ellard D, Rees K, Thorogood M. A systematic review of the effects of physical activity on physical functioning, quality of life and depression in older people with dementia. *Int J Geriatr Psychiatry.* 2011;26(10):1000–11.
69. Rhyner KT, Watts A. Exercise and depressive symptoms in older adults: a systematic meta-analytic review. *J Aging Phys Act.* 2016;24(2):234–46.
70. Rosenbaum S, Vancampfort D, Steel Z, Newby J, Ward PB, Stubbs B. Physical activity in the treatment of post-traumatic stress disorder: a systematic review and meta-analysis. *Psychiatry Res.* 2015;230(2):130–6.
71. Sallis JF, Cervero RB, Ascher W, Henderson KA, Kraft MK, Kerr J. An ecological approach to creating active living communities. *Annu Rev Public Health.* 2006;27:297–322.
72. Sallis JF, Linton L, Kraft MK. The first Active Living Research Conference: growth of a transdisciplinary field. *Am J Prev Med.* 2005;28(2 suppl 2):93–5.
73. Sallis JF, Owen N. Ecological models of health behavior. In: Glanz K, Rimer BK, Lewis FM, editors. *Health Behavior and Health Education: Theory, Research, and Practice.* 3rd ed. San Francisco (CA): Jossey-Bass; 2002. p. 462–84.
74. Saris WHM, Blair SN, van Baak MA, et al. How much physical activity is enough to prevent unhealthy weight gain? Outcome of the IASO 1st Stock Conference and Consensus statement. *Obes Rev.* 2003;4(2):101–14.
75. Sedentary Behaviour Research Network. Letter to the editor: standardized use of the terms "sedentary" and "sedentary behaviours." *Appl Physiol Nutr Metab.* 2012;37(3):540–2.
76. Sesso HD, Paffenbarger RS Jr, Lee IM. Physical activity and coronary heart disease in men: The Harvard Alumni Health Study. *Circulation.* 2000;102(9):975–80.
77. Shiroma EJ, Sesso HD, Lee IM. Physical activity and weight gain prevention in older men. *Int J Obes (Lond).* 2012;36(9):1165–9.
78. Stokols D. Establishing and maintaining healthy environments. Toward a social ecology of health promotion. *Am Psychol.* 1992;47(1):6–22.
79. Sun J-Y, Shi L, Gao X-D, Xu S-F. Physical activity and risk of lung cancer: a meta-analysis of prospective cohort studies. *Asian Pac J Cancer Prev.* 2012;13(7):3143–7.
80. Sun S, Schiller JH, Gazdar AF. Lung cancer in never smokers — a different disease. *Nat Rev Cancer.* 2007;7(10):778–90.
81. Swank AM. Clinical applications. A first step to health: just stand up and move. *ACSMs Health Fit J.* 2015;19(6):34–6.
82. Tardon A, Lee WJ, Delgado-Rodriguez M, et al. Leisure-time physical activity and lung cancer: a meta-analysis. *Cancer Causes Control.* 2005;16(4):389–97.
83. Taylor HL, Jacobs DR Jr, Schucker B, Knudsen J, Leon AS, Debacker G. A questionnaire for the assessment of leisure time physical activities. *J Chronic Dis.* 1978;31(12):741–55.

84. Trumbo P, Schlicker S, Yates AA, Poos M. Dietary reference intakes for energy, carbohydrate, fiber, fat, fatty acids, cholesterol, protein and amino acids. *J Am Diet Assoc.* 2002;102(11):1621–30.
85. U.S. Department of Agriculture, U.S. Department of Health and Human Services. *Dietary Guidelines for Americans, 2010* [Internet]. 7th ed. Washington (DC): U.S. Government Printing Office; [cited 2015 May 15] Available from: http://www.health.gov/dietaryguidelines/2010.asp
86. U.S. Department of Health and Human Services. *2008 Physical Activity Guidelines for Americans. Be Active, Healthy, and Happy!* Washington (DC): U.S. Department of Health and Human Services; 2008. 76 p.
87. U.S. Department of Health and Human Services. *Active Living* [Internet]. Washington (DC): U.S. Department of Health and Human Services, Office of the Surgeon General; [cited 2017 Oct 2]. Available from: http://www.surgeongeneral.gov/priorities/prevention/strategy/active-living.html
88. U.S. Department of Health and Human Services. *Physical Activity and Health: A Report of the Surgeon General.* Atlanta (GA): U.S. Department of Health and Human Services, Centers for Disease Control and Prevention, National Center for Chronic Disease Prevention and Health Promotion; 1996. 300 p.
89. U.S. Department of Health and Human Services. *Step It Up! The Surgeon General's Call to Action to Promote Walking and Walkable Communities.* Washington (DC): U.S. Department of Health and Human Services, Office of the Surgeon General; 2015. 72 p.
90. U.S. Department of Health and Human Services. *The Health Consequences of Smoking — 50 Years of Progress. A Report of the Surgeon General.* Washington (DC): U.S. Department of Health and Human Services; 2014. 1081 p.
91. U.S. Department of Health and Human Services. *The Surgeon General's Call to Action to Improve the Health and Wellness of Persons With Disabilities.* Washington (DC): U.S. Department of Health and Human Services, Office of the Surgeon General; 2005.
92. U.S. Department of Health and Human Services. *The Surgeon General's Vision for a Healthy and Fit Nation Fact Sheet.* Washington (DC): U.S. Department of Health and Human Services, Office of the Surgeon General; 2010.
93. Warburton DER, Charlesworth S, Ivey A, Nettlefold L, Bredin SSD. A systematic review of the evidence for Canada's physical activity guidelines for adults. *Int J Behav Nutr Phys Act.* 2010;7:39.
94. Ward BW, Schiller JS, Goodman RA. Multiple chronic conditions among US adults: a 2012 update. *Prev Chronic Dis.* 2014;11:E62.
95. Weinstein AR, Sesso HD, Lee IM, et al. The joint effects of physical activity and body mass index on coronary heart disease risk in women. *Arch Intern Med.* 2008;168(8):884–90.
96. Williams PT. Physical fitness and activity as separate heart disease risk factors: a meta-analysis. *Med Sci Sports Exerc.* 2001;33(5):754–61.
97. Wolin KY, Yan Y, Colditz GA, Lee IM. Physical activity and colon cancer prevention: a meta-analysis. *Br J Cancer.* 2009;100(4):611–6.
98. Woodcock J, Franco OH, Orsini N, Roberts I. Non-vigorous physical activity and all-cause mortality: systematic review and meta-analysis of cohort studies. *Int J Epidemiol.* 2011;40(1):121–38.
99. World Health Organization. *Global Recommendations on Physical Activity for Health.* Geneva (Switzerland): World Health Organization; 2010. 60 p.
100. World Health Organization. *Physical Activity Fact Sheet* [Internet]. Geneva (Switzerland): World Health Organization; [cited 2016 May 26]. Available from: http://www.who.int/topics/physical_activity/en/
101. World Health Organization. *The Top 10 Causes of Death* [Internet]. Geneva (Switzerland): World Health Organization; [cited 2016 May 26]. Available from: http://www.who.int/mediacentre/factsheets/fs310/en/
102. Zhao G, Ford ES, Li C, Balluz LS. Physical activity in U.S. older adults with diabetes mellitus: prevalence and correlates of meeting physical activity recommendations. *J Am Geriatr Soc.* 2011;59(1):132–7.

CHAPTER 2

The Health Consequences of Physical Inactivity and Sedentary Behavior

INTRODUCTION

Over the past century, technological advances have reduced the need for human movement throughout the day. Currently, fewer people in the United States participate in walking or biking for the purpose of active transport. Additionally, technological innovations have led to a lower level of required movement to perform **activities of daily living** and household management.

In the 1960s, more than half of all American workers had more labor-intensive jobs that require a significant amount of time spent in moderate- to vigorous-intensity activities (1). Over the past decades, those jobs have been largely replaced by jobs that require little movement. Currently, less than 20% of all jobs require moderate-intensity **physical activity** (20). Less active commuting and longer school days have also led to an increase in sitting among youth (79,119). In effect, we have moved from societies where a substantial amount of human movement was required for daily survival to societies in which the necessity for human movement is quite low, with the average American adult spending close to 8 hours of their waking time per day on average in sitting activities and less than 30 minutes per day on average in moderate- to vigorous-intensity activities (51,115).

High levels of inactivity and sitting behavior, as seen in the U.S. population, have been linked to numerous poor health outcomes, including, but not limited to, obesity, cardiovascular disease, diabetes, and certain cancers (27,66). Therefore, individuals for whom activity is not a compulsory part of the day may need to plan opportunities for physical activity that are not otherwise necessitated. Likewise, individuals who spend much of their time in sitting behaviors may benefit from activity plans that include strategies for reducing the amount of time they spend seated. This chapter continues the theme of the previous chapter and touches on both physical inactivity and sedentary behavior.

Physical Inactivity

Definition of Inactivity and Current U.S. Guidelines for Physical Activity

Physical inactivity describes individuals or groups of individuals who are not meeting a certain threshold of moderate to vigorous activity, often based on the established guidelines (41). The American College of Sports Medicine (ACSM) recommends moderate- to vigorous-intensity cardiorespiratory exercise training for ≥30 minutes per day on ≥5 days per week for a total of ≥150 minutes per week, vigorous-intensity cardiorespiratory exercise training for ≥20 minutes per day on ≥3 days per week (≥75 min · wk^{-1}), or a combination of the two to achieve a total energy expenditure (TEE) of ≥500–1,000 **metabolic equivalent (MET)** minutes per week. Additionally, resistance training, neuromotor, and **flexibility** exercises are also recommended (38). The Centers for Disease Control and Prevention (CDC) also recommends 60 minutes per day or more of moderate to vigorous activity for **children** and **adolescents** (ages 6–17 yr) (92). As seen in the previous chapter, there are many positive health effects of physical activity. As a result, physical inactivity is considered a risk factor for numerous poor health outcomes (66).

Deconditioning

Significant reduction or cessation in exercise and increases in inactivity results in partial or complete reversal of the physiological adaptions to exercise, known as **deconditioning**. Common causes for deconditioning are reductions in typical levels of physical activity, aging, casting, paralysis, and bed rest.

The process by which adaptations to exercise are gradually lost or reduced is commonly known as **detraining**. Because detraining relates specifically to exercise, it is the form of deconditioning that is most relatable to inactivity. The effects of detraining are most notable in muscle tissue, including the heart (50,86,110). Reduced metabolic function can also happen quickly in response to reductions in exercise (86,121). Additionally, decreases in exercise that are maintained over a longer period of time, in the form of an inactive lifestyle, can result in decreased bone mineral density, metabolic dysfunction, and neuromuscular complications (66,71). As a result, inactivity is linked to numerous poor health outcomes including certain cancers, diabetes, dyslipidemia, hypertension, immune deficiencies, metabolic syndrome, neurological disorders, depressive disorders, osteoporosis, overweight/obesity, oxidative stress, and **sarcopenia**, among others (66). Additionally, the World Health Organization (WHO) had estimated that inactivity is responsible for 3.3 million deaths a year, making it one of the most important underlying causes of death worldwide (126).

Prevalence of Inactivity

Rate estimates for physical inactivity vary across populations and may even differ within the same population depending on the measurement instrument used to capture physical activity. In the U.S. population, self-reported estimates of physical activity from questionnaires suggest that 45%–75% of adults and youth from large population-based surveys are inactive based on the CDC guidelines (32,62,74,116). Estimates of inactivity based on objectively collected data tend to be higher than those based on self-report. Accelerometer data collected from the National Health and Nutrition Examination Survey (NHANES) between 2003 and 2006 suggested that 58% of youth 6–11 years, >90% of adolescents aged 12–19 years, and >95% of adults aged 20 years or older would be considered inactive based on the CDC guidelines (115). Other studies using objective measures have reported similar results (60,116).

It is worth noting that differences in estimates of inactivity between subjective measures (like self-report recall questionnaires) and objective measures (like pedometer and accelerometers) may be due in part to inherent biases that differ across instruments (49,111). Although there are many validated self-report measures, these instruments are more prone to overestimate higher intensity activity and underestimate lower intensity activity due to various types of reporting bias (49). Although accelerometers are generally considered the most valid instrument for assessing time spent in different intensities of activity, they can underestimate nonambulatory activities such as bicycling, swimming, and upper body resistance training (depending on monitor placement) (111). Despite quantitative differences, the general agreement between measurement instruments provides stronger evidence to support the finding that the majority of Americans could be classified as inactive. With similar results being reported in other countries (44,67), reducing the prevalence of inactivity in the population has become a major area of focus in the chronic disease prevention efforts of the CDC and the WHO (15,125).

Exercise is Medicine

In response to the high prevalence of inactivity worldwide, the ACSM spearheaded the Exercise is Medicine® (EIM) (3) program as a global initiative to decrease population levels of inactivity. EIM calls for clinical inactivity screening and encourages physicians and other health care providers to include physical activity when designing treatment plans for patients by referring patients to evidence-based activity programs. The main premise behind the EIM initiative is based on the existing evidence for the importance of reducing physical inactivity in the prevention and treatment of certain health conditions and diseases. The primary stakeholders in the EIM campaign are health care providers, exercise professionals, and community resources (Table 2.1).

Table 2.1 Exercise is Medicine® Stakeholders

Stakeholder	Description	Role
Health care providers	Health care providers, organizations, and systems	Health care providers of all specialties are encouraged to take the Exercise is Medicine® (EIM) pledge to: ■ Promote physical activity in their health care setting. ■ Assess and record physical activity at visits. ■ Conclude visits with an **exercise prescription**/refer patients to an EIM certified exercise professional. ■ Be a champion for physical activity in their health care system.
Exercise professionals	NCCA-accredited fitness professionals Exercise scientists Exercise physiologists Kinesiologists	Exercise professionals are encouraged to serve as an extension of the existing health care system by: ■ Educating patients on the importance of physical activity ■ Advising patients on how to discuss ways to increase physical activity with primary care physicians ■ Learning to develop training programs for a variety of diseases ■ Learning to receive referrals from and provide feedback to health care providers
Community resources	EIM places: qualified places for hosting physical activity interventions	Programs offered within a community are to include: ■ Structured discussions on health/activity/diet ■ Lifestyle behavioral change programs based on the latest evidence-based strategies

NCCA, National Commission for Certifying Agencies.

Information from American College of Sports Medicine. *Exercise is Medicine®: A Global Health Initiative* [Internet]. Indianapolis (IN): American College of Sports Medicine; [cited 2016 Feb 29]. Available from: http://exerciseismedicine.org/

Large initiatives, like EIM, hope to reduce rates of inactivity by better identifying individuals who may benefit most from increasing activity and by making activity-related resources more accessible.

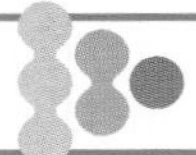

Sedentary Behavior

Definition and Measurement

The remainder of this chapter focuses on another component of movement that is separate from exercise and physical activity: sedentary behavior. First, it is necessary to establish the meaning of the term *sedentary*. Currently, two different definitions of sedentary continue to be used in the literature. In one definition, individuals or groups of individuals who are not meeting physical activity recommendations have been referred to as sedentary (10,89,91). Operationally, this definition would be the same as physical inactivity, and the two terms have been used interchangeably. A more recently established definition that better distinguishes *sedentary* from *inactive* would be those individuals or groups who perform high amounts of low energy expenditure activities, which have been referred to as *sedentary behaviors* (113). In this way, a person could be both sedentary and inactive but would not necessarily have to be both. Distinguishing the two terms is important because it allows for a greater understanding of the health consequences of being inactive versus being sedentary (vs. being both inactive and sedentary).

Sedentary behaviors have been more formally defined as waking behaviors that take place while in a sitting or reclined position and result in an energy expenditure of ≤1.5 METs; where 1 MET is the energy cost of resting quietly (often defined in terms of oxygen uptake as $3.5\ mL \cdot kg^{-1} \cdot min^{-1}$) (89,91,113). This definition focuses on both the postural and energy expenditure aspects of sedentary behavior while differentiating it from sleep. Based on this definition for sedentary behavior, **light-intensity activity** would then be defined as seated and nonseated activities with an energy expenditure between 1.5 and 3.0 METs.

Historically, feasibility concerns with direct observation have caused health-related studies of sedentary behavior to rely heavily on subjective self-report questionnaires which have been shown to do reasonably well at capturing certain domain-specific sedentary behaviors, such as watching television, sitting at a computer, or sitting while commuting. With the wider availability of objective measurement instruments, including accelerometers and **inclinometers**, it has become possible to gain more accurate and precise estimates of the total time a person spends in sedentary pursuits. Tremblay et al. (113) have suggested that sedentary behavior should be described in accordance with the SITT formula (similar to frequency, intensity, time, and type [FITT] for exercise) which includes **S**edentary behavior frequency (number of bouts), **I**nterruptions (or breaks), **T**ime (or duration), and **T**ype (or mode).

The subdiscipline of biology dedicated to the study of the body's response to short-term and long-term sedentary behavior with a particular focus on identifying unique mechanisms that are distinct from the biological basis of exercising is known as **sedentary physiology** (113), also sometimes referred to as *inactivity physiology* (46,47). Both sedentary behavior and exercise can be viewed as regions along a continuous scale of MET values, referred to as the *movement continuum* (Fig. 2.1). Because of this relationship on the continuum, some of the principles that apply to exercise physiology could also be seen as pertaining to sedentary physiology (*e.g.*, progression, individuality, specificity) (113). Therefore, deconditioning studies involving a downshift in the intensity of movement to the level of sedentary behavior, such as complete mobility loss (as with casting or paralysis) (43,94), bed rest (110,131), or loss of gravity (microgravity/space flight) (55,108) can be seen as providing evidence of the physiological effects of both inactivity and sedentary behavior.

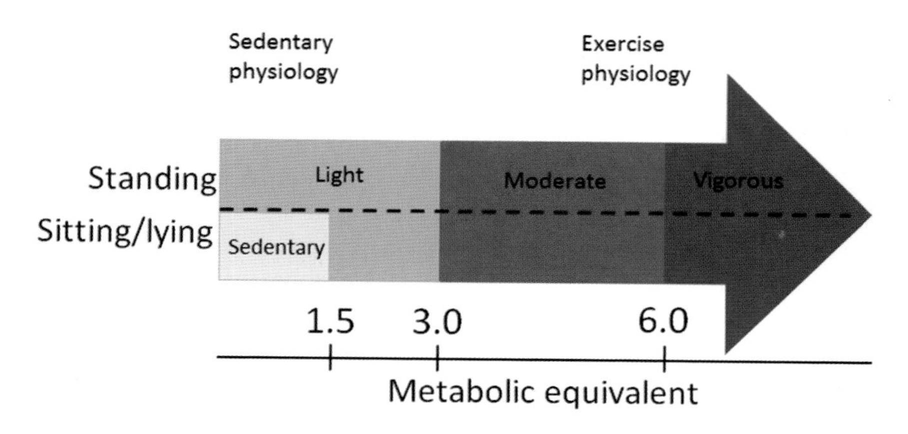

FIGURE 2.1. The movement continuum for waking movement with reference to sedentary and exercise physiology.

In light of the fact that sedentary behavior and exercise are often viewed as two parts of one continuum, it is important to note the physiological responses and adaptions to sedentary behavior are not necessarily the opposite of exercise adaptions or responses. This finding is likely due in part to the fact that the relationship (dose-response) between activity intensity and various disease outcomes is often not constant (linear) across the continuum (70). Additionally, there is evidence that sedentary behavior may negatively modify the effects of physical activity on health outcomes, essentially causing a shift in the dose-response curve between physical activity and certain disease outcomes so that more activity is necessary to reduce the disease risk when a person is also sedentary (28,63). There is also evidence that sedentary behavior and moderate- to vigorous-intensity physical activity may cause different physiological effects that contribute separately to certain disease pathways (47,48,113). Support for this observation can be seen in the fact that sedentary behavior has been shown to modify the effects of physical activity on health outcomes. Specific evidence from physiological research is presented in the next section of this chapter as it pertains to specific health outcomes.

Health Effects of Sedentary Behavior

Sedentary Behavior and Overall Mortality

Several studies have examined the connections between sedentary behavior and mortality, from either all causes or related to specific disease pathways (8,31,40,64,118,123). A meta-analysis of 18 studies that included over 700,000 individuals concluded that sedentary behavior was associated with a 49% increase in the risk of all-cause mortality (hazard ratio [HR] = 1.49; 95% confidence interval [CI] = [1.14, 2.03]) and a 90% increase in the risk of cardiovascular death (HR = 1.90; 95% CI = [1.36, 2.66]) (123). Another, more recent meta-analysis looking at 14 studies also found significant associations with all-cause mortality and cardiovascular mortality. That study also found that sedentary behavior was associated with a 13% increase in cancer mortality (HR = 1.13; 95% CI = [1.05, 1.21]) (8). The later study also examined the effect of sedentary behavior on all-cause mortality stratified by physical activity level. The results indicated that sedentary time was associated with a 30% lower risk for all-cause mortality in those with high physical activity levels when compared to those with low physical activity levels, suggesting that activity may attenuate some but not all of the association between sedentary behavior and all-cause mortality.

Another study that examined all-cause mortality in a large cohort of 40- to 79-year-old men and women with diabetes found that those individuals reporting more than 12 hours of sedentary behavior per day had a 21% increase in mortality risk (HR = 1.21; 95% CI = [1.08, 1.37]) compared with those individuals reporting less than 6 hours of sedentary behavior per day after controlling for physical activity levels (40). The study also found those individuals who were highly sedentary ($\geq$11 h · d^{-1}) and least active (<9.2 MET-h · d^{-1} of activity) had a 75% increased risk of all-cause mortality (HR = 1.75; 95% CI = [1.45, 2.11]) when compared with the least sedentary (<7 h · d^{-1}) and most active (≥20.5 MET-h · d^{-1}) individuals.

The vast majority of studies related to sedentary behavior and mortality examined all-cause mortality only. A smaller number of studies also looked at cardiovascular and cancer mortality. However, one study utilizing data from the National Institutes of Health and American Association of Retired Persons (NIH-AARP) Diet and Health Study (N = 221,426 individuals aged 50–71 yr; mean follow-up 14.1 yr) was able to examine associations between reported television watching and over a dozen of the leading causes of mortality in the United States (64). This study concluded that there were significant risk increases for death from cancer, heart disease, chronic obstructive pulmonary disease, diabetes, influenza/pneumonia, Parkinson disease, liver disease, and suicide with increased television watching.

Sedentary Behavior and Cardiovascular Disease

One of the earliest well-known studies in the field of physical activity epidemiology can been seen as providing early scientific evidence for the health effects of both physical inactivity and sedentary behavior on cardiovascular outcomes. This seminal study by Morris et al. (84) was conducted on a large cohort of London Transport Executive employees from 1949 to 1950. The results suggested the more sedentary bus drivers had close to twice the risk of fatal coronary heart disease as the bus conductors, whose job required both standing and walking to collect passenger tickets. Additional occupational studies followed that supported these findings (1,83,85,90,101).

Recently, there have been several review articles and meta-analyses that have summarized the evidence for the associations between sedentary behavior and the development of cardiovascular disease (8,26,35,123). The results of one meta-analysis suggested that for each 2 hours per day increase in screen time, there was a 17% increased risk for cardiovascular disease (HR: 1.17; 95% CI = [1.13, 1.20]) (35). When examined by comparing those individuals in the lowest category of screen time with those in the highest category of screen time, the researchers found that there was a risk increase for cardiovascular disease of 125% for those in the highest category after adjusting for important covariates including physical activity. Although not all studies included in these recent meta-analyses showed evidence for an association between cardiovascular disease and sedentary behavior, the pooled results from all four meta-analysis studies, respectively, suggested that overall, there were important, significant associations. A meta-analysis summarizing the results of studies examining the connections between sedentary behavior and cardiovascular mortality is discussed later in this chapter with other mortality outcomes.

Bed rest studies have been used to understand the biological relationship between sedentary behavior and cardiovascular disease outcomes. The results of bed rest studies indicate that prolonged periods of sedentary behavior are associated with deleterious changes in vascular function including reduced peripheral vascular function, increased blood pressure, and significant decreases in brachial artery diameter (12,25,45,97). Space simulation has also provided evidence for decreased endothelium-dependent vasodilation and increased endothelial cell damage in women after more than a month of head-down bed rest (25). That study also showed that the effects were mediated by physical activity, suggesting that the physiological connection between endothelial function and sedentary behavior could be the same as the physiological connection between exercise and endothelial function. It has also been proposed that sedentary behavior may be associated with cardiovascular disease through the effects on adiposity and obesity (47).

Sedentary Behavior and Obesity

Long-term weight gain, leading to obesity, results from a sustained positive energy balance that is achieved when caloric food intake exceeds TEE (24). The main components of TEE are basal metabolic rate, the thermic effect of food, and activity thermogenesis. Activity thermogenesis which may account for as much as 30% of TEE can be divided into exercise activity thermogenesis (EAT) and nonexercise activity thermogenesis (NEAT) (73).

NEAT is defined as all physical activities other than exercise for the purpose of **physical fitness** and typically accounts for more TEE than EAT (even in most individuals performing regular exercise) (73). Energy expenditure related to NEAT has been shown to vary by as much as 2,000 kcal per day between individuals (9). Differences in NEAT may be the result of differences in active transport, work-related activity, nonexercise leisure activity, and/or activities of daily living.

By definition, sedentary behaviors are those waking behaviors with the lowest energy expenditure. As a result, benefits to energy expenditure can be achieved by converting sedentary time to increased intensity activity (both exercise and nonexercise activities). In addition to the importance of sedentary behavior to energy balance, it has also been suggested that the deleterious effects of sedentary behavior on metabolic function and the association between certain sedentary behaviors, such as watching television, and excess caloric intake may also provide important connections between sedentary behaviors and obesity (11).

Currently, there are over a dozen review articles summarizing the association between sedentary behavior and weight gain, adiposity, and obesity (16,19,23,56,69,78,95,96,99,102,112,114,120,129). The majority of these studies have been conducted in children and adolescents. Two review studies in youth conducted meta-analyses examining the relationship of television watching and the development of obesity (114,129). Both of those studies reported positive associations between television watching and obesity. Odds ratios (ORs) reported in Zhang et al. (129) indicated that after controlling for other important variables, there was a 47% increased pooled odds of developing obesity in youth with the highest reported television watching versus those with the lowest (OR = 1.47; 95% CI = [1.33, 1.62]). Furthermore, they reported a linear dose-response relationship of a 13% increased risk of childhood obesity with every hour per day spent watching television ($p < .0001$).

Studies in adults examining the relationship between sedentary behavior and obesity have reported both positive and negative findings (96,112,120). An earlier study in Pima adults suggested that increased television watching ($\geq 3 \text{ h} \cdot \text{d}^{-1}$) was significantly associated with higher **body mass index (BMI)** in men but not in women (34). More recently, it has been suggested that there may be a bidirectional relationship between sedentary behavior and obesity-related variables, such that highly sedentary adults are prone to weight gain, whereas adults who are overweight and obese are prone to become more sedentary over time (37,42). A longitudinal study by Golubic et al. (42) suggested that after controlling for important covariates, objectively measured sedentary time was related to changes in fat mass. The authors also found that a 1.5-hour reduction in sedentary time was associated with a 1.4-kg reduction in body weight.

Sedentary Behavior and Diabetes/Metabolic Disease

In relation to impaired glucose tolerance and Type 2 diabetes mellitus, the results of several studies suggest that sedentary behavior has a strong influence on lipoprotein lipase (LPL) activity in skeletal muscles (7,46,47). LPL is an enzyme that is necessary for hydrolysis of the triglyceride contained in lipoproteins. LPL binds to circulating lipoproteins when present on the vascular endothelium. Higher circulating levels of LPL in skeletal muscle have been linked with higher plasma glucose levels (33,61). More specifically, higher levels of circulating LPL have been shown to cause preferential use of lipids as an energy source, which can lead to insulin resistance (33,106). One study in mice and rats showed that both acute and chronic sedentary behavior lead to a decrease in LPL activity in weight-bearing skeletal muscle. It has also been suggested that sedentary behavior may affect diabetes development through its influence on gene activation and deactivation (6) and on the regulation of β cell function (30).

Currently, there are numerous public health studies that have linked the amount of time spent watching television to diabetes-related outcomes and increased risk for diabetes development (29,31,36,57,58,100,122,128). An analysis of television watching time and the development of diabetes in the Diabetes Prevention Program suggested that in individuals at high risk for diabetes, there was a 3.4% increased risk for diabetes with each 1 hour per day of reported television watching (over ~3 yr of follow-up). However, this risk was attenuated when adjusting for body weight (100). Additionally, total sedentary behavior, obtained from accelerometer output, has also been linked to diabetes-related outcomes and the development of diabetes in several studies (22,30,52–54). Specifically, one study that examined the cross-sectional relationship between average total sedentary minutes per day from the accelerometer and cardiometabolic biomarkers in a representative sample of U.S. adults found that total sedentary minutes per day was positively associated with insulin, homeostasis model assessment of steady state beta cell function (HOMA-%B), and insulin sensitivity (HOMA-%S) ($p < .05$) (53).

Sedentary Behavior and Cancer

A **systematic review and meta-analyses** that included all forms of reported cancer suggested that individuals participating in higher amounts of sedentary behavior were at increased risk of developing cancer (HR = 1.13; 95% CI = [1.05, 1.21]) (44). There have also been a number of studies examining the connections between sedentary behavior and specific forms of cancer. The most examined associations have been with colorectal, breast, endometrial, ovarian, and prostate cancers (8,21,75–77,93,130).

Although the findings for an association with sedentary behavior for any one form of cancer have been mixed, recent large meta-analyses for women's breast cancer and for colon cancer suggest that overall, sedentary behavior may confer an increased risk for the development of these cancers (130). For women's breast cancer specifically, the pooled OR for developing breast cancer was 1.08 (95% CI = [1.04, 1.13]) across all 21 sites examined (130). The results were similar when only studies controlling for BMI or only studies controlling for physical activity were included. In the case of colon and rectal cancer, the meta-analyses included 23 studies, representing over 4 million individuals (21). The pooled **relative risk** (RR) of developing colon cancer was 1.30 (95% CI = [1.22, 1.39]) for sedentary individuals. Including only studies controlling for physical activity yielded similar results, whereas controlling for BMI gave attenuate but significant estimates of risk increase (RR = 1.24; 95% CI = [1.14, 1.35]) with higher sedentary behavior. Overall, the findings for an association between sedentary behavior and rectal cancer were not significant in that study.

The exact mechanisms by which sedentary behavior may be linked to the development of cancer are not completely understood. Some of the mechanisms that have been proposed include increased adiposity (98) and decreased insulin sensitivity/insulin resistance (39,80). It is plausible that different biological mechanisms may be involved with the formation of different cancers. For example, in the case of breast cancer, one study showed a positive association between sedentary behavior and increased breast density, a known risk factor for breast cancer, specifically (124).

Sedentary Behavior and Bone Mineral Density

Sedentary behavior has been shown to be related to reductions in bone mineral density (13,65,82,127,131). Results from studies of sedentary behavior and bone formation suggest that sedentary behavior does not lead to increased bone formation but causes rapid increases in bone absorption that leads to lower bone mineral density and increased risk of fracture or osteoporosis (59). Evidence for the effects of prolonged periods of sedentary behavior on bone mass has been gained from studies involving space flight and bed rest. One study, by Kim et al. (65), showed that in healthy males, markers of bone resorption including urinary calcium, deoxypyridinoline, and Type 1 collagen cross-linked *N*-telopeptides were increased during a 14-day period of bed rest. Other studies reporting similar results have shown that bouts of daily **aerobic** exercise did not offset the negative effects of bone metabolism that resulted from bed rest (108,131). In relation to this finding, the results of a literature review on the health effects of cycling, a form of exercise performed while sitting, suggests that road cycling does not confer significant osteogenic benefits (88). This conclusion was based on the findings of lower bone mineral density in key regions including the lumbar spine, pelvis, hip, and femoral neck.

A number of population-based studies have provided evidence for the link between sedentary behavior and reduced bone mass density and related poor health outcomes (17,18,81,87,107,109). One study in **older adults** (aged 55–83 yr) at high risk for physical frailty reported a 36% increased risk (HR = 1.36, CI = [1.02, 1.79], $p < .05$) of developing physical frailty over a 2-year follow-up for each hour per day of objectively recorded sedentary behavior at baseline, after controlling for important covariates including time spent in moderate to vigorous physical activity (109). Studies in adolescents have also provided evidence for the negative effects of sedentary behaviors on bone mineral density in younger populations. A study reporting on over 1,200 youth (aged 8–22 yr) from the NHANES suggested that the associations between sedentary behaviors and lower bone mineral density were not attenuated by time spent in moderate to vigorous activity but may be attenuated by reported frequency of **strength** training and vigorous play (17).

Sedentary Behavior and Physical Function in Older Adults

Physical independence has been associated with longer survival (4) and higher quality of life (68) in older adults. Several studies examining the associations between total time spent in sedentary behavior (measured objectively) and physical function in older adults concluded that there were important associations between higher levels of sedentary behavior and reduced physical function (72,103–105). One study found that there were significant negative associations between total sedentary time and a composite z score for function that was based on six function variables: chair stand, arm curl, 8-ft up and go, 6-minute walk test, chair sit and reach, and back scratch (103). These findings were significant after controlling for BMI, gender, age, register time, and minutes per day of moderate to vigorous activity. Another study (104) that specifically examined the effects of breaking up sedentary time on function in older adults found that breaking up sedentary time was associated with increased physical function, as determined through a composite z score based on results from a battery of tests (chair stand, arm curl, 8-ft up and go, 6-min walk test, chair sit and reach, and back scratch). This association was still significant after adjusting for time spent in moderate to vigorous activity and overall sedentary time.

Sedentary Behavior Goals and Guidelines

Just as sedentary physiology can be seen as a complementary field of research to exercise physiology, so can sedentary behavior reduction be seen as a complement to, without becoming a replacement for, setting exercise goals. Current evidence suggests that individuals who are highly sedentary even if they engage in prescribed levels of physical activity could benefit from reductions in sedentary behavior. Furthermore, for individuals who are finding it difficult to achieve physical activity goals due to health/physiological, psychological, or other reason, sedentary behavior reduction may provide a more accomplishable proximal goal toward increasing physical activity.

Currently, there are no standardized protocols for reducing sedentary behavior and the approaches used have typically been different than those taken to increase levels of moderate to vigorous physical activity. Whereas **exercise** is viewed as a planned moderate or vigorous activity done in bouts of 10 minutes or more, on *most* days, sedentary reduction is encouraged to take place throughout each day and can occur in short “microbursts” or longer bouts. Although health research provides evidence for both reducing total time spent sitting and breaking up long bouts of sitting, there are no specific guidelines for sedentary behavior as there are for physical activity (48).

Box 2.1 Adopted Sedentary Guidelines

Government or Organization	Guideline
American Academy of Pediatrics (2)	Limit children's media time to no more than 1–2 h of quality programming. Discourage television viewing for younger than age 2 yr. Remove television sets from bedrooms and encourage active alternatives.
Australia (5)	Screen time is not recommended for younger than 2 yr of age. 2–5 yr: Limit screen time to $1\ \text{h} \cdot \text{d}^{-1}$. Children younger than 5 yr should not be sedentary; bouts should be <1 h. 5–17 yr: Limit screen time to $<2\ \text{h} \cdot \text{d}^{-1}$ and break up prolonged periods of sitting. Adults: Minimize the amount of time spent in prolonged sitting and break up prolonged bouts of sitting.
Canada (14)	Screen time is not recommended for younger than 2 yr of age. 2–4 yr: Limit screen time to $1\ \text{h} \cdot \text{d}^{-1}$. 5–6 and 12–17 yr: Limit screen time to $<2\ \text{h} \cdot \text{d}^{-1}$. Limit stroller time in young children and motorized transport in older children and adolescents.
United Kingdom (117)	All children and young people should minimize the amount of time spent being sedentary (sitting) for extended periods.

However, some organizations and national governments have adopted general guidelines related to sedentary behavior (Box 2.1). Originally, these guidelines all focused around screen-based activities in children and adolescents. More recently, evidence gained from new research has allowed for some of the guidelines to be extended to adults and to other modes of sitting including transportation sitting (5,14). Currently, more evidence of the specific nature of the dose-response relationship between sedentary behavior and specific health outcomes is needed in order to create more explicit guidelines including those specific to different health outcomes.

SUMMARY

Inactivity, or the failure to perform a sufficient amount of physical activity, has been linked to numerous poor health outcomes and increases in mortality rates. Current evidence from population-based studies suggests that most American adults are not meeting the CDC physical activity recommendations. There is also evidence that spending too much time in very low-intensity activities, performed while sitting or lying down, is also a risk factor for poor health outcomes. Based on both biological and epidemiological evidence, it is likely that all individuals who spend excessive time in sedentary behaviors could benefit by decreasing sedentary time.

Unlike physical activity, there are currently no specific guidelines suggesting what amount of sedentary behavior is acceptable. A better understanding of the specific dose-response relationship between sedentary behavior and specific disease outcomes would be needed in order to identify a threshold for an acceptable level of daily sedentary behavior. However, the current literature suggests that both reducing total sedentary time and breaking up long periods of sedentary behavior throughout the day could lead to improved function and reductions in disease risk. Health care providers and exercise professionals, such as those certified through EIM, should consider working with individuals in all settings to both increase physical activity levels and decrease sedentary behavior.

REFERENCES

1. Alfredsson L, Hammar N, Hogstedt C. Incidence of myocardial infarction and mortality from specific causes among bus drivers in Sweden. *Int J Epidemiol.* 1993;22(1):57–61.
2. American Academy of Pediatrics. *Media and Children Communication Toolkit* [Internet]. Elk Grove Village (IL): American Academy of Pediatrics; [cited 2016 Feb 29]. Available from: https://www.aap.org/en-us/advocacy-and-policy/aap-health-initiatives/Pages/Media-and-Children.aspx
3. American College of Sports Medicine. *Exercise is Medicine®: A Global Health Initiative* [Internet]. Indianapolis (IN): American College of Sports Medicine; [cited 2016 Feb 29]. Available from: http://exerciseismedicine.org
4. Arai Y, Inagaki H, Takayama M, et al. Physical independence and mortality at the extreme limit of life span: supercentenarians study in Japan. *J Gerontol A Biol Sci Med Sci.* 2014;69(4):486–94.
5. Australian Government Department of Health. *Physical Activity and Sedentary Behaviour Guidelines.* Canberra (Australia): Commonwealth of Australia; [cited 2016 Feb 29]. Available from: http://www.health.gov.au/internet/main/publishing.nsf/Content/pasb
6. Bey L, Akunuri N, Zhao P, Hoffman EP, Hamilton DG, Hamilton MT. Patterns of global gene expression in rat skeletal muscle during unloading and low-intensity ambulatory activity. *Physiol Genomics.* 2003;13(2):157–67.
7. Bey L, Hamilton MT. Suppression of skeletal muscle lipoprotein lipase activity during physical inactivity: a molecular reason to maintain daily low-intensity activity. *J Physiol.* 2003;551(pt 2):673–82.
8. Biswas A, Oh PI, Faulkner GE, et al. Sedentary time and its association with risk for disease incidence, mortality, and hospitalization in adults: a systematic review and meta-analysis. *Ann Intern Med.* 2015;162(2):123–32.
9. Black AE, Coward WA, Cole TJ, Prentice AM. Human energy expenditure in affluent societies: an analysis of 574 doubly-labelled water measurements. *Eur J Clin Nutr.* 1996;50(2):72–92.
10. Blair SN, Cheng Y, Holder JS. Is physical activity or physical fitness more important in defining health benefits? *Med Sci Sports Exerc.* 2001;33(6 suppl):S379–99.
11. Blass EM, Anderson DR, Kirkorian HL, Pempek TA, Price I, Koleini MF. On the road to obesity: television viewing increases intake of high-density foods. *Physiol Behav.* 2006;88(4–5):597–604.
12. Bleeker MW, De Groot PC, Rongen GA, et al. Vascular adaptation to deconditioning and the effect of an exercise countermeasure: results of the Berlin Bed Rest study. *J Appl Physiol (1985).* 2005;99(4):1293–300.
13. Caillot-Augusseau A, Lafage-Proust MH, Soler C, Pernod J, Dubois F, Alexandre C. Bone formation and resorption biological markers in cosmonauts during and after a 180-day space flight (Euromir 95). *Clin Chem.* 1998;44(3):578–85.
14. Canadian Society for Exercise Physiology. *Canadian Physical Activity Guidelines. Canadian Sedentary Behaviour Guidelines* [Internet]. Ottawa (Canada): Canadian Society for Exercise Physiology; [cited 2016 Feb 29]. Available from: http://www.csep.ca/en/guidelines/get-the-guidelines
15. Centers for Disease Control and Prevention. *Chronic Disease Overview* [Internet]. Atlanta (GA): Centers for Disease Control and Prevention; [cited 2016 Aug 10]. Available from: https://www.cdc.gov/chronicdisease/overview/index.htm
16. Chastin SF, Egerton T, Leask C, Stamatakis E. Meta-analysis of the relationship between breaks in sedentary behavior and cardiometabolic health. *Obesity (Silver Spring).* 2015;23(9):1800–10.
17. Chastin SF, Mandrichenko O, Helbostadt JL, Skelton DA. Associations between objectively-measured sedentary behaviour and physical activity with bone mineral density in adults and older adults, the NHANES study. *Bone.* 2014;64:254–62.
18. Chastin SF, Mandrichenko O, Skelton DA. The frequency of osteogenic activities and the pattern of intermittence between periods of physical activity and sedentary behaviour affects bone mineral content: the cross-sectional NHANES study. *BMC Public Health.* 2014;14:4.
19. Chinapaw MJ, Proper KI, Brug J, van Mechelen W, Singh AS. Relationship between young peoples' sedentary behaviour and biomedical health indicators: a systematic review of prospective studies. *Obes Rev.* 2011;12(7):e621–32.
20. Church TS, Thomas DM, Tudor-Locke C, et al. Trends over 5 decades in U.S. occupation-related physical activity and their associations with obesity. *PLoS One.* 2011;6(5):e19657.
21. Cong YJ, Gan Y, Sun HL, et al. Association of sedentary behaviour with colon and rectal cancer: a meta-analysis of observational studies. *Br J Cancer.* 2014;110(3):817–26.
22. Cooper AR, Sebire S, Montgomery AA, et al. Sedentary time, breaks in sedentary time and metabolic variables in people with newly diagnosed Type 2 diabetes. *Diabetologia.* 2012;55(3):589–99.
23. Costigan SA, Barnett L, Plotnikoff RC, Lubans DR. The health indicators associated with screen-based sedentary behavior among adolescent girls: a systematic review. *J Adolesc Health.* 2013;52(4):382–92.
24. Daan S, Masman D, Strijkstra A, Verhulst S. Intraspecific allometry of basal metabolic rate: relations with body size, temperature, composition, and circadian phase in the kestrel, Falco tinnunculus. *J Biol Rhythms.* 1989;4(2):155–71.
25. Demiot C, Dignat-George F, Fortrat JO, et al. WISE 2005: chronic bed rest impairs microcirculatory endothelium in women. *Am J Physiol Heart Circ Physiol.* 2007;293(5):H3159–64.
26. de Rezende LF, Rey-López JP, Matsudo VK, do Carmo Luiz O. Sedentary behavior and health outcomes among older adults: a systematic review. *BMC Public Health.* 2014;14:333.
27. de Rezende LF, Rodrigues Lopes M, Rey-López JP, Matsudo VK, Luiz Odo C. Sedentary behavior and health outcomes: an overview of systematic reviews. *PLoS One.* 2014;9(8):e105620.

28. Dietz WH. The role of lifestyle in health: the epidemiology and consequences of inactivity. *Proc Nutr Soc.* 1996;55(3):829–40.
29. Dunstan DW, Barr EL, Healy GN, et al. Television viewing time and mortality: the Australian Diabetes, Obesity and Lifestyle Study (AusDiab). *Circulation.* 2010;121(3):384–91.
30. Dunstan DW, Kingwell BA, Larsen R, et al. Breaking up prolonged sitting reduces postprandial glucose and insulin responses. *Diabetes Care.* 2012;35(5):976–83.
31. Dunstan DW, Salmon J, Healy GN, et al. Association of television viewing with fasting and 2-h postchallenge plasma glucose levels in adults without diagnosed diabetes. *Diabetes Care.* 2007;30(3):516–22.
32. Fakhouri TH, Hughes JP, Burt VL, Song M, Fulton JE, Ogden CL. Physical activity in U.S. youth aged 12–15 years, 2012. *NCHS Data Brief.* 2014;141:1–8.
33. Ferreira LD, Pulawa LK, Jensen DR, Eckel RH. Overexpressing human lipoprotein lipase in mouse skeletal muscle is associated with insulin resistance. *Diabetes.* 2001;50(5):1064–8.
34. Fitzgerald SJ, Kriska AM, Pereira MA, de Courten MP. Associations among physical activity, television watching, and obesity in adult Pima Indians. *Med Sci Sports Exerc.* 1997;29(7):910–5.
35. Ford ES, Caspersen CJ. Sedentary behaviour and cardiovascular disease: a review of prospective studies. *Int J Epidemiol.* 2012;41(5):1338–53.
36. Ford ES, Schulze MB, Kröger J, Pischon T, Bergmann MM, Boeing H. Television watching and incident diabetes: findings from the European Prospective Investigation into Cancer and Nutrition-Potsdam Study. *J Diabetes.* 2010;2(1):23–7.
37. Friend DM, Devarakonda K, O'Neal TJ, et al. Basal ganglia dysfunction contributes to physical inactivity in obesity. *Cell Metab.* 2017;25(2):312–21.
38. Garber CE, Blissmer B, Deschenes MR, et al. American College of Sports Medicine position stand. Quantity and quality of exercise for developing and maintaining cardiorespiratory, musculoskeletal, and neuromotor fitness in apparently healthy adults: guidance for prescribing exercise. *Med Sci Sports Exerc.* 2011;43(7):1334–59.
39. Giovannucci E. Metabolic syndrome, hyperinsulinemia, and colon cancer: a review. *Am J Clin Nutr.* 2007;86(3):s836–42.
40. Glenn KR, Slaughter JC, Fowke JH, et al. Physical activity, sedentary behavior and all-cause mortality among Blacks and Whites with diabetes. *Ann Epidemiol.* 2015;25(9):649–55.
41. Go AS, Mozaffarian D, Roger VL, et al. Heart disease and stroke statistics — 2013 update: a report from the American Heart Association. *Circulation.* 2013;127(1):e6–e245.
42. Golubic R, Wijndaele K, Sharp SJ, et al. Physical activity, sedentary time and gain in overall and central body fat: 7-year follow-up of the ProActive trial cohort. *Int J Obes (Lond).* 2015;39(1):142–8.
43. Grana EA, Chiou-Tan F, Jaweed MM. Endplate dysfunction in healthy muscle following a period of disuse. *Muscle Nerve.* 1996;19(8):989–93.
44. Hallal PC, Andersen LB, Bull FC, Guthold R, Haskell W, Ekelund U. Global physical activity levels: surveillance progress, pitfalls, and prospects. *Lancet.* 2012;380(9838):247–57.
45. Hamburg NM, McMackin CJ, Huang AL, et al. Physical inactivity rapidly induces insulin resistance and microvascular dysfunction in healthy volunteers. *Arterioscler Thromb Vasc Biol.* 2007;27(12):2650–6.
46. Hamilton MT, Hamilton DG, Zderic TW. Exercise physiology versus inactivity physiology: an essential concept for understanding lipoprotein lipase regulation. *Exerc Sport Sci Rev.* 2004;32(4):161–6.
47. Hamilton MT, Hamilton DG, Zderic TW. Role of low energy expenditure and sitting in obesity, metabolic syndrome, Type 2 diabetes, and cardiovascular disease. *Diabetes.* 2007;56(11):2655–67.
48. Hamilton MT, Healy GN, Dunstan DW, Zderic TW, Owen N. Too little exercise and too much sitting: inactivity physiology and the need for new recommendations on sedentary behavior. *Curr Cardiovasc Risk Rep.* 2008;2(4):292–8.
49. Haskell WL. Physical activity by self-report: a brief history and future issues. *J Phys Act Health.* 2012;9(suppl 1):S5–10.
50. Hather BM, Adams GR, Tesch PA, Dudley GA. Skeletal muscle responses to lower limb suspension in humans. *J Appl Physiol (1985).* 1992;72(4):1493–8.
51. Healy GN, Clark BK, Winkler EA, Gardiner PA, Brown WJ, Matthews CE. Measurement of adults' sedentary time in population-based studies. *Am J Prev Med.* 2011;41(2):216–27.
52. Healy GN, Dunstan DW, Salmon J, et al. Breaks in sedentary time: beneficial associations with metabolic risk. *Diabetes Care.* 2008;31(4):661–6.
53. Healy GN, Matthews CE, Dunstan DW, Winkler EA, Owen N. Sedentary time and cardio-metabolic biomarkers in US adults: NHANES 2003–06. *Eur Heart J.* 2011;32(5):590–7.
54. Healy GN, Wijndaele K, Dunstan DW, et al. Objectively measured sedentary time, physical activity, and metabolic risk: the Australian Diabetes, Obesity and Lifestyle Study (AusDiab). *Diabetes Care.* 2008;31(2):369–71.
55. Hikida RS, Gollnick PD, Dudley GA, Convertino VA, Buchanan P. Structural and metabolic characteristics of human skeletal muscle following 30 days of simulated microgravity. *Aviat Space Environ Med.* 1989;60(7):664–70.
56. Hoare E, Skouteris H, Fuller-Tyszkiewicz M, Millar L, Allender S. Associations between obesogenic risk factors and depression among adolescents: a systematic review. *Obes Rev.* 2014;15(1):40–51.
57. Hu FB, Leitzmann MF, Stampfer MJ, Colditz GA, Willett WC, Rimm EB. Physical activity and television watching in relation to risk for Type 2 diabetes mellitus in men. *Arch Intern Med.* 2001;161(12):1542–8.
58. Hu FB, Li TY, Colditz GA, Willett WC, Manson JE. Television watching and other sedentary behaviors in relation to risk of obesity and Type 2 diabetes mellitus in women. *JAMA.* 2003;289(14):1785–91.

59. Inoue M, Tanaka H, Moriwake T, Oka M, Sekiguchi C, Seino Y. Altered biochemical markers of bone turnover in humans during 120 days of bed rest. *Bone.* 2000;26(3):281–6.
60. Jefferis BJ, Sartini C, Lee I-M, et al. Adherence to physical activity guidelines in older adults, using objectively measured physical activity in a population-based study. *BMC Public Health.* 2014;14:382.
61. Jensen DR, Schlaepfer IR, Morin CL, et al. Prevention of diet-induced obesity in transgenic mice overexpressing skeletal muscle lipoprotein lipase. *Am J Physiol.* 1997;273(2 pt 2):R683–9.
62. Kann L, Kinchen S, Shanklin S, Flint KH, Hawkins J, Harris WA. Youth Risk Behavioral Surveillance — United States 2013. *MMWR Surveil Summ.* 2014;63(4):35–7.
63. Katzmarzyk PT. Physical activity, sedentary behavior, and health: paradigm paralysis or paradigm shift? *Diabetes.* 2010;59(11):2717–25.
64. Keadle SK, Moore SC, Sampson JN, Xiao Q, Albanes D, Matthews CE. Causes of death associated with prolonged TV viewing: NIH-AARP Diet and Health Study. *Am J Prev Med.* 2015;49(6):811–21.
65. Kim H, Iwasaki K, Miyake T, Shiozawa T, Nozaki S, Yajima K. Changes in bone turnover markers during 14-day 6 degrees head-down bed rest. *J Bone Miner Metab.* 2003;21(5):311–5.
66. Knight JA. Physical inactivity: associated diseases and disorders. *Ann Clin Lab Sci.* 2012;42(3):320–37.
67. Kohl HW III, Craig CL, Lambert EV, et al. The pandemic of physical inactivity: global action for public health. *Lancet.* 2012;380(9838):294–305.
68. La Grow S, Yeung P, Towers A, Alpass F, Stephens C. The impact of mobility on quality of life among older persons. *J Aging Health.* 2013;25(5):723–36.
69. LeBlanc AG, Spence JC, Carson V, et al. Systematic review of sedentary behaviour and health indicators in the early years (aged 0–4 years). *Appl Physiol Nutr Metab.* 2012;37(4):753–72.
70. Lee I-M. Current issues in examining dose-response relationships between physical activity and health outcomes. In: Lee I-M, editor. *Epidemiologic Methods in Physical Activity Studies.* New York (NY): Oxford University Press; 2009. p. 56–76.
71. Lee I-M, Shiroma EJ, Lobelo F, Puska P, Blair SN, Katzmarzyk PT. Effect of physical inactivity on major non-communicable diseases worldwide: an analysis of burden of disease and life expectancy. *Lancet.* 2012;380(9838):219–29.
72. Lee J, Chang RW, Ehrlich-Jones L, et al. Sedentary behavior and physical function: objective evidence from the Osteoarthritis Initiative. *Arthritis Care Res (Hoboken).* 2015;67(3):366–73.
73. Levine JA. Nonexercise activity thermogenesis — liberating the life-force. *J Intern Med.* 2007;262(3):273–87.
74. Li C, Balluz LS, Okoro CA, et al. Surveillance of certain health behaviors and conditions among states and selected local areas — Behavioral Risk Factor Surveillance System, United States, 2009. *MMWR Surveill Summ.* 2011;60(9):1–250.
75. Lynch BM. Sedentary behavior and cancer: a systematic review of the literature and proposed biological mechanisms. *Cancer Epidemiol Biomarkers Prev.* 2010;19(11):2691–709.
76. Lynch BM, Dunstan DW, Healy GN, Winkler E, Eakin E, Owen N. Objectively measured physical activity and sedentary time of breast cancer survivors, and associations with adiposity: findings from NHANES (2003–2006). *Cancer Causes Control.* 2010;21(2):283–8.
77. Lynch BM, Dunstan DW, Winkler E, Healy GN, Eakin E, Owen N. Objectively assessed physical activity, sedentary time and waist circumference among prostate cancer survivors: findings from the National Health and Nutrition Examination Survey (2003–2006). *Eur J Cancer Care (Engl).* 2011;20(4):514–9.
78. Marshall SJ, Biddle SJ, Gorely T, Cameron N, Murdey I. Relationships between media use, body fatness and physical activity in children and youth: a meta-analysis. *Int J Obes Relat Metab Disord.* 2004;28(10):1238–46.
79. McDonald NC. Active transportation to school: trends among U.S. schoolchildren, 1969–2001. *Am J Prev Med.* 2007;32(6):509–16.
80. McKeown-Eyssen G. Epidemiology of colorectal cancer revisited: are serum triglycerides and/or plasma glucose associated with risk? *Cancer Epidemiol Biomarkers Prev.* 1994;3(8):687–95.
81. Moreno LA, Gottrand F, Huybrechts I, Ruiz JR, González-Gross M, DeHenauw S. Nutrition and lifestyle in European adolescents: the HELENA (Healthy Lifestyle in Europe by Nutrition in Adolescence) study. *Adv Nutr.* 2014;5(5):615S–23S.
82. Morey-Holton ER, Globus RK. Hindlimb unloading of growing rats: a model for predicting skeletal changes during space flight. *Bone.* 1998;22(5 suppl):83S–8S.
83. Morris JN, Heady JA, Raffle PA, Roberts CG, Parks JW. Coronary heart-disease and physical activity of work. *Lancet.* 1953;265(6795):1053–7.
84. Morris JN, Heady JA, Raffle PA, Roberts CG, Parks JW. Coronary heart-disease and physical activity of work. *Lancet.* 1953;265(6796):1111–20.
85. Netterstrøm B, Laursen P. Incidence and prevalence of ischaemic heart disease among urban busdrivers in Copenhagen. *Scand J Soc Med.* 1981;9(2):75–9.
86. Neufer PD. The effect of detraining and reduced training on the physiological adaptations to aerobic exercise training. *Sports Med.* 1989;8(5):302–20.
87. Oka H, Yoshimura N, Kinoshita H, Saiga A, Kawaguchi H, Nakamura K. Decreased activities of daily living and associations with bone loss among aged residents in a rural Japanese community: the Miyama study. *J Bone Miner Metab.* 2006;24(4):307–13.
88. Olmedillas H, González-Agüero A, Moreno LA, Casajus JA, Vicente-Rodríguez G. Cycling and bone health: a systematic review. *BMC Med.* 2012;10:168.
89. Owen N, Healy GN, Matthews CE, Dunstan DW. Too much sitting: the population health science of sedentary behavior. *Exerc Sport Sci Rev.* 2010;38(3):105–13.

90. Paffenbarger RS Jr, Laughlin ME, Gima AS, Black RA. Work activity of longshoremen as related to death from coronary heart disease and stroke. *N Engl J Med.* 1970;282(20):1109–14.
91. Pate RR, O'Neill JR, Lobelo F. The evolving definition of "sedentary." *Exerc Sport Sci Rev.* 2008;36(4):173–8.
92. Pate RR, Pratt M, Blair SN, et al. Physical activity and public health. A recommendation from the Centers for Disease Control and Prevention and the American College of Sports Medicine. *JAMA.* 1995;273(5):402–7.
93. Patel AV, Rodriguez C, Pavluck AL, Thun MJ, Calle EE. Recreational physical activity and sedentary behavior in relation to ovarian cancer risk in a large cohort of US women. *Am J Epidemiol.* 2006;163(8):709–16.
94. Pattullo MC, Cotter MA, Cameron NE, Barry JA. Effects of lengthened immobilization on functional and histochemical properties of rabbit tibialis anterior muscle. *Exp Physiol.* 1992;77(3):433–42.
95. Prentice-Dunn H, Prentice-Dunn S. Physical activity, sedentary behavior, and childhood obesity: a review of cross-sectional studies. *Psychol Health Med.* 2012;17(3):255–73.
96. Proper KI, Singh AS, van Mechelen W, Chinapaw MJ. Sedentary behaviors and health outcomes among adults: a systematic review of prospective studies. *Am J Prev Med.* 2011;40(2):174–82.
97. Purdy RE, Duckles SP, Krause DN, Rubera KM, Sara D. Effect of simulated microgravity on vascular contractility. *J Appl Physiol (1985).* 1998;85(4):1307–15.
98. Reeves GK, Pirie K, Beral V, Green J, Spencer E, Bull D. Cancer incidence and mortality in relation to body mass index in the Million Women Study: cohort study. *BMJ.* 2007;335(7630):1134.
99. Rey-López JP, Vicente-Rodríguez G, Biosca M, Moreno LA. Sedentary behaviour and obesity development in children and adolescents. *Nutr Metab Cardiovasc Dis.* 2008;18(3):242–51.
100. Rockette-Wagner B, Edelstein S, Venditti EM, et al. The impact of lifestyle intervention on sedentary time in individuals at high risk of diabetes. *Diabetologia.* 2015;58(6):1198–202.
101. Rosengren A, Anderson K, Wilhelmsen L. Risk of coronary heart disease in middle-aged male bus and tram drivers compared to men in other occupations: a prospective study. *Int J Epidemiol.* 1991;20(1):82–7.
102. Salmon J, Tremblay MS, Marshall SJ, Hume C. Health risks, correlates, and interventions to reduce sedentary behavior in young people. *Am J Prev Med.* 2011;41(2):197–206.
103. Santos DA, Silva AM, Baptista F, et al. Sedentary behavior and physical activity are independently related to functional fitness in older adults. *Exp Gerontol.* 2012;47(12):908–12.
104. Sardinha LB, Santos DA, Silva AM, Baptista F, Owen N. Breaking-up sedentary time is associated with physical function in older adults. *J Gerontol A Biol Sci Med Sci.* 2015;70(1):119–24.
105. Semanik PA, Lee J, Song J, et al. Accelerometer-monitored sedentary behavior and observed physical function loss. *Am J Public Health.* 2015;105(3):560–6.
106. Shimada M, Ishibashi S, Gotoda T, et al. Overexpression of human lipoprotein lipase protects diabetic transgenic mice from diabetic hypertriglyceridemia and hypercholesterolemia. *Arterioscler Thromb Vasc Biol.* 1995;15(10):1688–94.
107. Sioen I, Michels N, Polfliet C, et al. The influence of dairy consumption, sedentary behaviour and physical activity on bone mass in Flemish children: a cross-sectional study. *BMC Public Health.* 2015;15:717.
108. Smith SM, Davis-Street JE, Fesperman JV, et al. Evaluation of treadmill exercise in a lower body negative pressure chamber as a countermeasure for weightlessness-induced bone loss: a bed rest study with identical twins. *J Bone Miner Res.* 2003;18(12):2223–30.
109. Song J, Lindquist LA, Chang RW, et al. Sedentary behavior as a risk factor for physical frailty independent of moderate activity: results from the osteoarthritis initiative. *Am J Public Health.* 2015;105(7):1439–45.
110. Staron RS, Leonardi MJ, Karapondo DL, et al. Strength and skeletal muscle adaptations in heavy-resistance-trained women after detraining and retraining. *J Appl Physiol (1985).* 1991;70(2):631–40.
111. Strath SJ, Kaminsky LA, Ainsworth BE, et al. Guide to the assessment of physical activity: clinical and research applications: a scientific statement from the American Heart Association. *Circulation.* 2013;128(20):2259–79.
112. Thorp AA, Owen N, Neuhaus M, Dunstan DW. Sedentary behaviors and subsequent health outcomes in adults a systematic review of longitudinal studies, 1996–2011. *Am J Prev Med.* 2011;41(2):207–15.
113. Tremblay MS, Colley RC, Saunders TJ, Healy GN, Owen N. Physiological and health implications of a sedentary lifestyle. *Appl Physiol Nutr Metab.* 2010;35(6):725–40.
114. Tremblay MS, LeBlanc AG, Kho ME, et al. Systematic review of sedentary behaviour and health indicators in school-aged children and youth. *Int J Behav Nutr Phys Act.* 2011;8:98.
115. Troiano RP, Berrigan D, Dodd KW, Mâsse LC, Tilert T, McDowell M. Physical activity in the United States measured by accelerometer. *Med Sci Sports Exerc.* 2008;40(1):181–8.
116. Tucker JM, Welk GJ, Beyler NK. Physical activity in U.S.: adults compliance with the Physical Activity Guidelines for Americans. *Am J Prev Med.* 2011;40(4):454–61.
117. United Kingdom Department of Health. *UK Physical Activity Guidelines* [Internet]. London (United Kingdom): United Kingdom Department of Health; [cited 2016 Feb 29]. Available from: https://www.gov.uk/government/publications/uk-physical-activity-guidelines
118. van der Ploeg HP, Chey T, Korda RJ, Banks E, Bauman A. Sitting time and all-cause mortality risk in 222 497 Australian adults. *Arch Intern Med.* 2012;172(6):494–500.

119. van der Ploeg HP, Merom D, Corpuz G, Bauman AE. Trends in Australian children traveling to school 1971–2003: burning petrol or carbohydrates? *Prev Med.* 2008;46(1):60–2.
120. van Uffelen JG, Wong J, Chau JY, et al. Occupational sitting and health risks: a systematic review. *Am J Prev Med.* 2010;39(4):379–88.
121. Vukovich MD, Arciero PJ, Kohrt WM, Racette SB, Hansen PA, Holloszy JO. Changes in insulin action and GLUT-4 with 6 days of inactivity in endurance runners. *J Appl Physiol (1985).* 1996;80(1):240–4.
122. Wijndaele K, Healy GN, Dunstan DW, et al. Increased cardiometabolic risk is associated with increased TV viewing time. *Med Sci Sports Exerc.* 2010;42(8):1511–8.
123. Wilmot EG, Edwardson CL, Achana FA, et al. Sedentary time in adults and the association with diabetes, cardiovascular disease and death: systematic review and meta-analysis. *Diabetologia.* 2012;55(11):2895–905.
124. Wolin KY, Colangelo LA, Chiu BC, Ainsworth B, Chatterton R, Gapstur SM. Associations of physical activity, sedentary time, and insulin with percent breast density in Hispanic women. *J Womens Health (Larchmt).* 2007;16(7):1004–11.
125. World Health Organization. *Global Action Plan for the Prevention and Control of Noncommunicable Diseases 2013–2020* [Internet]. Geneva (Switzerland): World Health Organization; [cited 2016 Aug 10]. Available from: http://www.who.int/nmh/events/ncd_action_plan/en/
126. World Health Organization. *Global Health Risks* [Internet]. Geneva (Switzerland): World Health Organization; [cited 2016 Aug 10]. Available from: http://www.who.int/healthinfo/global_burden_disease/global_health_risks/en/index.html
127. Zerwekh JE, Ruml LA, Gottschalk F, Pak CY. The effects of twelve weeks of bed rest on bone histology, biochemical markers of bone turnover, and calcium homeostasis in eleven normal subjects. *J Bone Miner Res.* 1998;13(10):1594–601.
128. Zhang C, Solomon CG, Manson JE, Hu FB. A prospective study of pregravid physical activity and sedentary behaviors in relation to the risk for gestational diabetes mellitus. *Arch Intern Med.* 2006;166(5):543–8.
129. Zhang G, Wu L, Zhou L, Lu W, Mao C. Television watching and risk of childhood obesity: a meta-analysis. *Eur J Public Health.* 2016;26(1):13–8.
130. Zhou Y, Zhao H, Peng C. Association of sedentary behavior with the risk of breast cancer in women: update meta-analysis of observational studies. *Ann Epidemiol.* 2015;25(9):687–97.
131. Zwart SR, Hargens AR, Lee SM, et al. Lower body negative pressure treadmill exercise as a countermeasure for bed rest-induced bone loss in female identical twins. *Bone.* 2007;40(2):529–37.

PART II

Preparticipation Screening, Fitness Assessment, and Interpretation

CHAPTER 3

Preparticipation Screening

INTRODUCTION

The link between living a physically active lifestyle and the accompanying reduction in several chronic diseases is well established. **Physical activity** is beneficial in the primary prevention of cardiovascular disease (CVD), stroke, diabetes, obesity, osteoporosis, anxiety, depression, and some cancers (34). Should an individual decide to start participating in a more active lifestyle, it would be prudent to take certain precautions to minimize the possible risks associated with initiating or increasing **exercise**. Contemporary preparticipation screening guidelines have focused primarily on risk classification (*i.e.*, low, moderate, high) for individuals initiating exercise. This risk classification framework was based on the possible number of CVD risk factors or the presence of signs and symptoms and/or known cardiovascular, pulmonary, or metabolic disease. Thus, recommendations for a medical exam and exercise test were based on their risk classification and the proposed exercise **intensity** in an attempt to avoid exposing inactive individuals, with known or hidden CVD, to unaccustomed vigorous activity that may increase the risk of sudden cardiac death (SCD) and acute myocardial infarction (AMI).

Recent evidence suggests that this type of screening (39) may erroneously over-refer individuals to seek out **medical clearance** before exercise when, in fact, they do not require it and may inadvertently create a barrier for an individual to adopt a physically active lifestyle. Although the overall goal of exercise preparticipation screening has not changed (*i.e.*, identify those at risk for an adverse event during exercise), a new paradigm has been created that will encourage physical activity, while minimizing barriers, still ensuring the safety of the exercise participant.

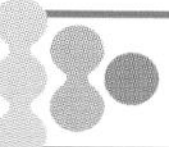

Preparticipation Health Screening

Exercise professionals should always incorporate some form of preparticipation screening or health appraisal prior to performing fitness testing or initiating an exercise program for an individual. The goals for preparticipation screening are (a) to identify who should receive medical clearance prior to initiating an exercise program or increasing the **frequency**, intensity, and/or volume of their current exercise program; (b) to identify those with clinically significant disease(s) to determine if they would benefit from participating in a medically supervised exercise program; and (c) to identify those with medical conditions who should be restricted from participating in an exercise program until their disease conditions are abated or better controlled. Based on these goals, the exercise professional will better understand and utilize the information from the preparticipation health screening algorithm (Fig. 3.1) by

- Determining an individual's current physical activity levels
- Identifying signs and symptoms underlying CVD, metabolic disease, and renal disease (Table 3.1) in that person
- Identifying individuals with diagnosed CVD and metabolic disease
- Using an individual's current level of exercise participation, disease history, signs and symptoms, and desired exercise program intensity to guide recommendations for preparticipation medical clearance.

It is important to note that an individual with pulmonary disease or a sign or symptom indicative of pulmonary disease will no longer be automatically referred for medical clearance. The presence of certain pulmonary diseases does not increase the risk of fatal or nonfatal cardiovascular complications during or immediately after exercise. It is believed that the risk of a cardiovascular complication in someone with pulmonary disease is not because of the disease but because of the person's sedentary lifestyle (15).

Two types of preparticipation screening will be presented in this chapter. The first will be directed toward the exercise professional working with a general, nonclinical population and the second for those professionals working in a clinical or cardiopulmonary rehabilitation setting. For those exercise professionals who are working in a nonclinical setting, it is important to understand that there is a new process for performing **preparticipation health screening**. Previous screening methods relied heavily on CVD risk factor assessment and subsequent risk classification. The new American College of Sports Medicine (ACSM) algorithm is based on (a) an individual's current level of physical activity; (b) the presence of signs or symptoms and/or known cardiovascular, metabolic, or pulmonary disease; and (c) the desired exercise intensity of the **exercise prescription** (ExR_x).

In the absence of a qualified exercise professional, the individual may use a self-screening method that will be explained later in this chapter. Also, if indicated during the screening process (see Fig. 3.1) that medical clearance should be sought from the appropriate health care provider, the manner of clearance should be determined by the health care provider using his or her clinical judgment. It is important to note that preparticipation health screening before initiating an exercise program should be distinguished from a periodic medical examination (34), which should be encouraged as part of routine health maintenance.

American College of Sports Medicine Preparticipation Screening Algorithm

The new ACSM preparticipation screening algorithm (29) is, in part, based on the knowledge that the **relative risk** for SCD and AMI in adults with underlying CVD is transiently increased during a bout of **vigorous intensity** exercise (24,32) but that the absolute risk during exercise

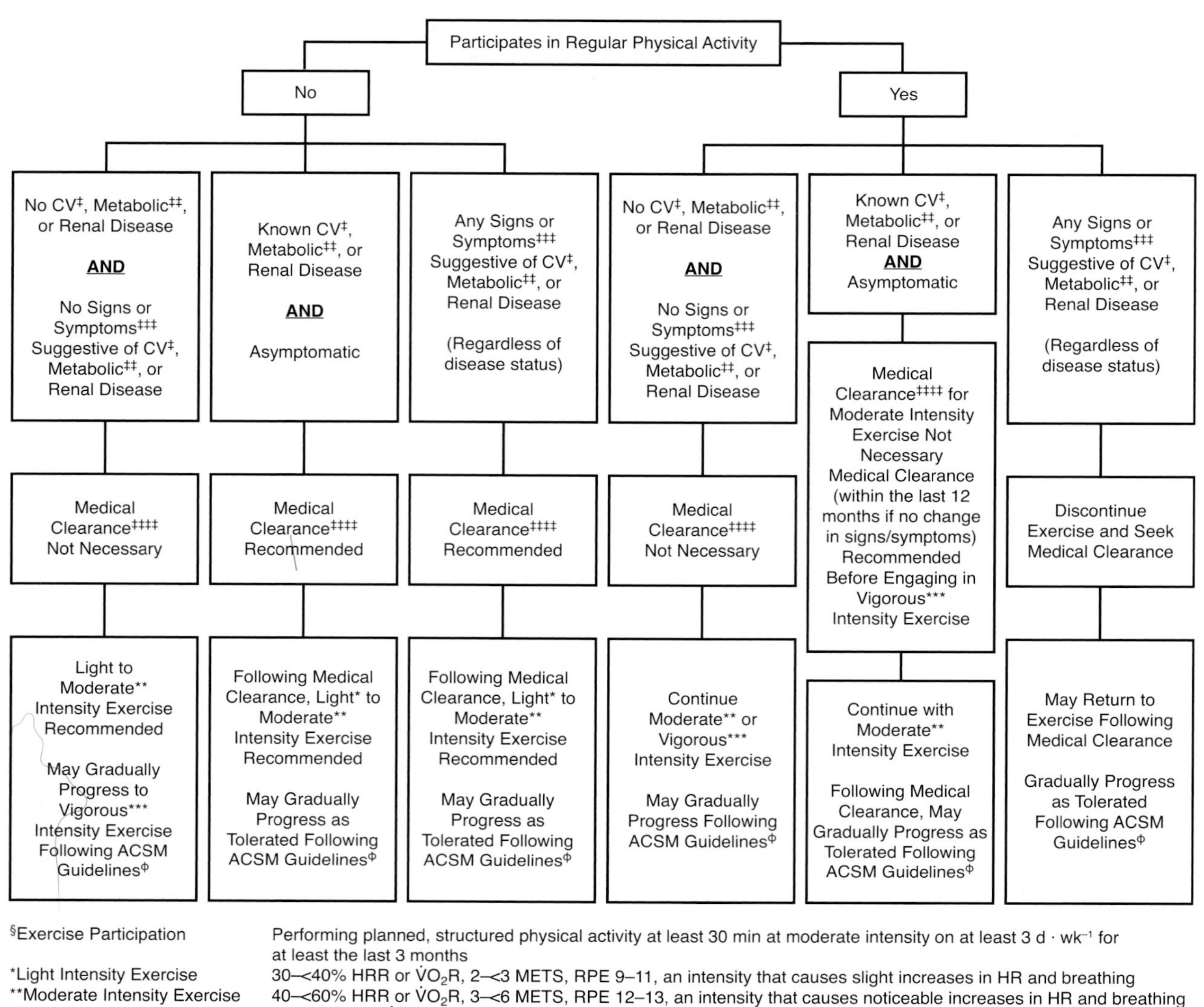

§Exercise Participation	Performing planned, structured physical activity at least 30 min at moderate intensity on at least 3 d · wk^{-1} for at least the last 3 months
*Light Intensity Exercise	30–<40% HRR or $\dot{V}O_2R$, 2–<3 METS, RPE 9–11, an intensity that causes slight increases in HR and breathing
**Moderate Intensity Exercise	40–<60% HRR or $\dot{V}O_2R$, 3–<6 METS, RPE 12–13, an intensity that causes noticeable increases in HR and breathing
***Vigorous Intensity Exercise	≥60% HRR or $\dot{V}O_2R$, ≥6 METS, RPE ≥14, an intensity that causes substantial increases in HR and breathing
‡Cardiovascular (CV) Disease	Cardiac, peripheral vascular, or cerebrovascular disease
‡‡Metabolic Disease	Type 1 and 2 diabetes mellitus
‡‡‡Signs and Symptoms	At rest or during activity. Includes pain, discomfort in the chest, neck, jaw, arms, or other areas that may result from ischemia; shortness of breath at rest or with mild exertion; dizziness or syncope; orthopnea or paroxysmal nocturnal dyspnea; ankle edema; palpitations or tachycardia; intermittent claudication; known heart murmur; unusual fatigue or shortness of breath with usual activities.
‡‡‡‡Medical Clearance	Approval from a healthcare professional to engage in exercise
ΦACSM Guidelines	See *ACSM's Guidelines for Exercise Testing and Prescription, 10th edition, 2018*

FIGURE 3.1. The American College of Sports Medicine Preparticipation Screening Algorithm. (From Riebe D, Franklin BA, Thompson PD, et al. Updating ACSM's recommendations for exercise preparticipation health screening. *Med Sci Sports Exerc.* 2015;47[8]:2473–9. Used with permission.)

is low in a healthy, asymptomatic individual (1,20,32,38). Evidence from the Physicians' Health Study and Nurses' Health Study suggest that SCD occurs every 1.5 million episodes of vigorous physical activity (1) and 36.5 million hours of moderate-to-vigorous physical activity in women (38). Exercise-related cardiovascular events are often preceded by warning signs and symptoms (32), and those events that ended in SCD were most often in people older than 35 years, where SCD could be attributed to underlying and often undiagnosed coronary artery disease (CAD) (21). Furthermore, physically inactive individuals are at a greater total risk for cardiac events compared with their active counterparts (11,34). Previous preparticipation screening included the assessment

Table 3.1 Major Signs and Symptoms Suggestive of Cardiovascular, Metabolic, and Renal Disease

Signs or Symptoms	Clarification/Significance
Pain; discomfort (or other anginal equivalent) in the chest, neck, jaw, arms, or other areas that may result from myocardial ischemia	One of the cardinal manifestations of cardiac disease, in particular, coronary artery disease
	Key features *favoring an ischemic origin* include the following: ▪ *Character*: constricting, squeezing, burning, "heaviness," or "heavy feeling" ▪ *Location*: substernal, across midthorax, anteriorly; in one or both arms, shoulders; in neck, cheeks, teeth; in forearms, fingers in interscapular region ▪ *Provoking factors*: exercise or exertion, excitement, other forms of stress, cold weather, occurrence after meals
	Key features *against an ischemic origin* include the following: ▪ *Character*: dull ache; "knifelike," sharp, stabbing; "jabs" aggravated by respiration ▪ *Location*: in left submammary area; in left hemithorax ▪ *Provoking factors*: after completion of exercise, provoked by a specific body motion
Shortness of breath at rest or with mild exertion	Dyspnea (defined as an abnormally uncomfortable awareness of breathing) is one of the principal symptoms of cardiac and pulmonary disease. It commonly occurs during strenuous exertion in healthy, well-trained individuals and during moderate exertion in healthy, untrained individuals. However, it should be regarded as abnormal when it occurs at a level of exertion that is not expected to evoke this symptom in a given individual. Abnormal exertional dyspnea suggests the presence of cardiopulmonary disorders, in particular, left ventricular dysfunction or chronic obstructive pulmonary disease.
Dizziness or syncope	Syncope (defined as a loss of consciousness) is most commonly caused by a reduced perfusion of the brain. Dizziness and, in particular, syncope *during* exercise may result from cardiac disorders that prevent the normal rise (or an actual fall) in cardiac output. Such cardiac disorders are potentially life-threatening and include severe coronary artery disease, hypertrophic cardiomyopathy, aortic stenosis, and malignant ventricular dysrhythmias. Although dizziness or syncope shortly *after* cessation of exercise should not be ignored, these symptoms may occur even in healthy individuals as a result of a reduction in venous return to the heart.
Orthopnea or paroxysmal nocturnal dyspnea	Orthopnea refers to dyspnea occurring at rest in the recumbent position that is relieved promptly by sitting upright or standing. Paroxysmal nocturnal dyspnea refers to dyspnea, beginning usually 2–5 h after the onset of sleep, which may be relieved by sitting on the side of the bed or getting out of bed. Both are symptoms of left ventricular dysfunction. Although nocturnal dyspnea may occur in individuals with chronic obstructive pulmonary disease, it differs in that it is usually relieved following a bowel movement rather than specifically by sitting up.
Ankle edema	Bilateral ankle edema that is most evident at night is a characteristic sign of heart failure or bilateral chronic venous insufficiency. Unilateral edema of a limb often results from venous thrombosis or lymphatic blockage in the limb. Generalized edema (known as *anasarca*) occurs in individuals with the nephrotic syndrome, severe heart failure, or hepatic cirrhosis.

(continued)

Table 3.1 Major Signs and Symptoms Suggestive of Cardiovascular, Metabolic, and Renal Disease *(continued)*

Signs or Symptoms	Clarification/Significance
Palpitations or tachycardia	Palpitations (defined as an unpleasant awareness of the forceful or rapid beating of the heart) may be induced by various disorders of cardiac rhythm. These include tachycardia, bradycardia of sudden onset, ectopic beats, compensatory pauses, and accentuated stroke volume resulting from valvular regurgitation. Palpitations also often result from anxiety states and high cardiac output (or hyperkinetic) states, such as anemia, fever, thyrotoxicosis, arteriovenous fistula, and the so-called *idiopathic hyperkinetic heart syndrome*.
Intermittent claudication	Intermittent claudication refers to the pain that occurs in the lower extremities with an inadequate blood supply (usually as a result of atherosclerosis) that is brought on by exercise. The pain does not occur with standing or sitting, is reproducible from day to day, is more severe when walking upstairs or up a hill, and is often described as a cramp, which disappears within 1–2 min after stopping exercise. Coronary artery disease is more prevalent in individuals with intermittent claudication. Patients with diabetes are at increased risk for this condition.
Known heart murmur	Although some may be innocent, heart murmurs may indicate valvular or other cardiovascular disease. From an exercise safety standpoint, it is especially important to exclude hypertrophic cardiomyopathy and aortic stenosis as underlying causes because these are among the more common causes of exertion-related sudden cardiac death.
Unusual fatigue or shortness of breath with usual activities	Although there may be benign origins for these symptoms, they also may signal the onset of or change in the status of cardiovascular disease or metabolic disease.

These signs or symptoms must be interpreted within the clinical context in which they appear because they are not all specific for cardiovascular disease.

Modified from Gordon SMBS. Health appraisal in the non-medical setting. In: Durstine JL, editor. *ACSM's Resource Manual for Guidelines for Exercise Testing and Prescription*. 2nd ed. Philadelphia (PA): Lippincott Williams & Wilkins; 1993. p. 219–28.

of CVD risk factors. There is insufficient evidence to suggest that the presence of one or more CVD risk factors, without underlying disease, confers any additional risk for an adverse event during exercise. With the high prevalence of CVD risk factors among adults (39) and the rarity of exercise-related SCD and AMI, the ability to predict cardiovascular events by assessing CVD risk factors becomes questionable, especially in otherwise healthy adults (32,33). Therefore, the new screening algorithm is based not on CVD risk factors but on whether or not the individual is sedentary or physically active.

The screening algorithm (see Fig. 3.1) starts by identifying whether or not the person presently participates in regular exercise. Individuals who are classified as currently exercising should have been physically active during the past 3 months for at least 30 minutes, on 3 or more days per week and exercising at a **moderate intensity** (40%–60% heart rate reserve [HRR] or 64%–76% maximal heart rate [HR_{max}]). The next level of classification is based on whether an individual has been told by a physician or other health care provider that he or she has a cardiovascular, metabolic, or renal disease or any signs or symptoms suggestive of cardiac, peripheral vascular, or cerebrovascular disease, Types 1 and 2 diabetes mellitus, or renal disease.

Once an individual's disease status has been determined, the exercise professional should shift attention to an assessment of any signs and symptoms suggestive of these diseases (see Table 3.1). The presence of signs and symptoms should be done to better identify those who have an undiagnosed disease. This part of the process can often be difficult because of the vague or ambiguous responses from people. The exercise professional should take the time to have a one-on-one conversation in order to clarify any such responses by asking additional questions to help better differentiate whether a response is actually because of a pathological condition or because of a misunderstanding of the signs or symptoms.

The final step in using the preparticipation screening algorithm is to determine the desired exercise intensity (see Fig. 3.1) for the individuals' ExR_x. It has been established that vigorous exercise is more likely to cause an acute cardiac event compared with light-to-moderate exercise in individuals (24,32). The exercise professional can utilize a health screening checklist (23) (Fig. 3.2) for guidance through this process. Once all the necessary information has been

Exercise Preparticipation Health Screening Questionnaire for Exercise Professionals

Assess your client's health needs by marking all *true* statements.

Step 1

SIGNS AND SYMPTOMS
Does your client experience:
____ chest discomfort with exertion
____ unreasonable breathlessness
____ dizziness, fainting, blackouts
____ ankle swelling
____ unpleasant awareness of a forceful, rapid or irregular heart rate
____ burning or cramping sensations in your lower legs when walking short distance
____ known heart murmur

If you **did** mark any of these statements under the symptoms, **STOP**, your client should should seek medical clearance before engaging in or resuming exercise. Your client may need to use a facility with a **medically qualified staff**.

If you **did not** mark any symptoms, continue to steps 2 and 3.

Step 2

CURRENT ACTIVITY
Has your client performed planned, structured physical activity for at least 30 min at moderate intensity on at least 3 days per week for at least the last 3 months?

Yes ☐ No ☐

Continue to Step 3.

Step 3

MEDICAL CONDITIONS
Has your client had or do they currently have:
____ a heart attack
____ heart surgery, cardiac catheterization, or coronary angioplasty
____ pacemaker/implantable cardiac defibrillator/rhythm disturbance
____ heart valve disease
____ heart failure
____ heart transplantation
____ congenital heart disease
____ diabetes
____ renal disease

Evaluating Steps 2 and 3:

- If you **did not mark any of the statements in Step 3**, medical clearance is not necessary.
- If you marked Step 2 "**yes**" and **marked any of the statements in Step 3**, your client may continue to exercise at light to moderate intensity without medical clearance. Medical clearance is recommended before engaging in vigorous exercise.
- If you marked Step 2 "**no**" and **marked any of the statements in Step 3**, medical clearance is recommended. Your client may need to use a facility with a **medically qualified staff**.

FIGURE 3.2. Exercise Preparticipation Health Screening Questionnaire for Exercise Professionals. (From Magal M, Riebe D. New preparticipation health screening recommendations: what exercise professionals need to know. *ACSM's Health Fitness J.* 2016;20[3]:22–7. Used with permission.)

collected, individuals are grouped into one of six categories (left to right) in the screening algorithm (see Fig. 3.1).

1. Individuals who do not participate in regular exercise; have no known cardiovascular, metabolic, or renal disease; and have no signs or symptoms suggestive of disease can begin an exercise program at a light-to-moderate intensity without medical clearance. The individual can increase beyond moderate intensity following the principle of progression and those guidelines outlined in Chapter 8.
2. Asymptomatic individuals who do not participate in regular exercise with a known cardiovascular, metabolic, or renal disease should obtain medical clearance before starting an exercise program. Once cleared to exercise, he or she should begin at a light-to-moderate intensity and progress to higher intensities as tolerated.
3. Individuals who are symptomatic and do not currently exercise should seek medical clearance before participating in exercise. Following medical clearance, the individual may start an exercise program of light-to-moderate intensity.
4. Those individuals who do participate in regular exercise and do not have any known disease or sign or symptom suggestive of disease do not need any medical clearance and may begin an exercise program starting at a moderate-to-vigorous intensity or continue with their current exercise program.
5. Individuals who participate in regular exercise and are asymptomatic but have a diagnosed cardiovascular, metabolic, or renal disease do *not* need medical clearance when starting a moderate-intensity exercise program. However, it is recommended that if the intensity of exercise increases to vigorous, the individual should seek medical clearance. In addition, if these individuals experience resting or exertional symptoms of disease or any change in health status, they should visit with their health care providers.
6. An individual who participates in regular exercise but experiences any signs or symptoms suggestive of cardiovascular, metabolic, or renal disease should discontinue the current exercise program and obtain medical clearance before continuing exercising at any intensity.

Should an individual be identified for needing medical clearance, he or she should be referred to an appropriate physician or health care provider. The type of medical clearance is left to the discretion of the provider. Because there is no standardized screening test, procedures may vary from practitioner to practitioner and may be as simple as a verbal consultation or more in-depth with a resting or stress electrocardiogram/echocardiogram, detection of coronary artery calcification via computed tomography, or even nuclear medicine imaging or angiography. It is suggested that the exercise professional request written clearance with special instructions or restrictions (*e.g.*, may not exercise over 8 **metabolic equivalents [METs]**). Continued communication between the provider and exercise professional is an essential component of this process and aids in the success of the individual's exercise program.

Self-Guided Methods

Traditionally, self-administered preparticipation health screening involved the use of the Physical Activity Readiness Questionnaire (PAR-Q) and the American Heart Association [AHA]/ACSM Health/Fitness Preparticipation Screening Questionnaire. With the advent of ACSM's new screening algorithm, the traditional questionnaires do not play as large a role in preparticipation screening because they relied heavily on risk factor classification. However, the PAR-Q was recently updated to the evidence-based Physical Activity Readiness Questionnaire for Everyone (PAR-Q+) (Fig. 3.3) and now includes a number of additional follow-up questions that guide the exercise professional in his or her preparticipation recommendations (36). The updated version was created to reduce barriers to exercise as well as to reduce the number of false positive screenings (17) and utilizes follow-up questions that allow the exercise professional to better tailor the ExR_x for the

2017 PAR-Q+

The Physical Activity Readiness Questionnaire for Everyone

The health benefits of regular physical activity are clear; more people should engage in physical activity every day of the week. Participating in physical activity is very safe for MOST people. This questionnaire will tell you whether it is necessary for you to seek further advice from your doctor OR a qualified exercise professional before becoming more physically active.

GENERAL HEALTH QUESTIONS

Please read the 7 questions below carefully and answer each one honestly: check YES or NO.	YES	NO
1) Has your doctor ever said that you have a heart condition ☐ OR high blood pressure ☐?	☐	☐
2) Do you feel pain in your chest at rest, during your daily activities of living, **OR** when you do physical activity?	☐	☐
3) Do you lose balance because of dizziness **OR** have you lost consciousness in the last 12 months? Please answer **NO** if your dizziness was associated with over-breathing (including during vigorous exercise).	☐	☐
4) Have you ever been diagnosed with another chronic medical condition (other than heart disease or high blood pressure)? **PLEASE LIST CONDITION(S) HERE:** ______	☐	☐
5) Are you currently taking prescribed medications for a chronic medical condition? **PLEASE LIST CONDITION(S) AND MEDICATIONS HERE:** ______	☐	☐
6) Do you currently have (or have had within the past 12 months) a bone, joint, or soft tissue (muscle, ligament, or tendon) problem that could be made worse by becoming more physically active? Please answer **NO** if you had a problem in the past, but it ***does not limit your current ability*** to be physically active. **PLEASE LIST CONDITION(S) HERE:** ______	☐	☐
7) Has your doctor ever said that you should only do medically supervised physical activity?	☐	☐

If you answered NO to all of the questions above, you are cleared for physical activity. Go to Page 4 to sign the PARTICIPANT DECLARATION. You do not need to complete Pages 2 and 3.

- Start becoming much more physically active – start slowly and build up gradually.
- Follow International Physical Activity Guidelines for your age (www.who.int/dietphysicalactivity/en/).
- You may take part in a health and fitness appraisal.
- If you are over the age of 45 yr and **NOT** accustomed to regular vigorous to maximal effort exercise, consult a qualified exercise professional before engaging in this intensity of exercise.
- If you have any further questions, contact a qualified exercise professional.

If you answered YES to one or more of the questions above, COMPLETE PAGES 2 AND 3.

Delay becoming more active if:

- You have a temporary illness such as a cold or fever; it is best to wait until you feel better.
- You are pregnant - talk to your health care practitioner, your physician, a qualified exercise professional, and/or complete the ePARmed-X+ at **www.eparmedx.com** before becoming more physically active.
- Your health changes - answer the questions on Pages 2 and 3 of this document and/or talk to your doctor or a qualified exercise professional before continuing with any physical activity program.

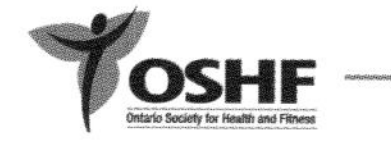

 1 / 4

01-01-2017

FIGURE 3.3. Physical Activity Readiness Questionnaire for Everyone (PAR-Q+). (Reprinted with permission from the PAR-Q+ Collaboration and the authors of the PAR-Q+ [Dr. Darren Warburton, Dr. Norman Gledhill, Dr. Veronica Jamnik, and Dr. Shannon Bredin].) *(continued)*

2017 PAR-Q+

FOLLOW-UP QUESTIONS ABOUT YOUR MEDICAL CONDITION(S)

1. Do you have Arthritis, Osteoporosis, or Back Problems?

If the above condition(s) is/are present, answer questions 1a-1c — If **NO** ☐ go to question 2

1a.	Do you have difficulty controlling your condition with medications or other physician-prescribed therapies? (Answer **NO** if you are not currently taking medications or other treatments)	**YES** ☐ **NO** ☐
1b.	Do you have joint problems causing pain, a recent fracture or fracture caused by osteoporosis or cancer, displaced vertebra (e.g., spondylolisthesis), and/or spondylolysis/pars defect (a crack in the bony ring on the back of the spinal column)?	**YES** ☐ **NO** ☐
1c.	Have you had steroid injections or taken steroid tablets regularly for more than 3 months?	**YES** ☐ **NO** ☐

2. Do you currently have Cancer of any kind?

If the above condition(s) is/are present, answer questions 2a-2b — If **NO** ☐ go to question 3

2a.	Does your cancer diagnosis include any of the following types: lung/bronchogenic, multiple myeloma (cancer of plasma cells), head, and/or neck?	**YES** ☐ **NO** ☐
2b.	Are you currently receiving cancer therapy (such as chemotheraphy or radiotherapy)?	**YES** ☐ **NO** ☐

3. Do you have a Heart or Cardiovascular Condition? *This includes Coronary Artery Disease, Heart Failure, Diagnosed Abnormality of Heart Rhythm*

If the above condition(s) is/are present, answer questions 3a-3d — If **NO** ☐ go to question 4

3a.	Do you have difficulty controlling your condition with medications or other physician-prescribed therapies? (Answer **NO** if you are not currently taking medications or other treatments)	**YES** ☐ **NO** ☐
3b.	Do you have an irregular heart beat that requires medical management? (e.g., atrial fibrillation, premature ventricular contraction)	**YES** ☐ **NO** ☐
3c.	Do you have chronic heart failure?	**YES** ☐ **NO** ☐
3d.	Do you have diagnosed coronary artery (cardiovascular) disease and have not participated in regular physical activity in the last 2 months?	**YES** ☐ **NO** ☐

4. Do you have High Blood Pressure?

If the above condition(s) is/are present, answer questions 4a-4b — If **NO** ☐ go to question 5

4a.	Do you have difficulty controlling your condition with medications or other physician-prescribed therapies? (Answer **NO** if you are not currently taking medications or other treatments)	**YES** ☐ **NO** ☐
4b.	Do you have a resting blood pressure equal to or greater than 160/90 mmHg with or without medication? (Answer **YES** if you do not know your resting blood pressure)	**YES** ☐ **NO** ☐

5. Do you have any Metabolic Conditions? *This includes Type 1 Diabetes, Type 2 Diabetes, Pre-Diabetes*

If the above condition(s) is/are present, answer questions 5a-5e — If **NO** ☐ go to question 6

5a.	Do you often have difficulty controlling your blood sugar levels with foods, medications, or other physician-prescribed therapies?	**YES** ☐ **NO** ☐
5b.	Do you often suffer from signs and symptoms of low blood sugar (hypoglycemia) following exercise and/or during activities of daily living? Signs of hypoglycemia may include shakiness, nervousness, unusual irritability, abnormal sweating, dizziness or light-headedness, mental confusion, difficulty speaking, weakness, or sleepiness.	**YES** ☐ **NO** ☐
5c.	Do you have any signs or symptoms of diabetes complications such as heart or vascular disease and/or complications affecting your eyes, kidneys, **OR** the sensation in your toes and feet?	**YES** ☐ **NO** ☐
5d.	Do you have other metabolic conditions (such as current pregnancy-related diabetes, chronic kidney disease, or liver problems)?	**YES** ☐ **NO** ☐
5e.	Are you planning to engage in what for you is unusually high (or vigorous) intensity exercise in the near future?	**YES** ☐ **NO** ☐

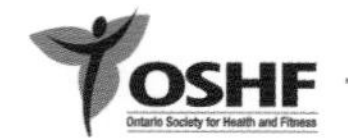

 2 / 4

01-01-2017

FIGURE 3.3. *(continued)*

2017 PAR-Q+

6. Do you have any Mental Health Problems or Learning Difficulties? *This includes Alzheimer's, Dementia, Depression, Anxiety Disorder, Eating Disorder, Psychotic Disorder, Intellectual Disability, Down Syndrome*

If the above condition(s) is/are present, answer questions 6a-6b — If **NO** ☐ go to question 7

6a.	Do you have difficulty controlling your condition with medications or other physician-prescribed therapies? (Answer **NO** if you are not currently taking medications or other treatments)	**YES** ☐ **NO** ☐
6b.	Do you have Down Syndrome **AND** back problems affecting nerves or muscles?	**YES** ☐ **NO** ☐

7. Do you have a Respiratory Disease? *This includes Chronic Obstructive Pulmonary Disease, Asthma, Pulmonary High Blood Pressure*

If the above condition(s) is/are present, answer questions 7a-7d — If **NO** ☐ go to question 8

7a.	Do you have difficulty controlling your condition with medications or other physician-prescribed therapies? (Answer **NO** if you are not currently taking medications or other treatments)	**YES** ☐ **NO** ☐
7b.	Has your doctor ever said your blood oxygen level is low at rest or during exercise and/or that you require supplemental oxygen therapy?	**YES** ☐ **NO** ☐
7c.	If asthmatic, do you currently have symptoms of chest tightness, wheezing, laboured breathing, consistent cough (more than 2 days/week), or have you used your rescue medication more than twice in the last week?	**YES** ☐ **NO** ☐
7d.	Has your doctor ever said you have high blood pressure in the blood vessels of your lungs?	**YES** ☐ **NO** ☐

8. Do you have a Spinal Cord Injury? *This includes Tetraplegia and Paraplegia*

If the above condition(s) is/are present, answer questions 8a-8c — If **NO** ☐ go to question 9

8a.	Do you have difficulty controlling your condition with medications or other physician-prescribed therapies? (Answer **NO** if you are not currently taking medications or other treatments)	**YES** ☐ **NO** ☐
8b.	Do you commonly exhibit low resting blood pressure significant enough to cause dizziness, light-headedness, and/or fainting?	**YES** ☐ **NO** ☐
8c.	Has your physician indicated that you exhibit sudden bouts of high blood pressure (known as Autonomic Dysreflexia)?	**YES** ☐ **NO** ☐

9. Have you had a Stroke? *This includes Transient Ischemic Attack (TIA) or Cerebrovascular Event*

If the above condition(s) is/are present, answer questions 9a-9c — If **NO** ☐ go to question 10

9a.	Do you have difficulty controlling your condition with medications or other physician-prescribed therapies? (Answer **NO** if you are not currently taking medications or other treatments)	**YES** ☐ **NO** ☐
9b.	Do you have any impairment in walking or mobility?	**YES** ☐ **NO** ☐
9c.	Have you experienced a stroke or impairment in nerves or muscles in the past 6 months?	**YES** ☐ **NO** ☐

10. Do you have any other medical condition not listed above or do you have two or more medical conditions?

If you have other medical conditions, answer questions 10a-10c — If **NO** ☐ read the Page 4 recommendations

10a.	Have you experienced a blackout, fainted, or lost consciousness as a result of a head injury within the last 12 months **OR** have you had a diagnosed concussion within the last 12 months?	**YES** ☐ **NO** ☐
10b.	Do you have a medical condition that is not listed (such as epilepsy, neurological conditions, kidney problems)?	**YES** ☐ **NO** ☐
10c.	Do you currently live with two or more medical conditions?	**YES** ☐ **NO** ☐

PLEASE LIST YOUR MEDICAL CONDITION(S) AND ANY RELATED MEDICATIONS HERE: ____________________

GO to Page 4 for recommendations about your current medical condition(s) and sign the PARTICIPANT DECLARATION.

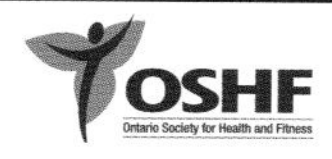

 3 / 4
01-01-2017

FIGURE 3.3. *(continued)*

2017 PAR-Q+

If you answered NO to all of the follow-up questions about your medical condition, you are ready to become more physically active - sign the PARTICIPANT DECLARATION below:

- It is advised that you consult a qualified exercise professional to help you develop a safe and effective physical activity plan to meet your health needs.
- You are encouraged to start slowly and build up gradually - 20 to 60 minutes of low to moderate intensity exercise, 3-5 days per week including aerobic and muscle strengthening exercises.
- As you progress, you should aim to accumulate 150 minutes or more of moderate intensity physical activity per week.
- If you are over the age of 45 yr and **NOT** accustomed to regular vigorous to maximal effort exercise, consult a qualified exercise professional before engaging in this intensity of exercise.

If you answered **YES** to **one or more of the follow-up questions** about your medical condition:

You should seek further information before becoming more physically active or engaging in a fitness appraisal. You should complete the specially designed online screening and exercise recommendations program - the **ePARmed-X+ at www.eparmedx.com** and/or visit a qualified exercise professional to work through the ePARmed-X+ and for further information.

Delay becoming more active if:

- You have a temporary illness such as a cold or fever; it is best to wait until you feel better.
- You are pregnant - talk to your health care practitioner, your physician, a qualified exercise professional, and/or complete the ePARmed-X+ **at www.eparmedx.com** before becoming more physically active.
- Your health changes - talk to your doctor or qualified exercise professional before continuing with any physical activity program.

- You are encouraged to photocopy the PAR-Q+. You must use the entire questionnaire and NO changes are permitted.
- The authors, the PAR-Q+ Collaboration, partner organizations, and their agents assume no liability for persons who undertake physical activity and/or make use of the PAR-Q+ or ePARmed-X+. If in doubt after completing the questionnaire, consult your doctor prior to physical activity.

PARTICIPANT DECLARATION

- All persons who have completed the PAR-Q+ please read and sign the declaration below.
- If you are less than the legal age required for consent or require the assent of a care provider, your parent, guardian or care provider must also sign this form.

I, the undersigned, have read, understood to my full satisfaction and completed this questionnaire. I acknowledge that this physical activity clearance is valid for a maximum of 12 months from the date it is completed and becomes invalid if my condition changes. I also acknowledge that a Trustee (such as my employer, community/fitness centre, health care provider, or other designate) may retain a copy of this form for their records. In these instances, the Trustee will be required to adhere to local, national, and international guidelines regarding the storage of personal health information ensuring that the Trustee maintains the privacy of the information and does not misuse or wrongfully disclose such information.

NAME ______________________ DATE ______________________

SIGNATURE ______________________ WITNESS ______________________

SIGNATURE OF PARENT/GUARDIAN/CARE PROVIDER ______________________

For more information, please contact
www.eparmedx.com
Email: eparmedx@gmail.com

Citation for PAR-Q+
Warburton DER, Jamnik VK, Bredin SSD, and Gledhill N on behalf of the PAR-Q+ Collaboration. The Physical Activity Readiness Questionnaire for Everyone (PAR-Q+) and Electronic Physical Activity Readiness Medical Examination (ePARmed-X+). Health & Fitness Journal of Canada 4(2):3-23, 2011.

The PAR-Q+ was created using the evidence-based AGREE process (1) by the PAR-Q+ Collaboration chaired by Dr. Darren E. R. Warburton with Dr. Norman Gledhill, Dr. Veronica Jamnik, and Dr. Donald C. McKenzie (2). Production of this document has been made possible through financial contributions from the Public Health Agency of Canada and the BC Ministry of Health Services. The views expressed herein do not necessarily represent the views of the Public Health Agency of Canada or the BC Ministry of Health Services.

Key References

1. Jamnik VK, Warburton DER, Makarski J, McKenzie DC, Shephard RJ, Stone J, and Gledhill N. Enhancing the effectiveness of clearance for physical activity participation; background and overall process. APNM 36(S1):S3-S13, 2011.
2. Warburton DER, Gledhill N, Jamnik VK, Bredin SSD, McKenzie DC, Stone J, Charlesworth S, and Shephard RJ. Evidence-based risk assessment and recommendations for physical activity clearance; Consensus Document. APNM 36(S1):S266-s298, 2011.
3. Chisholm DM, Collis ML, Kulak LL, Davenport W, and Gruber N. Physical activity readiness. British Columbia Medical Journal. 1975;17:375-378.
4. Thomas S, Reading J, and Shephard RJ. Revision of the Physical Activity Readiness Questionnaire (PAR-Q). Canadian Journal of Sport Science 1992;17:4 338-345.

OSHF Ontario Society for Health and Fitness

 4 / 4
01-01-2017

FIGURE 3.3. *(continued)*

individual based on medical history and possible signs and symptoms. The PAR-Q+ may be used as a self-guided tool, but because of the additional questions, it may be prudent to have a qualified exercise professional assess the results.

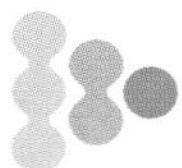

Risk Stratification for Those in Cardiac Rehabilitation and/or Medical Fitness Facilities

Exercise professionals who work with patients with known CVD in exercise-based cardiac rehabilitation settings or medical fitness facilities are advised to conduct a much more in-depth stratification process (40) that is different from the previously presented preparticipation screening for the general public. Risk stratification criteria outlined in Box 3.1 from the American Association of Cardiovascular and Pulmonary Rehabilitation (AACVPR) (2) provide a guideline to assist in the assessment of clinical populations. The AACVPR guidelines provide recommendations for telemetry monitoring and exercise supervision for patients' signs and symptoms or known disease. Clinical exercise professionals should be aware that the AACVPR guidelines do not take into account an individual with comorbidities (*e.g.*, Type 2 diabetes mellitus, morbid obesity, severe pulmonary disease, and debilitating neurological or orthopedic conditions) and how their condition may require a modification in the patient's monitoring or supervision during exercise. For example, a patient with CVD may require telemetry monitoring. If that same patient has Type 2 diabetes, the exercise professional would need to be aware of glucose monitoring as well as potential neuropathies.

Pre-exercise Evaluation

The following information will serve as bridge between preparticipation screening and fitness testing presented in subsequent chapters. The focus of this section is primarily on information for an exercise professional who is in a health/fitness setting, but the information can also benefit those that work in a clinical exercise setting. The pre-exercise process involves informed consent procedures, reviewing medical history and CVD risk factors, physical examination and laboratory tests, identification of contraindications to exercise, and participant instructions (patient preparation).

Informed Consent

The content and extent of an informed consent will vary based on the number and types of assessments being performed. Regardless, the consent should be comprehensive enough that the participant knows and understands both the risks and benefits associated with the test. The consent form should be verbally explained and should include a statement that says the individual has been given an opportunity to ask questions about the procedures and has sufficient information to give informed consent. Furthermore, the form must indicate that the participant is free to withdraw from the procedure at any time without any consequence. An essential element of the informed consent is the statement that "emergency procedures and equipment are available." The facility must ensure that there are appropriately trained individuals and written emergency policy and procedures and that emergency drills are practiced regularly (3). If the participant is a minor, a parent or legal guardian must provide consent, whereas the minor provides assent (*i.e.*, agreement to participate despite not giving consent because of age). Any information collected in the preparticipation and pre-exercise evaluation should be kept in a private, secure location as described in the Health Insurance Portability and Accountability Act (HIPAA) of 1996. In addition to informing the participant about what he or she will be doing, there are important ethical and legal considerations that go along with the informed consent. Figure 3.4 provides an example of an informed consent form for exercise testing.

Box 3.1 American Association of Cardiovascular and Pulmonary Rehabilitation Risk Stratification Criteria for Patients with Cardiovascular Disease

Lowest Risk

Characteristics of patients at lowest risk for exercise participation (all characteristics listed must be present for patients to remain at lowest risk):

- Absence of complex ventricular dysrhythmias during exercise testing and recovery
- Absence of angina or other significant symptoms (*e.g.*, unusual shortness of breath, light-headedness, or dizziness during exercise testing and recovery)
- Presence of normal hemodynamics during exercise testing and recovery (*i.e.*, appropriate increases and decreases in heart rate and systolic blood pressure with increasing workloads and recovery)
- Functional capacity ≥7 metabolic equivalents (METs)

Nonexercise Testing Findings

- Resting ejection fraction ≥50%
- Uncomplicated myocardial infarction or revascularization procedure
- Absence of complicated ventricular dysrhythmias at rest
- Absence of congestive heart failure
- Absence of signs or symptoms of post-event/post-procedure myocardial ischemia
- Absence of clinical depression

Moderate Risk

Characteristics of patients at moderate risk for exercise participation (any one or combination of these findings places a patient at moderate risk):

- Presence of angina or other significant symptoms (*e.g.*, unusual shortness of breath, light-headedness, or dizziness occurring only at high levels of exertion [≥7 METs])
- Mild-to-moderate level of silent ischemia during exercise testing or recovery (ST-segment depression <2 mm from baseline)
- Functional capacity <5 METs

Nonexercise Testing Findings

- Rest ejection fraction 40%–49%

Highest Risk

Characteristics of patients at high risk for exercise participation (any one or combination of these findings places a patient at high risk):

- Presence of complex ventricular dysrhythmias during exercise testing or recovery
- Presence of angina or other significant symptoms (*e.g.*, unusual shortness of breath, light-headedness, or dizziness at low levels of exertion [<5 METs] or during recovery)
- High level of silent ischemia (ST-segment depression ≥2 mm from baseline) during exercise testing or recovery
- Presence of abnormal hemodynamics with exercise testing (*i.e.*, chronotropic incompetence or flat or decreasing systolic blood pressure with increasing workloads) or recovery (*i.e.*, severe postexercise hypotension)

Nonexercise Testing Findings

- Rest ejection fraction <40%
- History of cardiac arrest or sudden death
- Complex dysrhythmias at rest
- Complicated myocardial infarction or revascularization procedure
- Presence of congestive heart failure
- Presence of signs or symptoms of post-event/post-procedure myocardial ischemia
- Presence of clinical depression

From Williams MA. Exercise testing in cardiac rehabilitation. Exercise prescription and beyond. *Cardiol Clin.* 2001;19(3):415–31.

Informed Consent for an Exercise Test

1. **Purpose and Explanation of the Test**
You will perform an exercise test on a cycle ergometer or a motor-driven treadmill. The exercise intensity will begin at a low level and will be advanced in stages depending on your fitness level. We may stop the test at any time because of signs of fatigue or changes in your heart rate, electrocardiogram, or blood pressure, or symptoms you may experience. It is important for you to realize that you may stop when you wish because of feelings of fatigue or any other discomfort.

2. **Attendant Risks and Discomforts**
There exists the possibility of certain changes occurring during the test. These include abnormal blood pressure; fainting; irregular, fast, or slow heart rhythm; and, in rare instances, heart attack, stroke, or death. Every effort will be made to minimize these risks by evaluation of preliminary information relating to your health and fitness and by careful observations during testing. Emergency equipment and trained personnel are available to deal with unusual situations that may arise.

3. **Responsibilities of the Participant**
Information you possess about your health status or previous experiences of heart-related symptoms (*e.g.*, shortness of breath with low-level activity; pain; pressure; tightness; heaviness in the chest, neck, jaw, back and/or arms) with physical effort may affect the safety of your exercise test. Your prompt reporting of these and any other unusual feelings with effort during the exercise test itself is very important. You are responsible for fully disclosing your medical history as well as symptoms that may occur during the test. You are also expected to report all medications (including nonprescription) taken recently and, in particular, those taken today to the testing staff.

4. **Benefits To Be Expected**
The results obtained from the exercise test may assist in the diagnosis of your illness, in evaluating the effect of your medications, or in evaluating what type of physical activities you might do with low risk.

5. **Inquiries**
Any questions about the procedures used in the exercise test or the results of your test are encouraged. If you have any concerns or questions, please ask us for further explanations.

6. **Use of Medical Records**
The information that is obtained during exercise testing will be treated as privileged and confidential as described in the Health Insurance Portability and Accountability Act of 1996. It is not to be released or revealed to any individual except your referring physician without your written consent. However, the information obtained may be used for statistical analysis or scientific purposes with your right to privacy retained.

7. **Freedom of Consent**
I hereby consent to voluntarily engage in an exercise test to determine my exercise capacity and state of cardiovascular health. My permission to perform this exercise test is given voluntarily. I understand that I am free to stop the test at any point if I so desire.

I have read this form, and I understand the test procedures that I will perform and the attendant risks and discomforts. Knowing these risks and discomforts, and having had an opportunity to ask questions that have been answered to my satisfaction, I consent to participate in this test.

____________________	______________________________
Date	Signature of Patient
____________________	______________________________
Date	Signature of Witness
____________________	______________________________
Date	Signature of Physician or Authorized Delegate

FIGURE 3.4. Sample of a consent form for symptom-limited exercise test. (From American College of Sports Medicine. *ACSM's Guidelines for Exercise Testing and Prescription.* 10th ed. Philadelphia [PA]: Wolters Kluwer; 2018. 480 p. Used with permission.)

Medical History and Cardiovascular Disease Risk Factor Assessment

The pre-exercise medical history should be comprehensive enough to provide the exercise professional an accurate view of the participant that will enable the professional to prescribe the appropriate level of exercise. Although CVD risk factor assessment is no longer a part of the preparticipation screening process, it continues to be important to assist in identifying and controlling CVD risk factors (Table 3.2) to aid in development of the individual's ExR_x, lifestyle modification, and disease prevention and management (9,14). A qualified exercise professional should complete a CVD risk factor assessment with a patient to determine if the patient meets any criteria for a positive risk factor from Table 3.2. If the participant does not know if he or she meets the criteria for the risk factor, it should be counted as a risk factor. The exercise professional should be reminded that because of the

Table 3.2 Atherosclerotic Cardiovascular Disease Risk Factors and Defining Criteria

Risk Factors[a]	Defining Criteria
Age	Men ≥45 yr; women ≥55 yr (13)
Family history	Myocardial infarction, coronary revascularization, or sudden death before 55 yr in father or other male first-degree relative or before 65 yr in mother or other female first-degree relative
Cigarette smoking	Current cigarette smoker or those who quit within the previous 6 mo or exposure to environmental tobacco smoke (35)
Physical inactivity	Not participating in at least 30 min of moderate-intensity physical activity (40%–59% $\dot{V}O_2R$) on at least 3 d of the week for at least 3 mo (27,34)
Obesity	Body mass index ≥30 $kg \cdot m^{-2}$ or waist girth >102 cm (40 in) for men and >88 cm (35 in) for women (Executive summary of the clinical guidelines on the identification, evaluation, and treatment of overweight and obesity in adults) (18)
Hypertension	Systolic blood pressure ≥140 mm Hg and/or diastolic ≥90 mm Hg, confirmed by measurements on at least two separate occasions, or on antihypertensive medication (7)
Dyslipidemia	Low-density lipoprotein (LDL) cholesterol ≥130 $mg \cdot dL^{-1}$ (3.37 $mmol \cdot L^{-1}$) or high-density lipoprotein[a] (HDL) cholesterol <40 $mg \cdot dL^{-1}$ (1.04 $mmol \cdot L^{-1}$) or on lipid-lowering medication. If total serum cholesterol is all that is available, use ≥200 $mg \cdot dL^{-1}$ (5.18 $mmol \cdot L^{-1}$) (26).
Diabetes	Fasting plasma glucose ≥126 $mg \cdot dL^{-1}$ (7.0 $mmol \cdot L^{-1}$) or 2-h plasma glucose values in oral glucose tolerance test (OGTT) ≥200 $mg \cdot dL^{-1}$ (11.1 $mmol \cdot L^{-1}$) or glycolated hemoglobin (HbA1C) ≥6.5% (4)
Negative Risk Factors Defining Criteria	
HDL ≥60 $mg \cdot dL^{-1}$ (1.55 $mmol \cdot L^{-1}$) cholesterol (HDL-C)[b]	

[a]If the presence or absence of a CVD risk factor is not disclosed or is not available, that CVD risk factor should be counted as a risk factor.
[b]High HDL-C is considered a negative risk factor. For individuals having high HDL ≥60 $mg \cdot dL^{-1}$ (1.55 $mmol \cdot L^{-1}$), one positive risk factor is subtracted from the sum of positive risk factors.
$\dot{V}O_2R$, oxygen uptake reserve.

Reprinted from American College of Sports Medicine. *ACSM's Guidelines for Exercise Testing and Prescription.* 10th ed. Philadelphia (PA): Wolters Kluwer; 2018. 480 p. Based on information from Mozaffaria D, Benjamin EJ, Go AS, et al. Heart disease and stroke statistics — 2015 update: a report from the American Heart Association. *Circulation.* 2015;131:e29–322; National Cholesterol Education Program Expert Panel on Detection, Evaluation, and Treatment of High Blood Cholesterol in Adults (Adult Treatment Panel III). Third report of the National Cholesterol Education Program (NCEP) Expert Panel on Detection, Evaluation, and Treatment of High Blood Cholesterol in Adults (Adult Treatment Panel III) final report. *Circulation.* 2002;106(25):3143–421; and U.S. Preventive Services Task Force. Screening for coronary heart disease: recommendation statement. *Ann Intern Med.* 2004;140(7):569–72.

cardioprotective effect of high-density lipoprotein cholesterol (HDL-C), it is considered a negative risk factor if the participant meets the threshold of >60 mg · dL^{-1} (1.55 mmol · L^{-1}) and to subtract that from the total number of positive risk factors.

Physical Examination/Laboratory Testing

If it is determined by the ACSM preparticipation screening algorithm that an individual requires a medical examination, it should be conducted by a physician or other qualified health care provider. However, a qualified exercise professional may assess an integral component of the pre-exercise evaluation: blood pressure (BP). In addition to a physical examination, the health care provider may request laboratory tests to assess lipids and lipoproteins, other blood chemistries, and pulmonary function. See Chapters 16 and 18 as well as the work of Bickley and Bates (6) for a detailed description of these assessments.

Blood Pressure

The measurement of resting BP is a vital component of any prescreening evaluation. It has been well established that the link between BP and the risk for a serious cardiovascular event is independent of other risk factors (22). Indeed, in individuals between the age of 40 and 70 years, an increase of just 20 mm Hg in systolic blood pressure (SBP) or 10 mm Hg in diastolic blood pressure (DBP) doubles the risk of that individual developing CVD (7). The main goal of BP treatment is to reach a BP of <140/90 mm Hg in most patients.

Currently, the 2014 Evidence-Based Guideline for the Management of High Blood Pressure in Adults (JNC 8) (16) does not address the classification of prehypertension or hypertension in adults but rather places focus on pharmacological treatment. Therefore, the framework proposed by the Seventh Report of the Joint National Committee on Prevention, Detection, Evaluation, and Treatment of High Blood Pressure (JNC 7) in 2004 remains a widely accepted classification scheme (37) where a normal BP (measured in millimeters of mercury [mm Hg]) is <120 SBP *and* <80 DBP, prehypertension is 120–139 SBP *or* 80–89 DBP, and stage 1 hypertension is 140–159 SBP *or* 90–99 DBP. For specific recommendations on medications used in the treatment and management of hypertension in adults, see JNC 8 (16) and the American Society of Hypertension and the International Society of Hypertension Clinical Practice Guidelines (37).

Lifestyle modification that includes increasing physical activity, weight reduction, eating plans (Dietary Approaches to Stop Hypertension [DASH]), decreased intake of dietary sodium (no more than 2 g sodium · d^{-1}), and moderation of alcohol remains the foundation of antihypertensive treatment. For additional information, see Chapter 15.

Blood pressure measurement The most accurate method for measuring BP is via direct intra-arterial measurement with a pressure transducer. Obviously, this procedure is very invasive, can only be performed by trained clinical professionals, and is not practical for most settings. Typically, resting BP is obtained indirectly by listening to the internal sounds of the body with a stethoscope via a technique termed *auscultation*. During auscultation for BP assessment, the exercise professional listens for the sounds of Korotkoff. In this technique, blood flow through the brachial artery is occluded with a cuff placed around the upper arm that has been inflated to a suprasystolic pressure. As the bladder in the cuff is gradually deflated, pulsatile blood flow is reestablished and is accompanied by sounds that can be heard with a stethoscope placed just below the cuff. Traditionally, there are five sounds that can be detected and are presented in Box 3.2. The sounds that can be heard are believed to originate from a combination of turbulent blood flow and oscillations of the arterial wall. To his credit, Korotkoff believed that the sounds were caused by the rushing of a small part of the pulse wave through the compressed area and vibrations from the "unsticking" vessel walls (30).

Box 3.2 Korotkoff Sounds

- Phase 1: The first initial sound or the onset of sound. Sounds like clear repetitive tapping. The sound may be faint at first and gradually increase in intensity of volume to phase 2. Phase 1 represents systole.
- Phase 2: Sounds are a soft tapping or murmur. They are often longer than the phase 1 sounds. These sounds have also been described as having a swishing component. The phase 2 sounds are typically 10–15 mm Hg after the onset of sound (phase 1).
- Phase 3: Sounds are like a loud tapping, high in both pitch and intensity. These sounds are crisper and louder than the phase 2 sounds.
- Phase 4: Sounds become muffled. The sounds become less distinct and less audible. Another way of describing this sound is as soft or blowing.
- Phase 5: Complete disappearance of sound. The true disappearance of sound usually occurs within 8–10 mm Hg of sound (phase 4) and is considered diastole.

Adapted from Kaminsky LA. *ACSM's Health-Related Physical Fitness Assessment Manual.* 4th ed. Baltimore (MD): Lippincott Williams & Wilkins; 2014. 192 p.

It is important to follow standard procedures for measuring BP, whether it is being assessed in the supine, sitting, or exercising positions prior to testing. Typically, the patient should be seated quietly and be wearing a short-sleeved or sleeveless garment. The actual measurement of BP should be taken twice allowing at least 1 minute between measurements. Appropriate procedures for measuring resting BP are presented in Box 3.3.

The type of instrument that is used for indirect BP measurement includes both ausculatory (manual) and oscillometric (automated) devices. Ausculatory devices include aneroid, mercury, and hybrid sphygmomanometers. Originally described by Rivia-Rocci in 1896, mercury manometers are based on gravity, leaving little room for measurement error. Despite the accuracy of mercury manometers, they are being phased out due to environmental concerns. Aneroid manometers measure pressure via a series of levers that register the pressure on a circular scale. These devices loose accuracy over time and require calibration at regular intervals. However, when calibrated, aneroid devices yield similar values to those measured by a mercury manometer (8). Although the possibility of an inaccurate measurement does exist when using an aneroid device, the possibility that there is observer error is also likely especially when devices with small dials are used. Hybrid sphygmomanometers combine the features of both oscillometric and ausculatory devices.

The use of automatic devices has increased in home and clinical settings. The variability and reliability of automated BP readings is often questioned. The AHA recommends automatic, cuff-style, upper arm monitors instead of wrist and/or finger monitors because of its decreased reliability. Further recommendations include choosing a validated monitor, ensuring that the monitor is validated for special needs (*e.g.*, pregnancy, **older adults**) and that the cuff fits appropriately. Skirton et al. (31) recommend the use of auscultatory devices over automatic devices in specific circumstances, such as management of hypertension, following trauma or where there is a potential for the individual's condition to deteriorate because of reduced reliability measures.

In addition to the type of device that is being used to measure BP, not following the appropriate procedures can lead to inaccurate measurements. Common errors when measuring BP are outlined in Box 3.4. When choosing a BP cuff, the cuff and bladder must fit appropriately. A bladder that is too small will lead to an overestimation of BP, whereas a bladder that is too large will lead to an underestimation of BP (28). Considerable BP variability can occur with breathing, emotion, exercise, meals, tobacco, alcohol, temperature, bladder distension, and pain. Furthermore, BP can

Box 3.3 Procedures for the Assessment of Resting Blood Pressure

1. The patient should be seated quietly for at least 5 minutes in a chair with back support and their feet on the floor. The arm that will be receiving the cuff should be bare. Patients should refrain from smoking cigarettes or ingesting caffeine at least 30 minutes before the measurement.
2. Select an appropriate cuff size to where the bladder in the cuff should encircle at least 80% of the upper arm.
3. Palpate the brachial artery pulse on the anteromedial aspect of the arm just below the belly of the biceps brachii and just above (2–3 cm or 1 in) the antecubital fossa. Firmly wrap the deflated cuff around the upper arm so the midline of the cuff is directly over the palpated brachial artery pulse. The bottom edge of the cuff should be at least 2.5 cm (1 in) above the antecubital fossa.
4. Locate and palpate the radial pulse. While palpating the radial pulse, rapidly inflate the cuff to 70 mm Hg and slowly increase the pressure by 10 mm Hg until the radial pulse disappears (estimate of systolic blood pressure [SBP]) and rapidly deflate the cuff.
5. Position the ear buds of the stethoscope so they are in line with the auditory canal and place the bell of the stethoscope just below the antecubital space over the brachial artery. Ensure that the diaphragm of the bell is in full contact with the skin. Do not place any part of the bell under the cuff.
6. Close the valve and rapidly inflate the cuff pressure to 20–30 mm Hg above the estimated SBP determined by palpation.
7. Slowly release the pressure at a rate of 2–3 mm Hg per second while listening for the first metallic tapping sound that corresponds to the first Korotkoff sound (phase 1).
8. Continue to release the pressure at an appropriate rate noting when the metallic sound becomes muffled (phase 4) and when the sound completely disappears (phase 5). Typically, the phase 5 sound represents the DBP, but both phases 4 and 5 should be noted.
9. At least two measurements should be made (a minimum of 1 min apart) and the average should be taken.
10. Blood pressure should be taken in both arms during a patient's first examination. The arm with the higher pressure (if they are not the same) should be used.

More detailed information can be found in Pickering et al. (28).

Modified from Reeves RA. The rational clinical examination. Does this patient have hypertension? How to measure blood pressure. *JAMA*. 1995;273(15):1211–8; Beevers G, Lip GY, O'Brien E. ABC of hypertension. Blood pressure measurement. Part I — sphygmomanometry: factors common to all techniques. *BMJ*. 2001:322(7292):981–5; and Beevers G, Lip GY, O'Brien E. ABC of hypertension. Blood pressure measurement. Part II — conventional sphygmomanometry: technique of ausculatory blood pressure measurement. *BMJ*. 2001:322(7293):1043–7.

be influenced by age, race, and circadian rhythm variation. Ideally, the individual should be relaxed in a quiet room at a comfortable temperature with a short rest period before BP measurement. The examination should include an appropriate measurement of BP, with verification in the contralateral arm (28). BP measurements may be taken in the lower extremity (*e.g.*, thigh or calf muscle) if an individual is suspected of having coarctation of the aorta or other type of obstructive aortic disease (12). Although measurements of BP can be taken in the lower extremity and forearm, the AHA contends that the accuracy of this procedure has not been verified (28).

The posture of the subject during BP measurement should be noted, whether it is supine, sitting, or standing. Sitting is most commonly used except when examining orthostatic tolerance. When the arm is supported at heart level, the BP should be similar in all three positions (provided a brief period has passed following a change in position to allow for baroreceptor reflex control of BP). To assess the possibility of orthostatic intolerance, BP is measured supine and then standing. A normal response is for the BP to not change (or rise slightly because of the muscular effort of standing).

Box 3.4 Potential Sources of Error in Blood Pressure Assessment

- Inaccurate sphygmomanometer
- Improper cuff size
- Auditory acuity of technician
- Rate of inflation or deflation of cuff pressure
- Experience of technician
- Faulty equipment
- Improper stethoscope placement or pressure
- Not having the cuff at heart level
- Certain physiological abnormalities (*e.g.*, damaged brachial artery, subclavian steal syndrome, arteriovenous fistula)
- Reaction time of technician[a]
- Background noise
- Allowing patient to hold treadmill handrails or flex elbow[a]

[a]Applies specifically during exercise testing.

From American College of Sports Medicine. *ACSM's Guidelines for Exercise Testing and Prescription.* 10th ed. Philadelphia (PA): Wolters Kluwer; 2018. 480 p.

A drop in BP in the standing position (sometimes accompanied by dizziness) indicates orthostatic intolerance (postural hypotension) and may be caused by antihypertensive medications and certain medical conditions (*e.g.*, diabetic autonomic neuropathy).

Supporting the arm during BP assessment is necessary to prevent possible increases (up to 10%) in DBP associated with an **isometric** muscle action of the unsupported arm (19). Furthermore, placing the arm in a dependent position below the level of the heart leads to an overestimation of SBP and DBP, whereas raising the arm leads to an underestimation of SBP and DBP, both caused by gravitationally derived hydrostatic pressure differences between the heart and the arm. Many BP devices are inaccurate if the wrist is not held at the heart level during measurement (5).

Patient Preparation

Each participant should be carefully prepared before all exercise testing. Ideally, a detailed set of instructions should be provided to the person when the testing appointment is made. Verbal and written instructions are recommended to reduce test anxiety and to standardize the response to testing. Instructions before testing should include avoiding eating and smoking for a minimum of 3 hours before testing and 8 hours before a nuclear imaging study. Individuals should wear comfortable footwear and loose-fitting clothing and should be instructed on whether medications should be tapered, discontinued, or continued for the test based on physician orders. Participants should avoid unusual physical efforts for at least 12 hours before testing (10,25).

A past medical history and physical examination that focuses on risk factors should be conducted before the exercise test to determine any risk factors or signs and symptoms of cardiovascular, pulmonary, metabolic, musculoskeletal, and neurological conditions (25). Furthermore, contraindications to testing should be determined before exercise testing (10). Contraindications to exercise testing are located in Chapter 4 (see Box 4.1). In addition, determining the individual's current physical activity level can aid in the selection of an appropriate testing protocol. Informed consent should be signed and included in the exercise test record. The informed consent must accurately describe all procedures and potential risks/benefits associated with these procedures.

Specific instructions should be given on how to perform the exercise test, purpose of the test, and a brief demonstration of the test procedure (*e.g.*, walking on treadmill, riding bicycle). Furthermore, any questions that the individual has should be addressed (10).

Protocol Selection

Selecting the appropriate exercise protocol is an important component in exercise testing. The exercise protocol should be based on the individual's past medical history, preparticipation screening, exercise history, and goals. The exercise professional must then determine what the appropriate mode of exercise will be (treadmill vs. cycle ergometer) and the appropriate exercise protocol. Detailed protocols to improve cardiovascular fitness may be found in Chapter 4.

SUMMARY

The purpose of preparticipation screening is to identify individuals who are at risk for experiencing an adverse exercise-related cardiovascular event. The new ACSM screening algorithm not only accomplishes this but also reduces the likelihood of creating additional barriers to the individual for adopting exercise. The screening algorithm is based on the following: There is a low risk of SCD and AMI associated with the adoption of a new exercise program, and the risk associated with vigorous exercise can be mitigated by the exercise professional starting the novice exerciser at a light- to moderate-intensity exercise (2–3 METs) and progressing over a 2- to 3-month period to a higher intensity, provided the person remains symptom-free (29).

In addition to utilizing an appropriate preparticipation screening tool (*e.g.*, **Physical Activity Readiness Questionnaire for Everyone [PAR-Q+]**), the exercise professional should administer a basic medical history that includes a CVD risk assessment. The additional information gained from the CVD assessment will assist the exercise professional in managing any CVD risk factors that may be present as well as writing an effective exercise program. Once an individual has gone through the screening process, an appropriate exercise mode and protocol should be chosen to assess any or all of the health-related components of fitness (**muscular strength** and **muscular endurance**, **cardiorespiratory fitness**, **flexibility**, **body composition**).

REFERENCES

1. Albert CM, Mittleman MA, Chae CU, Lee IM, Hennekens CH, Manson JE. Triggering of sudden death from cardiac causes by vigorous exertion. *N Engl J Med*. 2000;343(19):1355–61.
2. American Association of Cardiovascular and Pulmonary Rehabilitation. *Guidelines for Cardiac Rehabilitation and Secondary Prevention Programs*. 5th ed. Champaign (IL): Human Kinetics; 2013. 336 p.
3. American College of Sports Medicine position stand and American Heart Association. Recommendations for cardiovascular screening, staffing, and emergency policies at health/fitness facilities. *Med Sci Sports Exerc*. 1998;30(6):1009–18.
4. American Diabetes Association. 2. Classification and diagnosis of diabetes. *Diabetes Care*. 2015;38(suppl 1):S8–16.
5. Beevers G, Lip GY, O'Brien E. ABC of hypertension. Blood pressure measurement. Part I — sphygmomanometry: factors common to all techniques. *BMJ*. 2001:322(7292):981–5.
6. Bickley LS, Bates B. *Bates' Pocket Guide to Physical Examination and History Taking*. Baltimore (MD): Lippincott Williams & Wilkins; 2008. 416 p.
7. Chobanian AV, Bakris GL, Black HR, et al. Seventh Report of the Joint National Committee on Prevention, Detection, Evaluation, and Treatment of High Blood Pressure. *Hypertension*. 2003;42:1206–52.
8. Dorigatti F, Bonzo E, Zanier A, Palatini P. Validation of Heine Gamma G7 (G5) and XXL-LF aneroid devices for blood pressure measurement. *Blood Press Monit*. 2007;12(1):29–33.
9. Eckel RH, Jakicic JM, Ard JD, et al. 2013 AHA/ACC guideline on lifestyle management to reduce cardiovascular risk: a report of the American College of Cardiology/American Heart Association Task Force on Practice Guidelines. *J Am Coll Cardiol*. 2014;63:2960–84.

10. Fletcher GF, Ades PA, Kligfield P, et al. Exercise standards for testing and training: a scientific statement from the American Heart Association. *Circulation*. 2013;128:873–934.
11. Franklin BA, McCullough PA. Cardiorespiratory fitness: an independent and additive marker of risk stratification and health outcomes. *Mayo Clin Proc*. 2009;84(9):776–9.
12. Gardner AW. Exercise training for patients with peripheral artery disease. Activite physique pour des patients souffrant d arteriopathie. *Phys Sportsmed*. 2001;29(8):25,28, 31–2;35.
13. Gibbons RJ, Balady GJ, Bricker JT, et al. ACC/AHA 2002 guideline update for exercise testing: summary article. A report of the American College of Cardiology/American Heart Association Task Force on Practice Guidelines (Committee to Update the 1997 Exercise Testing Guidelines). *J Am Coll Cardiol*. 2002;40(8):1531–40.
14. Goff DC Jr, Lloyd-Jones DM, Bennett G, et al. 2013 ACC/AHA guideline on the assessment of cardiovascular risk: a report of the American College of Cardiology/American Heart Association Task Force on Practice Guidelines. *J Am Coll Cardiol*. 2014;63:2935–59.
15. Hill K, Gardiner P, Cavalheri V, Jenkins S, Healy G. Physical activity and sedentary behavior: applying lessons to chronic obstructive pulmonary disease. *Intern Med J*. 2015;45(5):474–82.
16. James PA, Oparil S, Carter BL, et al. 2014 Evidence-based guideline for the management of high blood pressure in adults: report from the panel members appointed to the Eighth Joint National Committee (JNC 8). *JAMA*. 2014;311:507–20.
17. Jamnik VK, Warburton DE, Makarski J, et al. Enhancing the effectiveness of clearance for physical activity participation: background and overall process. *Appl Physiol Nutr Metab*. 2011;36 suppl 1:S3–13.
18. Jensen MD, Ryan DH, Apovian CM, et al. 2013 AHA/ACC/TOS guideline for the management of overweight and obesity in adults: a report of the American College of Cardiology/American Heart Association Task Force on Practice Guidelines and The Obesity Society. *J Am Coll Cardiol*. 2014;63(25 pt B):2985–3023.
19. Kaminsky LA. *ACSM's Health-Related Physical Fitness Assessment Manual*. 4th ed. Baltimore (MD): Lippincott Williams & Wilkins; 2014. 192 p.
20. Kim JH, Malhotra R, Chiampas G, et al. Cardiac arrest during long-distance running races. *N Engl J Med*. 2012;366(2):130–40.
21. Kohl HW III, Powell KE, Gordon NF, Blair SN, Paffenbarger RS Jr. Physical activity, physical fitness, and sudden cardiac death. *Epidemiol Rev*. 1992;14:37–58.
22. Lewington S, Clarke R, Qizilbash N, Peto R, Collins R. Age-specific relevance of usual blood pressure to vascular mortality: a meta-analysis of individual data for one million adults in 61 prospective studies. *Lancet*. 2002;360(9349):1903–13.
23. Magal M, Riebe D. New preparticipation health screening recommendations: what exercise professionals need to know. *ACSM's Health Fitness J*. 2016;20(3):22–7.
24. Mittleman MA, Maclure M, Tofler GH, Sherwood JB, Goldberg RJ, Muller JE. Triggering of acute myocardial infarction by heavy physical exertion. Protection against triggering by regular exertion. Determinants of myocardial infarction onset study investigators. *N Engl J Med*. 1993;329(23):1677–83.
25. Myers J, Arena R, Franklin B, et al. Recommendations for clinical exercise laboratories: a scientific statement from the American Heart Association. *Circulation*. 2009;119:3144–61.
26. National Cholesterol Education Program Expert Panel on Detection, Evaluation, and Treatment of High Blood Cholesterol in Adults (Adult Treatment Panel III). Third report of the National Cholesterol Education Program (NCEP) Expert Panel on Detection, Evaluation, and Treatment of High Blood Cholesterol in Adults (Adult Treatment Panel III) final report. *Circulation*. 2002;106(25):3143–421.
27. Pate RR, Pratt M, Blair SN, et al. Physical activity and public health. A recommendation from the Centers for Disease Control and Prevention and the American College of Sports Medicine. *JAMA*. 1995;273(5):402–7.
28. Pickering TG, Hall JE, Appel LJ, et al. Recommendations for blood pressure measurement in humans and experimental animals: part 1: blood pressure measurement in humans: a statement for professionals from the Subcommittee of Professional and Public Education of the American Heart Association Council on High Blood Pressure Research. *Hypertension*. 2005;45:142–61.
29. Riebe D, Franklin BA, Thompson PD, et al. Updating ACSM's recommendations for exercise preparticipation health screening. *Med Sci Sports Exerc*. 2015;47(8):2473–9.
30. Shevchenko YL, Tsitlik JE. 90th Anniversary of the development by Nokolai S. Korotkoff of the ausculatory method of measuring blood pressure. *Circulation*. 1996;94(2):116–8.
31. Skirton H, Chamberlain W, Lawson C, Ryan H, Young E. A systematic review of variability and reliability of manual and automated blood pressure readings. *J Clin Nurs*. 2011;20(5–6):602–14.
32. Thompson PD, Franklin BA, Balady GJ, et al. Exercise and acute cardiovascular events placing the risks into perspective: a scientific statement from the American Heart Association Council on Nutrition, Physical Activity, and Metabolism and the Council on Clinical Cardiology. *Circulation*. 2007;115(17):2358–68.
33. Thompson PD, Stern MP, Williams P, Duncan K, Haskell WL, Wood PD. Death during jogging or running. A study of 18 cases. *JAMA*. 1979;242(12):1265–7.
34. U.S. Department of Health and Human Services. *Physical Activity Guidelines Advisory Committee Report*, 2008 [Internet]. Washington (DC): U.S. Department of Health and Human Services; 2008 [cited 2016 June 30]. 683 p. Available from: http://www.health.gov/paguidelines/Report/pdf/CommitteeReport.pdf

35. Verrill D, Graham H, Vitcenda M, Peno-Green L, Kramer V, Corbisiero T. Measuring behavioral outcomes in cardiopulmonary rehabilitation: an AACVPR statement. *J Cardiopulm Rehabil Prev.* 2009;29(3):193–203.
36. Warburton DE, Jamnik VK, Bredin SS, et al. Evidence-based risk assessment and recommendations for physical activity clearance: an introduction. *Appl Physiol Nutr Metab.* 2011;36(suppl 1):S1–2.
37. Weber MA, Schiffrin EL, White WB, et al. Clinical practice guidelines for the management of hypertension in the community: a statement by the American Society of Hypertension and the International Society of Hypertension. *J Clin Hypertens (Greenwich).* 2014;16(1):14–26.
38. Whang W, Manson JE, Hu FB, et al. Physical exertion, exercise, and sudden cardiac death in women. *JAMA.* 2006;295(12):1399–403.
39. Whitfield GP, Pettee Gabriel KK, Rahbar MH, Kohl HW III. Application of the American Heart Association/American College of Sports Medicine adult preparticipation screening checklist to a nationally representative sample of US adults aged ≥40 years from the National Health and Nutrition Examination Survey 2001 to 2004. *Circulation.* 2014;129:1113–20.
40. Williams MA. Exercise testing in cardiac rehabilitation. Exercise prescription and beyond. *Cardiol Clin.* 2001;19(3):415–31.

CHAPTER 4

Cardiorespiratory Fitness Assessment

INTRODUCTION

Cardiorespiratory fitness (CRF) is one of the five health-related components of **physical fitness** (CRF, **body composition**, **muscular strength**, **muscular endurance**, **flexibility**). It is characterized by the body's ability to perform moderate- to vigorous-intensity exercise using large muscle groups in a dynamic/rhythmic and continuous manner for prolonged periods of time. Thus, the ability to sustain this level of exertion is dependent on the integration of the respiratory, cardiovascular, and musculoskeletal systems. Higher levels of CRF are often associated with higher levels of **physical activity**, which are associated with a number of health benefits. This type of association can be characterized as a dose-response relationship. Low levels of CRF are associated with a marked increase in all-cause mortality (specifically from cardiovascular disease [CVD]). Increases in CRF result in a reduction in all-cause mortality (12,13,38,61,64). The assessment of CRF is, therefore, an important part of any primary or secondary prevention and rehabilitative program. The skills and knowledge required to complete the assessment, interpret the results, and write an appropriate **exercise prescription** (ExR_x) are an important responsibility of the exercise professional.

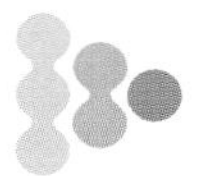

Measuring Cardiorespiratory Fitness and the Maximal Oxygen Uptake

Measurement (or assessment) of CRF can assist the professional by providing valuable information that can be used to determine the **intensity**, duration, and mode of **exercise** recommended as part of an exercise program. Additionally, the measurement of CRF following the initiation of an exercise training program can serve as motivation to the patient as reason for continuing with a regular exercise program and may encourage the addition of other modes of exercise to improve overall fitness. Last, the assessment of CRF can assist in identifying, diagnosing, and prognosis of comorbid conditions.

It is important to choose the test that best fits the patient's characteristics. The following are some of the factors to consider when choosing the appropriate type of test:

- What will the information be used for (functional capacity, ExR_x)?
- Whether physician supervision is required
- Health status of the participant
- Maximal or submaximal
- Length of the test
- Willingness of the participant
- Cost of the test to administer
- What personnel are needed (*i.e.*, qualifications)?
- What equipment and facilities are needed for the test?
- Whether there are any safety concerns

Maximal Oxygen Uptake (Absolute and Relative)

Maximal volume of oxygen consumed per unit of time ($\dot{V}O_{2max}$) is accepted as the criterion measure of CRF. This variable is typically expressed in absolute or relative terms. Absolute $\dot{V}O_{2max}$ is expressed in liters per minute ($L \cdot min^{-1}$) or milliliters per minute ($mL \cdot min^{-1}$) and provides a measure of energy expenditure for both non–weight- and weight-bearing activities such as arm or leg cycle ergometry and the treadmill. Absolute $\dot{V}O_{2max}$ is directly related to body mass or size and is typically greater in men compared with women. $\dot{V}O_{2max}$ is most often described relative to an individual's body weight; thus, relative $\dot{V}O_{2max}$ is expressed in milliliters per kilogram of body weight per minute ($mL \cdot kg^{-1} \cdot min^{-1}$) and is used to classify an individual's CRF level to allow for meaningful comparisons between/among individuals with differing body weight. Relative $\dot{V}O_2$ is often used to estimate energy expenditure of weight-bearing activities such as walking, running, and stair climbing. When expressing $\dot{V}O_{2max}$ simply as a linear function of body mass, CRF may be underestimated for heavier individuals (>75.4 kg) and overestimated for lighter individuals (<67.7 kg) (32).

Maximal Oxygen Consumption: Net and Gross Rates

It has been proposed that expressing $\dot{V}O_{2max}$ relative to an individual's fat-free mass ($mL \cdot kg\ FFM^{-1} \cdot min^{-1}$) would provide a more accurate estimate of his or her CRF and is independent of changes in body mass (19). The rate of oxygen consumption can also be expressed as gross $\dot{V}O_2$ or net $\dot{V}O_2$. Gross $\dot{V}O_2$ represents the *total* rate oxygen consumed (or caloric cost) at rest and during a bout of exercise. Net $\dot{V}O_2$, on the other hand, represents the rate of oxygen consumption in excess of an individual's resting $\dot{V}O_2$ and is used to describe the caloric cost of exercise. Both net and gross $\dot{V}O_2$ can be expressed in either absolute ($L \cdot min^{-1}$) or relative terms ($mL \cdot kg^{-1} \cdot min^{-1}$).

$\dot{V}O_{2max}$ is the product of the maximal cardiac output ($\dot{Q}$; $L\ blood \cdot min^{-1}$) and arterial–venous oxygen ($a\text{-}\bar{v}O_2$) difference ($mL\ O_2 \cdot L\ blood^{-1}$) or put more simply, delivery ($\dot{Q}$) and utilization ($a\text{-}\bar{v}O_2$ difference) and is illustrated in the following equation (Fick equation):

$$\dot{V}O_{2max} = \dot{Q}_{max} \times (a\text{-}\bar{v}O_2\ diff_{max})$$

Differences in $\dot{V}O_{2max}$ across populations and fitness levels result primarily from differences in $\dot{Q}$; therefore, $\dot{V}O_{2max}$ is closely related to the functional capacity of the heart (delivery). During exercise, the achievement of $\dot{V}O_{2max}$ implies that an individual's true physiological limit has been reached and a plateau in $\dot{V}O_2$ was observed between the final two work rates of a progressive exercise test. It is important to note that the intrinsic motivation of an individual as well as the test mode may influence their ability to achieve a "true" $\dot{V}O_{2max}$. Individuals with CVD or pulmonary disease rarely are able to achieve a plateau in $\dot{V}O_2$ despite exercising maximally. The term $\dot{V}O_{2peak}$ may be used instead when an individual is not able to achieve a plateau of $\dot{V}O_2$ during a maximal effort and is limited by local muscular factors or fatigue rather than central circulatory dynamics (44). $\dot{V}O_{2peak}$ is commonly used to describe CRF in these and other populations with chronic diseases and health conditions (3).

Open-Circuit Spirometry

Open-circuit spirometry, also known as *indirect calorimetry*, is the preferred method for the measurement of $\dot{V}O_{2max}$ and is measured during a graded incremental or ramp exercise test to exhaustion. During this procedure, the subject breathes through a mouthpiece, with the nose occluded (or through a facemask that covers the mouth and nose). This configuration allows pulmonary ventilation and expired fractions of oxygen (O_2) and carbon dioxide (CO_2) to be measured. An accurate assessment of anaerobic/ventilatory threshold and $\dot{V}O_{2max}$/$\dot{V}O_{2peak}$ can be achieved using open-circuit spirometry. Currently, there are a number of automated systems available that provide ease of use as well as mobility. Regardless of the type of automated system that is used, calibration of the unit is essential in order to obtain valid and reliable results (50). In addition, administration and interpretation of the test should be reserved for trained professionals. It is important to note that based on the health status of the patient, equipment costs, space, and required personnel, the direct measurement of $\dot{V}O_{2max}$ may not always be feasible and is often reserved for research or clinical settings.

Exercise Tests to Estimate $\dot{V}O_{2max}$

If $\dot{V}O_{2max}$ is not able to be directly measured, there are a variety of maximal and submaximal exercise tests that can be used to *estimate* $\dot{V}O_{2max}$. Exercise tests that estimate $\dot{V}O_{2max}$ have been validated by examining (a) the correlation between directly measured $\dot{V}O_{2max}$ and the $\dot{V}O_{2max}$ estimated from physiological responses to **submaximal** exercise (*e.g.*, heart rate [HR] at a specified power output) or (b) the correlation between directly measured $\dot{V}O_{2max}$ and field test performance (*e.g.*, time to run 1 or 1.5 mile [1.6 or 2.4 km]) or time to volitional fatigue using a standard **graded exercise test** protocol. It is important to understand that by estimating $\dot{V}O_{2max}$, there is a potential for error. Often, overestimation is more likely to occur with an exercise protocol that is chosen which is too aggressive for a given individual (*e.g.*, Bruce treadmill protocol in patients with heart failure) (3). Every effort should be taken to choose the appropriate exercise protocol given an individual's characteristics and minimize handrail use during testing on a treadmill (29).

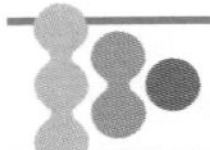

Contraindications to Exercise Testing

Prior to initiating an exercise test, the risk of performing the test must be weighed against the potential benefits. An exercise professional must understand both the relative and absolute contraindications to exercise testing (Box 4.1) (23). This emphasizes the importance of performing a thorough preexercise test evaluation in addition to carefully reviewing the patient's exercise history (as described in Chapter 3) to assist the exercise professional in identifying any potential contraindications to exercise testing. Individuals who are identified as having any absolute contraindications should

Box 4.1 Relative and Absolute Indications for Stopping an Exercise Test (1)

Contraindications to Symptom-Limited Maximal Exercise Testing

Absolute Contraindications

- Acute myocardial infarction within 2 d
- Ongoing unstable angina
- Uncontrolled cardiac arrhythmia with hemodynamic compromise
- Active endocarditis
- Symptomatic severe aortic stenosis
- Decompensated heart failure
- Acute pulmonary embolism, pulmonary infarction, or deep venous thrombosis
- Acute myocarditis or pericarditis
- Acute aortic dissection
- Physical disability that precludes safe and adequate testing

Relative Contraindications

- Known obstructive left main coronary artery stenosis
- Moderate to severe aortic stenosis with uncertain relationship to symptoms
- Tachyarrhythmias with uncontrolled ventricular rates
- Acquired advanced or complete heart block
- Recent stroke or transient ischemia attack
- Mental impairment with limited ability to cooperate
- Resting hypertension with systolic >200 mm Hg or diastolic >110 mm Hg
- Uncorrected medical conditions, such as significant anemia, important electrolyte imbalance, and hyperthyroidism

Reprinted with permission from Fletcher GF, Ades PA, Kligfield P, et al. Exercise standards for testing and training: a scientific statement from the American Heart Association. *Circulation*. 2013;128:873–934.

not be tested until the condition has been stabilized or adequately treated. Those who have relative contraindications may be tested only after a careful evaluation that has determined that the benefit involved in performing the test outweighs the associated risks.

Maximal versus Submaximal Exercise Testing

The decision to perform a maximal or submaximal exercise test depends largely on the reasons for the test, physical condition of the patient, and availability of appropriate equipment and personnel. **Maximal** exercise tests require participants to exercise to the point of volitional fatigue, which may be inappropriate for some individuals and may require the need for emergency equipment (23,50).

Exercise professionals often rely on submaximal exercise tests to assess CRF because maximal exercise testing is not always feasible in the health/fitness setting. The foundation of submaximal exercise testing is to determine the HR response to one or more submaximal work rates and to use the data to predict an individual's $\dot{V}O_{2max}$. In addition to predicting $\dot{V}O_{2max}$ from the HR–work rate relationship, the exercise professional should collect additional important physiological responses from the exercise test. The measurement of HR, blood pressure (BP), work rate, and rating of perceived exertion (RPE) can give valuable information to the exercise professional in regard to the patient's health and functional response to exercise. Combined with the patient's estimated $\dot{V}O_{2max}$, this information can be used to evaluate and track the patient's submaximal physiological responses over time and can be used to make modifications to his or her ExR_x.

To ensure an accurate estimation of $\dot{V}O_{2max}$ from a submaximal exercise test, all of the following assumptions must be met or achieved (34):

- A steady-state HR is obtained for each exercise work rate.
- A linear relationship exists between HR and work rate.
- The difference between actual and predicted maximal heart rate (HR_{max}) is minimal.
- Mechanical efficiency (*i.e.*, $\dot{V}O_2$ at a given work rate) is the same for everyone.
- The subject is not on any medications that may alter the HR response to exercise (*i.e.*, β-blockers).
- The subject is not using high quantities of caffeine, ill, or in a high-temperature environment, all of which may alter the HR response.

Guidelines for Exercise Testing

General Guidelines

Prior to any type of CRF testing, pertinent data such as preactivity screening (refer to Chapter 3), demographic, medical, and personal information should be gathered and reviewed to reduce the occurrence of unwanted or potentially harmful events that could occur during the exercise test. Once an individual has been properly screened and it has been determined he or she is safely able to undergo the CRF test, the exercise professional should ensure that the following pretest instructions are given the patient. These instructions should be provided to the patient at least 24 hours before the exercise test to ensure patient adherence as well as maximize patient safety and comfort.

- Review the patient's completed consent and screening forms.
- Have the appropriate data collection forms (data recording sheets, normative tables) ready prior to the exercise test.
- Calibrate all equipment (*e.g.*, cycle ergometer, treadmill, sphygmomanometer, skinfold calipers) at least monthly or more frequently based on usage.
- Assure a room temperature between 68°F and 72°F (20°C and 22°C) and a humidity of less than 60% with adequate ventilation (37). The testing environment can play a very important role in test validity and reliability.
- To minimize subject anxiety, the test procedures should be explained adequately and should not be rushed, and the test environment should be quiet and private.
- The room should be equipped with a comfortable seat and/or examination table to be used for resting BP and HR.
- The demeanor of personnel should be one of relaxed confidence to put the subject at ease.
- Finally, the exercise professional should be familiar with the emergency response plan.

When performing multiple assessments in one session, the sequence of testing is very important. Prior to any exertional assessments, resting measurements such as HR, BP, height, and body weight and body composition should be obtained. Once resting measurements have been taken, the following order can be followed for testing: cardiorespiratory, muscular fitness, and flexibility. Although an optimal order for testing multiple health-related components of fitness has not been determined, sufficient time should be allowed for HR and BP to return as close to baseline as possible between tests. For example, assessing CRF after a muscular fitness assessment (which can elevate HR) can influence the CRF results. Furthermore, the tester should be aware of and note any medications the participant is taking because some, such as β-blockers, can alter the HR response to exercise. In addition, the test sequence should be organized so that the same muscle groups will not be stressed repeatedly.

Pretest Instructions for Cardiorespiratory Fitness Assessment

To ensure the predictive accuracy for measuring CRF, reproducibility of the test, and ensure the safety of the patient, they should be presented with the following general instructions to standardize the test (23):

- The purpose for conducting the test should be clear to ensure diagnostic accuracy and patient safety.
- Patients should abstain from ingesting food, caffeine, alcohol, or tobacco products within 3 hours of testing (routine medications may be taken with small amounts of water).
- Appropriate, comfortable clothing and footwear should be worn.
- Strenuous exercise should not be performed at least 24 hours prior the test.
- If the exercise test is on an outpatient basis, the individual should be made aware that the fitness assessment is maximal and may cause fatigue. They may wish to have someone accompany them to drive home afterward.
- If the exercise test is performed for the diagnosis of ischemia, routine medications may be discontinued because some (β-blockers) can attenuate the HR and BP response to exercise as well as alter the hemodynamic response and reduce the sensitivity of an electrocardiogram (ECG, antianginal agents). No formal guidelines for medication tapering exist, but 24 hours or more could be required.
- If the exercise test is for functional or ExR_x purposes, individuals *should continue* their medication regimen so the exercise response will be consistent with responses expected during exercise (3).
- Participants should bring a list of their current medications that include dosage and frequency of administration and report when the last dose was taken.
- Ample fluid consumption 24 hours prior to the assessment is encouraged to ensure normal hydration.

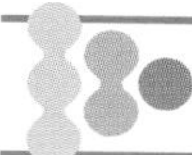

Cardiorespiratory Test Sequence and Measurements

Following the appropriate screening, measurements specific for CRF testing should be obtained prior to the start of the exercise test.

Position and Technique

At a minimum, preexercise HR and BP should be measured in the testing position. A preexercise HR should be obtained at the radial artery for 60 seconds. BP should be obtained following standardized procedures (see Chapter 3). During the exercise test, a minimum of HR, BP, RPE, and ECG should be measured at defined intervals while constant subjective measurements of signs or symptoms of cardiovascular or pulmonary disease are also recorded. These measurements should be obtained routinely during the exercise test and through recovery. Table 4.1 provides the recommended sequence for the measurement of HR, BP, RPE, and ECG during an exercise test.

HR can be measured either by palpitation, auscultation, or via HR monitors. The pulse palpation technique involves "feeling" the pulse by placing the second and third digits (*i.e.*, index and middle fingers) over the radial artery which is located on the thumb side of the wrist. The pulse is commonly counted for a 15-second time interval and then multiplied by 4 to determine the HR for 1 minute. During exercise, this 15-second method should be used to ensure that HR has reached a **steady state** (two measurements that are within four beats). To auscultate the HR, the bell of the stethoscope should be placed to the left of the sternum and just above the nipple. The exercise HR response should be a linear increase in work at a rate of approximately 10 ± 2 beats · MET^{-1}. HR_{max} decreases with age (64) and is decreased in patients on β-adrenergic receptor blockers along

Table 4.1 Best Practices for Monitoring during a Symptom-Limited Maximal Exercise Test (1)

Variable	Before Exercise Test	During Exercise Test	After Exercise Test
Electrocardiogram	Monitor continuously; record in supine position and position of exercise (*e.g.*, standing).	Monitor continuously; record during the last 5–10 s of each stage or every 2 min (ramp protocol).	Monitor continuously; record immediately postexercise, 60 s of recovery, and then every 2 min.
Heart rate[a]	Monitor continuously; record in supine position and position of exercise (*e.g.*, standing).	Monitor continuously; record during the last 5–10 s of each minute.	Monitor continuously; record during the last 5–10 s of each minute.
Blood pressure[a,b]	Monitor continuously; record in supine position and position of exercise (*e.g.*, standing).	Measure and record during the last 30–60 s of each stage or every 2 min (ramp protocol).	Measure and record immediately postexercise, 60 s of recovery, and then every 2 min.
Signs and symptoms	Monitored continuously; record as observed.	Monitor continuously; record as observed.	Monitor continuously; record as observed or as symptoms resolve.
Rating of perceived exertion	Explain scale.	Record during the last 5–10 s each stage or every 2 min (ramp protocol).	Obtain peak exercise shortly after exercise is terminated.

[a]In addition, heart rate and blood pressure should be assessed and recorded whenever adverse symptoms or abnormal electrocardiogram changes occur.
[b]An unchanged or decreasing systolic blood pressure with increasing workloads should be retaken (*i.e.*, verified immediately).

Adapted and used with permission from Brubaker PH, Kaminsky LA, Whaley MH. *Coronary Artery Disease: Essentials of Prevention and Rehabilitation Programs*. Champaign (IL): Human Kinetics; 2002. 364 p.

with the submaximal HR response. For an adult population, the most common equations to predict a patient's HR_{max} are as follows:

$$\text{Age-predicted } HR_{max} = 220 - \text{age (year)}$$
$$\text{Age predicted } HR_{max} = 208 - (0.7 \times \text{age})$$

BP, both preexercise and exercising, should be measured at heart level with the subject's arm supported and relaxed and not grasping the handrail (treadmill) or handlebar (cycle ergometer). Both systolic blood pressure (SBP) and diastolic blood pressure (DBP) measurements can be used to ensure that there is an appropriate exercise response and can be used as indicators for stopping an exercise test (Boxes 4.2 and 4.3). The normal SBP response to exercise should be to increase with increasing workloads of approximately 10 ± 2 mm Hg · MET^{-1} (23). On average, there is a greater response in men, increased with age, and in patients taking vasodilators, calcium channel blockers, angiotensin-converting enzyme inhibitors, and α- and β-adrenergic blockers. It is important for the exercise professional to understand what the appropriate response to exercise is, so he or she can correctly interpret what an inappropriate BP response to exercise is (Box 4.4).

Rating of Perceived Exertion

RPE can be a valuable indicator for monitoring the patient's exercise tolerance. Developed by Gunnar Borg, the RPE scale allows the exerciser to subjectively express his or her physical exertion during exercise (15) and correlates with exercising HR (16). However, there can be large interindividual

Box 4.2 General Indications for Stopping an Exercise Test[a]

- Onset of angina or angina-like symptoms
- Drop in SBP of ≥10 mm Hg with an increase in work rate or if SBP decreases below the value obtained in the same position prior to testing
- Excessive rise in BP: systolic pressure >250 mm Hg and/or diastolic pressure >115 mm Hg
- Shortness of breath, wheezing, leg cramps, or claudication
- Signs of poor perfusion: light-headedness, confusion, ataxia, pallor, cyanosis, nausea, or cold and clammy skin
- Failure of HR to increase with increased exercise intensity
- Noticeable change in heart rhythm by palpation or auscultation
- Subject requests to stop
- Physical or verbal manifestations of severe fatigue
- Failure of the testing equipment

[a]Assumes that testing is nondiagnostic and is being performed without electrocardiogram monitoring. For clinical testing, Box 4.3 provides more definitive and specific termination criteria.

Reprinted from American College of Sports Medicine. *ACSM's Guidelines for Exercise Testing and Prescription*. 10th ed. Philadelphia (PA): Wolters Kluwer; 2018. 480 p.

Box 4.3 Indications for Terminating a Symptom-Limited Maximal Exercise Test

Absolute Indications

- ST elevation (>1.0 mm) in leads without preexisting Q waves because of prior MI (other than aVR, aVL, or V_1)
- Drop in systolic blood pressure of >10 mm Hg, despite an increase in workload, when accompanied by other evidence of ischemia
- Moderate-to-severe angina
- Central nervous system symptoms (*e.g.*, ataxia, dizziness, or near syncope)
- Signs of poor perfusion (cyanosis or pallor)
- Sustained ventricular tachycardia or other arrhythmia, including second- or third-degree atrioventricular block, that interferes with normal maintenance of cardiac output during exercise
- Technical difficulties monitoring the ECG or systolic blood pressure
- The subject's request to stop

Relative Indications

- Marked ST displacement (horizontal or downsloping of >2 mm, measured 60 to 80 ms after the J point in a patient with suspected ischemia)
- Drop in systolic blood pressure >10 mm Hg (persistently below baseline) despite an increase in workload, *in the absence* of other evidence of ischemia
- Increasing chest pain
- Fatigue, shortness of breath, wheezing, leg cramps, or claudication
- Arrhythmias other than sustained ventricular tachycardia, including multifocal ectopy, ventricular triplets, supraventricular tachycardia, and bradyarrhythmias that have the potential to become more complex or to interfere with hemodynamic stability
- Exaggerated hypertensive response (systolic blood pressure >250 mm Hg or diastolic blood pressure >115 mm Hg)
- Development of bundle-branch block that cannot be distinguished from ventricular tachycardia
- S_pO_2 ≤80% (2)

Reprinted with permission from Gibbons RJ, Balady GJ, Bricker JT, et al. ACC/AHA 2002 guideline update for exercise testing: summary article. A report of the American College of Cardiology/American Heart Association Task Force on Practice Guidelines (Committee to Update the 1997 Exercise Testing Guidelines). *J Am Coll Cardiol*. 2002;40(8):1531–40.

Box 4.4 Abnormal Blood Pressure Responses to Exercise (1)

- Hypertensive response: An SBP >250 mm Hg is a relative indication to stop a test. An SBP ≥210 mm Hg in men and ≥190 mm Hg in women during exercise is considered an exaggerated response.
- Hypotensive response: A decrease of SBP below the pretest resting value or by >10 mm Hg after a preliminary increase, particularly in the presence of other indices of ischemia, is abnormal and often associated with myocardial ischemia, left ventricular dysfunction, and an increased risk of subsequent cardiac events.
- Blunted response: In patients with a limited ability to augment cardiac output ($\dot{Q}$), the response of SBP during exercise will be slower compared to normal.
- *Postexercise response*: SBP typically returns to preexercise levels or lower by 6 min of recovery. Studies have demonstrated that a delay in the recovery of SBP is highly related both to ischemic abnormalities and to a poor prognosis.
- Diastolic blood pressure (DBP) response during exercise: A peak DBP >90 mm Hg or an increase in DBP >10 mm Hg during exercise above the pretest resting value is considered an abnormal response.

variability in RPE reporting in healthy and patient populations (65). With this in mind, it is important to "anchor" the scale, that is, tell the participant what a "6" feels like or what "20" would feel like. A patient's ratings can be influenced by not only exercise but also psychological factors, mood states, environmental conditions (14), exercise modes, age (60), and thirst (58). Therefore, exercise professionals should not compare RPE responses across exercise modalities, nor across patients.

There are a number of RPE scales available and widely used. Most commonly used are the original Borg category scale (Fig. 4.1) which rates the exercise intensity from 6 to 20 and the category-ratio scale of 0–10 (CR-10). The revised CR-10 scale takes into account the nonlinear changes in blood lactate and ventilation during exercise along with the traditional linear rise in HR and $\dot{V}O_2$. Alternatively, an exercise professional could use the OMNI scales (Fig. 4.2) (59) to obtain their patient's RPE during various modes of exercise. These scales were originally designed to be used with **children** and **adolescents** using a picture system to illustrate intensity but have been modified to be used with adults engaging in exercise on a cycle ergometer, treadmill, stepper, and elliptical. The OMNI RPE values were correlated, as part of the validation testing, with HR and $\dot{V}O_2$ data. The validity coefficients for those modalities ranged from 0.82 to 0.95 and from 0.88 to 0.96 for HR and $\dot{V}O_2$, respectively (29,39,43,59). During exercise testing, the RPE can be used as an indicator for approaching/imminent fatigue where healthy adults reach their subjective limit of fatigue at an RPE of 18–19 (very, very, hard) on the category Borg scale or 9–10 (very, very strong) on the CR scale.

Test Termination Criteria

Graded exercise testing (GXT), whether maximal or submaximal, is considered safe when subjects are appropriately screened and testing guidelines are followed. Occasionally, the test may be terminated before the subject reaches his or her measured $\dot{V}O_{2max}/\dot{V}O_{2peak}$ based on the subject reaching volitional fatigue, experiencing sign or symptoms, or reaching a predetermined endpoint (*i.e.*, 50%–70% heart rate reserve [HRR] or 70%–85% age-predicted HR_{max}). Because of the inherent variation in HR_{max}, the upper limit of 85% of an estimated HR_{max} may, in fact, result in a maximal effort for some individuals and submaximal effort in others. General indications, those who do not rely on physician involvement and ECG monitoring, for stopping an exercise test are outlined previously in Box 4.2.

Rating of Perceived Exertion

Borg 6-20		
6	No exertion at all	
7	Extremely light	
8		
9	Very light	
10		
11	Light	
12		
13	Somewhat hard	
14		
15	Hard	(heavy)
16		
17	Very hard	
18		
19	Extremely hard	
20	Maximal exertion	

FIGURE 4.1. The original Borg category scale which rates the exercise intensity from 6–20. (© Gunnar Borg. Used with permission. *The scales with correct instructions can be obtained from Borg Perception* [http://borgperception.se/].)

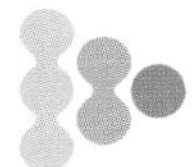

Procedures and Protocols for Maximal, Submaximal, and Field Exercise Tests

Modes of Testing

As previously stated, the mode that is chosen for the exercise test is dependent on the patient (and his or her goals), the setting, the available equipment, and the availability of trained personnel. Treadmills, cycle ergometers, steps, and field tests are the most commonly used for CRF testing. There are advantages and disadvantages of each exercise testing mode.

Field Tests

Field tests consist of walking or running for a predetermined time or distance (*i.e.*, 1.5-mile [2.4-km] walk/run test; 1-mile and 6-min walk test). The advantages of field tests are they are easy to administer to large numbers of individuals at one time and little equipment (*e.g.*, a stopwatch) is needed. It is important to note that a major disadvantage for field tests are that some can be near-maximal or maximal for some individuals, particularly in individuals with low **aerobic** fitness and potentially be unmonitored for test termination criteria (see Box 4.2) or BP and HR responses. Therefore, these tests may be inappropriate for sedentary individuals or individuals at increased risk for cardiovascular and/or musculoskeletal complications. An individual's level of motivation and pacing ability also can have a profound impact on test results.

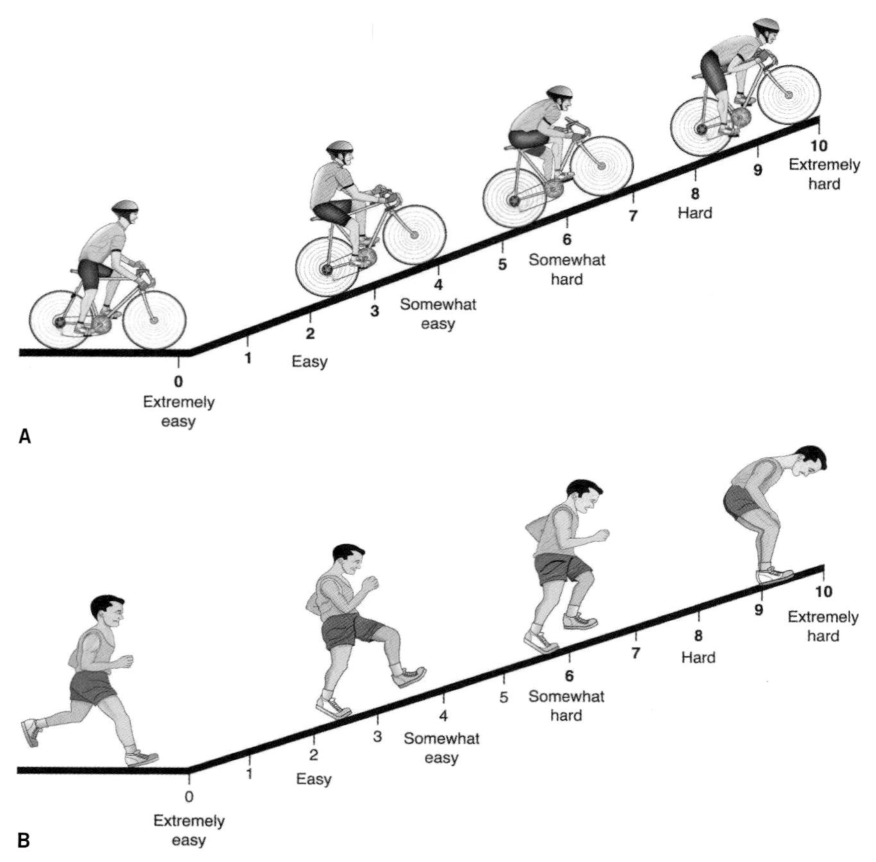

FIGURE 4.2. A. OMNI-Cycle Scale of perceived exertion for adults. (Reprinted from Robertson RJ, Goss FL, Dubé J, et al. Validation of the Adult OMNI Scale of Perceived Exertion for Cycle Ergometer Exercise. *Med Sci Sports Exerc.* 2004;36[1]:102–8.). **B.** OMNI-Walk/Run Scale of Perceived Exertion for Adults. (Reprinted from Utter AC, Robertson RJ, Green MJ, et al. Validation of the Adult OMNI Scale of Perceived Exertion for Walking/Running Exercise. *Med Sci Sports Exerc.* 2004;36[10]:1776–80.)

Motor-Driven Treadmills

Motor-driven treadmills can be used for submaximal and maximal testing and are often employed for diagnostic testing in the United States. They provide a familiar form of exercise to many and, if the correct protocol is chosen, can accommodate a wide range of fitness levels. Compared with field tests, treadmills can be expensive, not easily transportable, and potentially make some measurements (*e.g.*, BP) more difficult, particularly while an individual is running. Treadmills must be calibrated periodically to ensure the accuracy of the test when $\dot{V}O_2$ is not directly measured (47). In addition, holding on to the support rail(s) should be discouraged to ensure accuracy of metabolic work output, particularly when $\dot{V}O_2$ is estimated as opposed to directly measured. Frequent use of the handrail often leads to significant overestimation of $\dot{V}O_2$.

Mechanically Braked Cycle Ergometers

Mechanically braked cycle ergometers are also a viable test modality for submaximal and maximal testing and are frequently used for diagnostic testing, particularly in European laboratories (47). Advantages of this exercise mode include lower equipment expense, better transportability, and greater ease in obtaining BP and ECG (if appropriate) measurements. Cycle ergometers also provide a non–weight-bearing test modality in which work rates are easily adjusted in small increments.

The main disadvantage is cycling may be a less familiar mode of exercise to some individuals, often resulting in limiting localized muscle fatigue and an underestimation of $\dot{V}O_{2max}$. The cycle ergometer must be calibrated, and the subject must maintain the proper pedal rate because most tests require HR to be measured at specific work rates (47). Electronic cycle ergometers can deliver the same work rate across a range of pedal rates (*i.e.*, revolutions per minute [RPM]), but calibration might require special equipment not available in some laboratories. If a cycle ergometer cannot be calibrated for any reason, or if it does not provide a reasonable estimate of workload, it should not be used for fitness testing to predict CRF.

Step Testing

Step testing is an inexpensive modality for predicting CRF by measuring the HR response to stepping at a fixed rate and/or a fixed step height or by measuring postexercise recovery HR. Step tests require little or no equipment, steps are easily transportable, stepping skill requires little practice, the test usually is of short duration, and stepping is advantageous for mass testing (63). Postexercise (recovery) HR decreases with improved CRF, and test results are easy to explain to participants (36). Special precautions may be needed for those who have balance problems or are extremely deconditioned. Some single-stage step tests require an energy cost of 7–9 **metabolic equivalents (METs)**, which may exceed the maximal capacity of some participants (4). Therefore, the protocol chosen must be appropriate for the physical fitness level of the patient. In addition, inadequate compliance to the step cadence and excessive local muscular fatigue may diminish the value of a step test. Most tests do not monitor HR and BP while stepping because of the difficulty of these measures during the test.

Maximal Exercise Testing

Maximal exercise places the greatest demand on the body. Therefore, maximal exercise testing is, perhaps, the most challenging of all physical assessments for both the patient and the technician. This type of testing may also be referred to as a *GXT* or *stress test*. Regardless of the name, these tests use increases in workload until peak exertion or exhaustion is achieved. The maximal GXT has three main purposes and are as follows:

1. *Diagnosis*: most commonly to determine the presence of ischemic heart disease (IHD)
2. *Prognosis*: determine the risk for an adverse advent relative to disease history
3. *Evaluation* of the exercise response to help guide in their ExR_x

Common modes of testing are treadmill walking or running and stationary cycling. In the United States, the treadmill is most commonly used and elicits the greatest physiological response due to the use of a large muscle mass. Cycle ergometry, which is more commonly used in Europe, often produces a lower $\dot{V}O_{2max}$ due to localized muscle fatigue of the quadriceps muscle group and can result in a $\dot{V}O_{2peak}$ that can be 10%–20% lower than that of a treadmill test (49). Other modalities such as arm ergometry or total body recumbent stepping (10) may be more appropriate for those who have limited use of the lower extremities (paraplegia) or older individuals with balance deficits, respectively.

Exercise tests can be continuous or discontinuous. A *continuous* exercise test is performed with no rest between work increments and often varies in the duration of each exercise stage and in the increase in intensity (*e.g.*, increase in speed and grade). Most continuous exercise tests have multiple stages that last between 2 and 3 minutes, allowing individuals to reach a steady-state HR and $\dot{V}O_2$, and increase in intensity gradually (2–3 METs per stage). The currently recommended test duration is for the total exercise time to last between 6 and 12 minutes (18,23,47). Another form of continuous exercise test is a ramp test. Ramp exercise protocols increase intensity continuously (increase of 8, 15, 17, 25 W · min^{-1}) (22) to elicit a linear increase in $\dot{V}O_2$ and to bring the patient to volitional termination after approximately 10 minutes. Because there is a continual increase in work, plateaus in $\dot{V}O_2$ are rarely observed. However, the $\dot{V}O_{2peak}$ that is observed can be a valid index of $\dot{V}O_{2max}$ despite the lack of a plateau (20).

Discontinuous exercise tests are those where the workload is increased but the patient rests 5–10 minutes between workloads. Typically, each stage lasts 5–6 minutes allowing $\dot{V}O_2$ to reach a steady state. Because of the discontinuous nature of these tests and the lengthy stage times, the entire test can last 5 times longer compared to a continuous test with 2- to 3-minute stages. However, similar $\dot{V}O_{2max}$ values are obtained using a discontinuous protocol compared to a traditional continuous protocol (41).

Decisions concerning the use of a maximal GXT include the purpose of the test (diagnostic vs. functional), identification of who should have the test, whether a physical examination should be performed before the test, whether a physician should be present for the test, and what personnel will be needed to conduct the test. American College of Sports Medicine's (ACSM) revised recommendations for preparticipation screening (57) indicate that an individual should only be referred to seek **medical clearance** if they have a sign or symptom and/or known cardiovascular, metabolic, or pulmonary disease. Therefore, the use of a maximal exercise test is at the discretion of the health care provider.

Although maximal exercise tests are generally considered safe, the potential for an adverse event does exist based on the population being tested. In a clinical setting, the risk of complications (often defined as *death* or an *event requiring hospitalization*) is usually considered to be approximately 1/10,000 or a range of 0–5 per 100,000 tests (0.005%) (47). Over time, clinical exercise testing has migrated from being administered solely by physicians to nonphysicians, including allied health professionals such as clinical exercise physiologists, nurses, physical therapists, and physician assistants. Evidence supports these guidelines that exercise tests can be administered by allied health professionals working under a physician who is in the immediate vicinity (50).

Maximal testing performed in a preventive exercise setting (*e.g.*, health/fitness clubs) should follow established guidelines for emergency readiness and supervision by qualified health care providers (47). A joint statement from the American Heart Association (AHA) and the ACSM call for the following general guidelines to be followed: (a) Have written emergency plan that is rehearsed regularly, (b) ensure the presence of an automated external defibrillator, (c) and have trained staff who are able to recognize and abnormal physiological responses or signs and symptoms of IHD (8).

Maximal Treadmill Exercise Protocols

Traditionally, the treadmill has been the most used mode for GXT in the United States. Treadmill walking involves the use of a large muscle mass, enabling the subject to generally achieve a physiological maximum. The exercise test is performed on a motor-driven treadmill with variable speed and incline. Speed can increase up to 25 mph (40 kph) and a grade of 25% depending on the make of treadmill. Therefore, workload is usually expressed in miles per hour and percent grade.

Bruce and modified Bruce protocols The Bruce treadmill protocol is the most widely used exercise protocol in the United States (17,33) due to physician familiarity, availability of equations to predict functional capacity (25,46,48), and efficiency of time utilization for both the clinician and patient. The aerobic requirements (~5 METs) associated with the first stage of the Bruce protocol and the large increases (~3 METs) between stages may make it less than optimal for persons with a low functional capacity. In addition, the Bruce protocol encourages extensive handrail support, which results in over estimation of the patient's peak exercise capacity (31,46). In response to these limitations, modifications of the Bruce protocol and many other treadmill and cycle protocols have been developed, including patient-specific ramping protocols (24,36,48,51). A common recommendation is to choose a protocol that will result in test duration of 8–12 minutes (3).

The Bruce protocol consists of multiple 3-minute stages that begin at a walking pace of 1.7 mph (45.6 m · min^{-1}) and a 10% grade. Every stage, the speed and percent grade is increased. In the second stage (fourth to sixth minutes), the grade is increased to 12% and the speed is increased to 2.5 mph (67 m · min^{-1}). In subsequent stages, the grade is increased by 2% and the speed by either 0.8 or 0.9 mph (21.4 or 24.1 m · min^{-1}). $\dot{V}O_{2max}$ prediction equations (Table 4.2) have been developed utilizing the Bruce treadmill protocol in active and sedentary men and women, patients with CVD, and **older adults**.

The modified Bruce protocol (40) is more appropriate for high-risk or older adults. The protocol is similar to the standard Bruce with the exception of the first two stages. Stage 1 starts at 0% grade and 1.7 mph (45.6 m · min^{-1}) and progresses to a 5% grade while maintaining the same speed. In stage 3, the speed is maintained, but the grade is increased to 10%. At this point, the remainder of the protocol follows the standard Bruce.

Additional treadmill protocols The Balke and Ware (9) protocol is a multistage protocol consisting of 1-minute stages that begin at a speed of 3.4 mph (91.1 m · min^{-1}) at a grade of 0% during the first minute. The speed is maintained throughout the entire test, but the grade is increased by 1% every minute. Using the Balke equation from Table 4.2, the individual's $\dot{V}O_{2max}$ can be estimated. The Naughton (26) is another protocol that is best used for patients with CVD and patients who are high risk. The Naughton protocol consists of 2-minute stages starting at an initial speed of 1.0 mph (26.8 m · min^{-1}) and 0% grade. The second stage is at a 0% grade, but the speed is increased to 2.0 mph (53.6 m · min^{-1}). Hereafter, each stage increases by 2 mph (53.6 m · min^{-1}) and a grade of 3.5%.

The Modified Åstrand (56) is a protocol that can be used for highly trained individuals. There is an initial self-selected warm-up of 5 minutes. The test consists of 2-minute stages where the

Table 4.2 Treadmill $\dot{V}O_{2max}$ Estimation Equations

Protocol	Population	Equation	Reference
Balke	Active and sedentary men	$\dot{V}O_{2max}$ = 1.444 (time) + 14.99 SEE = 2.5 mL · kg^{-1} · min^{-1}	Pollock et al. (54)
	Active and sedentary women[a]	$\dot{V}O_{2max}$ = 1.38 (time) + 5.22 SEE = 2.2 mL · kg^{-1} · min^{-1}	Pollock et al. (55)
Bruce	Active and sedentary men	$\dot{V}O_{2max}$ = 14.76 − 1.379 (time) + 0.451 (time^2) − 0.012 (time^3) SEE = 3.35 mL · kg^{-1} · min^{-1}	Foster et al. (25)
	Active and sedentary women	$\dot{V}O_{2max}$ = 4.38 (time) − 3.90 SEE = 2.7 mL · kg^{-1} · min^{-1}	Pollock et al. (54)
	Patients with cardiac problem and older adults[b]	$\dot{V}O_{2max}$ = 2.282 (time) + 8.545 SEE = 4.9 mL · kg^{-1} · min^{-1}	McConnell, Foster, Conlin, and Thompson (46)
Modified Bruce[c]	High-risk, elderly	$\dot{V}O_2$ = 3.5 + (S × 0.1) + (S × G × 1.8)	ACSM (1)
Naughton	Male cardiac patients	$\dot{V}O_{2max}$ = 1.61 (time) + 3.6 SEE = 2.60 mL · kg^{-1} · min^{-1}	Foster et al. (26)

[a] For women, the Balke protocol begins at 3.0 mph and 0% grade for 3 minutes, increasing 2.5% every 3 minutes.
[b] This equation is used only for treadmill walking while holding the handrails.
[c] To estimate $\dot{V}O_2$ for the modified Bruce, the ACSM metabolic equation for walking can be used, where S is speed in m · min^{-1} (1 mph = 26.8 m · min^{-1}) and G is the percent grade expressed as a decimal (*e.g.*, 10% = 0.10).

speed remains constant (5 mph [134 m · min^{-1}]) but the grade increased by 2.5% every 2 minutes until exhaustion. Finally, Kaminsky and Whaley (36) developed a standard ramp protocol for assessing functional capacity in apparently healthy sedentary individuals. During the ramping protocol, the speed begins at 1.0 mph (26.8 m · min^{-1}) and increases gradually (0.1–0.4 mph, or 2.68–10.72 m · min^{-1} increments) every minute. The grade begins at 0% and can increase by 0%–5% each minute up to a maximal grade of 20%. Every 3 minutes, the work rate that is being performed on the ramp is equal to those of the traditional Bruce protocol.

Maximal Cycle Ergometer Exercise Protocols

Cycle ergometers are widely used in assessing CRF. Often, cycle ergometers are used when the patient has a condition that affects his or her ability to safely walk or jog on a treadmill or cycling is the patient's preferred modality and the patient is trained. On a friction-braked cycle ergometer, resistance is applied to a flywheel using a belt and weighted pendulum. The resistance is increased by tightening or loosening the brake belt by adjusting the workload adjustment knob. The resistance applied is expressed as kiloponds or kilograms (kp or kg). When determining work rate or power output, they are usually expressed in kilogram-meters per minute (kgm · min^{-1}) or watts (1 W ≈ 6 kgm · min^{-1}) and can be measured with the following equations:

Work rate = force × distance
Power = force × distance / time

where force is the resistance applied to the flywheel (kg) and the distance is the distance the flywheel travels per revolution times the number of RPM. On Monark and Bodyguard cycle ergometers, the flywheel travels 6 m per revolution. Therefore, if an individual was exercising on a Monark ergometer with a pedaling rate of 50 RPM and a resistance of 1.0 kg, he or she would have the following work rate (kgm · min^{-1}) and power (W):

Work = 1.0 kg × (6 m × 50 RPM) = 300 kgm · min^{-1}
Power = 300 / 6 = 50 W

The cadence that is selected for the exercise can greatly influence the amount of work that is performed and subsequently the $\dot{V}O_2$ response. Most protocols for untrained subjects use a pedaling rate of 60–90 RPM. However, trained cyclists can use higher pedaling rates (>80 RPM). In fact, a pedaling rate of 60 RPM produces the highest $\dot{V}O_{2max}$ when compared with rates of 50, 70, and 80 RPM (32).

The Åstrand protocol (5) is a continuous protocol that has 2- to 3-minute stages. To begin the test, subjects pedal at 50 RPM with an initial power output of 300 kgm · min^{-1} (50 W) for women and 600 kgm · min^{-1} (100 W) for men. Every 2–3 minutes, the power output should be increased in increments of 150 kgm · min^{-1} (25 W) and 300 kgm · min^{-1} (50 W) for women and men, respectively. The test is continued until exhaustion or the subject cannot maintain the pedaling rate of 50 RPM. To determine the individual's $\dot{V}O_{2max}$, use the final work rate and the ACSM metabolic equations for leg ergometry.

Developed by Fox (27), this cycle ergometer assessment is a discontinuous test. Each stage is 5 minutes long with 10 minutes of rest between. The starting workload is between 750 and 900 kgm · min^{-1} (125 and 150 W) for men and 450 and 600 kgm · min^{-1} (75 and 100 W) for women. How the workload is progressed is dependent on the patient's HR response. Typically, the workload is increased by 120–180 kgm · min^{-1} (20–30 W) per stage. The patient exercises until exhaustion or until unable to maintain the power output for at least 3 minutes that was 60–90 kgm · min^{-1} (10–15 W) higher than the previous workload. ACSM's metabolic equations for leg ergometry can be used to estimate $\dot{V}O_{2max}$ based on the last stage.

The Storer-Davis (62) protocol is a ramp style test that was developed to allow for a way to estimate $\dot{V}O_{2max}$ from a cycle ergometer test. After an initial warm-up period of 4 minutes at 0 W, the workload is increased 15 W · min^{-1} at a recommended RPM of 60. The following equations can then be used to estimate the subject's $\dot{V}O_{2max}$.

Men:
$\dot{V}O_{2max}$ (mL · min^{-1}) = (10.51 × watts) + (6.35 × kg) − (10.49 − age) + 519.3

Women:
$\dot{V}O_{2max}$ (mL · min^{-1}) = (9.39 × watts) + (7.7 × kg) − (5.88 × age) + 136.7

Submaximal Exercise Testing

Directly measuring an individual's functional CRF for aerobic fitness classification and for ExR_x is ideal but not always practical because of the associated cost and time, not to mention patient motivation, to perform a maximal test. Therefore, submaximal exercise testing can be a valid and reliable method for predicting CRF. These exercise tests are either single or multistage tests and involve a treadmill, cycle ergometer, or bench stepping exercises for the prediction of CRF. During the test, HR, BP, and RPE are monitored. Box 4.5 provides general procedures for submaximal exercise testing using a cycle ergometer.

Box 4.5 General Procedures for Submaximal Cardiorespiratory Fitness Testing

1. Obtain resting HR and BP immediately prior to exercise in the exercise posture.
2. The patient should be familiarized with the ergometer. If using a cycle ergometer, properly position the patient on the ergometer (*i.e.*, upright posture, ~25-degree bend in the knee at maximal leg extension, and hands in proper position on handlebars) (52,53).
3. The exercise test should begin with a 2–3 min warm-up to acquaint the patient with the mode of exercise and prepare him or her for the exercise intensity in the first stage of the test.
4. A specific protocol should consist of 2- or 3-min stages with appropriate increments in work rate.
5. HR should be monitored at least two times during each stage, near the end of the second and third minutes of each stage. If HR is >110 beats · min^{-1}, steady state HR (*i.e.*, two HRs within 5 beats · min^{-1}) should be reached before the workload is increased.
6. BP should be monitored in the last minute of each stage and repeated (verified) in the event of a hypotensive or hypertensive response.
7. RPE (using either the Borg category or category-ratio scale [see Fig. 4.1]) and additional rating scales should be monitored near the end of the last minute of each stage.
8. Patient's appearance and symptoms should be monitored and recorded regularly.
9. The test should be terminated when the subject reaches 70% heart rate reserve (85% of age-predicted HR_{max}), fails to conform to the exercise test protocol, experiences adverse signs or symptoms, requests to stop, or experiences an emergency situation.
10. An appropriate cool-down/recovery period should be initiated consisting of either
    a. Continued exercise at a work rate equivalent to that of the first stage of the exercise test protocol or lower or
    b. A passive cool-down if the subject experiences signs of discomfort or an emergency situation occurs
11. All physiologic observations (*e.g.*, HR, BP, signs and symptoms) should be continued for at least 5 min of recovery unless abnormal responses occur, which would warrant a longer posttest surveillance period. Continue low-level exercise until HR and BP stabilize but not necessarily until they reach preexercise levels.

Reprinted from American College of Sports Medicine. *ACSM's Guidelines for Exercise Testing and Prescription*. 10th ed. Philadelphia (PA): Wolters Kluwer; 2018. 480 p.

Submaximal exercise tests rely on the assumption that there is a linear relationship between $\dot{V}O_2$ and HR and work rate. To this end, it is essential that a steady-state HR is achieved during each exercise work rate. To estimate $\dot{V}O_{2max}$, two submaximal HRs can be plotted against work rate (*i.e.*, HR–$\dot{V}O_2$ relationship) and extrapolated to HR_{max} to estimate $\dot{V}O_{2max}$. This linear relationship holds true during light- to moderate-intensity exercise but becomes curvilinear and higher during very low intensities. Typically, HR is obtained by palpation; however, the accuracy of this method varies with the experience and technique of the fitness professional. Alterations to palpation that may increase accuracy of HR measurement include the use of an ECG, HR monitor, or a stethoscope. Additionally, submaximal HR response can be altered by several environmental (*i.e.*, heat and humidity), dietary (*i.e.*, caffeine, time since last meal), and behavioral (*i.e.*, anxiety, smoking, previous activity) factors (see pretest instructions earlier in this chapter) that must be controlled for, as previously discussed.

Assumptions and Sources of Error in Submaximal Prediction of Cardiorespiratory Fitness

The following list of assumptions is specific to submaximal testing:

- A linear (straight line) relationship exists between $\dot{V}O_2$ and HR within the range of 110–150 bpm. It is at this point that stroke volume has reached a plateau (approximately 40%–50% of max) and the HR and oxygen consumption track linearly.
- HR_{max} is similar for individuals of similar ages. Unfortunately, a large variation (±11 bpm) (40) exists in the age prediction ($HR_{max} = 220 - \text{age}$) of HR_{max}, and this assumption may provide for the greatest source of error (±10%–15%) in the submaximal prediction of $\dot{V}O_{2max}$.
- A steady-state HR can be achieved in 3–4 minutes at a constant, submaximal work output. A steady-state HR is ensured by consecutive HR measurements being within five beats of each other.
- A cadence of 50 RPM is typically considered comfortable and mechanically efficient in most individuals. It is assumed that each subject expends the same amount of energy and has the same absolute oxygen requirements at the same work output on the cycle. Maintaining a constant pedal rate on a mechanically braked ergometer is essential to ensure a constant power output.
- The HR at two separate work outputs can be plotted as the HR–$\dot{V}O_2$ relationship and extrapolated to the estimated HR_{max}. The Bruce submaximal treadmill protocol is an example of a multistage test that utilize a minimum of two stages to predict CRF. The Åstrand protocol prediction is based on the steady-state HR at a single-work stage.

In addition to the assumptions that are made with submaximal testing (that can introduce possible sources of error), these types of tests require predetermined endpoints for completion of the test. The exercise professional should be familiar with the indications for stopping an exercise test that can be found in Box 4.2. In addition to terminating the test because of completion of the protocol or meeting one of the requirements in Box 4.2, the exercise professional should consider terminating the test if the patient exceeds 70% of his or her HRR or 85% age-predicted HR_{max}. Continuing the exercise test past these thresholds can potentially expose the patient to near-maximal levels of exertion and possibly increase the risk for cardiovascular complications.

As discussed previously in this chapter, various modes of exercise can be used in the completion of submaximal exercise tests. The most common modes of exercise for laboratory-based exercise testing include the treadmill and the mechanically braked cycle ergometer. Although both provide adequate mechanisms for completion of submaximal testing, each has inherent advantages and disadvantages that must be considered. Regardless of the mode of exercise, following standardized procedures (see Box 4.5) will help ensure an accurate test.

To estimate $\dot{V}O_{2max}$ with a multistage model, the use of two submaximal HRs and their associated workloads is required. The steady-state HR should be ≥110 bpm but less than 70% HRR (85% age-predicted HR_{max}) for two consecutive stages. The following equations can be used to estimate $\dot{V}O_{2max}$:

$$\dot{V}O_{2max} = SM_2 + b\,(HR_{max} - HR_2)$$
$$b = (SM_2 - SM_1)\,/\,(HR_2 - HR_1)$$

The slope (b) can be calculated by finding the ratio in the differences between the two submaximal workloads (SM) (predicted from ACSM metabolic equations in Chapter 8) and the corresponding HRs.

An example is provided in the following text:
Submaximal data from cycle ergometer protocol for a 72-kg 38-year-old male
Age-predicted HR_{max}: 220 − age = 182 bpm
ACSM cycle ergometer $\dot{V}O_2$ metabolic equation: $\dot{V}O_2 = 3.5 + 3.5 + (1.8 \times WR) / BM$

	Workload (kgm · min^{-1})	Steady-state HR (bpm)
Stage 1	150	104
Stage 2	300	118
SM_1 $\dot{V}O_2 = 3.5 + 3 + (1.8 \times 300) / 72 = 14.5$ mL · kg^{-1} · min^{-1}		
Stage 3	450	130
SM_2 $\dot{V}O_2 = 3.5 + 3.5 + (1.8 \times 450) / 72 = 18.25$ mL · kg^{-1} · min^{-1}		

Slope (b) = (SM_2 − SM_1) / (HR_2 − HR_1)
$b = (18.25 - 14.5) / (130 - 118)$
$b = 3.75 / 12$
$b = 0.31$

$\dot{V}O_{2max}$ = SM_2 + b (HR_{max} − HR_2)
$= 18.25 + 0.31\,(182 - 118)$
$= 18.25 + 19.84$
$\dot{V}O_{2max} = 38.09$ mL · kg^{-1} · min^{-1}

Submaximal Single-Stage Treadmill Protocols

Ebbeling et al. (21) developed a single-stage walking treadmill test suitable for estimating $\dot{V}O_{2max}$ in adults with low-risk health between the ages of 20 and 59 years old. Walking speed is individualized for this protocol and ranges from 2.0 to 4.5 mph (53.6–120.6 m · min^{-1}) depending on the individual's age, sex, and fitness level. A warm-up period of 4 minutes, at a comfortable walking page at 0% grade, should be used to elicit an HR within 50%–70% of the subjects age-predicted HR_{max}. The actual test consists of a single 4-minute stage conducted at a brisk walk at a 5% grade. A steady-state HR should be recorded in third to fourth minute to be used in the $\dot{V}O_{2max}$ estimation equation:

$$\dot{V}O_{2max}\ (mL \cdot kg^{-1} \cdot min^{-1}) = 15.1 + (21.8 \times \text{speed in mph}) - (0.327 \times HR) - (0.263 \times \text{speed} \times \text{age}) + (0.00504 \times HR \times \text{age}) + (5.48 \times \text{sex});\ \text{females} = 0,\ \text{males} = 1$$

For younger adults (18–28 yr), a single-stage jogging protocol was developed (28) to estimate $\dot{V}O_{2max}$. Subjects should select a comfortable jogging pace between 4.3 and 7.5 mph (115.2 and 201 m · min^{-1}) and no more than 6.5 mph (174.2 m · min^{-1}) for women and 7.5 mph (201 m · min^{-1}) for men. The subject should jog at this pace for 3 minutes and not have a steady-state HR exceed 180 bpm:

$$\dot{V}O_{2max}\ (mL \cdot kg^{-1} \cdot min^{-1}) = 54.07 - (0.1938 \times \text{weight in kg}) + (4.47 \times \text{speed in mph}) - (0.1453 \times HR) + 7.062\ (\text{sex});\ \text{females} = 0,\ \text{males} = 1$$

Submaximal Cycle Ergometer Protocols

The Åstrand-Ryhming cycle ergometer test is a single-stage test lasting 6 minutes (6). The pedal rate is set at 50 RPM with the goal of obtaining HR values between 125 and 170 bpm, with HR measured during the fifth and sixth minute of work. The average of the two HRs is then used to estimate $\dot{V}O_{2max}$ from a nomogram (Fig. 4.3). The suggested work rate is based on sex and an individual's fitness status as follows:

Men, unconditioned: 300 or 600 kgm · min^{-1} (50 or 100 W)
Men, conditioned: 600 or 900 kgm · min^{-1} (100 or 150 W)
Women, unconditioned: 300 or 450 kgm · min^{-1} (50 or 75 W)
Women, conditioned: 450 or 600 kgm · min^{-1} (75 or 100 W)

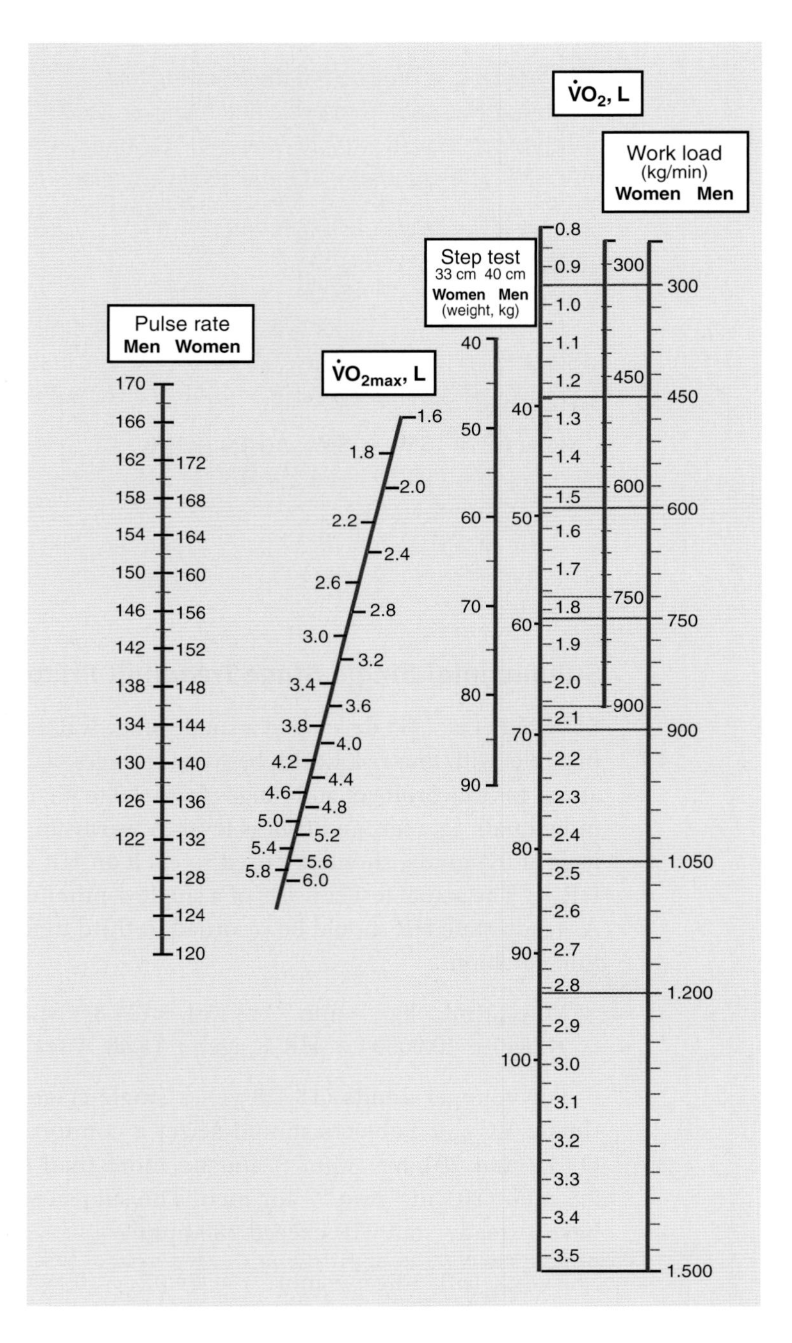

FIGURE 4.3. Modified Åstrand-Ryhming nomogram. (Reprinted from Åstrand PO, Ryhming I. A nomogram for calculation of aerobic capacity (physical fitness) from pulse rate during sub-maximal work. *J Appl Physiol.* 1954;7:218–21).

Table 4.3 Åstrand-Ryhming Age Correction Factors

Age	Correction Factor
15	1.10
25	1.00
35	0.87
40	0.83
45	0.78
50	0.75
55	0.71
60	0.68
65	0.65

The value from the nomogram must then be adjusted for age because HR_{max} decreases with age by multiplying the $\dot{V}O_{2max}$ value by the correction factors in Table 4.3 (4).

Fox (27) was able to modify the maximal protocol to one that can predict $\dot{V}O_{2max}$. The patient performs a single workload at 900 kgm · min^{-1} (150 W) for 5 minutes. To estimate $\dot{V}O_{2max}$, use the measured HR at the end of fifth minute in the following equation:

$$\dot{V}O_{2max}\ (mL \cdot min^{-1}) = 6{,}300 - (19.26 \times HR)$$

In contrast with the Åstrand-Ryhming and Fox cycle ergometer single-stage tests, a multistage cycle ergometer was proposed by Wyndham and colleagues (66) and refined by Maritz et al. (42). This multistage test was devised to test HR during a series of submaximal work rates and extrapolated the assumed linear HR response to the subject's age-predicted HR_{max}, which will allow for the estimation of the individual's $\dot{V}O_{2max}$. This multistage method is a well-known assessment technique to estimate $\dot{V}O_{2max}$.

Submaximal Bench Stepping Protocols

Two popular bench stepping protocols are those by Åstrand-Ryhming and McArdle et al. (45). The Åstrand-Ryhming protocol can predict $\dot{V}O_{2max}$ using the same nomogram (see Fig. 4.3) as the cycle ergometer but using HR and body weight during bench stepping. For this test, the patient steps at a rate of 22.5 steps per minute for 5 minutes. The step height is set at 13 in (33 cm) for women and 15.75 in (40 cm) for men. Immediately after exercise (15–30 s), the 15-second postexercise HR should be taken to be used in the nomogram. The Queens College step test devised by McArdle et al. (44) is 3 minutes long and uses a step rate of 22 steps per minute for females and 24 steps per minute for males. The step height is constant at 16.25 in (41.3 cm). Five seconds after stopping, take a 15-second HR. The following equation can be used to estimate $\dot{V}O_{2max}$ with a standard prediction error of ±16%:

Men: $\dot{V}O_{2max}\ (mL \cdot kg^{-1} \cdot min^{-1}) = 111.33 - (0.42 \times HR)$

Women: $\dot{V}O_{2max}\ (mL \cdot kg^{-1} \cdot min^{-1}) = 65.81 - (0.1847 \times HR)$

Additional Submaximal Exercise Tests

Recumbent stepper protocol Often found in rehabilitation settings, total body recumbent steppers may be an appropriate alternative to a cycle ergometer or treadmill protocol. Billinger et al. (11) devised a protocol using a commercially available recumbent stepper (NuStep T5xr) that has

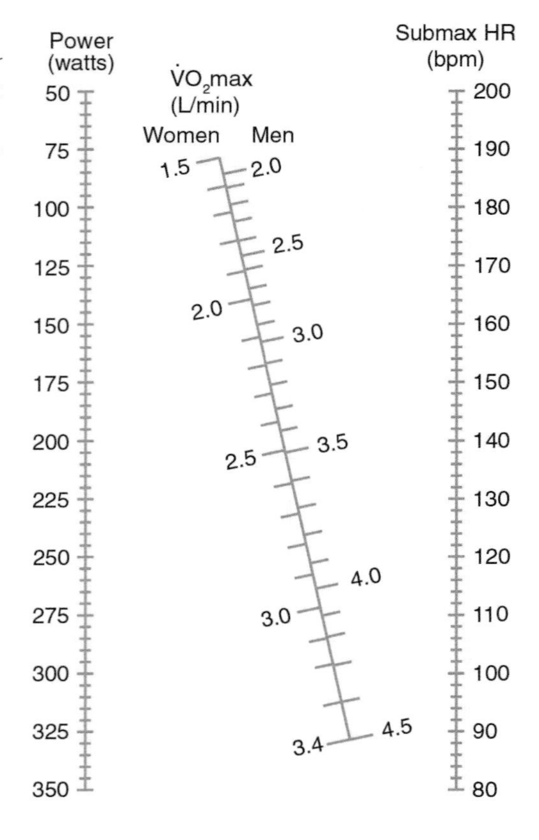

FIGURE 4.4. Åstrand-Ryhming age correction factors. From *Concept II Rowing Ergometer Nomogram for Prediction of Maximal Oxygen Consumption* by Dr. Fritz Hagerman, Ohio University, Athens, OH. The nomogram is not appropriate for use with non-Concept II ergometers and is designed to be used by noncompetitive or unskilled rowers participating in aerobic conditioning programs. Adapted by permission of Concept II, Inc., RR1, Box 110, Morrisville, VT. (800) 245-5676.

10 settings ranging from 50 to 290 W. The protocol starts with an initial warm-up of 2 minutes at a setting of 30 W, and the resistance was increased every 3 minutes based on their protocol. During the test, a cadence of 100 steps per minute should be maintained to estimate $\dot{V}O_{2peak}$:

$$\dot{V}O_{2peak}\ (mL \cdot kg^{-1} \cdot min^{-1}) = 125.707 + (-0.476 \times age) + (7.686 \times sex) + (-0.451 \times weight) + (0.179 \times watts) + (-0.415 \times HR)$$

Age = years; sex: 0 = female, 1 = male; weight = kg; watts and HR should correspond to ending submaximal values

Rowing ergometer To estimate $\dot{V}O_{2max}$ on a Concept II rowing ergometer, Hagerman (30) developed a protocol where the patient can sustain the self-selected intensity for 5–10 minutes without the HR exceeding 170 bpm (Fig. 4.4). HR should be measured at the end of each minute until the patient reaches a steady-state HR. A nomogram can then be used to estimate $\dot{V}O_{2max}$ from the submaximal work rate (watts) and HR.

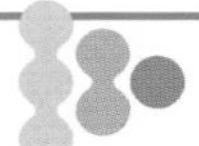

Field Tests for Cardiorespiratory Fitness Tests

Two of the most widely used run/walk tests (subjects may run, walk, or use a combination of both to complete the test) for assessing CRF are the 1.5-mile (2.4-km) test for time and the Cooper 12-minute test. The objective of the former test for time is to cover the 1.5 mile in the shortest period of time. The Cooper 12-minute test is based on covering the greatest distance in the allotted time period. $\dot{V}O_{2max}$ can be estimated from using the following equations:

1.5-mile run/walk test

$$\dot{V}O_{2max}\ (mL \cdot kg^{-1} \cdot min^{-1}) = 3.5 + 483 / 1.5\text{-mile time (min)}$$

12-minute walk/run test
$\dot{V}O_{2max}$ (mL · kg^{-1} · min^{-1}) = (distance in meters − 504.9) / 44.73

The Rockport One-Mile Fitness Walking Test is another well-recognized field test for estimating CRF. In this test, an individual walks 1 mile (1.6 km) as fast as possible, preferably on a track or a level surface, and HR is obtained in the final minute. An alternative is to measure a 10-second HR immediately on completion of the 1-mile (1.6-km) walk, but this may overestimate the $\dot{V}O_{2max}$ compared with when HR is measured during the walk. $\dot{V}O_{2max}$ is estimated using the following regression equation (37):

$\dot{V}O_{2max}$ (mL · kg^{-1} · min^{-1}) = 132.853 − (0.1692 × body mass in kg) − (0.3877 × age in yr) + (6.315 × gender) − (3.2649 × time in min) − (0.1565 × HR)
(standard error of estimate [SEE] = mL · kg^{-1} · min^{-1}; gender = 0 for female, 1 for male)

In addition to independently predicting morbidity and mortality (19,59), the 6-minute walk test has been used to evaluate CRF in populations considered to have reduced CRF such as older adults and some clinical patient populations (*e.g.*, individuals with CHF or pulmonary disease). The American Thoracic Society has published guidelines on 6-minute walk test procedures and interpretation (7). Even though the test is considered submaximal, it may result in near-maximal performance for those with low physical fitness levels or disease (35). Patients completing less than 300 m (~984 ft) during the 6-minute walk demonstrate a poorer short-term survival compared with those surpassing this threshold (19). Several multivariate equations are available to predict $\dot{V}O_{2peak}$ from the 6-minute walk; however, the following equation requires minimal clinical information (19):

$\dot{V}O_{2peak}$ = $\dot{V}O_2$ mL · kg^{-1} · min^{-1} = (0.02 × distance [m]) − (0.191 × age [yr]) − (0.07 × weight [kg]) + (0.09 × height [cm]) + (0.26 × RPP [× 10^{-3}]) + 2.45
where m = meter; yr = year; kg = kilogram; cm = centimeter; RPP = rate pressure product (HR × systolic BP [SBP] in mm Hg); SEE = 2.68

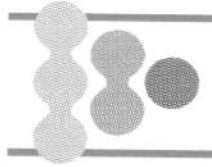

Criterion-Referenced Standards versus Normative Data

Upon completion of an exercise test, the results should be interpreted by comparing the test results with established standards or norms (Table 4.4). Traditionally, two sets of standards are used for comparisons: criterion-referenced standards and normative standards. Criterion-referenced standards are those that are considered desirable to achieve based on external criteria and may use adjectives such as "excellent" or "poor" in the data interpretation tables. Criterion-referenced standards exist mostly in CRF evaluations and in body fat analyses. These standards, however, are open to subjective interpretation, and disagreement is present among experts regarding what these results truly mean when used for interpretation.

Normative standards (norms) are based on previous performances by a similar group of individuals. Norms compare how the patient performed versus other like individuals, and the data are presented using percentile values to assist in identifying level of fitness. Evaluative decisions about a patient's health-related physical fitness can be based on either criterion-referenced standards or normative standards.

Interpretation of Results from Submaximal Exercise Testing

Although submaximal exercise testing is not as precise as maximal exercise testing, it provides a general reflection of an individual's CRF at a lower cost, potentially reduces risk for adverse events, and may require less time and effort on the part of the subject. It is important to keep in mind

Table 4.4 Cardiorespiratory Fitness Classifications ($\dot{V}O_{2max}$) by Age and Sex (1)

$\dot{V}O_{2max}$ ($mL\ O_2 \cdot kg^{-1} \cdot min^{-1}$) — MEN

		Age Group (yr)				
Percentile		20–29 (*n* = 513)	30–39 (*n* = 963)	40–49 (*n* = 1,327)	50–59 (*n* = 1,078)	60–69 (*n* = 593)
95	Superior	66.3	59.8	55.6	50.7	43.0
90	Excellent	61.8	56.5	52.1	45.6	40.3
85		59.3	54.2	49.3	43.2	38.2
80		57.1	51.6	46.7	41.2	36.1
75	Good	55.2	49.2	45.0	39.7	34.5
70		53.7	48.0	43.9	38.2	32.9
65		52.1	46.6	42.1	36.3	31.6
60		50.2	45.2	40.3	35.1	30.5
55	Fair	49.0	43.8	38.9	33.8	29.1
50		48.0	42.4	37.8	32.6	28.2
45		46.5	41.3	36.7	31.6	27.2
40		44.9	39.6	35.7	30.7	26.6
35	Poor	43.5	38.5	34.6	29.5	25.7
30		41.9	37.4	33.3	28.4	24.6
25		40.1	35.9	31.9	27.1	23.7
20		38.1	34.1	30.5	26.1	22.4
15	Very Poor	35.4	32.7	29.0	24.4	21.2
10		32.1	30.2	26.8	22.8	19.8
5		29.0	27.2	24.2	20.9	17.4

$\dot{V}O_{2max}$ ($mL\ O_2 \cdot kg^{-1} \cdot min^{-1}$) — WOMEN

		Age Group (yr)				
Percentile		20–29 (*n* = 410)	30–39 (*n* = 608)	40–49 (*n* = 843)	50–59 (*n* = 805)	60–69 (*n* = 408)
95	Superior	56.0	45.8	41.7	35.9	29.4
90	Excellent	51.3	41.4	38.4	32.0	27.0
85		48.3	39.3	36.0	30.2	25.6
80		46.5	37.5	34.0	28.6	24.6
75	Good	44.7	36.1	32.4	27.6	23.8
70		43.2	34.6	31.1	26.8	23.1
65		41.6	33.5	30.0	26.0	22.0
60		40.6	32.2	28.7	25.2	21.2
55	Fair	38.9	31.2	27.7	24.4	20.5
50		37.6	30.2	26.7	23.4	20.0
45		35.9	29.3	25.9	22.7	19.6
40		34.6	28.2	24.9	21.8	18.9

Table 4.4 Cardiorespiratory Fitness Classifications ($\dot{V}O_{2max}$) by Age and Sex (1) *(continued)*

$\dot{V}O_{2max}$ (mL $O_2 \cdot kg^{-1} \cdot min^{-1}$) — WOMEN

		Age Group (yr)				
Percentile		20–29 (*n* = 410)	30–39 (*n* = 608)	40–49 (*n* = 843)	50–59 (*n* = 805)	60–69 (*n* = 408)
35	Poor	33.6	27.4	24.1	21.2	18.4
30		32.0	26.4	23.3	20.6	17.9
25		30.5	25.3	22.1	19.9	17.2
20		28.6	24.1	21.3	19.1	16.5
15	Very Poor	26.2	22.5	20.0	18.3	15.6
10		23.9	20.9	18.8	17.3	14.6
5		21.7	19.0	17.0	16.0	13.4

Percentiles from cardiopulmonary exercise testing on a treadmill with measured $\dot{V}O_{2max}$ (mL $O_2 \cdot kg^{-1} \cdot min^{-1}$). Data obtained from the FRIEND (Fitness Registry and the Importance of Exercise National Database) Registry for men and women who were considered free from known CVD.

that some of the assumptions inherent in a submaximal test are more easily met (*e.g.*, steady-state HR can be verified), whereas others (*e.g.*, estimated HR_{max}) introduce errors into the prediction of $\dot{V}O_{2max}$. When using submaximal testing to look for improvements in CRF, over the course of repeated submaximal tests, the HR response at a given work rate will decrease independent of the accuracy of the $\dot{V}O_{2max}$ prediction. This is one of the physiological hallmarks to adaption in CRF. Despite differences in test accuracy and methodology, virtually all evaluations can establish a baseline and be used to track relative progress during exercise training.

SUMMARY

The assessment of an individual's CRF is an important component in any primary or secondary prevention or rehabilitative programs. Prior to the assessment, it is important to determine if the participant is able to perform the exercise test as well as what CRF test would be most appropriate. The exercise professional can choose from simple field tests to more involved cycler ergometer or treadmill protocols to predict the individuals CRF. It is important to keep in mind that the CRF exercise protocol should be based on the patient's goals, current health status, and familiarity with the testing modality.

After the CRF assessment, the exercise professional should debrief the patient as to how they performed in the CRF assessment as well as what their fitness classification is to give them (a) an idea of what their current level of CRF is and (b) a starting point for their exercise program. The exercise professional can then use the data collected from the CRF assessment to designing a safe, effective, and individualized exercise program.

REFERENCES

1. American College of Sports Medicine. *ACSM's Guidelines for Exercise Testing and Prescription*. 10th ed. Philadelphia (PA): Wolters Kluwer; 2018. 480 p.
2. American Thoracic Society, American College of Chest Physicians. ATS/ACCP statement on cardiopulmonary exercise testing. *Am J Respir Crit Care Med*. 2003;167(2):211–77.

3. Arena R, Myers J, Williams MA, et al. Assessment of functional capacity in clinical and research settings: a scientific statement from the American Heart Association Committee on Exercise, Rehabilitation, and Prevention of the Council on Clinical Cardiology and the Council on Cardiovascular Nursing. *Circulation*. 2007;116(3):329–43.
4. Åstrand P-O. Aerobic work capacity in men and women with special reference to age. *Acta Physiol Scandl*. 1960;49(169):45–60.
5. Åstrand P-O. *Work Tests With the Bicycle Ergometer*. Varberg (Sweden): AB Cykelfabriken Monark; 1965.
6. Åstrand P-O, Ryhming I. A nomogram for calculation of aerobic capacity (physical fitness) from pulse rate during sub-maximal work. *J Appl Physiol*. 1954;7(2):218–21.
7. ATS Committee on Proficiency Standards for Clinical Pulmonary Function Laboratories. ATS statement: guidelines for the six-minute walk test. *Am J Respir Crit Care Med*. 2002;166(1):111–7.
8. Balady GJ, Chaitman B, Driscoll D, et al. AHA/ACSM joint position statement: recommendations for cardiovascular screening, staffing, and emergency policies at health/fitness facilities. *Med Sci Sports Exerc*. 1998;30(6):1009–18.
9. Balke B, Ware R. An experimental study of physical fitness of Air Force personnel. *U S Armed Forces Med J*. 1959;10:675–88.
10. Billinger SA, Loudon JK, Gajewski BJ. Validity of a total upper body recumbent stepper exercise test to assess cardiorespiratory fitness. *J Strength Cond Res*. 2008;22:1556–62.
11. Billinger SA, Van Swearingen E, McClain M, Lentz AA, Good MB. Recumbent stepper submaximal exercise test to predict peak oxygen uptake. *Med Sci Sports Exerc*. 2012;44(8):1539–44.
12. Blair SN, Kohl HW III, Barlow CE, Paffenbarger RS Jr, Gibbons LW, Macera CA. Changes in physical fitness and all-cause mortality. A prospective study of healthy and unhealthy men. *JAMA*. 1995;273(14):1093–8.
13. Blair SN, Kohl HW III, Paffenbarger RS Jr, Clark DG, Cooper KH, Gibbons LW. Physical fitness and all-cause mortality. A prospective study of healthy men and women. *JAMA*. 1989;262(17):2395–401.
14. Borg G. *Borg's Perceived Exertion and Pain Scales*. Champaign (IL): Human Kinetics; 1998. 104 p.
15. Borg GA. Psychophysical bases of perceived exertion. *Med Sci Sports Exerc*. 1982;14(5):377–81.
16. Borg GV, Linderholm H. Perceived exertion and pulse rate during graded exercise in various age groups. *Acta Med Scand*. 1967;472(suppl):S194–206.
17. Bruce RA, Kusumi F, Hosmer D. Maximal oxygen intake and nomographic assessment of functional aerobic impairment in cardiovascular disease. *Am Heart J*. 1973;85(4):546–62.
18. Buchfuhrer MJ, Hansen JE, Robinson TE, Sue DY, Wasserman K, Whipp BJ. Optimizing the exercise protocol for cardiopulmonary assessment. *J Appl Physiol Respir Environ Exerc Physiol*. 1983;55:1558–64.
19. Cahalin LP, Mathier MA, Semigran MJ, Dec GW, DiSalvo TG. The six-minute walk test predicts peak oxygen uptake and survival in patients with advanced heart failure. *Chest*. 1996;110(2):325–32.
20. Day JR, Rossiter HB, Coats EM, Skasick A, Whipp BJ. The maximally attainable $\dot{V}O_2$ during exercise in humans: the peak vs. maximum issue. *J Appl Physiol*. 2003;95(5):1901–7.
21. Ebbeling C, Ward A, Puleo EM, Widrick J, Ripple J. Development of a single-stage submaximal treadmill walking test. *Med Sci Sports Exerc*. 1991;23:966–73.
22. Fairshter RD, Walters J, Salness K, Fox M, Minh VD, Wilson AF. A comparison of incremental exercise test during cycle and treadmill ergometry. *Med Sci Sports Exerc*. 1983;15(6):549–54.
23. Fletcher GF, Ades PA, Kligfield P, et al. Exercise standards for testing and training: a scientific statement from the American Heart Association. *Circulation*. 2013;128:873–934.
24. Foster C, Crowe AJ, Daines E, et al. Predicting functional capacity during treadmill testing independent of exercise protocol. *Med Sci Sports Exerc*. 1996;28(6):752–6.
25. Foster C, Jackson AS, Pollock ML, et al. Generalized equations for predicting functional capacity from treadmill performance. *Am Heart J*. 1984;107(6):1229–34.
26. Foster C, Pollock ML, Rod JL, Dymond DS, Wible G, Schmidt DH. Evaluation of functional capacity during exercise radionuclide angiography. *Cardiology*. 1983;70:85–93.
27. Fox EL. A simple, accurate technique for predicting maximal aerobic power. *J Appl Physiol*. 1973;35:914–6.
28. George J, Vehrs P, Allsen P, Fellingham G, Fisher G. $\dot{V}O_{2max}$ estimation from a submaximal 1-mile track jog for fit college-age individuals. *Med Sci Sports Exerc*. 1993;25:401–6.
29. Guidetti L, Sgadari A, Buzzachera CF, et al. Validation of the OMNI-Cycle Scale of Perceived Exertion in the elderly. *J Aging Phys Act*. 2011;19(3):214–24.
30. Hagerman F. *Concept II Rowing Ergometer Nomogram for Prediction of Maximal Oxygen Consumption* [Abstract]. Morrisville (VT): Concept II; 1993.
31. Haskell WL, Savin W, Oldridge N, DeBusk R. Factors influencing estimated oxygen uptake during exercise testing soon after myocardial infarction. *Am J Cardiol*. 1982;50(2):299–304.
32. Heil DP. Body mass scaling of peak oxygen uptake in 20- to 79-yr-old adults. *Med Sci Sports Exerc*. 1997;29(12):1602–8.
33. Hermansen L, Saltin B. Oxygen uptake during maximal treadmill and bicycle exercise. *J Appl Physiol*. 1969;26(1):31–7.
34. Heyward VA, Gibson AL. *Advanced Fitness Assessment and Exercise Prescription*. 7th ed. Champaign (IL): Human Kinetics; 2014. 552 p.
35. Jetté M, Campbell J, Mongeon J, Routhier R. The Canadian Home Fitness Test as a predictor for aerobic capacity. *Can Med Assoc J*. 1976;114(8):680–2.

36. Kaminsky LA, Whaley MH. Evaluation of a new standardized ramp protocol: the BSU/Bruce Ramp protocol. *J Cardiopulm Rehabil.* 1998;18(6):438–44.
37. Kingma B, Frijns A, van Marken Lichtenbelt W. The thermoneutral zone: implications for metabolic studies. *Front Biosci (Elite Ed).* 2012;4:1975–85.
38. Kodama S, Saito K, Tanaka S, et al. Cardiorespiratory fitness as a quantitative predictor of all-cause mortality and cardiovascular events in healthy men and women: a meta-analysis. *JAMA.* 2009;301(19):2024–35.
39. Krause MP, Goss FL, Robertson RJ, et al. Concurrent validity of an OMNI rating of perceived exertion scale for bench stepping exercise. *J Strength Cond Res.* 2012;26(2):506–12.
40. Lerman J, Bruce RA, Sivarajan E, Pettet G, Trimble S. Low-level dynamic exercises for earlier cardiac rehabilitation: aerobic and hemodynamic responses. *Arch Phys Med Rehabil.* 1976;57:355–60.
41. Maksud MG, Coutts KD. Comparison of a continuous and discontinuous graded treadmill test for maximal oxygen uptake. *Med Sci Sports.* 1971;3:63–5.
42. Maritz JS, Morrison JF, Peter J, Strydom NB, Wyndham CH. A practical method of estimating an individual's maximal oxygen intake. *Ergonomics.* 1961;4(2):97–122.
43. Mays RJ, Goss FL, Schafer MA, Kim KH, Nagle-Stilley EF, Robertson RJ. Validation of adult OMNI perceived exertion scales for elliptical ergometry. *Percept Mot Skills.* 2010;111(3):848–62.
44. McArdle WD, Katch FI, Katch VL. *Exercise Physiology: Nutrition, Energy, and Human Performance.* Philadelphia (PA): Wolters Kluwer; 2015. 1028 p.
45. McArdle WD, Katch FI, Pechar GS, Jacobson L, Ruck S. Reliability and interrelationships between maximal oxygen intake, physical work capacity and step-test scores in college women. *Med Sci Sports.* 1972;4(4):182–6.
46. McConnell TR, Foster C, Conlin NC, Thompson NN. Prediction of functional capacity during treadmill testing: effect of handrail support. *J Cardiopulm Rehabil.* 1991;11(4):255–60.
47. Myers J, Arena R, Franklin B, et al. Recommendations for clinical exercise laboratories: a scientific statement from the American Heart Association. *Circulation.* 2009;119(24):3144–61.
48. Myers J, Bellin D. Ramp exercise protocols for clinical and cardiopulmonary exercise testing. *Sports Med.* 2000;30(1):23–9.
49. Myers J, Buchanan N, Walsh D, et al. Comparison of the ramp versus standard exercise protocols. *J Am Coll Cardiol.* 1991;17(6):1334–42.
50. Myers J, Forman DE, Balady GJ, et al. Supervision of exercise testing by nonphysicians: a scientific statement from the American Heart Association. *Circulation.* 2014;130:1014–27.
51. Peterson MJ, Pieper CF, Morey MC. Accuracy of VO2(max) prediction equations in older adults. *Med Sci Sports Exerc.* 2003;35(1):145–9.
52. Peveler WW. Effects of saddle height on economy in cycling. *J Strength Cond Res.* 2008;22(4):1355–9.
53. Peveler WW, Pounders JD, Bishop PA. Effects of saddle height on anaerobic power production in cycling. *J Strength Cond Res.* 2007;21(4):1023–7.
54. Pollock ML, Bohannon RL, Cooper KH, et al. A comparative analysis of four protocols for maximal treadmill testing. *Am Heart J.* 1976;92:39–46.
55. Pollock ML, Foster C, Schmidt D, Hellman C, Linnerud AC, Ward A. Comparative analysis of physiologic responses to three different maximal graded exercise test protocols in healthy women. *Am Heart J.* 1982;103:363–73.
56. Pollock ML, Wilmore JH, Fox SM III. *Health and Fitness Through Physical Activity.* New York (NY): Wiley; 1978. 357 p.
57. Riebe D, Franklin BA, Thompson PD, et al. Updating ACSM's recommendations for exercise preparticipation health screening. *Med Sci Sports Exerc.* 2015;47(11):2473–9.
58. Riebe D, Maresh CM, Armstrong LE, et al. Effects of oral and intravenous rehydration on ratings of perceived exertion and thirst. *Med Sci Sports Exerc.* 1997;29:117–24.
59. Robertson RJ. *Perceived Exertion for Practitioners: Rating Effort With the OMNI Picture System.* Champaign (IL): Human Kinetics; 2004. 171 p.
60. Robertson RJ, Noble BJ. Perception of physical exertion: methods, mediators, and applications. *Exerc Sport Sci Rev.* 1997;25:407–52.
61. Sesso HD, Paffenbarger RS Jr, Lee I-M. Physical activity and coronary heart disease in men: The Harvard Alumni Health Study. *Circulation.* 2000;102(9):975–80.
62. Storer TW, Davis HA, Caiozzo VJ. Accurate prediction of VO2max in cycle ergometry. *Med Sci Sports Exerc.* 1990;22:704–12.
63. Swain DP, editor. *ACSM's Resource Manual for Guidelines for Exercise Testing and Prescription.* 7th ed. Philadelphia (PA): Wolters Kluwer; 2014. 896 p.
64. Wang CY, Haskell WL, Farrell SW, et al. Cardiorespiratory fitness levels among US adults 20–49 years of age: findings from the 1999–2004 National Health and Nutrition Examination Survey. *Am J Epidemiol.* 2010;171(4):426–35.
65. Whaley MH, Brubaker PH, Kaminsky LA, Miller CR. Validity of rating of perceived exertion during graded exercise testing in apparently healthy adults and cardiac patients. *J Cardiopulm Rehabil.* 1997;17(4):261–7.
66. Wyndham CH, Strydom NB, Maritz JS, Morrison JF, Peter J, Potgieter ZU. Maximum oxygen intake and maximum heart rate during strenuous work. *J Appl Physiol.* 1959;14:927–36.

CHAPTER 5

Muscle Strength Assessment

INTRODUCTION

The human body has over 600 muscles that are used for work, for play, and to accomplish **activities of daily living (ADL)**. Skeletal muscle across the age continuum has the ability to adapt to the circumstances of its use and disuse (76). This ability to adapt (muscle plasticity) can be assessed through changes in muscle size, muscle architecture, enzyme activity, or isoform expression as well as organelle and extracellular structures (76).

Health-related **physical fitness** includes the characteristics of functional capacity and is affected by the **physical activity** level and other lifestyle factors (10,13,14,37,43–45, 100,102,103,109,117). Maintaining an appropriate level of health-related physical fitness is necessary for a person to meet emergencies, reduce the risk of disease and injury (3,6,8,11,18,19,23,25,28,32,37,46,47,63,87,105,109,115), work efficiently (15,31), and participate and enjoy physical activity (4,5,15,21,24,26–28,30,39,40,66,84,86,110,112,122), (sports, recreation, leisure). A high health-related physical fitness level focuses on optimum health and prevents the onset of disease and problems associated with inactivity at all ages (15,40,42,87,90,92,102,103,108,112,119).

Minimal levels of **muscular strength**, **muscular endurance**, and **muscular power** (muscular fitness) are required to perform ADL, maintain functional independence during aging, and be able to participate in leisure time physical activities without undue fatigue or risk of injury (49,50,54,55,77,79,91,101,111,116,121). Musculoskeletal fitness requires muscle strength and endurance as well as bone strength (having the necessary bone mineral content and density to withstand repeated loads placed upon muscle insertion) (12,55,63). Adequate levels of muscular fitness may reduce the risk of low back problems, osteoporotic fractures, and musculoskeletal injuries (49,55,91,116).

Resistance training is performed with various **exercise** modalities including exercise machines, free weights, or the use of gravity acting on the participant's body mass. Most resistance training (**strength**) programs are based on a system of exercise to a

one repetition maximum (1-RM) as presented in the mid-1940s by Delorme (33) for use in physical medicine and rehabilitation. Every time the athlete/participant performs a particular exercise, the bout (or set) is performed for the maximum number of repetitions possible (repetition maximum or RM), and this number is recorded along with the mass lifted or opposing force imposed by an exercise machine (a range from 1-RM to 15-RM). The 1-RM is commonly utilized to accurately determine maximum strength for a specific movement, and this value is used to calculate percentages of one's 1-RM depending on the desired **exercise prescription** goals. For example, calculating 50% of the 1-RM would give the exercise professional a target weight to incorporate into an exercise prescription for muscular endurance. Determination of the 1-RM is explained in more detail in Box 5.1 (69).

Muscular strength assessment has many purposes and has been safely administered across the age continuum (2,6,8,15,16,18,19,21,25–28,30,32,34–36,38–40,43–45, 47,50,51,57,63,70). Muscle strength data collected in **children** and **adolescents** provide meaningful information and understanding of growth, **maturation**, effects of acute and regular response to physical activity, trainability, variation within normal patterns, and secular trends (27,30,36,39,40,51,56,69,77,82,84,89,105,107). Muscular strength assessment allows the exercise physiologist to identify strengths and weaknesses (baseline) and to set specific attainable goals (12,55,63). Furthermore, muscular strength assessment allows for tracking strength changes (improvements/decrements) over time allowing for adjustments in the exercise prescription that will bring about a positive physiological response (15,17,45,47,57,66,70,87,110,122).

Aging is associated with a decrease in **skeletal muscle mass** and muscle strength (**sarcopenia**) (19,20,37) and power (77) which may lead to lower physical function in ADL (chair stand, ascending stairs) (43–45,48,50,102,103,109). Low physical performance (strength and cardiorespiratory) has been demonstrated to predict both mobility and disability (96), nursing home admission, and mortality in community-dwelling **older adults** (50,109).

Muscular fitness testing can be conducted with persons of all ages, levels of physical conditioning, and training experience; however, protocols and techniques should be individualized to accommodate each patient's levels of experience and strength (2,15,38–40,43–45,48,50,52,64,65,67,70,73,102–104). The evaluation must consider various musculoskeletal fitness parameters and be age-appropriate in order to ensure that valid and reliable measurements are obtained (15,38–40,102,103).

The goal of the strength or endurance test selected is for the assessment to be reliable (similar results twice), valid (truly measures what test claims to measure), and objective (correct results no matter who the tester). Furthermore, metabolic energy system (64,68,70,72,101,103,111,116) and biomechanical movement pattern specificity (64,68,70,99,106) are essential components of test selection because they simulate the energy demands and movement patterns of the participant's ADL.

Box 5.1 One Repetition Maximum Testing Procedure

1. Tester demonstrates and explains the proper mechanics of the intended movement using only the bar (if applicable). Provide as much detail as is necessary based on previous resistance training experience by the lifter.
2. Practice the intended movement (*e.g.*, the bench press, utilize a hooked-thumb grip) with the bar only until movement technique is correct according to the technician.
3. Two warm-up trials are recommended in obtaining a safe and accurate 1-RM.
4. For the first warm-up trial, the tester instructs the lifter to complete 5–10 repetitions with a load that the lifter reports as "easy" using correct form and movement velocity, followed by a 1-minute rest (51). The 1-minute rest interval should have the lifter perform 30 seconds of active flexibility movements within his or her full, available range of motion for the muscle group being assessed.
5. The second warm-up trial requires the lifter to complete three to five repetitions of the exercise movement at 60%–80% of the estimated 1-RM load and is followed by a 2-minute rest interval of active recovery inclusive of flexibility. For example, if the estimated 1-RM was 100 lb, then the second warm-up trial should be completed using 60–80 lb.
6. The third warm-up trial requires the lifter to complete two to three repetitions of the exercise movement at ~90%–95% of the estimated 1-RM. For example, if the estimated 1-RM was 100 lb, then the third warm-up trial should be completed using 90–95 lb. The lifter attempts two to three repetitions with correct form. Upon completion, the lifter rests 2–4 minutes or longer if necessary with active recovery inclusive of flexibility (51).
7. The technician increases the load equivalent to the lifter's estimated 1-RM determined by the following 1-RM prediction equation:

   1-RM = 100 · rep wt / (102.78 − 2.78 · reps) (22)
8. The lifter attempts only one repetition with this load. A successful or unsuccessful lift will require the lifter to rest 2–4 minutes to allow for a full recovery before attempting another 1-RM effort at the next higher or lower weight increment, respectively (51). For example, if the 100 lb was successfully lifted, an additional 2.5%–5% load should be added for the next 1-RM trial. If the 1-RM attempt was unsuccessful, the load should be reduced 2.5%–5% (51).
9. Continue the process described in step 8 until the participant fails to complete the exercise movement in the correct form. The 1-RM is generally achieved in three to five trials.
10. Record the 1-RM value as the maximum weight lifted with correct form.

From Abadie BR, Altorfer GL, Schuler PB. Does a regression equation to predict maximal strength in untrained lifters remain valid when the subjects are technique trained? *J Strength Cond Res.* 1999;13(3):259–63; Beam WC, Adams GM. *Exercise Physiology Laboratory Manual.* New York (NY): McGraw-Hill; 2011. 320 p.; Haff GG, Triplett NT, editors. *Essentials of Strength Training and Conditioning.* 4th ed. Champaign (IL): Human Kinetics; 2016. 752 p.; Heyward VH, Gibson AL. *Advanced Fitness Assessment and Exercise Prescription.* 7th ed. Champaign (IL): Human Kinetics; 2014. 552 p.; Kraemer WJ, Fry AC. Strength testing: development and evaluation of methodology. In: Maud PJ, Foster C, editors. *Physiological Assessment of Human Fitness.* Champaign (IL): Human Kinetics; 1995. p. 115–38; Levinger I, Goodman C, Hare DL, Jerums G, Toia D, Selig S. The reliability of the 1RM strength test for untrained middle-aged individuals. *J Sci Med Sport.* 2009;12(2):310–6; and Rontu JP, Hannula MI, Leskinen S, Linnamo V, Salmi JA. One-repetition maximum bench press performance estimated with a new accelerometer method. *J Strength Cond Res.* 2010;24(8):2018–25.

Dynamic Strength (Isotonic)

Dynamic exercise involves both **concentric** and **eccentric** muscle actions when the muscles are shortened or lengthened (12). The force-generating capacity of the muscle varies throughout the movement during dynamic movements. Dynamic strength is limited to the load that can be lifted by the weakest point within the specific joint system **range of motion** (66). Common free- and machine-weight exercises utilized as dynamic strength tests are the bench press and the back squat/leg press. Depending on the controlled or standardized conditions of these two tests, one could classify them as a field or laboratory tests (12).

Free-weight and constant-resistance weight machines are recommended for muscular fitness testing. Free-weight testing will require more neuromuscular coordination to both stabilize and maintain body balance by the participant and thus may be used with individuals with more resistance training experience. Utilization of machines for muscular fitness testing reduces the need for spotting (guarding) during the test and may be more appropriate with individuals who have limited resistance training experience or are unfamiliar with resistance training movements. However, use of such machine devices may limit the range of motion and the direction of the movement. Additional limitations of constant-resistance machines include weight increments that are too large and the inability to accommodate various body sizes (55). A common field test for lower extremity power is the vertical jump test (12). Furthermore, Faigenbaum and colleagues (40) have conducted similar research with children and found such muscular fitness assessment to be safe and appropriate; however, they had specialized equipment sized to youth participants. Beam and Adams (12) suggest that one of the most operational definitions of dynamic strength is expressed as the 1-RM for the specific movement tested (bench press, leg press, and back squat are commonly assessed): The highest load that can be lifted through a full range of motion utilizing correct form is the 1-RM. The 1-RM can be directly measured (see Box 5.1) through some trial and error or indirectly estimated from a **submaximal** effort for a summary of both test procedures. The 1-RM may be estimated by determining the number of submaximal repetitions completed to fatigue. Brzycki (22) and others (59,60,65,82) suggest that estimations of 1-RM using prediction equations are best suited using a load that allows no more than 10 repetitions to fatigue (~75% 1-RM). A sample 1-RM prediction equation is included in Box 5.1.

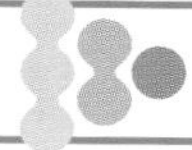

Muscular Endurance Strength

A component of muscular strength, **muscular endurance**, is the ability of a muscle group to execute repeated muscle contractions (58,63,97). Muscular endurance is important for many ADL including numerous household activities such as house cleaning, painting, lawn mowing (rotary push mower), and snow shoveling. Muscular endurance tests such as the 1-minute sit-up test and the push-up tests have traditionally been components of physical fitness assessments of youth (83,97), the military (U.S. Army), and other professionals to either compare with normative data previously collected (Aerobics Institute, Dallas, TX) or determine one's readiness for a particular job's specific task. There is no functional utility in the timed sit-up or push-up test; however, they are commonly used as measures of physical fitness. These movements do not comprise specific movement patterns that are used in ADL or in the workplace. The 10th edition of the American College of Sports Medicine (ACSM) guidelines has recently eliminated the timed 1-minute sit-up test. One can make a case that such assessments serve little functional utility and that other functional assessments found later in this chapter are more useful.

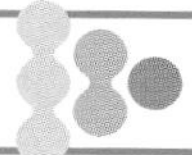

Isometric (Static) Strength–Handgrip Strength

The functional and clinical importance of **isometric** handgrip strength cannot be underestimated. The utility of this test spans the age continuum (7,46,52,62–64,68,71,77,85,88,119,123). Adequate handgrip strength represents the muscles of the forearm and has been associated with lower mortality (46,63,100), reduced risk of falling, and other ADL. Moreover, Ortega et al. (94) suggested that a low level of muscular strength in late adolescence, as measured by knee extension and handgrip strength tests, was associated with all-cause premature mortality to a similar extent as classic risk factors such as **body mass index** or blood pressure indicating the need for strength assessment in adolescents (52,94). Wind et al. (123) found that grip strength was strongly correlated with total muscle strength (r = .736–.890), suggesting that grip strength could be used as a general indicator for overall muscle strength.

Handgrip strength (r = .60) is related to muscle mass in older adults (63), and others have found higher correlations (53,80).

One of the common handgrip dynamometers, the Jamar (manufactured by Jamar Performance Products, Lafayette, IN), utilizes a sealed hydraulic system to activate its force indicator during static muscle action. Strength is often measured in units of force or torque. Isometric dynamometry expresses force in newtons (N); however, kilograms and pounds are commonly found on the dials of many handgrip dynamometers (12).

Isometric strength assessment may be made on many muscles using a cable tensiometer, but only the isometric handgrip strength test is described in Box 5.2.

The Jamar manual suggests a sit or stand position; however, Balogun et al. (9) indicated that the standing position produced higher handgrip strength than the seated position. Mathiowetz et al. (80) found that handgrip strength was highest when the arm was held at a 90° angle in a small sample of women (n = 29). Box 5.2 emphasizes the importance of consistent verbal instruction prior to and during the **maximal** effort. Following such directions enhances the reliability of the handgrip test (78). Most investigators use the best of two or three trials (53,81). See Box 4.6 and Table 4.8 in the *ACSM's Guidelines for Exercise Testing and Prescription, 10th edition*, for isometric handgrip strength evaluation.

Box 5.2 Procedures for Isometric Handgrip Dynamometer

1. The participant is in the standing position.
2. The participant's head is in the mid-position (facing straight ahead).
3. The grip size may need to be adjusted so the third digit's second phalanx is approximately at a right angle.
   a. Grip adjustments of 1.3 cm (~0.5 in) on the Jamar dynamometer are made by removing the moveable handle and repositioning grip into one of the five manufactured slots; slot 1 = innermost position for the smallest grip size; slot 5 = slot at the outside position for the largest grip size.
   b. Grip adjustments up to 4 cm for other dynamometers (Lafayette) are possible.
4. The grip setting (1–5 for Jamar) is recorded by the technician.
5. The participant's forearm is placed at any angle between 90° and 180° of the upper arm (right angle to straight).
6. The participant's wrist and forearm are positioned in the mid-prone position.
7. The participant is instructed to exert maximally and quickly after hearing the technician's following instructions:
   a. "Are you ready?"
   b. "Squeeze as hard as you can." As the participant begins the technician says, "Harder! . . . Harder! . . . Relax."
8. The participant will be asked to complete two or three trials, alternatively with each hand.
9. The participant will be given a 30-second or up to a 1-minute rest between trials for the same hand.
10. The technician records the force in kilogram and then converts the circled best score to newtons by multiplying the kilogram value by 9.8066.
11. The technician resets the dynamometer's pointer to 0 after each trial.

Beam WC, Adams GM. *Exercise Physiology Laboratory Manual*. New York (NY): McGraw-Hill; 2011. 320 p.

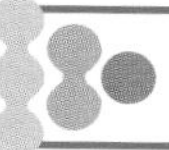

Rate of Force Development

The rate of rise in contractile force from resting state represents the "explosive" muscle strength which is indicated by the **rate of force development** (RFD) assessed during the early phase of skeletal muscle contraction (1). RFD is critically important for athletes participating in high-intensity activities requiring fast movements, and peak RFD has been correlated to the vertical jump (r = .68) and peak force (r = .51) (83). Furthermore, adults across the age continuum require rapid RFD when conducting many ADL, for example, rising from a chair, climbing stairs, and crossing a street. RFD has been examined primarily in isometric (91,92) and plyometric settings (83), utilizing a variety of resistance training protocols typically designed to emulate testing conditions, suggestive of motor learning. RFD is a critical component of optimal muscle function across the age continuum; yet, more research is required to demonstrate clinical utility of RFD.

Isokinetic Strength Assessment

Isokinetic exercise is a dynamic form of resistance exercise (124) that was first developed in 1967 (56,118) and requires a device that provides resistance to limb movement so that a limb segment cannot accelerate beyond the machine's preset angular speed (106). Therefore, the isokinetic dynamometer does not provide resistance or measure torque until the moving limb segment reaches the preset velocity, which is often referred to as *accommodating resistance* (106,124). Therefore, theoretically, when the moving limb segment achieves the preset velocity and attempts to accelerate, the limb will move at a constant speed (106). Isokinetic dynamometers (Cybex II, Biodex) are often used to assess muscular strength, power, and endurance in a variety of performance and health-related areas including geriatrics research (41,43,44,108) and rehabilitation (29). These isokinetic instruments are found in athletic training and research facilities to assess training-induced changes in muscle function (16,90). The accuracy of isokinetic exercise testing has been researched intensively, and the results have demonstrated high levels of reliability and validity (16). Perrin (98) reported reliability coefficients for knee extension peak torque at 60° per second and 180° per second ranged from r = .84 to .93. These reliability coefficients were lower than those reported by Johnson and Siegel (61), where the reliability coefficients for power and total work assessed at a 180° per second for knee flexion and extension ranged from r = .90 to .95. Feiring et al. (41) reported intraclass correlation coefficients (ICCs) ranging from .82 to .98 for isokinetic peak torque and single repletion work at 60°, 180°, 240°, and 300° per second. The suggested testing procedure summary in Box 5.3 is applicable to the Biodex (Biodex Medical, Shirley, NY), Humac (CSMI, Stoughton, MA), Kin-Com (Chattecx, Chattanooga, TN), Cybex II+ (Computer Sports Medicine, Inc., Stoughton, MA), and other dynamometers still in use. There may be differences in the number of trials, duration of the rest interval, and calibration processes. The procedures described in Box 5.3 apply to all joints that can be isokinetically tested; however, the procedures will address the knee joint and knee extension and flexion movements. Evaluation of the knee typically utilizes isokinetic velocities of 60°, 180°, and 300° per second, commonly referred to as the *slow*, *medium*, and *fast velocities*, respectively.

The result of an isokinetic strength evaluation includes peak torque (highest of the three to five trials) (ft-lb or N-m) for both knee extension and knee flexion for both legs at the three velocities tested, relative torque (ft-lb · lb^{-1} body weight or N-m · kg^{-1}), the ratios of flexion to extension strength (flexion peak torque/extension peak torque), and the bilateral percentage deficit for knee extension and knee flexion at all three velocities (12).

Box 5.3 Isokinetic Testing Procedures

Instrument Procedures

1. Follow calibration procedures for both torque and angle.
2. Most dynamometers are computer-assisted; therefore, basic participant information is entered into the device's computer program prior to the start of testing.

Participant Preparation

1. Remove shoes to help minimize gravity effect on torque output.
2. The participant sits with the hips flexed at a 90° angle in an upright position.
3. The technician adjusts the seat location (up or down; forward or backward) until the lateral epicondyle (knee joint axis of rotation) is visually aligned with the dynamometer axis where input device attaches to dynamometer.
4. The technician adjusts the length of the lever arm so that the distal edge of protective pad (shin pad) is secured immediately above the medial and lateral malleoli of the ankle. The technician will pull the strap firmly to secure the strap (often made of Velcro).
5. The technician will secure all straps around various parts of the participant's body to ensure minimal recruitment of other muscle groups to assist with knee flexion or extension. These straps may vary across instruments but may include ankle (shin), thigh, abdomen (seat belt), and shoulder straps applied diagonally across the shoulders and secured to the opposite side.
6. The participant will flex the knee at least 90° or as limited by the chair apparatus and participant range of motion. Depending on dynamometer type, range of motion limits may be set at this time followed by completing the gravity correction procedure.
7. The participant will cross their arms across their chest during both the warm-up and the test protocol. The participant should not be allowed to grab onto the side of the chair.
8. The technician demonstrates and explains the movements required for proper completion of the strength test. Furthermore, the technician makes sure the participant recognizes that each repetition is a maximal effort. Each laboratory and/or testing facility will determine whether or not verbal encouragement is given.
9. The participant will warm up by completing 5–10 submaximal flexion and extension repetitions (~50% of maximal voluntary contraction). Beginning velocity is 60° per second and ending with 300° per second.
10. Beginning with the 60° per second, the participant will be instructed to complete three to five maximal contractions (extension and flexion = one repetition) followed by a 60-second rest.
11. The participant completes three to five maximal contractions at 180° per second followed by a 60-second rest.
12. The participant completes three to five maximal contractions 300° per second followed by the participant's setup is rearranged to test the opposite leg. The range of motion limits and gravity correction procedures are followed as mentioned earlier, and the warm-up and testing steps are repeated.
13. When test is complete, the data are saved in the device's software and a report is printed out for the participant.

Functional Strength Assessments

One of the primary goals of a clinical assessment tool is to provide a time-efficient, cost-effective, and easy-to-implement method for identifying factors that may limit musculoskeletal performance or function. Moreover, as the number of older adults as a percentage of the population continues to increase, preserving mobility and independence through the maintenance of strength, endurance, agility, and balance is critical. The ability of a clinician to identify limitations in movement stability and mobility can provide him or her with markers for interventions that can aid safety (3–5,11,48,74,75) and performance development (17,18,51,54,79,93,103). The Functional Movement Screen (FMS), the Fullerton Senior Fitness Test (SFT), timed up and go (TUG), and the short physical performance battery (SPPB) are assessments clinicians and practitioners alike may use to establish a patient's baseline functional strength from which an appropriate exercise prescription targeting muscular strength/power development may be formulated.

Functional Movement Screen

The FMS (see Chapter 7 for details of FMS) was designed to identify functional movement deficits and asymmetries or imbalances that may be predictive of musculoskeletal conditions and potential future injuries. Identified deficits may be targeted through a careful/thoughtful, individualized exercise prescription.

The FMS consists of seven functional movement tests that are scored on a scale of 0–3, with the sum creating a composite score with a range of 0–21 points. The seven movement patterns assessed include the deep squat, in-line lunge, hurdle step, shoulder mobility, active straight-leg raise, trunk stability push-up, and quadruped rotary stability (114,116) (http://www.functionalmovement.com). These movement patterns are designed to provide subjective, observable performance of basic locomotor, manipulative, and stabilizing movements by requiring the participant to attain/assume extreme body positions that enhance the technician's ability to observe weaknesses, limitations, or imbalances (http://www.functionalmovement.com).

The Fullerton SFT (102) assesses lower body strength and power (30-s chair stand), upper body strength (30-s arm curl), **aerobic** endurance, lower body **flexibility**, upper body flexibility, and agility. See Rikli and Jones (103) for normative data on Fullerton SFT.

The "get-up and go" test (79), also known as the TUG, requires the participant to stand from a chair, walk a short distance, turn around, return, and sit down. The TUG is a simple, short-duration, and widely used performance-based assessment of lower extremity function, functional mobility (9,48,74,75,111,120), and fall risk (48,54). Numerous governing bodies recommend the use of the TUG as a screening tool indicative of fall risk including the American and British Geriatric Societies (50) and the society of Nordic geriatricians (113). A brief description of the TUG procedure can be found in Box 5.4.

Box 5.4 Time Up and Go Test

1. Participants stand from a standard chair (seat height between 44 and 47 cm [17.3 and 18.5 in]).
2. Walk a 3-m distance (usually marked on floor) at a comfortable pace.
3. Turn, walk back to chair, ands sit down.
4. Participants may use walking aids; however, they may not use their arms to stand.
5. The test is timed with a stopwatch.
6. The test begins on the command "go" and ends when the participant's back is positioned against the seatback after sitting.
7. The test is performed two times.

Herman T, Giladi N, Hausdorff JM. Properties of the "Timed Up and Go" test: more than meets the eye. *Gerontology.* 2011;57:203–10.

Box 5.5 Short Physical Performance Battery

Standing Balance

Participants are asked to maintain side-by-side, semitandem position (heel of one foot beside the "great" toe of the other foot), and tandem (heel of one foot directly in front of the opposite foot).

Participant earns a score of 1 for holding side-by-side position for 10 seconds but was unable to hold semitandem standing position for 10 seconds. Participants earn a score of 2 for holding semitandem standing position for 10 seconds but were not able to maintain full tandem for 10 seconds. Participants earn a score of 3 for holding the tandem stand position for 3–9 seconds. A score of 4 is earned for holding the tandem stand position for 10 seconds.

Walking

A 2.4-m (8-ft) walking track is marked on the floor. The participants are instructed to walk at their "normal" pace. This walk will be timed and participants are allowed two trial walks. The faster of the two walks is used for the walk score. The scoring is as follows: ≥5.7 seconds = 1; 4.1–5.6 seconds = 2; 3.2–4.0 seconds = 3; ≤3.1 seconds = 4.

Repeated Chair Stand

Participants are instructed to fold their arms across the chest and stand up from a seated position one time, and if successful, they were instructed to stand up and sit down five times as fast as possible. The scores for the length of time required for the stand-to-sit task are as follows: ≥16.7 seconds = 1; 13.7–16.6 seconds = 2; 11.2–13.6 seconds = 3; ≤11.1 seconds = 4. A summary SPPB performance score is determined by summing the scores for standing balance, walking speed, and repeated chair rise tests. Possible score range is 3–12.

The SPPB is a composite measure of lower extremity function utilizing standing balance, walking speed, and ability to rise from a chair measures. The assessments can be carried out at home or in a clinic (Box 5.5). Low scores in the SPPB have predictive value for a wide range of health outcomes: mobility loss, disability, hospitalization, length of hospital stay, nursing home admission, and death (50). Reliability of the SPPB has been shown to be remarkably high in the U.S. populations, with ICC values ranging between .88 and .92 (95).

Strength Evaluation

A key factor in preserving mobility and independence in later years is maintaining the fitness capacity (*e.g.*, strength, endurance, power, agility, and balance) needed to perform normal everyday activities. These activities include simple housework, climbing steps, lifting and carrying objects, getting in and out of chairs or transportation vehicles, and walking far enough in and around stores, buildings, and parking lots to do one's own shopping and errands (104,125). Exercise professionals need to properly assess fundamental movements to determine the specific muscle strengthening exercises for a given participant. A structured, moderate-intensity exercise program compared with a health education program reduced major mobility disability over 2.6 years among older adults at risk for disability (96). These findings suggest mobility benefits from such a program in vulnerable older adults (96). Although the LIFE study performed resistance training, strength changes were not a primary outcome. However, previous research (19,32,37,43–45,47,50,51,63,71,80,87,96,103,105,108,114) suggests that strength training has significant positive benefits for all ages (15,26–28,36,39,40,57,74,75,100,110,112,122).

SUMMARY

This chapter presented evidence-based tests and normative data for a variety of muscular strength and functional strength testing procedures. The relevance of each test and the population served are also presented.

REFERENCES

1. Aagaard P, Simonsen EB, Andersen JL, Magnusson P, Dyhre-Poulsen P. Increased rate of force development and neural drive of human skeletal muscle following resistance training. *J Appl Physiol.* 2002;93:1318–26.
2. Abadie BR, Altorfer GL, Schuler PB. Does a regression equation to predict maximal strength in untrained lifters remain valid when the subjects are technique trained? *J Strength Cond Res.* 1999;13(3):259–63.
3. Ades PA, Savage P, Cress ME, Brochu M, Lee NM, Poehlman ET. Resistance training on physical performance in disabled older female cardiac patients. *Med Sci Sports Exerc.* 2003;35(8):1265–70.
4. American College of Sports Medicine. American College of Sports Medicine position stand. Progression models in resistance training for healthy adults. *Med Sci Sports Exerc.* 2009;41(3):687–708.
5. American College of Sports Medicine. American College of Sports Medicine position stand. The recommended quantity and quality of exercise for developing and maintaining cardiorespiratory and muscular fitness, and flexibility in healthy adults. *Med Sci Sports Exerc.* 1998;30(6):975–91.
6. American Geriatrics Society, British Geriatrics Society, American Academy of Orthopaedic Surgeons Panel on Falls Prevention. Guideline for the prevention of falls in older persons. *J Am Geriatr Soc.* 2001;49:664–72.
7. Arnold CM, Warkentin KD, Chilibeck PD, Magnus CR. The reliability and validity of handheld dynamometry for the measurement of lower-extremity muscle strength in older adults. *J Strength Cond Res.* 2010;24(3):815–24.
8. Baker MK, Atlantis E, Singh MAF. Multi-modal exercise programs for older adults. *Age Ageing.* 2007;36(4):375–81.
9. Balogun JA, Adenlola SA, Akinloye AA. Grip strength normative data for the Harpenden dynamometer. *J Orthop Sports Phys Ther.* 1991;14(4):155–60.
10. Barry E, Galvin R, Keogh C, Fahey T. Is the Timed Up and Go test a useful predictor of risk of falls in community dwelling older adults: a systematic review and meta-analysis. *BMC Geriatr.* 2014;14(1):14.
11. Bassey EJ, Rothwell MC, Littlewood JJ, Pye W. Pre- and postmenopausal women have different bone mineral density responses to the same high-impact exercise. *J Bone Miner Res.* 1998;13(12):1805–13.
12. Beam WC, Adams GM. *Exercise Physiology Laboratory Manual.* New York (NY): McGraw-Hill; 2011. 320 p.
13. Bean JF, Kiely DK, LaRose S, Alian J, Frontera WR. Is stair climb power a clinically relevant measure of leg power impairments in at-risk older adults? *Arch Phys Med Rehabil.* 2007;88(5):604–9.
14. Beauchet O, Annweiler C, Dubost V, et al. Stops walking when talking: a predictor of falls in older adults? *Eur J Neurol.* 2009;16(7):786–95.
15. Behm DG, Faigenbaum AD, Falk B, Klentrou P. Canadian society for exercise physiology position paper: resistance training in children and adolescents. *Appl Physiol Nutr Metab.* 2008;33(3):547–61.
16. Bemben MG, Grump KJ, Massey BH. Assessment of technical accuracy of the Cybex II isokinetic dynamometer and analog recording system. *J Orthop Sports Phys Ther.* 1988;10(1):12–7.
17. Binder EF, Yarasheski KE, Steger-May K, et al. Effects of progressive resistance training on body composition in frail older adults: results of a randomized, controlled trial. *J Gerontol A Biol Sci Med Sci.* 2005;60(11):1425–31.
18. Blumenthal JA, Babyak MA, Moore KA, et al. Effects of exercise training on older patients with major depression. *Arch Intern Med.* 1999; 159:2349–56.
19. Borst SE. Interventions for sarcopenia and muscle weakness in older people. *Age Ageing.* 2004;33(6):548–55.
20. Bortz WM II. A conceptual framework of frailty: a review. *J Gerontol A Biol Sci Med Sci.* 2002;57A(5):M283–8.
21. Brown DW, Brown DR, Heath GW, et al. Associations between physical activity dose and health-related quality of life. *Med Sci Sports Exerc.* 2004;36(5):890–6.
22. Brzycki M. Strength testing — predicting a one-rep max from reps-to-fatigue. *J Health Phys Educ Recr Dance.* 1993;64:88–90.
23. Buchner DM, Larson EB, Wagner EH, Koepsell TD, de Lateur BJ. Evidence for a non-linear relationship between leg strength and gait speed. *Age Ageing.* 1996;25(5):386–91.
24. Campbell WW, Leidy HJ. Dietary protein and resistance training effects on muscle and body composition in older persons. *J Am Coll Nutr.* 2007;26(6):696S–703S.
25. Carter ND, Kannus P, Khan K. Exercise in the prevention of falls in older people: a systematic literature review examining the rationale and the evidence. *Sports Med.* 2001;31(6):427–38.

26. Castro-Piñero J, González-Montesinos JL, Mora J, et al. Percentile values for muscular strength field tests in children aged 6 to 17 years: influence of weight status. *J Strength Cond Res.* 2009;23(8):2295–310.
27. Castro-Piñero J, Ortega FB, Artero EG, et al. Assessing muscular strength in youth: usefulness of standing long jump as a general index of muscular fitness. *J Strength Cond Res.* 2010;24(7):1810–7.
28. Chang JT, Morton SC, Rubenstein LZ, et al. Interventions for the prevention of falls in older adults: systematic review and meta-analysis of randomised clinical trials. *BMJ.* 2004;328(7441):680.
29. Costill DL, Fink WJ, Habansky AJ. Muscle rehabilitation after knee surgery. *Phys Sportsmed.* 1977;5:71–4.
30. Cox KF. Investigating the impact of strength-based assessment on youth with emotional or behavioral disorders. *J Child Fam Stud.* 2006;15(3):278–92.
31. Cronin JB, Jones JV, Hagstrom JT. Kinematics and kinetics of the seated row and implications for conditioning. *J Strength Cond Res.* 2007;21(4):1265–70.
32. Danforth KN, Shah AD, Townsend MK, et al. Physical activity and urinary incontinence among healthy, older women. *Obstet Gynecol.* 2007;109(3):721–7.
33. Delorme TL. Restoration of muscle power by heavy-resistance exercises. *J Bone Joint Surg Am.* 1945;27:645–67.
34. Desgorces FD, Berthelot G, Dietrich G, Testa MS. Local muscular endurance and prediction of 1 repetition maximum for bench in 4 athletic populations. *J Strength Cond Res.* 2010;24(2):394–400.
35. de Vos NJ, Singh NA, Ross DA, Stavrinos TM, Orr R, Fiatarone Singh MA. Optimal load for increasing muscle power during explosive resistance training in older adults. *J Gerontol A Biol Sci Med Sci.* 2005;60(5):638–47.
36. Docherty D. *Measurement in Pediatric Exercise Science.* Champaign (IL): Human Kinetics; 1996. 344 p.
37. Dutta C, Hadley EC. The significance of sarcopenia in old age. *J Gerontol A Biol Sci Med Sci.* 1995;50A:1–4.
38. Eston R, Evans HJL. The validity of submaximal ratings of perceived exertion to predict one repetition maximum. *J Sports Sci Med.* 2009;8(4):567–73.
39. Faigenbaum AD, Kraemer WJ, Blimkie CJ, et al. Youth resistance training: updated position statement paper from the National Strength and Conditioning Association. *J Strength Cond Res.* 2009;23:S60–79.
40. Faigenbaum AD, Milliken LA, Westcott WL. Maximal strength testing in healthy children. *J Strength Cond Res.* 2003;17(1):162–6.
41. Feiring DC, Ellenbecker TS, Derscheid GL. Test-retest reliability of the Biodex isokinetic dynamometer. *J Orthop Sports Phys Ther.* 1990;11(7):298–300.
42. Fenter PC, Bellew JW, Pitts TA, Kay RE. Reliability of stabilised commercial dynamometers for measuring hip abduction strength: a pilot study. *Br J Sports Med.* 2003;37(4):331–4.
43. Fiatarone MA, Marks EC, Ryan ND, Meredith CN, Lipsitz LA, Evans WJ. High-intensity strength training in nonagenarians. Effects on skeletal muscle. *JAMA.* 1990;263:3029–34.
44. Fiatarone MA, O'Neill EF, Ryan ND, et al. Exercise training and nutritional supplementation for physical frailty in very elderly people. *N Engl J Med.* 1994;330(25):1769–75.
45. Frontera WR, Hughes VA, Fielding RA, Fiatarone MA, Evans WJ, Roubenoff R. Aging of skeletal muscle: a 12-yr longitudinal study. *J Appl Physiol.* 2000;88:1321–6.
46. Gale CR, Martyn CN, Cooper C, Sayer AA. Grip strength, body composition, and mortality. *Int J Epidemiol.* 2007;36(1):228–35.
47. Granacher U, Muehlbauer T, Gruber M. A qualitative review of balance and strength performance in healthy older adults: impact for testing and training. *J Aging Res.* 2012;2012:708905.
48. Greene BR, O'Donovan A, Romero-Ortuno R, Cogan L, Scanaill CN, Kenny RA. Quantitative falls risk assessment using the Timed Up and Go test. *IEEE Trans Biomed Eng.* 2010;57(12):2918–26.
49. Gribble PA, Brigle J, Pietrosimone BG, Pfile KR, Webster KA. Intrarater reliability of the functional movement screen. *J Strength Cond Res.* 2013;27(4):978–81.
50. Guralnik JM, Simonsick EM, Ferrucci L, et al. A short physical performance battery assessing lower extremity function: association with self-reported disability and prediction of mortality and nursing home admission. *J Gerontol.* 1994;49:M85–94.
51. Haff GG, Triplett NT, editors. *Essentials of Strength Training and Conditioning.* 4th ed. Champaign (IL): Human Kinetics; 2016. p. 752.
52. Häger-Ross C, Rösblad B. Norms for grip strength in children aged 4–16 years. *Acta Paediatr.* 2002;91(6):617–25.
53. Hamilton GF, McDonald C, Chenier TC. Measurement of grip strength: validity and reliability of the sphygmomanometer and Jamar grip dynamometer. *J Orthop Sports Phys Ther.* 1992;16(5):215–9.
54. Herman T, Giladi N, Hausdorff JM. Properties of the "Timed Up and Go" test: more than meets the eye. *Gerontology.* 2011;57:203–10.
55. Heyward VH, Gibson AL. *Advanced Fitness Assessment and Exercise Prescription.* 7th ed. Champaign (IL): Human Kinetics; 2014. 552 p.
56. Hislop HJ, Perrine JJ. The isokinetic concept of exercise. *Phys Ther.* 1967;47:114–7.
57. Hosking JP, Bhat US, Dubowitz V, Edwards RH. Measurements of muscle strength and performance in children with normal and diseased muscle. *Arch Dis Child.* 1976;51(12):957–63.
58. Housh TJ, Cramer JT, Weir JP, Beck TW, Johnson GO. *Laboratory Manual for Exercise Physiology, Exercise Testing, and Physical Fitness.* Scottsdale (AZ): Holcomb Hathaway; 2016. p. 336.
59. Jaric S. Muscle strength testing: use of normalisation for body size. *Sports Med.* 2002;32(10):615–31.

60. Jidovtseff B, Harris NK, Crielaard JM, Cronin JB. Using the load-velocity relationship for 1RM prediction. *J Strength Cond Res.* 2011;25(1):267–70.
61. Johnson J, Siegel D. Reliability of an isokinetic movement of the knee extensors. *Res Q.* 1978;49(1):88–90.
62. Johnson MJ, Friedl KE, Frykman PN, Moore RJ. Loss of muscle mass is poorly reflected in grip strength performance in healthy young men. *Med Sci Sports Exerc.* 1994;26(2):235–40.
63. Kallman DA, Plato CC, Tobin JD. The role of muscle loss in the age-related decline of grip strength: cross-sectional and longitudinal perspectives. *J Gerontol.* 1990;45:M82–8.
64. Kelln BM, McKeon PO, Gontkof LM, Hertel J. Hand-held dynamometry: reliability of lower extremity muscle testing in healthy, physically active, young adults. *J Sport Rehabil.* 2008;17(2):160–70.
65. Kim PS, Mayhew JL, Peterson DF. A modified YMCA bench press test as a predictor of 1 repetition maximum bench press strength. *J Strength Cond Res.* 2002;16(3):440–5.
66. Knuttgen HG. Force, work, and power in athletic training. *Sports Sci Exchange.* 1995;8(4):1–5.
67. Knutzen KM, Brilla LR, Caine D. Validity of 1-RM prediction equations for older adults. *J Strength Cond Res.* 1999;13(3):242–46.
68. Kolber MJ, Beekhuizen K, Cheng MSS, Fiebert IM. The reliability of hand-held dynamometry in measuring isometric strength of the shoulder internal and external rotator musculature using a stabilization device. *Physiother Theory Pract.* 2007;23(2):119–24.
69. Komi PV. *Strength and Power in Sport.* Oxford (United Kingdom): Blackwell; 2003. 544 p.
70. Kraemer WJ, Fry AC. Strength testing: development and evaluation of methodology. In: Maud PJ, Foster C, editors. *Physiological Assessment of Human Fitness.* Champaign (IL): Human Kinetics; 1995. p. 115–38.
71. Kuh D, Hardy R, Butterworth S, et al. Developmental origins of midlife grip strength: findings from a birth cohort study. *J Gerontol A Biol Sci Med Sci.* 2006;61(7):702–6.
72. Larsson L, Grimby G, Karlsson J. Muscle strength and speed of movement in relation to age and muscle morphology. *J Appl Physiol Respir Environ Exerc Physiol.* 1979;46(3):451–6.
73. Levinger I, Goodman C, Hare DL, Jerums G, Toia D, Selig S. The reliability of the 1RM strength test for untrained middle-aged individuals. *J Sci Med Sport.* 2009;12(2):310–6.
74. Lindemann U, Claus H, Stuber M, et al. Measuring power during the sit-to-stand transfer. *Eur J Appl Physiol.* 2003;89(5):466–70.
75. Lord SR, Murray SM, Chapman K, Muron B, Tiedemann A. Sit-to-stand performance depends on sensation, speed, balance, and psychological status in addition to strength in older people. *J Gerontol A Biol Sci Med Sci.* 2002;57(8):M539–43.
76. MacIntosh BR, Gardiner PF, McComas AJ. *Skeletal Muscle: Form and Function.* 2nd ed. Champaign (IL): Human Kinetics; 2006. 432 p.
77. Maffiuletti NA, Aagaard P, Blazevich AJ, Folland J, Tillin N, Duchateau J. Rate of force development: physiological and methodological considerations. *Eur J Appl Physiol.* 2016;116:1091–116.
78. Martin HJ, Yule V, Syddall HE, Dennison EM, Cooper C, Aihie Sayer A. Is hand-held dynamometry useful for the measurement of quadriceps strength in older people? A comparison with the gold standard Biodex dynamometry. *Gerontology.* 2006; 52(3):154–9.
79. Mathias S, Nayak US, Isaacs B. Balance in elderly patients: the "get-up and go" test. *Arch Phys Med Rehabil.* 1986;67(6):387–9.
80. Mathiowetz V, Rennells C, Donahoe L. Effect of elbow position on grip and key pinch strength. *J Hand Surg Am.* 1985;10(5):694–7.
81. Mathiowetz V, Wiemer DM, Federman SM. Grip and pinch strength: norms for 6- to 19-year-olds. *Am J Occup Ther.* 1986;40(10):705–11.
82. Mayhew JL, Prinster JL, Ware JS, Zimmer DL, Arabas JR, Bemben MG. Muscular endurance repetitions to predict bench press strength in men of different training levels. *J Sports Med Phys Fitness.* 1995;35:108–13.
83. McLellan CP, Lovell DI, Gass GC. The role of rate of force development on vertical jump performance. *J Strength Cond Res.* 2011;25(2):379–85.
84. Milliken LA, Faigenbaum AD, Loud RL, Westcott WL. Correlates of upper and lower body muscular strength in children. *J Strength Cond Res.* 2008;22(4):1339–46.
85. Molenaar HM, Zuidam JM, Selles RW, Stam HJ, Hovius SE. Age-specific reliability of two grip-strength dynamometers when used by children. *J Bone Joint Surg Am.* 2008;90(5):1053–9.
86. Neiman D. *Exercise Testing and Prescription: A Health-Related Approach.* 7th ed. New York (NY): McGraw-Hill; 2011. 774 p.
87. Nelson ME, Rejeski WJ, Blair SN, et al. Physical activity and public health in older adults: recommendation from the American College of Sports Medicine and the American Heart Association. *Circulation.* 2007;116(9):1094–105.
88. Newman DG, Pearn J, Barnes A, Young CM, Kehoe M, Newman J. Norms for hand grip strength. *Arch Dis Child.* 1984;59(5):453–9.
89. Oberg T, Karsznia A, Oberg K. Basic gait parameters: reference data for normal subjects, 10-79 years of age. *J Rehabil Res Dev.* 1993;30:210–23.
90. Oh-Park M, Wang C, Verghese J. Stair negotiation time in community-dwelling older adults: normative values and association with functional decline. *Arch Phys Med Rehabil.* 2011;92(12):2006–11.
91. Oliveira AS, Corvino RB, Caputo F, Aagard P, Denadai BS. Effects of fast-velocity eccentric resistance training on early and late rate of force development. *Eur J Sport Sci.* 2016;16(2):199–205.
92. Oliveira FB, Oliveira AS, Rizatto GF, Denadai BS. Resistance training for explosive and maximal strength: effects on early and late rate of force development. *J Sports Sci Med.* 2013;12(3):402–8.
93. Onate JA, Dewey T, Kollock RO, et al. Real-time intersession and interrater reliability of the functional movement screen. *J Strength Cond Res.* 2012;26(2):408–15.

94. Ortega FB, Silventoinen K, Tynelius P, Rasmussen F. Muscular strength in male adolescents and premature death: cohort study of one million participants. *BMJ.* 2012;345:e7279.
95. Ostir GV, Volpato S, Fried LP, Chaves P, Guralnik JM. Reliability and sensitivity to change assessed for a summary measure of lower body function: results from the Women's Health and Aging Study. *J Clin Epidemiol.* 2002;55(9):916–21.
96. Pahor M, Guralnik JM, Ambrosius WT, et al. Effect of structured physical activity on prevention of major mobility disability in older adults: the LIFE study randomized clinical trial. *JAMA.* 2014;311(23):2387–96.
97. Pate RR, Burgess ML, Woods JA, Ross JG, Baumgartner T. Validity of field tests of upper body muscular strength. *Res Q Exerc Sport.* 1993;64(1):17–24.
98. Perrin DH. Reliability of isokinetic measures. *Athletic Training.* 1986;21:319–321.
99. Pincivero DM, Lephart SM, Karunakara RA. Reliability and precision of isokinetic strength and muscular endurance for the quadriceps and hamstrings. *Int J Sports Med.* 1997;18(2):113–7.
100. Rantanen T, Harris T, Leveille SG, et al. Muscle strength and body mass index as long-term predictors of mortality in initially healthy men. *J Gerontol A Biol Sci Med Sci.* 2000;55(3):M168–73.
101. Ries JD, Echternach JL, Nof L, Gagnon Blodgett M. Test–retest reliability and minimal detectable change scores for the timed "up & go" test, the six-minute walk test, and gait speed in people with Alzheimer disease. *Phys Ther.* 2009;89(6):569–79.
102. Rikli RE, Jones CJ. Development and validation of a functional fitness test for community-residing older adults. *J Aging Phys Act.* 1999;7:129–61.
103. Rikli RE, Jones CJ. Development and validation of criterion-referenced clinically relevant fitness standards for maintaining physical independence in later years. *Gerontologist.* 2013;53(2):255–67.
104. Rontu JP, Hannula MI, Leskinen S, Linnamo V, Salmi JA. One-repetition maximum bench press performance estimated with a new accelerometer method. *J Strength Cond Res.* 2010;24(8):2018–25.
105. Rosano C, Aizenstein H, Brach J, Longenberger A, Studenski S, Newman AB. Special article: gait measures indicate underlying focal gray matter atrophy in the brain of older adults. *J Gerontol A Biol Sci Med Sci.* 2008;63(12):1380–8.
106. Rothstein JM, Lamb RL, Mayhew TP. Clinical uses of isokinetic measurements. Critical issues. *Phys Ther.* 1987;67(12):1840–4.
107. Safrit MJ, Wood TM. *Introduction to Measurement in Physical Education and Exercise Science.* 3rd ed. St. Louis (MO): Mosby; 1995. 717 p.
108. Salem GJ, Wang MY, Young JT, Marion M, Greendale GA. Knee strength and lower- and higher-intensity functional performance in older adults. *Med Sci Sports Exerc.* 2000;32(10):1679–84.
109. Schoene D, Wu SM, Mikolaizak AS, et al. Discriminative ability and predictive validity of the timed up and go test in identifying older people who fall: systematic review and meta-analysis. *J Am Geriatr Soc.* 2013;61(2):202–8.
110. Sewall L, Micheli LJ. Strength training for children. *J Pediatr Orthop.* 1986;6(2):143–6.
111. Shumway-Cook A, Brauer S, Woollacott M. Predicting the probability for falls in community-dwelling older adults using the timed up & go test. *Phys Ther.* 2000;80(9):896–903.
112. Sirard JR, Pate RR. Physical activity assessment in children and adolescents. *Sports Med.* 2001;31(6):439–54.
113. Sletvold O, Tilvis R, Jonsson A, et al. Geriatric work-up in the Nordic countries. The Nordic approach to comprehensive geriatric assessment. *Dan Med Bull.* 1996;43:350–9.
114. Smith CA, Chimera NJ, Wright NJ, Warren M. Interrater and intrarater reliability of the functional movement screen. *J Strength Cond Res.* 2013;27(4):982–7.
115. Steffen TM, Hacker TA, Mollinger L. Age- and gender-related test performance in community-dwelling elderly people: six-minute walk test, Berg Balance Scale, timed up & go test, and gait speeds. *Phys Ther.* 2002;82(2):128–37.
116. Teyhen DS, Shaffer SW, Lorenson CL, et al. The functional movement screen: a reliability study. *J Orthop Sports Phys Ther.* 2012;42(6):530–40.
117. The RM prescription. *Penn State Sports Med Newsl.* 1992;1(2):7.
118. Thistle HG, Hislop HJ, Moffroid MT, Lowman E. Isokinetic contraction: a new concept of resistive exercise. *Arch Phys Med Rehabil.* 1967;48:279–82.
119. Verschuren O, Ketelaar M, Takken T, Van Brussel M, Helders PJ, Gorter JW. Reliability of hand-held dynamometry and functional strength tests for the lower extremity in children with cerebral palsy. *Disabil Rehabil.* 2008;30(18):1358–66.
120. Wall JC, Bell C, Campbell S, Davis J. The timed get-up-and-go test revisited: measurement of the component tasks. *J Rehabil Res Dev* . 2000;37(1):109–13.
121. Williams EN, Carroll SG, Reddihough DS, Phillips BA, Galea MP. Investigation of the timed 'up & go' test in children. *Dev Med Child Neurol.* 2005;47(8):518–24.
122. Wilmore JH, Costill DL. *Training for Sport and Activity: The Physiological Basis of the Conditioning Process.* Dubuque (IA): Wm. C. Brown; 1988. 420 p.
123. Wind AE, Takken T, Helders PJ, Engelbert RH. Is grip strength a predictor for total muscle strength in healthy children, adolescents, and young adults? *Eur J Pediatr.* 2010;169(3):281–7.
124. Wyatt MP, Edwards AM. Comparison of quadriceps and hamstring torque values during isokinetic exercise. *J Orthop Sports Phys Ther.* 1981;3(2):48–56.
125. Yim-Chiplis PK, Talbot LA. Defining and measuring balance in adults. *Biol Res Nurs.* 2000;1(4):321–31.

CHAPTER 6

Body Composition Assessment

INTRODUCTION

Body composition describes the amount and relative proportions of fat mass (FM) and fat-free mass (FFM) in the human body. Once considered as only descriptive, the study of body composition is evolving into functional body composition as evidence emerges that there is "cross-talk" between body components acting as regulatory systems that affects body functions and metabolic processes via hormones, cytokines, and metabolites (5,43).

Measurement of body composition is a standard component of testing and evaluation for exercise professionals (28,59). Valuable information regarding percent body fat (PBF), fat distribution, body segment girth, and bone density may be gained through body composition assessment and utilized for reducing health risks associated with disease (63) and for designing safe and effective training programs that optimize athletic performance (39). This chapter discusses body composition assessment and compares commonly used measurement techniques.

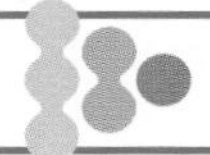

Rationale for Body Composition Assessment

The assessment of body composition in **children** and **adolescent** (70), adult, **older adults** (15), special populations such as pregnant (76) and postmenopausal women (32), and individuals with intellectual disability (10) has many benefits. PBF estimation provides vital information concerning health and fitness. An excess amount of body fat, or obesity, is linked to several diseases including Type 2 diabetes mellitus, hypertension, hyperlipidemia, cardiovascular disease (CVD) (44), associated increased morbidity and mortality from CVD (69), and certain types of cancer (6). In addition, increased PBF has been linked to increased risk of musculoskeletal symptoms due to increased mechanical stress (71) and to osteoarthritis possibly due to proinflammatory mediators activated by an increased level of adipokines secreted by adipose tissue (54). Because of the current epidemic of obesity in adults 18 years and older (~35%), in children and adolescents (~17%) in the United States (47), and on a global scale more than half a billion adults (46,77), detection of obesity is of primary importance for health and exercise science professionals (43,55). Assessment of body composition also plays a critical role in determining if interventions such as **exercise** may be effective in modifying disease risks associated with accumulation of excess adipose tissue without requiring significant weight loss (55).

Body composition assessment is useful for those individuals with a low, as well as high, PBF. During times of malnutrition (*e.g.*, eating disorders) and in some weight-sensitive sports, body fat levels and water content can fall to dangerously low levels (1,39). Meyer et al. (39) state that weight-sensitive sports "are those in which extreme dieting, low PBF, frequent mass fluctuation and eating disorders have been reported in both literature and practice" (p. 1046). These include gravitational sports (*e.g.*, long-distance running, road cycling, high jumping, pole vaulting), weight class sports (*e.g.*, wrestling, judo boxing, weightlifting), and aesthetic sports (*e.g.*, figure skating, rhythmic and artistic gymnastics, and bodybuilding) (39). Such sports require athletes to compete at either low weight or with minimal body fat. Measurement of FFM and bone mineral density (BMD) has several important ramifications. In the clinical setting, assessment of FFM and BMD can be used to assess the effects of aging (15) and disease (4,18,63). A progressive reduction in BMD, that is, osteopenia and osteoporosis, may occur with aging, **physical inactivity**, and overtraining. In addition, **sarcopenia**, the degenerative loss of **skeletal muscle mass** and **strength** as a result of aging, reduced **physical activity**, and certain diseases, can be assessed (43,51). Sarcopenia reduces the ability to perform **activities of daily living (ADL)**; alters metabolism, muscle, and bone function; and increases the risk of musculoskeletal injury. Thus, body composition assessment in the clinical setting can be used to monitor the progression of disease or muscle/bone enhancement as a result of therapeutic or pharmaceutical intervention (43,63).

Also, assessment of body composition may assist in the diagnosis of diseases obscured in individuals with a normal weight but a high PBF and decreased FFM (*e.g.*, sarcopenic obesity) and/or decreased BMD (43). In hospitalized patients, nutritional status is assessed on a regular basis. Body composition assists in documenting the efficiency of nutritional support (63). Assessment of body composition is also an essential tool in helping manage the treatment of cancer survivors who frequently experience extremely altered body composition such as muscle wasting, a central feature of cancer cachexia (4,18,43,63).

Furthermore, in apparently healthy individuals, assessment of body composition can be used to quantify changes in FM, FFM, and BMD as a result of weight training and weight loss and weight gain (25,52). These measurements may be used for individualization of **exercise prescriptions** and for the evaluation of an exercise conditioning program. In the athletic population, body composition assessment can be used to quantify changes in FFM and BMD as a result of physical training and aid in distinguishing healthy from unhealthy weight loss and weight gain (1,39). In this regard, overtraining combined with low energy availability in both women (31) and men (62) can negatively affect the athlete's body composition and health acutely and over the long term. The International Olympic Committee's consensus statement on relative energy deficiency in sport (RED-S) addresses the complexities involved as they pertain to both female and male athletes (42). In addition, concern has been expressed that the focus on body mass and composition in sport may have unintended negative effects on the athlete (*e.g.*, body image issues, disordered eating/eating disorders, dehydration) (39).

Body Composition Models

Body composition methods can be categorized as being direct, indirect, or doubly indirect (1,59,60). The direct method initially (~1945) employed cadaver dissection and the subsequent chemical analysis in vitro (13). More modern approaches at the direct method use in vivo methods such as magnetic resonance imaging (MRI), computed tomography (CT), and neutron activation analysis (13,22). Indirect methods measure one parameter to estimate another (1). For instance, **hydrostatic weighing** (HW) is used to measure body volume and then PBF is estimated based on assumed values for the density of FM and FFM (1,13,28). Doubly indirect methods (*e.g.*, skinfolds), which uses one indirect measure to predict another indirect measure, were primarily derived from the indirect method, HW. Due to technological advances over the past two decades, equations to convert skinfold thickness to PBF are being derived from methods that directly measure values of body composition in vivo and thus are theoretically more accurate (22).

Different models have been proposed for characterizing human body composition by discrete compartments with the sum totaling the individual's body mass. The *two-compartment (2C) model* partitions body mass into FM and FFM (1,22,28) and has the widest application to body composition analysis. This model is limited by the assumptions that water and mineral contents of the body remain constant throughout life and between all individuals and that the density of FFM is constant among all individuals. However, FFM composition is known to be altered by age, sex, pregnancy, weight loss/gain, race/ethnic differences (22,52), some states of disease (*e.g.*, osteoporosis, sarcopenia), and in highly trained athletes (22,40).

Multicompartment models have been developed because of violation of the inherent assumptions of the **2C model**. These models divide the body into more than two compartments and require fewer assumptions about the composition of the FFM. Thus, multicompartment models provide more accurate results (1,22,24,28,59,63). The 3C model includes FM but also partitions FFM into total body water (TBW) and dry FFM. The 4C model partitions body mass into FM, TBW, BMD, and the residual dry FFM. Thus, the addition of BMD (via dual-energy x-ray absorptiometry [DXA]) is added to the 3C model. In addition, 4C models often serve as the criterion model for body composition measurement in validation studies (1,22,52). The measurement of soft tissue mineral content (via in vivo neutron analysis or by using a prediction equation based on neutron analysis) has been added to 4C models to generate a criterion 5C model. The choice of an appropriate model depends on the component of FFM that is expected to vary the most from population norms.

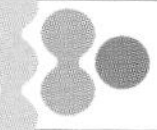

Methodologies in Body Composition Assessment

Direct in vivo methods are used on a limited basis due to the paucity of specially trained personnel, high costs associated with instrumentation, and, in general, lack of portability. Therefore, most body composition measurements involve indirect assessment or estimation. The decision on which method to use depends on several factors, including the needs of the individual, purpose of the evaluation, cost of the measurements or equipment needed, availability of each assessment tool, and the technician's expertise (1,22,24,28,37,57,59,65). In regard to the latter, body composition assessment certification for anthropometric techniques only exists from the International Society for the Advancement of Kinanthropometry (ISAK) (38,39,59). The following is a brief summary of basic and selected advanced methods to assess body composition.

Height, Body Mass, and Body Mass Index

Height

Anthropometry is the measurement of the human body using simple physical techniques. Height should be assessed with a stadiometer (a vertical ruler mounted on a wall with a wide horizontal headboard). Standard procedures for height measurements include no shoes, heels together, erect posture, head level looking straight ahead, after a deep inhalation, and holding breath. Height can vary slightly throughout the day with variations in fluid content of the spine's intervertebral discs and is affected by activity level (upright, weight-bearing exercise increases spinal disc compression, which can slightly reduce height). Height is typically greatest in the morning (when intervertebral disc fluid content is highest), so selecting a standard time and monitoring preactivity level increases reliability when multiple measures are taken from the same individual over time (38,59).

Body Mass

Body mass is best measured on a calibrated scale. Ideally, measurements should be completed with minimal clothing. Facilities should adopt the most reasonable clothing policy for their population (60). Body mass can change at various times of day because of meal/beverage consumption, urination, defecation, and potential dehydration/water loss. Thus, a standard time (*e.g.*, early in the morning) relative to exercise and nutritional intake will increase the consistency of measurements (38,59).

Body Mass Index

Body mass index (BMI) is used to assess an individual's mass relative to height (BMI = body mass / height squared; $kg \cdot m^{-2}$). The primary advantages of BMI are that it is a relatively easy measure to obtain and it is useful for categorizing the extent of overweight and obesity in large populations (30,49,70). In this regard, the American College of Cardiology and the American Heart Association's classification of overweight and obesity is based on BMI (29). Adult BMI is a reasonably generalizable height-independent measure of body shape and composition for comparisons across sex and race/ethnic groups (27). In a prospective study of approximately 1 million African Americans and White men and women, the risk of premature mortality was higher in those classified as underweight and overweight/obese categories (3, Table 4.1) when compared with the lower end of normal weight (50). Recently, a 15-year longitudinal study with approximately 30,000 participants found BMI to be significantly better than PBF in predicting mortality from CVD (49). The data from this study also suggest that "excess body *weight* is a stronger predictor of CVD than is an excess of body fat" (49). One should be cautious when using BMI as the sole indicator of cardiometabolic health, a practice some employers have selected to determine employee health insurance costs. An analysis of National Health and Nutrition Examination Survey (NHANES) data from 2005 to 2012 determined that 29% of individuals with obesity based on BMI were metabolically healthy, whereas 30% of normal weight individuals classified by BMI were cardiometabolically unhealthy (64). The former finding is supported by an extensive review of the metabolically healthy but obese (MHO) phenotype (48). The review reported that the percentage of adults in the United States and Europe combined that are obese (BMI $\geq$30) and meet 0 of the metabolic syndrome (MetS) criteria is estimated to be ~12%–17% (48).

Recent findings indicate that the association between all-cause mortality and BMI may be affected by race. For instance, BMI and mortality are strongly related among White Americans but not very robust in African Americans (34). However, African Americans' mortality risk increased with an elevated waist circumference (WC) compared with those with a low WC (34).

BMI is a relatively poor predictor of PBF (2). Additionally, BMI may result in inaccurate classifications (normal, overweight, obese) for some individuals particularly those who are muscular (51). This shortcoming is because BMI presumes that excessive weight is solely due to increased adiposity (38). However, misclassification of body weight is not prevalent in nonathletic adult populations who are weight stable or who have gained weight in their adult years. Thus, BMI should provide a reasonably accurate classification of weight status in these individuals (38). Finally, BMI can be used for estimating ideal body weight and body weight (49): $\text{Wt (lb)} = [5 \cdot \text{BMI} + (\text{BMI} \cdot 5^{-1})] \cdot (\text{Ht} - 60\ \text{in})$. For application of the equation to weight loss management and for the metric version of the equation, see Peterson et al. (51).

Circumferences

Circumferences, or girths, are used to estimate body composition and provide specific reference to the distribution of fat in the body. The pattern of body fat distribution is an important predictor of the health risks associated with obesity. Increased fat distribution on the trunk (android obesity) increases the risk of hypertension, MetS, Type 2 diabetes, dyslipidemia, coronary artery disease, and premature death when compared with individuals whose fat is distributed in the hip and thigh region (gynoid obesity) (16,17).

Using circumference measures as a means for estimating body composition has the advantage of being easy to learn, quick to complete, and inexpensive. Various translational equations are available for men and women to convert girth measurements to body fat estimations across a range of ages and percentage of body fat (22,65,66,75). Accuracy of circumference measures vary but can range within 2.5%–4.0% of the body composition derived from hydrostatic densitometry. Circumferences also provide information about growth and frame size (24,28). Briefly, measurement technique consists of using an inelastic tape measure placed in a horizontal plane or perpendicular to the length of the segment being measured. Tension on the tape should be snug but not so tight as to compress the subcutaneous fat layer (24,28,59,65). Duplicate measurements are obtained in a rotational order instead of consecutively (3, Box 4.1) (24,28).

Waist Circumference

The WC has been advocated for use as a "vital sign" in clinical practice because research has demonstrated that the distribution of body fat is more important in determining CVD risk than excess total body fat (17). In this regard, WC represents subcutaneous adipose tissue (SAT) as well as visceral adipose tissue (VAT). VAT is closely associated with increased cardiometabolic risk, although the exact mechanism(s) have yet to be fully elucidated (16). As such, the relationship should not be considered a cause-and-effect one (16). Furthermore, racial differences exist in abdominal depot-specific body fatness with African American men and women having lower amounts of VAT for a given amount of total body fat than White Americans (9,33). Thus, WC alone as a simple marker of visceral adiposity is limited (16). However, WC alone has been used an indicator of CVD risk (3, Table 4.2) (7,29). Ethnic- or country-specific WC cutoff points for risk of metabolic complications are available from the World Health Organization (WHO) and the International Diabetes Federation (77). It is more effective to use the WC and the BMI together as factors indicative of cardiometabolic risk (Table 6.1) (3, Table 4.1) (17,29) as well as mortality risk (11,56). Additionally, WC and BMI together may also be used in public health to assist an individual in determining his or her PBF by a simple charting method (35).

Table 6.1 Cardiometabolic Risk Score Values across Tertiles of Waist Circumference within Each of the Three Body Mass Index Categories[a]

	WC Tertiles					
Men	**T1**		**T2**		**T3**	
BMI <25 kg · m^{-2}	WC ≤ 84 cm	2.1 ± 0.1	84 cm < WC ≤ 90 cm	$2.5 \pm 0.1^{**}$	WC > 90 cm	$2.7 \pm 0.1^{***}$
25 kg · m^{-2} ≤ BMI <30 kg · m^{-2}	WC ≤ 95 cm	2.7 ± 0.1	95 cm < WC ≤ 101 cm	$3.3 \pm 0.1^{**}$	WC > 101 cm	$3.6 \pm 0.1^{***}$
BMI ≥30 kg · m^{-2}	WC ≤ 108 cm	3.7 ± 0.1	108 cm < WC ≤ 116 cm	$4.1 \pm 0.1^{*}$	WC > 116 cm	$4.5 \pm 0.1^{**\dagger}$
	WC Tertiles					
Women	**T1**		**T2**		**T3**	
BMI <25 kg · m^{-2}	WC ≤ 76 cm	1.5 ± 0.1	76 cm < WC ≤ 83 cm	$1.9 \pm 0.1^{**}$	WC > 83 cm	$2.7 \pm 0.1^{***\dagger\dagger\dagger}$
25 kg · m^{-2} ≤ BMI <30 kg · m^{-2}	WC ≤ 87 cm	2.5 ± 0.1	87 cm < WC ≤ 93 cm	$3.3 \pm 0.1^{***}$	WC > 93 cm	$3.8 \pm 0.1^{***\dagger\dagger}$
BMI ≥30 kg · m^{-2}	WC ≤ 100 cm	3.4 ± 0.1	100 < WC ≤ 108 cm	3.8 ± 0.1	WC > 108 cm	$4.6 \pm 0.1^{**\dagger\dagger}$

$^{*}p < .05$. $^{**}p < .01$. $^{***}p < .0001$ denote significantly different from the first WC tertile group within the same BMI category, and $^{\dagger}p < .05$. $^{\dagger\dagger}p < 0.01$. $^{\dagger\dagger\dagger}p < .0001$ denote significantly different from the middle WC tertile group within the same BMI category. T1, T2, and T3 are the WC tertile groups. All statistical analyses were adjusted for age, ethnicity, physician's specialty, smoking status, and educational level.
[a]Data are given for men and women separately, as means ± standardized error of the means (SEMs).

Source: Nazare JA, Smith J, Borel AL, et al. Usefulness of measuring both body mass index and waist circumference for the estimation of visceral adiposity and related cardiometabolic risk profile (from the INSPIRE ME IAA study). *Am J Cardiol.* 2015;115:307–15.

The exact site used for measurement of the WC has been reported to vary considerably (52) with one study finding 14 different descriptions of the WC measurement sites in the literature (72). Wang et al. (72) compared WC measurements at four commonly used sites (Table 6.2) with body fat measured in 74 subjects using DXA. They found that the four WC measurements were not all similar in value because the narrowest waist was significantly less than the WC values at the other three sites. However, they found that WC values measured at the four sites are almost equally associated with total body fat and trunk fat in both females and males (72). Ross et al. (53) convened a panel of experts to systematically review the WC measurement protocol in 120 studies. They determined that WC measurement protocol had no substantial influence on the association of WC with all-cause and CVD mortality, CVD, and diabetes. Based on practical considerations for reliable measurement of WC, the expert panel recommended using either the WHO guidelines or the National Institutes of Health (NIH) guidelines (see Table 6.2). Of the two protocols, the panel singled out the NIH protocol for adoption. The NIH method uses an easily located landmark, the superior border of the iliac crest, to aid in accurately locating the waist and thus eliminates potential errors (53). Interestingly, Wang et al.'s (72) study found the NIH WC site to have the highest correlation with percentage of body fat. These investigators also noted that the NIH WC site is close to L4–L5 which is where MRI and CT single-slice measurements are performed to measure VAT (72).

Table 6.2 The Four Most Commonly Measured Waist Circumference Sites Defined by Specific Anatomic Landmarks

Measurement Sites	Comment
Immediately below the lowest rib	
At the narrowest waist	ASM site[a]
Midpoint between the lowest rib and the iliac crest	WHO site[b]
Immediately above the iliac crest	NIH and NHANES III site[c]

[a]Recommended in the *Anthropometric Standardization Reference Manual* (ASM).
[b]Recommended in the WHO guidelines.
[c]Recommended in the NIH guidelines and applied in the third National Health and Nutrition Examination Survey (NHANES III).

Source: Wang J, Thornton JC, Bari S, et al. Comparisons of waist circumferences measured at 4 sites. *Am J Clin Nutr.* 2003;77:379–84.

Hip Circumference

Hip circumference, considered individually, and not as ratio with WC, is also emerging as an important factor to consider in risk models for CVD, diabetes, and mortality (6). Hip circumference is inversely related to CVD, diabetes, and mortality (8). The protective effects of larger hips may be brought about by regulation of free fatty acid release and uptake and a beneficial adipokine profile related to the gluteofemoral SAT (8).

Waist-to-Hip Ratio

The waist-to-hip ratio (WHR) is a ratio measurement of the circumference of the waist to that of the hip and is an indicator of body fat distribution. A high WHR may indicate visceral obesity. Visceral obesity increases the risk of hypertension, Type 2 diabetes, hyperlipidemia, MetS, and CVD. Multiple measurements are taken until each is within 5 mm (~0.20 in) of each other. Young adults are at a very high risk for disease when WHR values are >0.95 for men and 0.86 for women. These values rise to 1.03 and 0.90, respectively, for ages 60–69 years. WHO has established WHR cutoff points for "substantially increased risk of metabolic complications" as follows: ≥0.90 (men) and ≥0.85 (women) (77).

Hydrodensitometry

Underwater or HW (also known as *hydrodensitometry*) was considered the criterion method for body composition. It is a direct method for determining the volume of the body but is an indirect method for predicting PBF. HW is based on Archimedes principle for determining body density (BD). Archimedes principle states that a body immersed in water is subjected to a buoyant force that results in a loss of weight equal to the weight of the displaced water. Subtracting the body weight measured while submersed in water from the body weight measured on land provides the weight of the displaced water. Body fat contributes to buoyancy because the assumed density of fat ($0.9007\ g \cdot cm^{-3}$) is less than water ($1\ g \cdot cm^{-3}$), whereas FFM (assumed to average $1.100\ g \cdot cm^{-3}$) exceeds the density of water. Density is inversely related to body fat. Thus, HW is based on the equation: $BD = mass \cdot volume^{-1}$. A volumetric analysis of the body is possible with HW because body volume can be determined via hydrodensitometry. BD is then converted to PBF using a 2C (fat and FFM) model equation, such as the Siri or Brozek BD equations (22,23). Detailed methods used in HW are reviewed elsewhere (22,24,26,28,59,60). Although the density of lean tissue is assumed to be 1.100 g · cm^{-3} for all subjects in the Siri and Brozek equations, this value differs in African Americans (>1.10 g · cm^{-3}) and in children and older adults (<1.10 g · cm^{-3}), which is a major source of error if population-specific equations are not used with these groups (13,22). Critical limitations of HW are discussed elsewhere (13).

Skinfold Measurement

One of the more popular and practical methods used to estimate PBF is the skinfold thickness measurement (24,28,38,39). Skinfold measurement is relatively simple and noninvasive and predicts PBF reasonably well if performed properly by a trained technician using a high-quality skinfold caliper (*e.g.*, a Lange or Harpenden caliper) (24,28). However, skinfold analysis provides only an estimate of PBF, and over the past 20 years, analysis has shifted from regression equations based on a 2C model (*e.g.*, HW) to equations developed from 3C (*e.g.*, DXA) and 4C models. Skinfold analysis is based on the principle that the amount of subcutaneous fat (fat immediately below the skin) is directly proportional to the total amount of body fat. The proportion of subcutaneous to total fat varies with sex, age, race/ethnicity, and other factors.

Taking the Measurements

The skinfold sites to be measured are determined by the regression equation selected (*i.e.*, two-, three-, four-, or seven-site skinfold). As a standard, all measurements are taken on the right side of the body. Each site is marked by measuring an established distance from a prominent anatomical landmark(s) corresponding to the description of the skinfold site (24,28,38). Next, a short line is marked directly over the center of the grasped (described in the following text) skinfold in the proximity of the aforementioned marked landmark. The convergence of these two marks designates the measurement site (3, Box 4.2, for sites and procedures). The thumb and forefinger of the left hand are separated about 8 cm (3.15 in) and placed 1 cm (0.39 in) above the skinfold site. A double fold of skin and subcutaneous fat is then firmly grasped between the thumb and index finger on a line perpendicular to the long axis of the skinfold and lifted away from the body while the subject is relaxed. For individuals with obesity, a large grasping area (*i.e.*, >8 cm) may be needed. With the caliper dial facing up, the jaws of the caliper are opened and slipped over the skinfold with the caliper tips perpendicular to the mark designating the measurement site. The tips of the caliper should then be placed halfway between the base and the crest of the fold and 1 cm below the fingers. The pressure of the caliper tips should be applied slowly to the skinfold to prevent discomfort. To ensure equal pressure on each side of the fold, the caliper tips should be parallel and not be twisted on the skinfold. The skinfold thickness measurement is subsequently recorded within 2–3 seconds while the tester's left hand maintains the grasp of the skinfold.

To ensure accuracy, measurements are obtained in duplicate and recorded to the nearest 0.5 mm. If there is more than a 2-mm difference between readings, a third measurement is needed. It is important to rotate through the measurement sites as opposed to taking two or three measurements sequentially from the same site (see Fig. 6.1 for a picture of selected skinfold sites) (24,28,38). The measurements for each site are then averaged. The average thickness is then entered into a regression equation to estimate PBF. Care must be taken to match the exact location and orientation of the skinfold. For instance, the orientation of the abdominal skinfold may be vertical or horizontal depending what the investigators used to establish the regression equation (24).

Potential Disadvantages

The major limitations to the skinfold procedure are the amount of technician training in equation selection, accuracy of skinfold site location, selection of appropriate calipers, and measurement technique (38,39). ISAK emphasizes using the raw data (*e.g.*, individual skinfolds, sum of skinfolds)

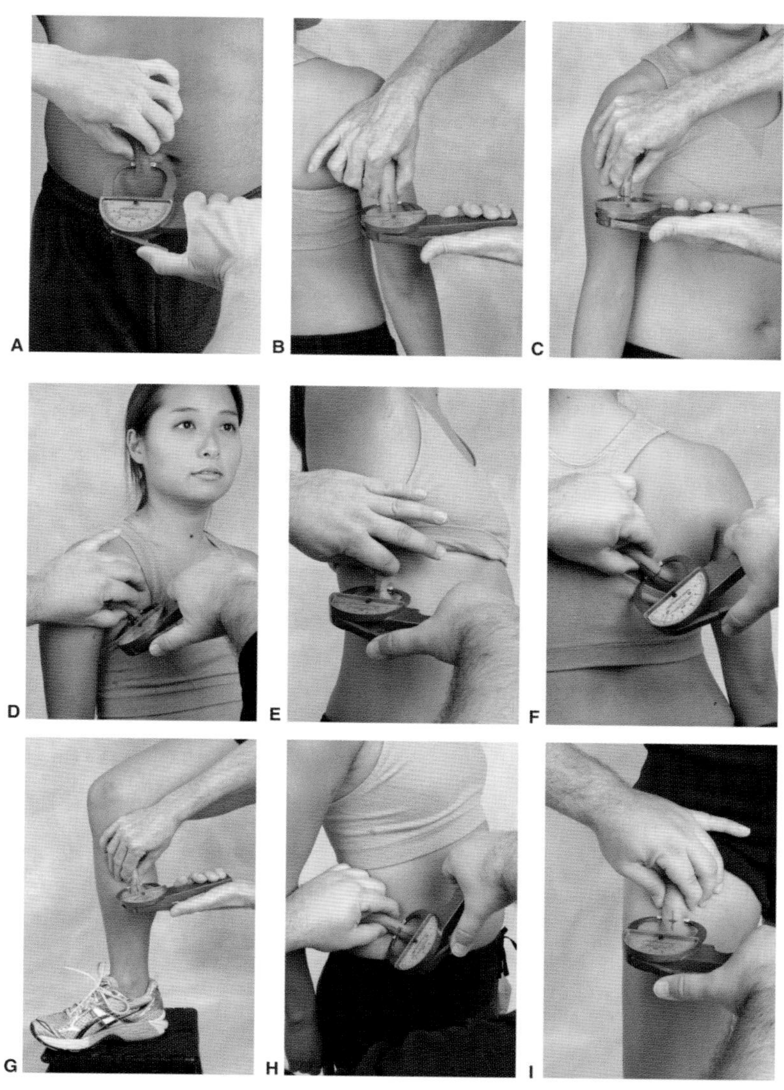

FIGURE 6.1. Common sites for skinfold measurements. (Reprinted from Bushman B, editor. *ACSM's Resources for the Personal Trainer.* 4th ed. Philadelphia [PA]: Wolters Kluwer; 2014. Figure 12.6.)

directly (*i.e.*, used to construct a "skinfold map," calculate ratios) (38,39). Communication with the patient is a must because some patients may feel uncomfortable having someone in such close contact with their body (59). They may prefer to have someone of the same sex perform the skinfolds or observe the measurements. Common sites and detailed instruction for measurement can be found in Box 4.1 of *ACSM's Guidelines for Exercise Testing and Prescription, 10th edition* (*GETP10*) (3) and elsewhere (24,28,38,39,59). In those with abdominal subcutaneous fat that is not easily grasped because of marked abdominal obesity, skinfold assessment may not be accurate, and thus, other body composition assessment techniques may be required.

Bioelectrical Impedance

Bioelectrical impedance analysis (BIA) is a noninvasive and easy-to-administer body composition assessment tool (22,24,28,59,60). A small electrical current is sent through the body (from ankle to wrist, or from hand to hand, or foot to foot), and the impedance to that current is measured.

The theory underlying BIA is that lean tissue (mostly water and electrolytes) is a good electrical conductor (low impedance), whereas fat is a poor electrical conductor and acts as impedance to electrical current. BIA estimates TBW and uses equations for PBF (using a 3C model) based on assumptions about hydration levels and the exact water content of various tissues. A single-frequency (50 kHz), low-level current (500 mA) is used to measure whole-body impedance using electrodes placed on two distant peripheral sites. Unlike lower frequency current (<50 kHz), which flows through the extracellular fluid, higher frequencies penetrate the cell membranes and flow through both the intracellular and extracellular fluid. Thus, total body impedance at the constant frequency of 50 kHz primarily reflects the volumes of water (intracellular and extracellular fluid) and muscle compartments constituting the FFM.

Potential Disadvantages

Potential limitations to single-frequency BIA analyzers are that they cannot distinguish between intracellular and extracellular water components, and they assume the body to be a single cylinder with constant resistivity (22,59). Other BIA analyzers have been developed to address these limitations. Multifrequency BIA analyzers (also known as *bioimpedance spectroscopy*) allow for partitioning intracellular and extracellular components as a range from low to high frequencies are used (1,22). Common analyzers studied typically use ~50 frequencies ranging from 5 to 1,000 kHz, whereas newer models use up to ~256 frequencies ranging from 4 to 1,000 kHz. They may be less affected by hydration status and may provide a better estimate of FFM. Multifrequency BIA may enhance the clinical application of BIA to assess changes and shifts between intracellular and extracellular fluid compartments associated with certain diseases as well as accurate measurements of hydration status (59,63). Both have been shown to provide accurate assessment of TBW compared with deuterium dilution (41). A multiple-frequency BIA device that is incorporated into a smartphone is currently being developed (12). Preliminary results indicate that the body fat estimates from the smartphone do not differ significantly from measurements utilizing DXA (12). A review of the use of BIA on athletes recommends using generalized BIA equations (provided in the article) until athlete-specific BIA equations are developed from a multiple-component model that includes TBW (40). However, there is a limitation of using BIA to assess or monitoring body composition of athletes because accurate measurements call for abstaining from exercise (1).

Air Displacement Plethysmography

Body volume can be measured by air displacement rather than water displacement. Air displacement plethysmography (ADP) is usually a quick and comfortable assessment; is noninvasive; and accommodates infants, children, adults, obese, older adults, and individuals with disabilities. ADP is performed with the BOD POD system (Life Measurement Instruments, Concord, CA), which uses a dual-chamber (*e.g.*, 450 L for the subject test chamber, 300 L for the reference chamber) plethysmograph that measures body volume via changes in air pressure using Boyle's law ($P_1 \cdot P_2 = V_2 \cdot V_1$). The volume of air displaced is equal to body volume and is calculated indirectly by subtracting the volume of air remaining in the chamber when the subject is inside from the volume of air in the chamber when it is empty. A diaphragm (which separates the two internal chambers) oscillates back and forth to create volume changes that produce pressure changes in the two chambers. Thoracic gas volume is measured or derived from a published prediction equation. Corrected body volume (raw body volume − thoracic gas volume) is then calculated (24).

Potential Disadvantages

A major disadvantage for ADP is initial cost of purchasing the ADP unit. Sources of error include (a) interlaboratory variation, (b) variations in testing conditions, (c) test performance while not in a fasting state, (d) air that is not accounted for in the lungs or that is trapped within clothing and bodily hair, and (e) body moisture and/or increased body temperature. Most prediction equations used to convert BD to PBF using ADP are similar to HW. As such, error results when assumptions associated with the density of FFM are violated. More details can be found elsewhere (1,22,24,28,59).

Ultrasound

Ultrasound imaging is a fast, portable, noninvasive, relatively inexpensive technique to measure tissue (*e.g.*, fat, muscle) thickness that does not expose the subject to ionizing radiation risks (5,26,59). Ultrasound provides sonic energy at frequencies between 3 and 22 MHz (1). The pulse is propagated through the tissues at a specific velocity. The pattern produced depends on its wavelength (frequency) and the density of the tissues (24). Part of the energy is reflected, whereas the rest is refracted where the tissue density dictates the magnitude of reflection (23). In A-mode (amplitude mode) ultrasound, a pulse is sent from the probe through the subject and back (similar to an echo), and the depth (time of echo) is visually displayed. B-mode (brightness-modulation) ultrasonography collects similar information but converts the echoes into dots where the brightness emulates the amplitude of the reflected signal in a two-dimensional image (59). B-mode is the most frequently used ultrasound technique (22). Ultrasound has been shown to be reliable and valid for measuring VAT (5). Furthermore, studies utilizing needle puncture measurements, MRI, and CT have confirmed the accuracy of SAT depth measured by ultrasound (5,26). Measurements may be taken at the same sites as skinfolds (5); however, ultrasound measurements are not directly equivalent to skinfolds (59). Skinfold's thickness represent a compressed double layer of adipose tissue and skin, whereas the ultrasound thickness represents a single uncompressed layer of adipose tissue and skin (59). SAT thicknesses determined by ultrasound may then be used to estimate BD. BD is then used to estimate PBF via regression equations developed by utilizing PBF determined by a criterion method such as DXA.

Potential Disadvantages

Critical to reliable ultrasonic measurement is an experienced and skillful technician as well as the creation of a standardized technique (*i.e.*, exact locations of measurement, procedures and techniques for the application of a uniform and constant pressure on the probe) (5,24,59).

Dual-Energy X-Ray Absorptiometry

DXA is based on a 3C model of total body mineral stores, FFM, and FM (1,22,59,60). DXA has been used since 1999 by NHANES to conduct full body scans to develop a body composition data base (45). DXA is routinely used in clinical practice for the measurement of BMD and increasingly utilized clinically and in research for assessment of body composition (63).

The principle of absorptiometry is based on exponential attenuation of x-rays at two energies as they pass through the body. DXA machines are commonly used in hospitals and research facilities. X-rays are generated at two energies via a low-current x-ray tube located underneath the DXA machine. A detector positioned overhead on the scanning arm and interface with a computer is necessary for scanning the image. A DXA scan generates pertinent information regarding the masses (grams) of fat, lean tissue, and bone mineral content and density for the total body and for specific regions (*e.g.*, the head, trunk, limbs).

Advantages and Potential Disadvantages

DXA has many advantages as it is easy to administer and subjects have a higher comfort level compared with other techniques such as HW. DXA uses low-level radiation and is safe, fast, and accurate. DXA has been shown to correlate highly with HW and other multicompartment models

(4C) in athletes and in young, middle-aged, or older adult men and women. Regional measurement of FFM is also useful for examining the effects of various exercise programs, such as resistance training on muscular hypertrophy (26).

There are some limitations associated with DXA measurements. An individual's size is of some concern. A very tall person or individual of large weight (*e.g.*, >300 lb) whose body extends beyond the measurable range on the scanner table may have to maintain a cramped position, which can distort regional measurements. Often, individuals with morbid obesity may not be able to be scanned due to such limitations. Furthermore, because of its emission of low-level radiation, several states require a physician's prescription in order to perform DXA scans. This requirement, in addition to cost and lack of portability, could limit the use of DXA primarily to the clinical and research settings. To circumvent these limitations, DXA is being used as a criterion measure to develop reference values using easy-to-obtain anthropometric measurements such as height, weight, BMI, skinfolds, and circumferences.

Body Composition Assessment in Children and Adolescents

The prevalence of obesity in children and adolescents aged 2–18 years is increasing in both developing and developed countries (46,77). However, in the United States, obesity, as defined by an age- and gender-specific BMI ≥95th percentile (47,70), has stabilized at approximately 17% (12.5 million) (45,47). Associated with obesity in these populations is an increased risk of developing cardiometabolic diseases (23,73) as well as premature mortality in adulthood (69). Thus, body composition assessment has become a very important public health tool and is also increasingly being used in the clinical setting (23,70,73). However, these populations can be difficult to assess because of the effects of growth/**maturation** on FFM, FM, and hydration state (37,73). As such, reference data in the form of body composition growth charts for FM and FFM, hydration, and density of lean tissue are being developed from a 4C model (73). BMI is an easy-to-obtain index and used clinically to screen children and adolescents even though it does not always accurately distinguish FM from FFM in these populations (23,70). Nevertheless, *z* scores for BMI and another easily obtained ratio, the WHR, were found to be significantly related to *z* scores for PBF determined by DXA in a large (<5,000), nationally representative sample of 8- to 19-year-old U.S. children enrolled in NHANES 2001–2004 (68). This study also revealed that WC and triceps skinfold were in close agreement to PBF (68). Additionally, a retrospective study of 2.3 million adolescents found that an increased BMI in late adolescents was strongly associated in cardiovascular mortality in young adulthood or midlife (69).

Skinfolds are commonly used to determine PBF in these populations, but the results have been mixed. Selection of the appropriate equation is critical as a multitude of specific equations have been developed for children and adolescents, but few have correlated well with DXA (57,67). However, PBF predicted from equations for 8- to 17-year-old American girls and boys, which utilized NHANES data, exhibit strong correlations of .91 and .94, respectively, with PBF as determined by DXA (57). Furthermore, these equations utilize measurements that are easy to obtain in the field (Table 6.3) and were developed using a large (3,334 boys and 2,040 girls) race/ethnicity diverse sample. Skinfold measures from triceps and subscapular sites have also been used to establish the relationship between PBF and chronic disease risk factors based on a sample over 12,000 6- to 18-year-old boys and girls enrolled in NHANES 1994–1998 and 1999–2004 (23).

Use of ADP for infants weighing up to 17.6 lb has been show using a 4C model to provide accurate and reliable body composition data using the Pea Pod (Life Measurement Instruments, Concord, CA) (19). For children 2–6 years old, use of a pediatric seat placed in the BOD POD has been found to have a standard error of estimate (SEE) of 2.09 PBF compared to a 4C model (20). The 4C model has also served as a reference to develop accurate prediction equations for the use of ADP in children and adolescents with obesity that are moderately better than DXA (74).

Table 6.3 Percent Body Fat Prediction Equation for 8- to 17-Year-Old American Children[a]

Gender	Equation[b]	R^2	Adj. R^2	RMSE
Girls	%BF = 31.836841 − 0.609018 × (menses) + 0.003317 × (age − 161) − 0.975391 × (Race1) + 0.499227 × (Race2) + 0.602171 × (Race3) + 0.173877 × (Race4) + 0.053756 × (weight − 56) − 18.641446 × (height − 1.58) + 0.218830 × (waist − 76) + 0.744310 × (triceps − 15) − 0.018648 × (triceps − 15)^2 − 0.194114 × (menses) × (triceps − 15) + 0.005748 × (menses) × (triceps)^2	0.829	0.828	2.744
Boys	%BF = 28.009373 − 0.038460 × (age − 161) − 0.425327 × (Race1) + 0.350376 × (Race2) − 0.238080 × (Race3) − 0.106154 × (Race4) − 0.113560 × (weight − 56) − 10.010607 × (height − 1.58) + 0.353623 × (waist − 76) + 0.690984 × (triceps − 15) − 0.016657 × (triceps − 15)^2 − 0.000852 × (age − 161) × (weight − 56)	0.888	0.888	2.624

RMSE, root mean square error; %BF, percent body fat.

[a]Intercept and coefficient values were calculated using the full dataset.

[b]Menses = menarche status (girls) is 0 if have not started period and 1 if started periods; Race1 = 1 if non-Hispanic African American and 0 if not non-Hispanic African American; Race2 = 1 if Mexican American and 0 if not Mexican American; Race3 = 1 if other Hispanic and 0 if not other Hispanic; Race4 = 1 if other non-Hispanic race group including non-Hispanic multiracial and 0 if not other non-Hispanic race group; weight = weight in kilograms; height = height in meters; waist = waist circumference in centimeters; triceps = triceps skinfolds in millimeters.

Source: Stevens J, Cai J, Truesdale KP, Cuttler L, Robinson TN, Roberts AL. Percent body fat prediction equations for 8- to 17-year-old American children. *Pediatr Obes*. 2013;9:261–71.

BIA estimates of PBF in children and adolescents compared with PBF determined by either 3C or 4C models have found BIA to be a practical method to use in these populations but susceptible to considerable measurement error (61). When compared with a 4C model, HW has been shown to underestimate PBF in children because of the difficulty in following the procedures of being submerged underwater and exhaling completely (21). Overall, much progress is being made to practically and accurately assess body composition of children and adolescents (23,36,37,57,61,68,70,73).

Body Fat Prediction Equation Selection

Regression equations are used to convert data collected from either skinfold, BIA, or ultrasound measurements to PBF. Presently, no clear guidelines exist to direct their development (2). Generalized equations, developed from heterogeneous samples, account for differences in age, sex, ethnicity, and other characteristics by including these variables as predictors in the equation and can be applied to diverse populations (24,28,60). In this regard, 28 equations have recently been developed to predict PBF in Americans 8 years and older using easily obtained demographic and anthropometric measures that can be entered into a Web site (American Body Composition Calculator: http://ABCC.sph.unc.edu) to calculate PBF (58). PBF from these equations compared with 1999–2006 NHANES PBF data derived from DXA resulted in an R^2 that ranged from 0.664 to 0.845 in males and from 0.748 to 0.809 in females (58). Additionally, equations using simple anthropometric measurements (*e.g.*, height, weight, WC) have been validated (men R^2 = 0.79; women R^2 = 0.84) using MRI as the reference method to predict adipose tissue mass and total FM (2).

In contrast with generalized equations, population-specific equations that account for differences in the density of FFM are developed from homogeneous samples based on a restricted combination of age, sex, race or ethnicity, sport status, or a clinical condition resulting in a more accurate estimate of PBF when applied to this distinctive population (28,58). The validity of existing specific and generalized equations was recently examined using a large (~10,000 adults), diverse sample from the 1994–2004 NHANES data that included PBF determined by DXA (14). Box 4.3 of *GETP10* (3) lists generalized equations that allow calculation of body composition from skinfolds, whereas population-specific equations are provided in Table 4.3 of *GETP10* (3).

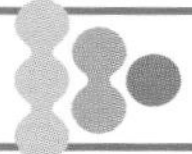

Interpretation of Body Fat Percentage Estimates

Interpretation of body fat percentage estimates is complicated by three factors: (a) lack of established and accepted universal standards for PBF; (b) all methods of measurement are indirect, so error needs to be considered; and (c) there is no universally accepted criterion measurement method. The American College of Sports Medicine (ACSM) in *GETP10* (3) states, "A consensus opinion for an exact PBF value associated with optimal health risk has yet to be defined; however, a range of 10%–22% and 20%–32% for men and women, respectively, has long been viewed as satisfactory for health." Standards may be based on health or physical performance, but only sex is considered a differentiating factor in PBF classifications (Fig. 6.2).

The *GETP10* (3) includes the normative-based standards developed by The Cooper Institute in Dallas, Texas. These norms were revised in 1994 and were developed using skinfold measurements to estimate body fat percentage in a population of predominately White and college-educated men and women (3, Tables 4.4 and 4.5).

Measurement Error Considerations

A major concern in interpreting body fat percentage values is the relatively large SEE of the measurements (*e.g.*, ±3.5% for skinfold equations) (58). For example, a 45-yr-old woman

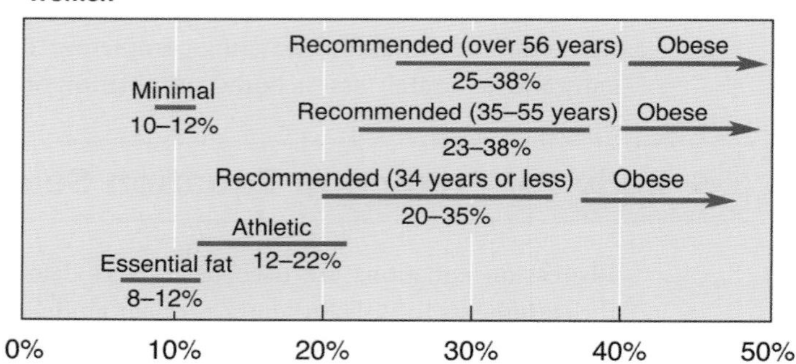

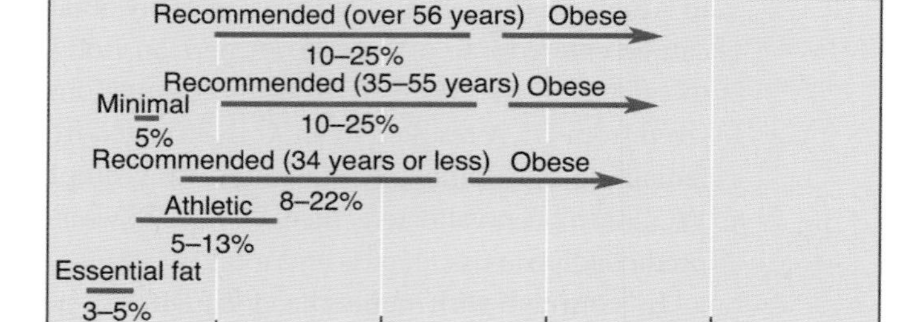

FIGURE 6.2. Percent body fat standards for men and women. (Reprinted from American College of Sports Medicine. *ACSM's Resource Manual for Exercise Testing and Prescription*. 7th ed. Philadelphia [PA]: Wolters Kluwer; 2014. Figure 18.3.)

who had a PBF of 28.5% based on skinfold measurements (35th percentile) could be as low as 21.5% (70th percentile) or as high as 35.5% (10th percentile) when considering the 95% confidence interval (CI) (±2 SEE). Because of the lack of accepted national standards and the large SEE, interpretation of PBF estimates needs to be done with caution and shared with patients only after careful explanation of the meaning of the values. The most appropriate use of these estimates may be for serial measurements over time to evaluate responses to diet or physical activity where the same measurement procedure (*i.e.*, instrument and technician) is used.

SUMMARY

Assessing body composition is essential for determining and tracking health status and aids in optimizing physical performance; therefore, it is of great importance for health care providers, fitness practitioners, and athletic personnel to be knowledgeable about the advantages as well as the limitations, of various body composition methods.

In most healthy, nonathletic adults, a reasonable assessment of excess weight status can be determined from simple measurements of height, weight, and waist circumference. These measurements are easy to obtain, do not require extensive training to perform, and do not require expensive equipment.

Skinfold measurements, underwater weighing, BIA and ADP are routinely utilized.

More advanced body composition methods such as DXA, CT, positron emission tomography, MRI, ultrasound, and isotopic dilution may be employed when more specific information is needed, and the financial resources, equipment, and highly trained personnel are available.

REFERENCES

1. Ackland TR, Lohman TG, Sundgot-Borgen J, et al. Current status of body composition assessment in sport: review and position statement on behalf of the Ad Hoc Research Working Group on Body Composition Health and Performance, under the auspices of the I.O.C. Medical Commission. *Sports Med.* 2012:42(3):227–49.
2. Al-Gindan YY, Hankey CR, Govan L, Gallagher D, Heymsfield SB, Lean ME. Derivation and validation of simple anthropometric equations to predict adipose tissue mass and total fat mass with MRI as the reference method. *Br J Nutr.* 2015;114:1852–67.
3. American College of Sports Medicine. *ACSM's Guidelines for Exercise Testing and Prescription.* 10th ed. Philadelphia (PA): Wolters Kluwer; 2018. 480 p.
4. Battaglini C, Naumann F, Groff D, Shields E, Hackney AC, Peppercorn J. Comparison of body composition assessment methods in breast cancer survivors. *Oncol Nurs Forum.* 2011;38(4):E283–90.
5. Bazzocchi A, Filonzi G, Ponti F, Albisinni U, Guglielmi G, Battista G. Ultrasound: which role in body composition? *Eur J Radiol.* 2016;85(8):1469–80.
6. Bhaskaran K, Douglas I, Forbes H, dos-Santos-Silva I, Leon DA, Smeeth L. Body-mass index and risk of 22 specific cancers: a population-based cohort study of 5.24 million UK adults. *Lancet.* 2014;384:755–65.
7. Bray GA. Don't throw the baby out with the bath water. *Am J Clin Nutr.* 2004;79:347–9.
8. Cameron AJ, Magliano DJ, Söderberg SC. A systematic review of the impact of including both waist and hip circumference in risk models for cardiovascular diseases, diabetes and mortality. *Obes Rev.* 2013;14:86–94.
9. Camhi SM, Bray GA, Bouchard C, et al. The relationship of waist circumference and BMI to visceral, subcutaneous, and total body fat: sex and race differences. *Obesity (Silver Spring).* 2011;19:402–8.
10. Casey AF. Measuring body composition in individuals with intellectual disability: a scoping review. *J Obes.* 2013;2013:628428.
11. Cerhan JR, Moore SC, Jacobs EJ, et al. A pooled analysis of waist circumference and mortality in 650,000 adults. *Mayo Clin Proc.* 2014;89(3):335–45.
12. Choi A, Kim JY, Jo S, et al. Smartphone-based bioelectrical impedance analysis devices for daily obesity management. *Sensors (Basel).* 2015;15:22151–66.
13. Clarys JP, Scafoglieri A, Provyn S, Sesboüé B, Van Roy P. Hazards of hydrodensitometry. *J Sports Med Phys Fitness.* 2011;51:95–102.

14. Cui Z, Truesdale KP, Cai J, Stevens J. Evaluation of anthropometric equations to assess body fat in adults: NHANES 1999-2004. *Med Sci Sports Exerc.* 2014;46(6):1147–58.
15. Decaria JE, Sharp C, Petrella RJ. Scoping review report: obesity in older adults. *Int J Obes (Lond).* 2012;36:1141–50.
16. Després JP. Body fat distribution and risk of cardiovascular disease: an update. *Circulation.* 2012;126:1301–13.
17. Després JP. Waist circumference as a vital sign in cardiology 20 years after its initial publication in the *American Journal of Cardiology*. *Am J Cardiol.* 2014;114:320–3.
18. Di Sebastiano KM, Mourtzakis M. A critical evaluation of body composition modalities used to assess adipose and skeletal muscle tissue in cancer. *Appl Physiol Nutr Metab.* 2012;37:811–21.
19. Ellis KJ, Yao M, Shypailo RJ, Urlando A, Wong WW, Heird WC. Body-composition assessment in infancy: air-displacement plethysmography compared with a reference 4-compartment model. *Am J Clin Nutr.* 2007;85(1):90–5.
20. Fields DA, Allison DB. Air-displacement plethysmography pediatric option in 2–6 years old using the four-compartment model as a criterion method. *Obesity (Silver Spring).* 2012;20(8):1732–7.
21. Fields DA, Goran MI. Body composition techniques and the four-compartment model in children. *J Appl Physiol.* 2000;89(2): 613–20.
22. Fosbøl MØ, Zerahn B. Contemporary methods of body composition measurement. *Clin Physiol Funct Imaging.* 2015;35:81–97.
23. Going SB, Lohman TG, Cussler EC, Williams DP, Morrison JA, Horn PS. Percent body fat and chronic disease risk factors in U.S. children and youth. *Am J Prev Med.* 2011;41(4 suppl 2):S77–86.
24. Graves JE, Kanaley JA, Garzarella L, Pollock ML. Anthropometry and body composition measurement. In: Maud PJ, Foster C, editors. *Physiological Assessment of Human Fitness.* 2nd ed. Champaign (IL): Human Kinetics; 2006. p. 185–225.
25. Heymsfield SB, Gonzalez MCC, Shen W, Redman L, Thomas D. Weight loss composition is one-fourth fat-free mass: a critical review and critique of this widely cited rule. *Obes Rev.* 2014;15(4):310–21.
26. Heymsfield SB, Lohman TG, Wang Z, Going SB, editors. *Human Body Composition.* 2nd ed. Champaign (IL): Human Kinetics; 2005. 356 p.
27. Heymsfield SB, Peterson CM, Thomas DM, et al. Scaling of adult body weight to height across sex and race/ethnic groups: relevance to BMI. *Am J Clin Nutr.* 2014;100:1455–61.
28. Heyward VH, Gibson AL. Assessing body composition. In: Heyward VH, Gibson AL, editors. *Advanced Fitness Assessment and Exercise Prescription.* 7th ed. Champaign (IL): Human Kinetics; 2014. p. 219–65.
29. Janssen I, Katzmarzyk PT, Ross R. Waist circumference and not body mass index explains obesity-related health risk. *Am J Clin Nutr.* 2004;79:379–84.
30. Jensen MD, Ryan DH, Apovian CM, et al. 2013 AHA/ACC/TOS guideline for the management of overweight and obesity in adults: a report of the American College of Cardiology/American Heart Association Task Force on Practice Guidelines and The Obesity Society. *J Am Coll Cardiol.* 2014;63(25 pt B):2985–3023.
31. Joy E, De Souza MJ, Nattiv A, et al. 2014 Female Athlete Triad Coalition consensus statement on treatment and return to play of the female athlete triad. *Curr Sports Med Rep.* 2014;13(4):219–32.
32. Kanellakis S, Manios Y. Validation of five simple models estimating body fat in White postmenopausal women: use in clinical practice and research. *Obesity (Silver Spring).* 2012;20:1329–32.
33. Katzmarzyk PT, Bray GA, Greenway FL, et al. Racial differences in abdominal depot-specific adiposity in White and African American adults. *Am J Clin Nutr.* 2010;91:7–15.
34. Katzmarzyk PT, Mire E, Bray GA, Greenway FL, Heymsfield SB, Bouchard C. Anthropometric markers of obesity and mortality in White and African American adults: the Pennington Longitudinal Study. *Obesity (Silver Spring).* 2013;21(5):1070–5.
35. Lee WS. Body fatness charts based on BMI and waist circumference. *Obesity (Silver Spring).* 2016;24(1):245–9.
36. Lohman TG, Hingle M, Going SB. Body composition in children. *Pediatr Exerc Sci.* 2013;25:573–90.
37. Malina RM, Geithner CA. Body composition of young athletes. *Am J Lifestyle Med.* 2011;5:262–78.
38. Marfell-Jones M, Nevill AM, Steward AD. Anthropometric surrogates for fatness and health. In: Stewart AD, Sutton L, editors. *Body Composition in Sport, Exercise and Health.* London (United Kingdom): Routledge; 2012. p. 126–46.
39. Meyer NL, Sundgot-Borgen J, Lohman TG, et al. Body composition for health and performance: a survey of body composition assessment practice carried out by the Ad Hoc Research Working Group on Body Composition, Health and Performance under the auspices of the IOC Medical Commission. *Br J Sports Med.* 2013;47:1044–53.
40. Moon JR. Body composition in athletes and sports nutrition: an examination of bioimpedance analysis technique. *Eur J Clin Nutr.* 2013;67(suppl 1):S54–9.
41. Moon JR, Tobkin SE, Roberts MD, et al. Total body water estimations in healthy men and women using bioimpedance spectroscopy: a deuterium oxide comparison. *Nutr Metab (Lond).* 2008;5:7.
42. Mountjoy M, Sundgot-Borgen J, Burke L, et al. The IOC consensus statement: beyond the Female Athlete Triad — relative energy deficiency in sport (RED-S). *Br J Sports Med.* 2014;48:491–7.
43. Müller MJ, Baracos V, Bosy-Westphal A, et al. Functional body composition and related aspects in research on obesity and cachexia: report on the 12th Stock Conference held on 6 and 7 September 2013 in Hamburg, Germany. *Obes Rev.* 2014;15(8):640–56.
44. Nakamura K, Fuster JJ, Walsh K. Adipokines: a link between obesity and cardiovascular disease. *J Cardiol.* 2014;63(4):250–9.
45. National Center for Health Statistics. *National Health and Nutrition Examination Survey* [Internet]. Atlanta (GA): Centers for Disease Control and Prevention; [cited 2017 Jan 29]. Available from: http://www.cdc.gov/nchs/nhanes.htm

46. Ng M, Fleming T, Robinson M, et al. Global, regional, and national prevalence of overweight and obesity in children and adults 1980-2013: a systematic analysis. *Lancet*. 2014;384(9945):766–81.
47. Ogden CL, Carroll MD, Kit BK, Flegal KM. Prevalence of childhood and adult obesity in the United States, 2011-2012. *JAMA*. 2014;311(8):806–14.
48. Ortega FB, Lavie CJ, Blair SN. Obesity and cardiovascular disease. *Circ Res*. 2016;118:1752–70.
49. Ortega FB, Sui X, Lavine CJ, Blair SN. Body mass index, the most widely used but also widely criticized index: would a criterion standard measure of total body fat be a better predictor of cardiovascular disease mortality? *Mayo Clin Proc*. 2016;91(4):443–55.
50. Patel AV, Hildebrand JS, Gapstur SM. Body mass index and all-cause mortality in a large prospective cohort of White and Black U.S. adults. *PLoS One*. 2014;9(10):e109153.
51. Peterson CM, Thomas DM, Blackburn GL, Heymsfield SB. Universal equation for estimating ideal body weight and body weight at any BMI. *Am J Clin Nutr*. 2016;103:1197–203.
52. Pourhassan M, Schautz B, Braun W, Gluer CC, Bosy-Westphal A, Müller MJ. Impact of body-composition methodology on the composition of weight loss and weight gain. *Eur J Clin Nutr*. 2013;67:446–54.
53. Ross R, Berentzen T, Bradshaw AJ, et al. Does the relationship between waist circumference, morbidity and mortality depend on measurement protocol for waist circumference? *Obes Rev*. 2008;9:312–25.
54. Roy B, Curtis ME, Fears LS, Nahashon SN, Fentress HM. Molecular mechanisms of obesity-induced osteoporosis and muscle atrophy. *Front Physiol*. 2016;7:439.
55. Seabolt LA, Welch EB, Silver HJ. Imaging methods for analyzing body composition in human obesity and cardiometabolic disease. *Ann N Y Acad Sci*. 2015;1353:41–59.
56. Sharma S, Batsis JA, Coutinho T, et al. Normal-weight central obesity and mortality risk in older adults with coronary artery disease. *Mayo Clin Proc*. 2016;9(3):343–51.
57. Stevens J, Cai J, Truesdale KP, Cuttler L, Robinson TN, Roberts AL. Percent body fat prediction equations for 8- to 17-year-old American children. *Pediatr Obes*. 2013;9:261–71.
58. Stevens J, Ou F-S, Cai J, Heymsfield SB, Truesdale KP. Prediction of percent body fat measurements in Americans 8 years and older. *Int J Obes (Lond)*. 2016;40:587–94.
59. Stewart AD, Sutton L, editors. *Body Composition in Sport, Exercise and Health*. London (United Kingdom): Routledge; 2012. 218 p.
60. Swain DP, editor. Body composition status and assessment. In: DP Swain, editor. *ACSM's Resource Manual for Guidelines for Exercise Testing and Prescription*. 7th ed. Philadelphia (PA): Lippincott Williams & Wilkins; 2014. p. 287–308.
61. Talma H, Chinapaw MJM, Bakker B, HiraSing RA, Terwee CB, Altenburg TM. Bioelectrical impedance analysis to estimate body composition in children and adolescents: a systematic review and evidence appraisal of validity, responsiveness, reliability and measurement error. *Obes Rev*. 2013;14:895–905.
62. Tenforde AS, Barrack MT, Nattiv A, Fredericson M. Parallels with the female athlete triad in male athletes. *Sports Med*. 2016; 46:171–82.
63. Thibault R, Genton L, Pichard C. Body composition: why, when and for who? *Clin Nutr*. 2012;31:435–47.
64. Tomiyama AJ, Hunger JM, Nguyen-Cuu J, Wells C. Misclassification of cardiometabolic health when using body mass index categories in NHANES 2005–2012. *Int J Obes*. 2016;40(5):883–6.
65. Tran ZV, Weltman A. Generalized equation for predicting body density of women from girth measurements. *Med Sci Sports Exerc*. 1989;21(1):101–4.
66. Tran ZV, Weltman A. Predicting body composition of men from girth measurements. *Hum Biol*. 1988;60(1):167–75.
67. Truesdale KP, Roberts A, Cai J, Berge JM, Stevens J. Comparison of eight equations that predict percent body fat using skinfolds in American youth. *Child Obes*. 2016;12(4):314–23.
68. Tuan NT, Wang Y. Adiposity assessments: agreement between dual-energy X-ray absorptiometry and anthropometric measures in U.S. children. *Obesity (Silver Spring)*. 2014;22(6):1495–504.
69. Twig G, Yaniv G, Levine H, et al. Body-mass index in 2.3 million adolescents and cardiovascular death in adulthood. *N Engl J Med*. 2016;374(25):2430–40.
70. U.S. Preventive Services Task Force. Screening for obesity in children and adolescents: US Preventive Services Task Force recommendation statement. *Pediatrics*. 2010;125(2):361–7.
71. Viester L, Verhagen EA, Oude Hengel KM, et al. The relationship between body mass index and musculoskeletal symptoms in the working population. *BMC Musculoskelet Disord*. 2013;14:238.
72. Wang J, Thornton JC, Bari S, et al. Comparisons of waist circumferences measured at 4 sites. *Am J Clin Nutr*. 2003;77:379–84.
73. Wells JC. Toward body composition reference data for infants, children, and adolescents. *Adv Nutr*. 2014;5:320S–9S.
74. Wells JCK, Haroun D, Williams JE, et al. Evaluation of lean tissue density for use in air displacement plethysmography in obese children and adolescents. *Eur J Clin Nutr*. 2011;65:1094–101.
75. Weltman A, Levine S, Seip RL, Tran ZV. Accurate assessment of body composition in obese females. *Am J Clin Nutr*. 1988; 48(5):1179–83.
76. Widen EM, Gallagher D. Body composition changes in pregnancy: measurement, predictors and outcomes. *Eur J Clin Nutr*. 2014; 68:643–52.
77. World Health Organization. *Waist Circumferences and Waist-hip Ratio: Report of WHO Expert Consultation*. Geneva (Switzerland): World Health Organization; 2008. 39 p.

CHAPTER 7

Flexibility and Functional Movement Assessments

INTRODUCTION

Assessments for flexibility and **functional movement ability** have historically been treated as less significant than muscular and cardiovascular assessments in determining the overall fitness level of an individual. This finding is evident in both the low number of flexibility assessments reported in previous texts and the lack of development of newer assessments. Likewise, the widespread use of functional movement assessments by sport coaches and personal trainers, and inclusion of these assessments in the determination of fitness, prompted their inclusion in this text. Given that an individual's ability to move through a **range of motion (ROM)** will determine if that person can properly complete other fitness-related assessments (**muscular strength**, **muscular endurance** test, or cardiovascular assessment), it is appropriate to properly assess both flexibility and functional movement as equal in importance to muscular and cardiovascular ability. Flexibility assessment is important because there is an associated decrease in performance of **activities of daily living (ADL)** with inadequate flexibility. Consequently, maintaining flexibility of all joints facilitates movement and may prevent injury; in contrast, when an activity moves the structures of a joint beyond its full ROM, tissue damage can occur.

This chapter covers commonly used assessments, their strengths and limitations, and available normative data.

Flexibility

Labeling an individual as "flexible" is a misnomer because flexibility is joint specific just as muscular strength and endurance is specific to the muscles involved. **Flexibility** is not a general term but rather depends on the muscle and joint that is being evaluated, the distensibility of the joint capsule, presence of an adequate warm-up, muscle viscosity, and the tightness of surrounding ligaments and tendons. Therefore, no single test can characterize overall flexibility, but measurements taken at several joints will give an overall impression of flexibility or lack thereof.

Sit-and-Reach Test

The sit-and-reach test is the most widely utilized test for assessment of flexibility mainly because of its simplicity and ability to be performed by just about anyone. The sit-and-reach test is performed either with a sit-and-reach box, a properly placed tape measure, or in a modified manner in a chair and is valid and reliable for evaluating flexibility of the hamstrings, hip, and lower back, which is important to the prevention of chronic lower back pain and the promotion of a healthy lifestyle (9,11).

The sit-and-reach test has been commonly used to assess low back and hamstring flexibility; however, its relationship to predict the incidence of low back pain is limited (4). The sit-and-reach test is suggested to be a better measure of hamstring flexibility than low back flexibility (7). The relative importance of hamstring flexibility to ADL and sports performance supports the inclusion of the sit-and-reach test for health-related fitness testing until a criterion measure evaluation of low back flexibility is available.

The most important limitation of the sit-and-reach test is that it only measures flexibility at a single joint and movement (hip flexion), and although it is an important measure, it cannot be used to generalize overall flexibility of the individual because no other joints are measured. Many fitness batteries use only the sit-and-reach test to measure flexibility, thereby providing an incomplete assessment of overall flexibility. Furthermore, it is not uncommon to see the results of the fitness assessment interpreted as overall flexibility, although only a single flexibility assessment was utilized. This inaccurate interpretation of the results cannot provide an indication of overall flexibility.

The procedure for performing the Canadian trunk forward flexion test, which is measured in centimeters, is provided in Box 7.1. Fitness categories by age groups and gender for the Canadian trunk forward flexion test are provided in Table 7.1. The protocol for the Young Men's Christian Association (YMCA) sit-and-reach test and fitness data are published elsewhere (6).

Individual Joint Measurements

Every joint in the body has an acceptable and normal ROM, which is dependent on various factors, including genetics, orthopedic health, muscular tension, and strength. Laboratory tests usually quantify flexibility in terms of ROM expressed in degrees as measured with either a goniometer or an inclinometer (Fig. 7.1). Measurement of ROM is particularly useful in athletic training, rehabilitation, and conditioning settings; however, the measurements can be misleading if performed without standard procedures, calibration, and instruments. A precise measurement of joint ROM can be assessed at most anatomic joints following the procedures outlined in Box 7.2 and compared with norms provided in Table 7.2.

As with **strength** testing, consistency and accuracy during flexibility assessment are critical for obtaining meaningful data. Several factors that may compromise accuracy if not performed

Box 7.1 Canadian Trunk Forward Flexion (Sit-and-Reach) Test Procedures

Pretest: Participants should perform a short warm-up prior to this test and include some stretches. It is also recommended that the participant refrain from fast, jerky movements, which may increase the possibility of an injury. The participant's shoes should be removed.

1. The participant sits with the soles of their feet flat against a sit-and-reach box with the zero mark at the 26 cm. Inner edges of the soles should be 6 in (15.2 cm) apart. (Note the zero point at the foot/box interface and use the appropriate norms.)
2. The participant should slowly reach forward with both hands as far as possible, holding this position approximately 2 seconds. Be sure that the participant keeps the hands parallel and does not lead with one hand, or bounce. Fingertips can be overlapped and should be in contact with the measuring portion of the sit-and-reach box.
3. The score is the most distant point (cm) reached with the fingertips. The better of two trials should be recorded. To assist with the best attempt, the participant should exhale and drop their head between the arms when reaching. Testers should ensure that the knees of the participant stay extended; however, the participant's knees should not be pressed down. The participant should breathe normally during the test and should not hold their breath at any time.

Norms for the Canadian test are presented in Table 7.1. Note that these norms use a sit-and-reach box in which the "zero" point is at the 26 cm mark. If a box is used in which the zero point is set at 23 cm (*e.g.*, FitnessGram), subtract 3 cm from each value in this table.

Reprinted with permission from Canadian Society for Exercise Physiology. *Canadian Society for Exercise Physiology — Physical Activity Training for Health (CSEP-PATH) Resource Manual*. Ottawa (Canada): Canadian Society for Exercise Physiology; 2013.

Table 7.1 Fitness Categories for Canadian Trunk Forward Flexion Test Using a Sit-and-Reach Box (cm) by Age and Sex

	Age (yr)									
Category	20–29		30–39		40–49		50–59		60–69	
Sex	M	W	M	W	M	W	M	W	M	W
Excellent	≥40	≥41	≥38	≥41	≥35	≥38	≥35	≥39	≥33	≥35
Very good	34–39	37–40	33–37	36–40	29–34	34–37	28–34	33–38	25–32	31–34
Good	30–33	33–36	28–32	32–35	24–28	30–33	24–27	30–32	20–24	27–30
Fair	25–29	28–32	23–27	27–31	18–23	25–29	16–23	25–29	15–19	23–26
Poor	≤24	≤27	≤22	≤26	≤17	≤24	≤15	≤24	≤14	≤22

M, men; W, women.
These norms are based on a sit-and-reach box in which the "zero" point is set at 26 cm. When using a box in which the zero point is set at 23 cm, subtract 3 cm from each value in this table.

Reprinted with permission from the Canadian Society for Exercise Physiology. *Canadian Society for Exercise Physiology — Physical Activity Training for Health (CSEP-PATH) Resource Manual*. Ottawa (Canada): Canadian Society for Exercise Physiology; 2013.

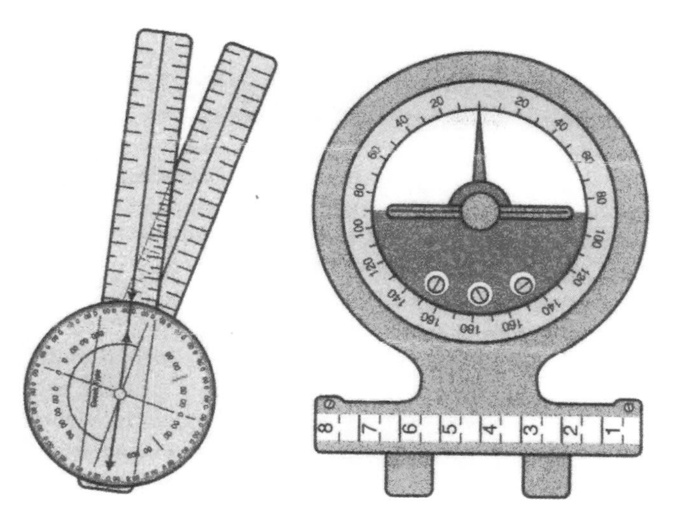

FIGURE 7.1. Devices used for measuring joint range of motion. **A.** Standard goniometer *(left)*. **B.** Mechanical inclinometer *(right)*. (From Swain DP. *ACSM's Resource Manual for Guidelines for Exercise Testing and Prescription.* 7th ed. Philadelphia [PA]: Wolters Kluwer; 2014. Fig. 22.5.)

Table 7.2 Range of Motion of Select Single Joint Movements in Degrees

	Degrees		Degrees
Shoulder Girdle Movement			
Flexion	90–120	Extension	20–60
Abduction	80–100		
Horizontal abduction	30–45	Horizontal adduction	90–135
Medial rotation	70–90	Lateral rotation	70–90
Elbow Movement			
Flexion	135–160		
Supination	75–90	Pronation	75–90
Trunk Movement			
Flexion	120–150	Extension	20–45
Lateral flexion	10–35	Rotation	20–40
Hip Movement			
Flexion	90–135	Extension	10–30
Abduction	30–50	Adduction	10–30
Medial rotation	30–45	Lateral rotation	45–60
Knee Movement			
Flexion	130–140	Extension	5–10
Ankle Movement			
Dorsiflexion	15–20	Plantar flexion	30–50
Inversion	10–30	Eversion	10–20

Adapted from Norkin CC, Levangie PK. *Joint Structure and Function: A Comprehensive Analysis.* 5th ed. Philadelphia (PA): F.A. Davis; 2011. 588 p.

Box 7.2 Procedures for Measuring Range of Motion with a Goniometer

1. Place the patient in the recommended testing position.
2. Stabilize the proximal joint component.
3. Move the distal joint component through the available ROM. Make sure the ROM is performed slowly and that the end of the range is attained and end-feel determined.
4. Return distal joint component to the starting position.
5. Palpate bony anatomic landmarks.
6. Align the goniometer, placing the stabilization and movement arms so that they are centered along each body segment according to the landmarks for each joint measurement.
7. Read and record the starting position.
8. Stabilize proximal joint segment.
9. Move the distal component through the full ROM.
10. Read and record ROM.

consistently include anatomic landmark identification, positioning and stabilization of the body, application and stabilization of the measurement device, consistency in technique and protocol, appropriate recording of measures, and recognition of limiting factors or situations during recording. In order for a specific joint ROM to be compared with available norms, standardized landmarks for each measurement should be identified and used whenever possible.

Several commonly measured joints have standard landmarks identified and should be used consistently when measuring ROM. Inaccurate identification of bony or surface landmarks is a common source of error during assessment; therefore, knowledge of surface anatomy is required before accurate measurements can be recorded. In addition to stabilizing body segments, the measurement device must also be properly positioned to ensure data accuracy. The technician should be familiar with the device being used as well as the methodology and biomechanics. Inappropriate placement and use of the device represents a major source of error in many studies examining ROM (4).

Goniometer

The most common instrument used for measuring joint ROM is the two-arm **goniometer** (see Fig. 7.1). This device is portable, relatively easy to use, and inexpensive. Moreover, the measurements obtained are highly reproducible. The transparent plastic device includes two arms with a protractor for measuring degrees of joint displacement. One arm remains fixed to the proximal articulating segment (*e.g.*, upper arm), and the other adjusts through the ROM with the distal segment (*e.g.*, forearm), measuring the resulting degree of movement. The center of the protractor remains fixed at the joint's axis of rotation.

Limitations of the conventional goniometer include difficulty stabilizing moving segments and visually determining a vertical axis; however, higher validity and reliability are demonstrated when proper procedures are followed (4). When using a goniometer, the proximal segment of the joint should be stabilized, and the distal segment remains freely moveable. Body position should be conducive to the movement being measured and comfortable for the subject. Joints can be measured in varied positions; however, reliability depends on reproducibility of the position. The patient should be able to maintain the reference position without performing extraneous movement during the measurement.

A newer alternative to the traditional goniometer is a goniometer "app" available for most smartphones (available at the App Store). These apps act as a digital gravity inclinometer by using the accelerometer chip built into most smartphones to calculate the angle of rotation and measure ROM. Several goniometer apps such as Goniometer, MyKnee, and Goniometer Pro (G-Pro) are available for most smartphones. Each has different applications, uses, and price, but all measure angles to within 0.1°. Of particular interest are those apps such as Goniometer for English that allow you to measure angles achieved during movement using video clips you have taken of the individual.

Inclinometer

Spinal and other complex movements, including supination, pronation, ankle inversion, and eversion, are difficult if not impossible to assess with a traditional goniometer. Such data are more accurately measured using an **inclinometer** (see Fig. 7.1). Inclinometers use a universal center of gravity to establish a starting point that remains constant from test to test. The pendulum-weighted inclinometer indicates degrees of motion using a weighted needle and protractor. As with the goniometer, careful placement of the inclinometer is crucial to obtaining an accurate measurement. The American Medical Association (1) suggests that ROM should be measured using the average of three consecutive trials.

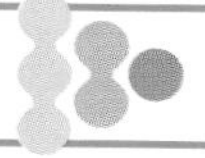

Functional Movement Assessments

Functional movement assessments, or movement screens, are commonly used by both clinicians and practitioners in order to determine an individual's movement proficiency, predict potential injury, and design appropriate training and rehabilitation programs (3–5,8). Until recently, movement screens have been largely based on the qualitative assessment. However, in recent years, a growing body of research has attempted to quantify movement quality in order to allow a more efficient and consistent method for establishing one's current movement efficiency and to provide a consistent rating system to gauge improvement in movement ability over time (4,5). Although more research is needed on many of these assessments, they provide the practitioner and clinician with some foundational tools to assess quality of movement and prescribe appropriate training **exercise**. In turn, this may reduce muscular imbalances/asymmetries and determine readiness to participate in certain weight training activities.

The Functional Movement Screen

The Functional Movement Screen (FMS) is a series of seven tests and three clearing assessments developed to provide the practitioner with a basic snapshot of potential movement constraints that may also predict injury (5). This test is scored on a scale of 0–3, with 3 = being optimal, 2 = being satisfactory, 1 = being unsatisfactory, and 0 = being the score if pain is present while performing a movement (3,4). Traditionally, the acceptable score for the FMS is a minimum of 14 points; however, if the participant receives a low score (<2) on any single test or unequal scores on tests that assess each side of the body (*i.e.*, a score of 2 on the left side and 3 on the right side), additional tests to address deficits may be needed (2,8).

Although some researchers have investigated the ability of the FMS to predict performance, this practice likely should be avoided because this screen was specifically designed to identify areas of deficiency in mobility and stability that may lead to injury in individuals who are asymptomatic and has not been found to relate to predictors of athletic success (3,4,12). When performed by trained individuals, the FMS has demonstrated good reliability (10,13). Box 7.3 provides instructions for administering the FMS.

Box 7.3 Functional Movement Screen

1. Deep Squat

The deep squat assessment is used to assess bilateral, symmetrical, and functional mobility of the hips, knees, and ankles. Additionally, the use of the dowel held overhead during this assessment helps in determining bilateral, symmetrical mobility of the shoulders as well as the thoracic spine.

Instructions:

- Stand with the feet pointing straight ahead and approximately shoulder width apart.
- While holding the dowel with both hands, place it directly on top of the head and position the arms so the elbows are bent at approximately 90°.
- Extend both arms to press the dowel straight up over the head.
- Squat as low as possible while keeping the dowel aligned over the feet.
- If the individual is unable to achieve a rating of 3 on this assessment, the individual should elevate the heels by placing them on a 2 × 6 board.

Scoring:

3 = The following criteria must be met:
- Upper torso and tibia should be parallel to one another, or torso is near vertical.
- The femur should be below horizontal in relation to the ground.
- The feet should be straight ahead, and the knees should be aligned over the feet while keeping the heels in full contact with the ground.
- The dowel should be aligned over the feet.

2 = All of the previous criteria to score a 3 must be met; however, the individual had to elevate the heels on a 2 × 6 board.

1 = Individual was unable to perform the movement even after they were allowed to elevate the heels.

0 = If any pain was experienced by the individual while performing this movement

2. Hurdle Step

The hurdle step assesses bilateral functional mobility and stability of the hips, knees, and ankles while attempting to replicate proper stride mechanics during a stepping motion.

Instructions:

- To create the hurdle, place a strip of masking tape across an open doorway at the height of the participant's tibial tuberosity.
- Hold the dowel across shoulder blades as when performing a back squat; place the feet approximately hip width apart. Stand with toes directly under the tape.
- Once in position, lift one foot up and over the hurdle, tap the heel to the ground on the opposite side, and return to the starting position without touching the hurdle.
- Repeat with other foot.
- Score both movements independently.
- The final score for this assessment should be the lowest of the raw scores.

Scoring:

3 = All of the following criteria must be met:
- The hips, knees, and ankles should remain aligned in the sagittal plane.
- Minimal, or no, movement is noted in the lumbar spine.
- The dowel should remain parallel in relation to the hurdle.

2 = The individual performs the movement with some compensation.

1 = Was unable to perform the movement, was unable to maintain balance, or contact between the foot and hurdle occurs

0 = If any pain was experienced by the individual while performing this movement

3. Inline Lunge

The inline lunge assesses hip and ankle mobility and stability, quadriceps flexibility, and knee stability while forcing the individual to resist rotation and maintain proper trunk alignment.

Instructions:

- Cut a piece of masking tape the length of the lower leg (from the tibial tuberosity to the floor). Place this tape on the floor.
- The toes of the back foot should be placed on the back end of the tape while keeping the heel flat and the foot pointed straight ahead.
- The heel of the front foot should be positioned at the other end of the tape.
- Hold the dowel so it is in contact with the back of the head, upper back, and buttocks. If the left foot is in front, hold the top of the dowel with the right hand, and the other hand positioned against the lumbar spine. Vice versa if right foot is in front.
- Without moving the feet, bend both knees to lower the rear knee toward the front heel. Do not touch the knee to the floor. Return to starting position and repeat twice more.
- Switch the feet and arm positions and then perform this movement on the opposite side.
- Score both movements independently.
- The final score for this assessment should be the lowest of the raw scores.

Scoring:

3 = The following criteria must be met:
  - Front foot must remain flat on the floor; heel cannot lift.
  - Rear knee must come in contact with front heel.
  - Cannot lean upper body forward, left or right

2 = Individual performs this movement with some compensation.

1 = Unable to perform the movement; was unable to maintain balance

0 = If any pain was experienced by the individual while performing this movement

4. Shoulder Mobility

The shoulder mobility screen assesses bilateral shoulder ROM. This screen may also be used to assess normal scapular mobility and thoracic spine extension.

Instructions:

- Measure the distance between the base of the palm and the end of the middle finger.
- Stand with the feet together and arms hanging comfortably.
- Make two fists, so that the fingers are around the thumbs, and extend both arms directly out to the sides at shoulder level.
- In one smooth motion, place the right fist overhead and down the back as far as possible while simultaneously taking the left fist up the back as far as possible.
- Do not "creep" the hands closer after their initial placement or attempt to get greater ROM by arching the back.
- Score this movement by measuring the distance between both fists.
- Perform this same motion with the left fist on top and right fist on bottom and repeat this assessment in the same manner.
- Score both movements independently.
- The final score for this assessment should be the lowest of the raw scores.

(continued)

Box 7.3 Functional Movement Screen *(continued)*

Scoring: Score the movement and then perform the Shoulder Clearing Test as described in the following text:

3 = Fists are within 1 hand length of one another (as measured in step 1).
2 = Fists are within 1 ½ hand lengths away from one another.
1 = Fists are greater than 1 ½ hand lengths away from one another.
0 = If any pain was experienced by the individual while performing this movement

Shoulder Clearing Test:

- Stand tall with the feet together and the arms hanging comfortably at the sides.
- Place the palm of the right hand completely flat, on the front of the left shoulder.
- While maintaining the position of the palm, raise the elbow as high as possible.
- Perform this movement in the same manner with the left arm.
- If no pain is experienced, the individual "passes" the test. If any pain is experienced, the individual would "fail" the clearing test and receive a "0" for the shoulder mobility assessment.

5. Active Straight-Leg Raise

The active straight-leg raise assesses active hamstring flexibility and gastrocnemius-soleus flexibility. This assessment also focuses on ability to maintain a stable pelvis while simultaneously raising the lead leg and keeping active extension on the opposite leg.

Instructions:

- Participant should lie flat on his or her back within an open doorway so that the doorframe contacts the thigh midway between the hip and knee.
- Place arms on the floor out to the sides with the palms facing upward.
- Keep both legs straight. Lift outer leg as high as possible while keeping the other leg on the floor.
- Lower the leg and repeat for the other side.
- Score both movements independently.
- The final score for this assessment should be the lowest of the raw scores.

Scoring:

3 = The following criteria must be met:
  - The leg is lifted high enough for the ankle to pass through the doorway.
  - Lifted leg remains straight with no flexion of knee.
  - Other leg remains in contact with the floor with no flexion of the knee.

2 = The ankle was only lifted high enough to be above the knee.
1 = The ankle was not lifted above the height of the knee.
0 = If any pain was experienced by the individual while performing this movement

6. Trunk Stability Push-Up

Trunk stability push-up assesses the ability to maintain rigidity of the torso and resist anterior/posterior movement.

Instructions:

- Lie face down on the floor, feet and legs together, toes pointing toward the floor, hands shoulder width apart and in line with the forehead. Point elbows out to the sides.
- While maintaining a rigid torso, push the body upward as one unit into a push-up position.
- If unable to perform this movement, the following compensations should be allowed:
  - Males: Pull the hands down so that they are in line with the chin and reattempt.
  - Females: Pull the hands down so that they are in line with clavicle and reattempt.

Scoring: Score the movement and then perform the Spinal Extension Clearing Test as described in the following text:

3 = Able to perform a repetition with no sag in the spine with the initial described hand position
2 = Able to perform a repetition with no sag in the spine using the modified hand position
1 = Unable to perform a proper repetition using the modified hand position
0 = If any pain was experienced by the individual while performing this movement

Spinal Extension Clearing Test

- Lie face down and place the hands next to the shoulders.
- While keeping the lower body in contact with the ground, push upward to lift the chest off the ground until the elbows are straight.
- If an individual experiences pain during this movement, he or she will receive a final score of "0" on the trunk stability push-up assessment; however, both scores should be documented for future reference.

7. Rotary Stability

The rotary stability test assesses multiplane trunk stability and neuromuscular control during combined upper and lower extremity movement.

Instructions:

- Kneel on hands and knees, with approximately 6 in of space between the hands and between the knees. A 2 × 6 board can be placed under the participant to ensure proper placement.
- Position the hands so that they are under the shoulders and the knees directly under the hips. Toes should be pulled toward the shins so toes are pointed into the floor.
- Simultaneously extend the right arm and right leg at the same time so they are pointed directly in front and behind.
- Without touching the floor, bring the right elbow to the right knee.
- Return to the extended position and then back to the start position.
- Repeat this process on the left side.

If unable to perform this movement, the following compensations should be allowed:

- Perform the same action using a diagonal pattern (*i.e.*, right arm to left knee/left arm to right knee).
- Score both movements independently.
- The final score for this assessment should be the lowest of the raw scores.

Scoring: Score the movement and then have the individual perform the Spinal Flexion Clearing Test as described in the following text:

3 = Able to perform a correct unilateral pattern
2 = Able to perform a correct diagonal pattern
1 = Unable to perform a diagonal pattern
0 = If any pain was experienced by the individual while performing this movement

Spinal Flexion Clearing Test

- Kneel on the floor on the hands and knees.
- Rock back and touch the buttocks to the heels and the chest to the thighs.
- If an individual experiences pain during this movement, he or she will receive a final score of "0" on the rotary stability assessment; however, both scores should be documented for future reference.

Functional Movement Screen instructions have been adapted from Cook G. *Movement: Functional Movement Systems: Screening, Assessment, and Corrective Strategies.* Aptos (CA): On Target; 2010. 407 p.; and Cook G, Burton L, Hoogenboom B. Pre-participation screening: the use of fundamental movements as an assessment of function — part 1. *N Am J Sports Phys Ther.* 2006;1(2):62–72.

Contraindications to Range of Motion and Functional Assessment

There are some situations where ROM assessments are contraindicated. These include any time immediately after an injury has occurred or when surgery causes disruption of tissue, while on medication for pain, while taking muscle relaxants, in regions of osteoporosis or bone fragility, and in joints with dislocation or unhealed fracture. Additionally, ROM assessments that cause pain or discomfort during the movement should be terminated immediately.

SUMMARY

Evaluation of the flexibility and functional movement ability of individuals should be an integral part of a full fitness assessment and can be used to determine functional deficiencies that may be addressed in the **exercise prescription**. A full evaluation of flexibility will include measurement of ROM at several major joints and will not rely on a single test to determine an overall flexibility score or rating.

REFERENCES

1. American Medical Association. *Guides to the Evaluation of Permanent Impairment*. 4th ed. Chicago (IL): American Medical Association; 1993. 339 p.
2. Chorba RS, Chorba DJ, Bouillon LE, Overmyer CA, Landis JA. Use of a functional movement screening tool to determine injury risk in female collegiate athletes. *N Am J Sports Phys Ther*. 2010;5(2):47–54.
3. Cook G, Burton L, Hoogenboom B. Pre-participation screening: the use of fundamental movements as an assessment of function — part 1. *N Am J Sports Phys Ther*. 2006;1(2):62–72.
4. Cook G, Burton L, Hoogenboom B. Pre-participation screening: the use of fundamental movements as an assessment of function — part 2. *N Am J Sports Phys Ther*. 2006;1(3):132–9.
5. Frost DM, Beach TA, Callaghan JP, McGill SM. Using the Functional Movement Screen™ to evaluate the effectiveness of training. *J Strength Cond Res*. 2012;26(6):1620–30.
6. Golding LA, Myers CR, Sinning WE. *Y's Way to Physical Fitness: The Complete Guide to Fitness Testing and Instruction*. 3rd ed. Chicago (IL): Human Kinetics; 1989. 202 p.
7. Jackson AW, Baker AA. The relationship of the sit and reach test to criterion measures of hamstring and back flexibility in young females. *Res Q Exerc Sport*. 1986;57(3):183–6.
8. Kiesel K, Plisky PJ, Voight ML. Can serious injury in professional football be predicted by a preseason functional movement screen? *N Am J Sports Phys Ther*. 2007;2(3):147–58.
9. Liemohn WP, Sharpe GL, Wasserman JF. Lumbosacral movement in the sit-and-reach and in Cailliet's protective-hamstring stretch. *Spine (Phila Pa 1976)*. 1994;19(18):2127–30.
10. Minick KI, Kiesel KB, Burton L, Taylor A, Plisky P, Butler RJ. Interrater reliability of the functional movement screen. *J Strength Cond Res*. 2010;24(2):479–86.
11. Minkler S, Patterson P. The validity of the modified sit-and-reach test in college-age students. *Res Q Exerc Sport*. 1994;65(2):189–92.
12. Parchmann CJ, McBride JM. Relationship between functional movement screen and athletic performance. *J Strength Cond Res*. 2011;25(12):3378–84.
13. Teyhen DS, Shaffer SW, Lorenson CL, et al. The Functional Movement Screen: a reliability study. *J Orthop Sports Phys Ther*. 2012;42(6):530–40.

PART III

Exercise Prescription

CHAPTER 8

General Principles of Exercise Prescription

INTRODUCTION

Common sense, the ancients, modern research, and practice all point toward the indisputable fact that an important part of a healthy lifestyle is physical activity. Conversely, **sedentary behaviors** are counterproductive to health. Various forms of physical activity have been shown to increase longevity as well as the quality of that increased lifespan. Countless physical and mental health benefits have been attributed to increased physical activity. Despite all the research and the increased public awareness concerning physical activity and/or exercise, millions of Americans continue to avoid regular physical activity (2). Several recent national standards emphasize the benefits of regular **aerobic** physical activity and/or exercise and encourage all of us (no matter our age) to engage in at least 20–60 minutes of these behaviors for a minimum of 3 days per week (2,6,9,11,12). In addition, it is important to consider other components of a healthy lifestyle such as resistance, **flexibility**, and neuromotor training. Most individuals can begin a formal physical activity program without consultation with a health care provider. However, high-risk individuals, specifically those with symptoms of disease, may require medical evaluation and clearance prior to initiation of physical activity.

This chapter addresses specific guidelines for physical activity and/or exercise programming. This chapter also presents the new guidelines from the American College of Sports Medicine (ACSM) as published in the 10th edition of the *ACSM's Guidelines for Exercise Testing and Prescription* (GETP10) (2).

Exercise Prescription for All

In 1975, the ACSM defined **exercise prescription** in the first edition of the *GETP* as follows (4):

> Exercise prescription includes the type, intensity, duration, frequency and progression of physical activity. These five components are applicable to the development of exercise programs for persons regardless of age, functional capacity, and presence or absence of CHD [coronary heart disease] risk factors or CHD.

In the current (10th) edition of the *GETP10* (2), these five components of exercise prescription are reported as **F**requency, **I**ntensity, **T**ime, and **T**ype (**FITT**) with the **V**olume of exercise added along with the **P**rogression component to produce the acronym **FITT-VP**. In addition, the ACSM has also added the component of the pattern of the activity to be an important consideration in exercise programming (2).

A recent PubMed search performed by the authors of this chapter using the past 40 years as a time frame and searching the term *exercise and chronic disease* returned over 18,000 research articles that have been published regarding the effects of exercise/physical activity as an intervention in the prevention of, management of, and rehabilitation for many chronic diseases (often known as *Special Populations*) since the publication of the first edition of the *GETP* (4). What much of the research in this area over the past 40+ years has elucidated is that physical activity and/or exercise plays a key role in the prevention, management, and rehabilitation of disease processes in conjunction with other healthy lifestyle behaviors. The *Domains*, as listed in Box 8.1, describe the broad realm of the involvement in achieving overall health of the whole person. Exercise programs clearly have the preponderance of their effectiveness in the Physical Health Domain, but the interactions between the components of all of the domains are undeniable. Exercise has been demonstrated to have a positive impact on many of the aspects of the domains outside of Physical Health (2,7). The exercise professional must be cognizant that an exercise program is just one element contributing to the overall health of a person. Recognition of the other domains in the development of a total program equips the exercise professional with a significant tool in knowing when to refer an individual to other health care providers for healthy lifestyle guidance that lies outside the exercise professional's scope of practice.

The development and administration of an exercise program lies within the Physical Health Domain. As characterized in Table 8.1, the Physical Health Domain consists of Health-Related, Skill-Related, and Medical-Related Components. The degree of impact and overlap of the individual components of a specific domain is greater within that domain as illustrated in Figure 8.1 for the Physical Health Domain. The evidence supporting the importance of regular physical activity and/or exercise in the prevention and treatment of chronic diseases prompted the ACSM and the American Medical Association to co-launch in 2007 the initiative *Exercise is Medicine*. This initiative has called for exercise/physical activity to be a standard part of disease prevention and medical treatment (7).

In examining the role of exercise as an intervention with Special Populations, the basic FITT-VP principle continues to apply with the caveat that the exercise professional must know the limitations

Box 8.1 The Five Domains of Health

1. Emotional Health
2. Social Health
3. Physical Health
4. Mental Health
5. Spiritual Health

Table 8.1 Examples of Individual Elements of Health-Related, Skill-Related, and Medical-Related Components

Health-Related Components	Skill-Related Components	Medical-Related Components
Cardiorespiratory	Agility	Integumentary
Muscular strength	Balance	Musculoskeletal
Muscular endurance	Coordination	Cardiovascular/lymphatic
Body composition	Power	Respiratory
Flexibility	Speed	Neurologic
	Reaction time	Endocrine
		Digestive/excretory/urinary
		Immune
		Reproductive

and contraindications of exercise within each population. The aspects of an exercise program have historically been divided into targeting exercises that address Health-Related and/or Skill-Related Components of the Physical Health Domain. Program designs for the general population typically prioritize targeting the Health-Related Components of Physical Health Domain. The broad spectrum of target components in developing a total program requires the exercise professional to prioritize the specific components of Physical Health that should be the focus of the patient's exercise program. Although focusing on exercises that address the Health-Related Components have been demonstrated to benefit many of the high-profile chronic diseases, some of the Special Populations may benefit to a greater degree by equally prioritizing some of the Skill-Related Components, such as balance and coordination, with the Health-Related Components in the development of their exercise programs. The following chapters in this book can serve as a guide to the exercise professional in deciding which exercises to incorporate and prioritize for a number of individual Special Populations.

This chapter serves as a guide for general evidenced-based principles in designing exercise prescriptions for all populations. The foundation to developing an effective exercise prescription is the exercise professional's knowledge of the indications and contraindications of exercise for the intended population and the appropriate use of the "common thread" principles of FITT-VP.

Physical activity is considered to be any bodily movement, whereas **exercise** is a subset of physical activity that is both regular and structured. Perhaps, the difference between physical activity and exercise is best viewed on an individual-by-individual basis. One individual may find the term *physical activity* more appealing, whereas another is more interested in increasing exercise. Physical activity can also be thought of as a continuum from light to moderate to vigorous (1).

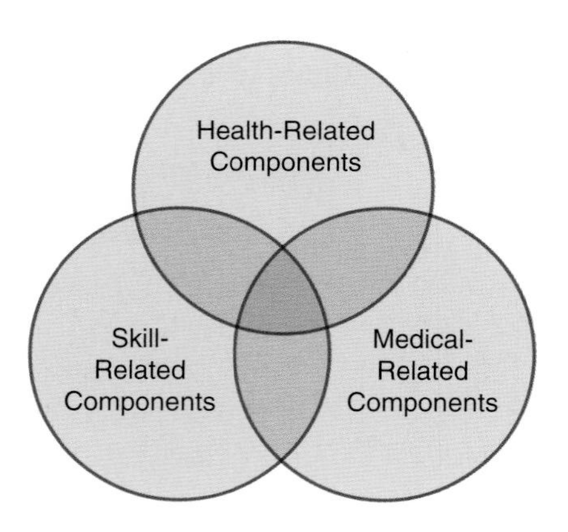

FIGURE 8.1. The interactions of health-related, skill-related, and medical-related components.

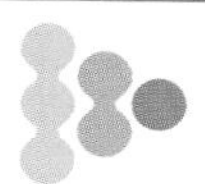

Current FITT-VP Recommendations from the American College of Sports Medicine

Physical activity and/or exercise recommendations in the United States have been on the national scene since the 1950s. An exercise professional should be aware of and stay current with the evolving nature of these recommendations. It is important to remember that a comprehensive program that supports a healthy lifestyle through physical activity and/or exercise is the overall goal. A summary of the most recent aerobic, resistance, flexibility, and neuromotor training guidelines from the ACSM published in 2018 can be found in Table 8.2 (2,7).

The traditional, structured approach to exercise prescription described by the ACSM involves specific recommendations regarding mode or type, frequency, intensity and time, or duration of activity often known as the *FITT* components. The variables of volume of exercise and the progression of the program are also important to the whole exercise prescription process. Addressing the components of muscular fitness, flexibility, and neuromotor training contributes to the whole program.

As a way to involve more individuals who are sedentary, recent physical activity recommendations have adopted a lifestyle approach to increasing physical activity. This newer approach to exercise prescription is sometimes referred to as the *public health approach* (9). In essence, the concept used with the progression of exercise ("start low and go slow") can be applied to the overall program when working with a patient who may be deconditioned from years of inactivity and is at an early stage of change that has significant barriers and obstacles to initiating an exercise program.

Overall, the ACSM considers the following five points (2):

1. All individuals should engage in at least 20–60 minutes of aerobic physical activity of at least a moderate intensity on at least 5 days per week.
2. Additional health and fitness benefits can be achieved by adding more time in moderate-intensity activity or by substituting more vigorous activity.
3. Previously inactive men and women and people at risk for heart, metabolic (diabetes), and renal diseases should first consult a health care provider before initiating a program of vigorous physical activity to which they are unaccustomed.
4. Persons with symptomatic heart, diabetes, or renal disease who would like to increase their physical activity should be evaluated by a health care provider and provided an exercise program appropriate for their clinical status.
5. Muscular strength–developing activities (resistance training) should be performed at a minimum of two times per week. Also, flexibility and neuromotor exercises should be included in a prudent overall program.

Note: Points 3 and 4 were previously discussed in Chapter 2.

Aerobic Frequency

Frequency of exercise (*i.e.*, the number of days per week) is an important contributor to health/fitness benefits that result from an aerobic program. Aerobic exercise is recommended on 3–5 days per week for most adults, with the frequency varying with the **intensity** of exercise. Improvements in **cardiorespiratory fitness** (CRF) are lessened with exercise frequencies less than 3 days per week and plateau in improvement with exercise performed greater than 5 days per week. Vigorous-intensity exercise performed greater than 5 days per week might increase the incidence of musculoskeletal injury, so this amount of vigorous-intensity exercise is not recommended for

Table 8.2 Summary of the American College of Sports Medicine FITT-VP Components

Aerobic frequency	≥5 d · wk^{-1} of moderate exercise OR ≥3 d · wk^{-1} of vigorous exercise OR A combination of moderate and vigorous exercise on ≥3–5 d · wk^{-1}	See Intensity for moderate and vigorous definitions
Aerobic intensity	Moderate and/or vigorous exercise Note: light-to-moderate exercise for deconditioned individuals	Moderate = 40%–59% heart rate reserve (HRR) or oxygen uptake reserve ($\dot{V}O_2R$) Vigorous = 60%–89% HRR or $\dot{V}O_2R$
Aerobic time or duration	30–60 min · d^{-1} for moderate 20–60 min · d^{-1} for vigorous OR A combination of moderate and vigorous Note: <20 min · d^{-1} for previously sedentary	
Aerobic type or mode	Regular, purposeful exercise that involves major muscle groups and is continuous and rhythmic in nature	
Aerobic volume	Target of 500–1,000 MET-min · wk^{-1} Note: a pedometer step count of 7,000 · d^{-1} Note: Exercising below this may be beneficial for some.	MET-min · wk^{-1} = METs of activity times the number of minutes per week That is, 3 METs walk performed for 45 min 5 d · wk^{-1} = 675 MET-min · wk^{-1}
Aerobic pattern	One or multiple (≥10 min) sessions · d^{-1} Note: Sessions less than 10 min may yield favorable results.	
Aerobic progression	A gradual progression of increasing exercise time, frequency, and intensity "Start low and go slow"	Depends on functional capacity, health status, age, preferences, goals, and needs of patient
Resistance training	At least 2–3 d · wk^{-1} 2–4 sets 60%–70% 1-RM 8–12 repetitions	
Flexibility training	At least 2–3 times per wk 10–30 s per stretch — up to a total of 60 s 2–4 repetitions per stretch	
Neuromotor training	≥2–3 d · wk^{-1} ≥20–30 min · d^{-1}	

Created from information found in American College of Sports Medicine. *ACSM's Guidelines for Exercise Testing and Prescription.* 10th ed. Philadelphia (PA): Wolters Kluwer; 2018. 480 p.; and Garber CE, Blissmer B, Deschenes MR, et al. American College of Sports Medicine position stand. Quantity and quality of exercise for developing and maintaining cardiorespiratory, musculoskeletal, and neuromotor fitness in apparently healthy adults: guidance for prescribing exercise. *Med Sci Sports Exerc.* 2011;43(7):1334–59.

adults who are not well conditioned. Nevertheless, if a variety of exercise modes placing different impact stresses on the body (*e.g.*, running, cycling), or using different muscle groups (*e.g.*, swimming, running), are included in the exercise program, daily vigorous-intensity exercise may be recommended for some individuals. Alternatively, a weekly combination of 3–5 days per week of moderate- and vigorous-intensity exercise can be performed, which may be more suitable for some individuals (2,7).

Health/fitness benefits can occur in some individuals who exercise only once or twice per week at moderate-to-vigorous intensity, especially with large volumes of exercise. Exercising one to two times per week is not recommended for most adults because the risk of musculoskeletal injury and adverse cardiovascular events are higher in individuals who are not physically active on a regular basis and those who engage in unaccustomed exercise (2,7,9).

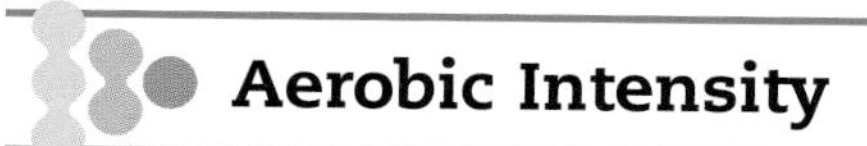

Aerobic Intensity

There is a positive dose response of health/fitness benefits that results from increasing exercise intensity. The overload principle of training states exercise below a minimum intensity, or *threshold*, will not challenge the body sufficiently to result in changes in physiologic parameters, including increased **maximal oxygen consumption** ($\dot{V}O_{2max}$). However, the minimum threshold of intensity for benefit seems to vary depending on an individual's current CRF level and other factors such as age, health status, physiologic differences, genetics, habitual physical activity, and social and psychological factors (10). Therefore, precisely defining an exact threshold to improve CRF may be difficult.

Writing the Aerobic Exercise Intensity

It is important to realize that the exact or precise intensity of exercise is an issue with measurement error, especially in the age prediction of maximal heart rate (HR_{max}) (standard formula for age-predicted maximal heart rate [APMHR] = 220 − age; standard deviation = ± 12 − 15 bpm). There is the potential for significant error in all of the APMHR formulas. The exercise professional should consider these potential errors because the vast majority of exercise prescriptions are done on individuals involving predominately the prediction of HR_{max} by one's age rather than knowing precisely the HR_{max} (as determined from a maximal exercise test).

Exercise Intensity Prescription Calculation Examples from Heart Rate

The following is a bullet summary of some different methods that may be employed in the prescription of exercise intensity by target heart rate (THR). It is common to use a percentage, or range of percentages, to calculate a THR: for example, 50%–85% of $\dot{V}O_2$ or 60%–90% of HR_{max}.

- **Percentage of APMHR**

  Using the 220 − age = APMHR formula.

For example: If your patient's age is 45 years old, his or her APMHR is 175 bpm (220 − 45 = 175 bpm).

  60% of 175 = 105; 90% of 175 = 156 bpm; THR = 105–156 bpm

- **Karvonen formula**

The popular Karvonen formula was developed by the cardiologist Marti Karvonen in the 1950s and essentially considers heart rate reserve (HRR). The Karvonen formula can be written as [(220 − age) − resting HR] × (% intensity desired / 100) + resting HR. Note you can use any well-supported formula for APMHR such as the one from Gellish et al. (8): APMHR = 206.7 − 0.67 × age. For example: If your patient is 45 years old and has a resting HR of 72 bpm, then the solution to the Karvonen formula would be (using 60% and 89% of HRR)

[(220 − 45) − 72] × (60 / 100) + 72 = 133.8 bpm
[(220 − 45) − 72] × (89 / 100) + 72 = 163.7 bpm
THR = 134–164 bpm (rounded off)

■ **Modified Karvonen formula**

Finally, you can use the Karvonen HRR formula but taking into account a known HR_{max} as measured from a maximal **graded exercise test**.

$$[(HR_{max} - \text{resting HR}) \times (\% \text{ intensity desired} / 100)] + \text{resting HR}$$

For example: age = 45 years; measured HR_{max} = 179 bpm; resting HR = 72 bpm

$[(179 - 72) \times 60 / 100] + 72 = 136.2$ bpm
$[(179 - 72) \times 89 / 100] + 72 = 167.2$ bpm
THR = 136–167 bpm (rounded off)

Heart rate is not the only monitoring tool that can be used to determine exercise intensity. Workloads and **metabolic equivalents (METs)** are two other popular forms of intensity setting parameters for individuals, and there are a few other minor-intensity monitoring parameters such as the rating of perceived exertion (RPE), the talk test, and systolic blood pressure (6). RPEs and other affective scales have been proven through the literature and are a staple in many health and fitness settings (10). Several of these techniques for determining exercise intensity have been summarized in Box 8.2.

Another method to alter the exercise intensity involves interval training. Interval training involves varying the exercise intensity at fixed intervals during a single exercise session, which can increase the total volume and/or average exercise intensity performed during that session. Improvements in CRF and cardiometabolic biomarkers with short-term (≤3 mo) interval training are similar or superior to **steady state** moderate- to vigorous-intensity exercise in healthy adults and individuals with metabolic, cardiovascular, or pulmonary disease (2).

During interval training, several aspects of the aerobic program can be varied depending on the goals of the training session and **physical fitness** level of the patient. These variables include the number, duration, and intensity of the work and recovery intervals; the number of repetitions of the intervals; and the duration of the between-interval rest period. Studies of high-intensity interval training (HIIT) and sprint interval training (SIT) demonstrate improvements in CRF,

Box 8.2 Summary of Methods for Prescribing Exercise Intensity Using Heart Rate (HR), Oxygen Uptake (O_2), and Metabolic Equivalents (METs)

- HRR method: Target HR (THR) = $[(HR_{max/peak}{}^{a} - HR_{rest}) \times \%$ intensity desired$] + HR_{rest}$
- $\dot{V}O_2R$ method: Target $\dot{V}O_2R^{c} = [(\dot{V}O_{2max/peak}{}^{b} - \dot{V}O_{2rest}) \times \%$ intensity desired$] + \dot{V}O_{rest}$
- HR method: Target HR = $HR_{max/peak}{}^{a} \times \%$ intensity desired
- $\dot{V}O_2$ method: Target $\dot{V}O_2{}^{c} = \dot{V}O_{2max/peak}{}^{b} - \%$ intensity desired
- MET method: Target $MET^{c} = [(\dot{V}O_{2max/peak}{}^{b}) / 3.5 \text{ mL} \cdot \text{kg}^{-1} \cdot \text{min}^{-1}] \times \%$ intensity desired

$HR_{max/peak}$, maximal or peak heart rate; HRR, heart rate reserve; HR_{rest}, resting heart rate; $\dot{V}O_{2max/peak}$, maximal or peak volume of oxygen consumed per unit of time; $\dot{V}O_2R$, oxygen uptake reserve; $\dot{V}O_{2rest}$, resting volume of oxygen consumed per unit of time.

[a] $HR_{max/peak}$ is the highest value obtained during maximal/peak exercise or it can be estimated by 220 − age or some other prediction equation.

[b] $\dot{V}O_{2max/peak}$ is the highest value obtained during maximal/peak exercise or it can be estimated from a submaximal exercise test.

[c] Activities at the target $\dot{V}O_2$ and MET can be determined using the compendium of physical activities.

Reprinted from American College of Sports Medicine. *ACSM's Guidelines for Exercise Testing and Prescription.* 10th ed. Philadelphia (PA): Wolters Kluwer; 2018. Box 6.2.

cardiometabolic biomarkers, and other fitness- and health-related physiological variables when including repeated alternating short (<45–240 s) bouts of vigorous- to near-maximal intensity exercise followed by equal or longer bouts (60–360 s) of light- to moderate-intensity aerobic exercise. Training responses to HIIT have been reported across a wide range of modalities, work:active recovery interval ratios, and series durations, and the individualized interval training exercise prescription will depend on the desired fitness and health goals and personal characteristics (2).

Aerobic Time (Duration)

Exercise time/duration is prescribed as the amount of time exercise is performed (*i.e.*, time per session). Most adults are recommended to accumulate 30–60 minutes per day (≥150 min $\cdot$ wk^{-1}) of moderate-intensity exercise, 20–60 minutes per day (≥75 min $\cdot$ wk^{-1}) of vigorous-intensity exercise, or a combination of moderate- and vigorous-intensity exercise per day to attain the volumes of exercise recommended in the following discussion. However, less than 20 minutes of exercise per day can be beneficial, especially in individuals who are previously sedentary. For weight management, longer durations of exercise (≥60–90 min per session) may be needed, especially in individuals who spend large amounts of time in sedentary behaviors (5). The recommended time/duration of exercise may be performed continuously (*i.e.*, one session) or intermittently and can be accumulated over the course of a day in one or more sessions that total at least 10 minutes (2,12). Exercise bouts of less than 10 minutes may yield favorable adaptations in very deconditioned individuals or when done as part of a high-intensity aerobic interval program, but further study is needed to confirm the effectiveness of these shorter durations of exercise (2,7).

Aerobic Type (Mode)

Rhythmic, aerobic type exercises involving large muscle groups are recommended for improving CRF. The modes of exercise that result in improvement and maintenance of CRF are found in Table 8.3. The principle of specificity of training should be kept in mind when selecting the exercise modalities to be included in the aerobic program. The specificity principle states that the physiologic adaptations to exercise are specific to the type of exercise performed (10).

Table 8.3 shows aerobic or cardiorespiratory endurance exercises categorized by the intensity and skill demands:

- *Type A exercises* are recommended for all adults, require little skill to perform, and the intensity can easily be modified to accommodate a wide range of physical fitness levels.
- *Type B exercises* are typically performed at a **vigorous intensity** and are recommended for individuals who are at least of average physical fitness and who have been doing some exercise on a regular basis.
- *Type C exercises* require skill to perform and therefore are best for individuals who have reasonably developed motor skills and physical fitness to perform the exercises safely.
- *Type D exercises* are recreational sports that can improve physical fitness but which are generally recommended as ancillary physical activities performed in addition to recommended conditioning physical activities. Type D physical activities are recommended only for individuals who possess adequate motor skills and physical fitness to perform the sport; however, many of these sports may be modified to accommodate individuals of lower skill and physical fitness levels (2,7).

Table 8.3 Modes of Aerobic Exercises to Improve Physical Fitness

Exercise Group	Exercise Description	Recommended for	Examples
A	Endurance activities requiring minimal skill or physical fitness to perform	All adults	Walking, leisurely cycling, aqua-aerobics, slow dancing
B	Vigorous intensity endurance activities requiring minimal skill	Adults (as per the preparticipation screening guidelines in Chapter 2) who are habitually physically active and/or at least average physical fitness.	Jogging, running, rowing, aerobics, spinning, elliptical exercise, stepping exercise, fast dancing
C	Endurance activities requiring skill to perform	Adults with acquired skill and/or at least average physical fitness levels	Swimming, cross-country skiing, skating
D	Recreational sports	Adults with a regular exercise program and at least average physical fitness	Racquet sports, basketball, soccer, down-hill skiing, hiking

From Garber CE, Blissmer B, Deschenes MR, et al. American College of Sports Medicine position stand. Quantity and quality of exercise for developing and maintaining cardiorespiratory, musculoskeletal, and neuromotor fitness in apparently healthy adults: guidance for prescribing exercise. *Med Sci Sports Exerc*. 2011;43(7):1334–59.

Reprinted from American College of Sports Medicine. *ACSM's Guidelines for Exercise Testing and Prescription.* 10th ed. Philadelphia (PA): Wolters Kluwer; 2018. 480 p. Table 6.4.

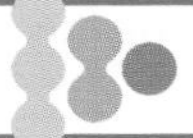

Aerobic Volume

Exercise volume is the product of **F**requency, **I**ntensity, and **T**ime (duration). Evidence (2,7) supports the important role of exercise volume in realizing health/fitness outcomes, particularly with respect to **body composition** and weight management. Thus, exercise volume may be used to estimate the gross energy expenditure of an individual's aerobic program. MET-minutes per week and kilocalories per week can be used to estimate exercise volume in a standardized manner. Box 8.3 shows the definition and calculations for METs, MET-minutes, and kilocalories per minute for a wide array of physical activities. These variables can also be estimated using published tables. MET-minutes and kilocalories per minute can then be used to calculate MET-minutes per week and kilocalories per week that are accumulated as part of an exercise program to evaluate whether the exercise volume is sufficient to result in health/fitness benefits (2,7).

The results of epidemiologic studies and randomized clinical trials have demonstrated a dose-response *association* between the volume of exercise and health/fitness outcomes (*i.e.*, with greater amounts of exercise, the health/fitness benefits also increase). Whether or not there is a minimum or maximum amount of exercise that is needed to attain health/fitness benefits is not clear. However, a total energy expenditure of at least 500–1,000 MET-minutes per week is consistently associated with lower rates of cardiovascular disease and premature mortality. Thus, at least 500–1,000 MET-minutes per week is a reasonable target volume for most adults. The conversion from a better known standard of kilocalories per week to MET-minutes per week is to multiply the kilocalories per week by about 0.82 to get MET-minutes per week (*e.g.*, an exercise at 8 METs of light jogging by a 70-kg person for 30 min three times a week would be about 882 kcal · wk^{-1} or 720 MET-min · wk^{-1}). Lower volumes of exercise (*i.e.*, 4 kcal · kg^{-1} · wk^{-1} or 330 kcal · wk^{-1}) can result in health/fitness benefits in some individuals, especially in those who are deconditioned. Even lower volumes of exercise may have benefit, but evidence is lacking to make definitive recommendations (2,5,7).

Box 8.3 Calculation of METs, MET-Min^{-1}, and kcal · Min^{-1}

Metabolic equivalents (METs): An index of energy expenditure (EE). "A MET is the ratio of the rate of energy expended during an activity to the rate of energy expended at rest. . . . [One] MET is the rate of EE while sitting at rest . . . by convention [1 MET is equal to] an oxygen uptake of 3.5 [mL · kg^{-1} · min^{-1}]."

MET-min: An index of EE that quantifies the total amount of physical activity performed in a standardized manner across individuals and types of activities. Calculated as the product of the number of METs associated with one or more physical activities and the number of minutes the activities were performed (*i.e.*, METs × min); usually standardized per week or per day as a measure of exercise volume.

Kilocalorie (kcal): The energy needed to increase the temperature of 1 kg of water by 1° C. To convert METs to kcal · min^{-1}, it is necessary to know an individual's body weight, kcal · min^{-1} = [(METs × 3.5 mL · kg^{-1} · min^{-1} × body wt in kg) ÷ 1,000)] × 5. Usually standardized as kilocalorie per week or per day as a measure of exercise volume.

Example:
Jogging (at ~7 METs) for 30 min on 3 d · wk^{-1} for a 70-kg male:
7 METs × 30 min × 3 times per week = 630 MET-min · wk^{-1}
[(7 METs × 3.5 mL · kg^{-1} · min^{-1} × 70 kg) ÷ 1,000)] × 5 = 8.575 kcal · min^{-1}
8.575 kcal · min^{-1} × 30 min × 3 times per week = 771.75 kcal · wk^{-1}

Pedometers are effective tools for promoting physical activity and can be used to approximate exercise volume in steps per day. The goal of 10,000 steps per day is often cited, but achieving a pedometer step count of at least 5,400–7,900 steps per day can meet recommended exercise targets. To achieve step counts of 5,400–7,900 steps per day, one can estimate total exercise volume by considering the following: (a) walking 100 steps per minute provides a very rough approximation of moderate-intensity exercise; (b) walking 1 mile per day yields about 2,000 steps per day; and (c) walking at a moderate intensity for 30 minutes per day yields about 3,000–4,000 steps per day. Higher step counts are necessary for weight management. A population-based study estimated men may require 11,000–12,000 steps per day and women 8,000–12,000 steps per day, to maintain a normal weight. Because of the substantial errors of prediction when using pedometer step counts, it is recommended using steps per minute *combined with* currently recommended time/durations of exercise (12).

Aerobic Progression

The recommended rate of progression in an exercise program depends on the individual's health status, physical fitness, training responses, and exercise program goals. Progression may consist of increasing any of the components of the FITT-VP principle of aerobic exercise as tolerated by the individual. During the initial phase of the exercise program, applying the principal of "start low and go slow" is prudent to reduce risks of adverse cardiovascular events and musculoskeletal injury as well as to enhance adoption and adherence to exercise. Initiating exercise at a light-to-moderate intensity in currently inactive individuals and then increasing exercise time/duration as tolerated is recommended. An increase in exercise time/duration per session of 5–10 minutes every 1–2 weeks over the first 4–6 weeks of an exercise training program is reasonable for the average adult. After the individual has been exercising regularly for at least 1 month, the FITT-VP of exercise is gradually adjusted upward over the next 4–8 months — or longer for **older adults** and individuals who are very deconditioned — to meet the recommended quantity and quality of exercise presented in *GETP* (10). Any progression in the FITT-VP principle of aerobic program should be made gradually, avoiding large increases in any of the FITT-VP components to minimize risks of muscular soreness, injury, undue fatigue, and the long-term risk of overtraining. Following any adjustments in the aerobic program, the individual should be monitored for any adverse effects of the increased volume, such as excessive shortness of breath, fatigue, and muscle soreness, and downward adjustments should be made if the exercise is not well tolerated (2,7).

In addition, exercise may be performed in one (continuous) session per day or in multiple sessions of 10 minutes or more to accumulate the desired duration and volume of exercise per day. Exercise bouts of less than 10 minutes may yield favorable adaptations in deconditioned individuals.

Resistance Components

For adults, the research has shown that a health-related resistance training program can (a) make **activities of daily living (ADL)** less stressful physiologically and (b) effectively manage, attenuate, and even prevent chronic diseases and health conditions such as osteoporosis, Type 2 diabetes mellitus, and obesity. For these reasons, although resistance training is important across the age span, its importance becomes even greater with age (3).

Resistance training of each major muscle group 2–3 days per week with at least 48 hours separating the exercise training sessions for the same muscle group is recommended for all adults. Many types of resistance training equipment can effectively be used to improve muscular fitness. Both multijoint and single-joint exercises targeting agonist and antagonist muscle groups are recommended for all adults as part of a comprehensive resistance training program (2,7).

Ideally, adults should train each muscle group for a total of two to four sets with 8–12 repetitions per set with a rest interval of 2–3 minutes between sets to improve muscular fitness. However, even a single set per muscle group will significantly improve **muscular strength**, particularly among novice weightlifters. Older adults or deconditioned individuals should begin a training regimen with at least one set of 10–15 repetitions of very light to light-intensity (*i.e.*, 40%–50% **one repetition maximum**, or **1-RM**) resistance exercise for muscular fitness improvements (2,7).

All individuals should perform resistance training using correct technique. Proper resistance exercise techniques employ controlled movements through the full **range of motion (ROM)** and involve **concentric** (*i.e.*, shortening) and **eccentric** (*i.e.*, lengthening) muscle actions.

As muscles adapt to a resistance exercise training program, the participant should continue to subject them to overload to continue to increase muscular strength and mass by gradually increasing resistance, number of sets, or frequency of training (2,3,7).

Flexibility Components

Flexibility exercises improve the ROM of the muscle tendon unit (or joints) involved. Flexibility exercises are most effective when the muscle temperature has risen some by doing some light exercise previously. Flexibility exercises may acutely reduce power and **strength**, so it is recommended that flexibility exercises be performed after an exercise and sport where strength and power are important to overall performance. A series of flexibility exercises targeting the major joints should be performed. A variety of static, dynamic, and proprioceptive neuromuscular facilitation (PNF) flexibility exercises can improve the ROM around that joint.

A total of 60 seconds of flexibility exercise per joint is generally recommended. Holding a single flexibility exercise for 10–30 seconds to the point of tightness or slight discomfort is effective. Older adults may benefit from holding each stretch for 30–60 seconds. A 20%–75% maximum voluntary contraction held for 3–6 seconds followed by 10–30 seconds of a partner-assisted stretch is recommended for PNF techniques. Performing flexibility exercises at least 2–3 days per week is recommended with daily flexibility exercise being most effective (2,7).

Neuromotor Components

Neuromotor exercises involving balance, agility, coordination, and gait are recommended on at least 2–3 days per week for older adults and are likely beneficial for younger adults as well. The optimal duration or number of repetitions of these exercises is not yet known for improvement, but neuromotor exercise routines lasting at least 20–30 minutes in duration for a total of at least 60 minutes each week may be effective. The actual exercises that might compose a neuromotor training program are not yet delineated. Further research in this area is needed. Neuromotor training may also be known as functional fitness training and may have elements that overlap with other established training exercises such as resistance training (2,7).

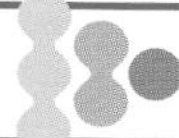

Setting Up a Program

Process

Figure 8.2 addresses one suggested process of interviewing a patient and preparing an exercise program. The individual should be interviewed to address his or her past and present history with health in general and physical activity/exercise in particular. With the appropriate forms, such as a health history questionnaire and informed consent, the exercise professional will determine the need for medical intervention (with a health care provider) with the help of the preactivity

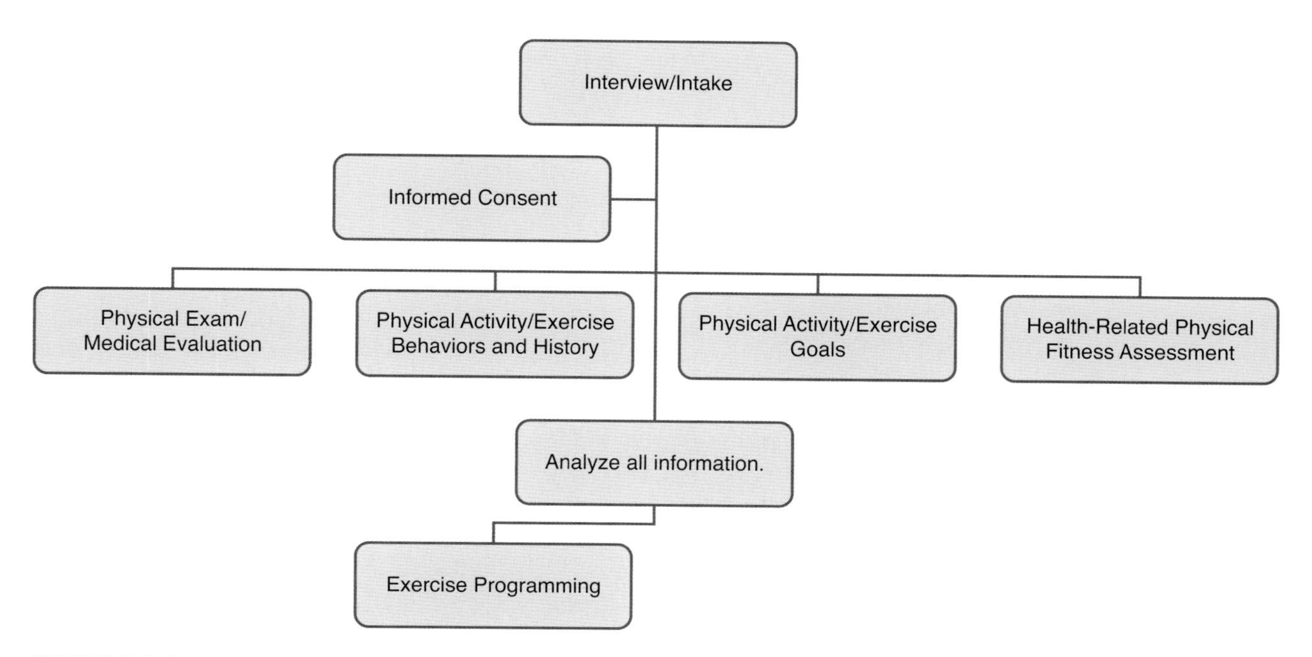

FIGURE 8.2. Components of developing an individualized exercise program.

Box 8.4 Checklist for Healthy (Exercise) Lifestyle Program

- Organize intake session: questions, forms, and equipment.
- Interview patient.
  - Basic demographics — age, sex, etc.
  - Past medical and health history (see Health History Questionnaire)
  - Current medical and health behaviors: signs and symptoms
  - Past and present physical activity/exercise history
  - Future physical activity/exercise goals
  - Perform informed consent.
- Perform resting assessments.
  - Heart rate
  - Blood pressure
  - ACSM risk classification
- Perform *needed*, *appropriate* health-related physical fitness assessments.
  - Cardiorespiratory fitness
    - Field testing
    - Submaximal testing
    - Maximal testing
  - Body composition
    - Anthropometry
    - Composition
    - Weight management
  - Muscular fitness
    - Muscular strength
    - Muscular endurance
    - Flexibility
  - Balance and posture
- Analyze all intake/assessment data: Compare with normative data and decide on patient's needs (prioritize).
- Compose cardiorespiratory fitness program through physical activity/exercise.
  - FITT principle
    - Frequency
    - Intensity
    - Duration (time)
    - Mode (type)
  - Supervision and monitoring needs
  - Address warm-up/conditioning/cool-down needs
  - Overall volume
  - Pattern and progression
- Compose muscular fitness program.
  - Exercise mode: free weights, machines
  - Number and names of exercises
  - Intensity: weight
  - Repetitions
  - Sets
  - Progressive resistance: overload

- Compose flexibility program.
  - Flexibility type: static, dynamic, PNF
  - Number and names of exercises
  - Intensity
  - Repetitions
  - Sets
- Compose neuromotor program.
  - Names of exercises
- Address behavior change issues for patient.
  - Address stage of change.
  - Address common adherence issues and solutions: motivators and barriers.
  - Address relapse prevention.

screening process (see Chapter 2). The patient also should be interviewed for his or her physical activity and exercise goals. Finally, the exercise professional will design a tailored physical fitness assessment battery for his or her patient. All this information needs to be summarized and used in the development of a comprehensive program.

Box 8.4 presents a checklist (similar to Fig. 8.2) that can be used to be sure all aspects necessary to design a successful program for your patient are addressed.

Screening/Evaluation

There is a need to understand some basic features about a patient such as past (medical and health history) as well as present medical status and health behaviors. In addition, it is important to discuss with a patient his or her history and current practice regarding physical activity and exercise. There are a number of forms available for this. These forms are often termed *health history questionnaires*. Exercise professionals should assess the current and past physical activity/exercise habits of patients as well as the following:

- Current motivation and barriers to physical activity/exercise
- Preferred forms of physical activity/exercise
- Beliefs about benefits and risks of physical activity/exercise
- Risk factors for coronary heart disease (CHD) (hypertension, diabetes mellitus, hyperlipidemia, smoking, inactivity, obesity, family history of heart disease, etc.)
- Physical limitations precluding certain physical activities
- Physical activity–induced symptoms
- Concurrent disease (cardiac, pulmonary, musculoskeletal, vascular, psychiatric, etc.)
- Social support for physical activity/exercise participation
- Physical activity/exercise time and scheduling considerations
- Current medical status

Developing the Individualized Exercise Program

A suggested form (Fig. 8.3) has been provided to use as a template for developing an individualized exercise program. The form represents the science of exercise prescription using the state of science as described by the ACSM in its seminal publication of the *GETP10* (2). The art of exercise prescription is in the individualizing of the program for your patient to achieve the goals of enhancing health through a sustainable physical activity program.

CLIENT: ______

Health/Medical History Considerations: ______

Physical Activity/Exercise Considerations: ______

Aerobic

	Frequency	Time	Type	Volume	Pattern	Progression
GOAL	≥5 d · wk^{-1} of mod ex - OR - ≥3 d · wk^{-1} of vig ex - OR - Combo	30–60 min mod ex - OR - 20–60 min vig ex - OR - Combo	Regular, purposeful, major muscle groups, continuous and rhythmic	500–1000 MET-min · wk^{-1}	1 or multiple (≥10 min) bouts	Gradual progression: increasing time, frequency, and intensity
CLIENT						

- Mod ex: 40%–59% HRR or $\dot{V}O_2R$
- Vig ex: 60%–89% HRR or $\dot{V}O_2R$

Aerobic Intensity techniques

			40%	60%	89%
HRR	Age = RHR =	APMHR =			
METs ($\dot{V}O_2R$)	…				
Workloads	TM sp/gr &/or cycle kpm				

Resistance

	Exercises	Days per week	Intensity	Reps	Sets
GOAL	Each major muscle group	≥2–3 d · wk^{-1}	60%–70% 1 RM*	8–12 reps	2–4 sets
CLIENT					

*Age group and goal dependent

Flexibility

	Exercises	Days per week	Intensity	Reps	Time
GOAL	Each major muscle-tendon unit	≥2–3 d · wk^{-1}	Tightness or slight discomfort	2–4 reps per stretch	10–30 s per stretch–up to a total of 60 s
CLIENT					

Neuromotor

	Exercises	Days per week	Intensity	Time
GOAL		≥2–3 d · wk^{-1}		≥20–30 min · d^{-1}
CLIENT				

Personal Limitations: ______

Personal Barriers: ______

FIGURE 8.3. A suggested form for an individualized exercise program.

SUMMARY

The evidence-based science of designing a program for a patient is addressed in this chapter. This science has been well addressed by many other resources available to us all through the print media as well as the Internet. The art of getting an individual to understand, engage, and maintain recommendations toward physical activity and/or exercise needs to be a give-and-take process. The exercise professional will succeed by working with the patient to develop a relationship that allows the patient to win in adopting a healthy exercise lifestyle program.

RECOMMENDED RESOURCES

ACSM Positions stands: http://www.acsm-msse.org/
Centers for Disease Control and Prevention: http://www.cdc.gov/
Exercise Prescription on the Net: http://www.exrx.net
U.S. Government Portal on Physical Activity: http://www.health.gov/PAGuidelines/

REFERENCES

1. Ainsworth BE, Haskell WL, Whitt MC, et al. Compendium of physical activities: an update of activity codes and MET intensities. *Med Sci Sports Exerc.* 2000;32(9 suppl):S498–504.
2. American College of Sports Medicine. *ACSM's Guidelines for Exercise Testing and Prescription.* 10th ed. Philadelphia (PA): Wolters Kluwer; 2018. 480 p.
3. American College of Sports Medicine. American College of Sports Medicine position stand. Progression models in resistance training for healthy adults. *Med Sci Sports Exerc.* 2009;41(3):687–708.
4. American College of Sports Medicine. *Guidelines for Graded Exercise Testing and Exercise Prescription.* Philadelphia (PA): Lea & Febiger; 1975. 116 p.
5. Donnelly JE, Blair SN, Jakicic JM, Manore MM, Rankin JW, Smith BK. American College of Sports Medicine position stand. Appropriate physical activity intervention strategies for weight loss and prevention of weight regain. *Med Sci Sports Exerc.* 2009;41(2):459–71.
6. Fletcher GF, Ades PA, Kligfield P, et al. Exercise standards for testing and training: a scientific statement from the American Heart Association. *Circulation.* 2013;128(8):873–934.
7. Garber CE, Blissmer B, Deschenes MR, et al. American College of Sports Medicine position stand. Quantity and quality of exercise for developing and maintaining cardiorespiratory, musculoskeletal, and neuromotor fitness in apparently healthy adults: guidance for prescribing exercise. *Med Sci Sports Exerc.* 2011;43(7):1334–59.
8. Gellish RL, Goslin BR, Olson RE, McDonald A. Russia GDP, Moudgil UK. Longitudinal modeling of the relationship between age and max heart rate. *Med Sci Sports Exerc.* 2007;39:822–829.
9. Haskell WL, Lee IM, Pate RR, et al. Physical activity and public health: updated recommendation for adults from the American College of Sports Medicine and the American Heart Association. *Med Sci Sports Exerc.* 2007;39(8):1423–34.
10. Swain DP, editor. *ACSM's Resource Manual for Guidelines for Exercise Testing and Prescription.* 7th ed. Philadelphia (PA): Wolters Kluwer; 2014. 896 p.
11. U.S. Department of Health and Human Services. *2008 Physical Activity Guidelines for Americans* [Internet]. Washington (DC): U.S. Department of Health and Human Services; [cited 2016 Mar 28]. Available from: http://www.health.gov/paguidelines/pdf/paguide.pdf
12. U.S. Department of Health and Human Services. *Exercise and Physical Activity* [Internet]. Bethesda (MD): National Institute on Aging, National Institutes of Health; [cited 2016 Mar 28]. Available from: http://www.nia.nih.gov/HealthInformation/Publications/ExerciseGuide

CHAPTER 9

Special Considerations across the Lifespan: Pregnancy, Children and Youth, and Older Adults

INTRODUCTION

This chapter addresses **exercise** testing, prescription, and progression considerations for three conditions that may occur across the lifespan including pregnancy, children and youth, and older adults. Online case studies are available for each of these conditions.

PREGNANCY

Pregnancy is characterized by profound physiological and anatomical adaptations that ensure optimal accommodations to the increasing metabolic demands of both mother and fetus (5,26,43,51,91). Pregnancy involves a gestational period, typically between 38 and 40 weeks divided into trimesters, each characterized by unique physiological and anatomical adaptations (27,43,91). A thorough understanding of the physiological and anatomical adaptations that occur with pregnancy allows the fitness professional to safely and effectively design an exercise program.

Many of the physiological and anatomical adaptations that occur during pregnancy are related to increased plasma and tissue concentrations of hormones, growth factors, prostanoids, and other substances (43,51,91). Hemodynamic adaptations include an increase in total blood volume of approximately 30%–50% (43,51) associated with an increase in cardiac output of approximately 1,500 mL (51). The disproportionate increase in plasma volume (1,000 mL) compared with erythrocyte volume (500 mL) commonly results in dilutional anemia and fatigue (51). Resting heart rate (HR) increases by approximately 16 bpm and maximal HR decreases by approximately 4 bpm through the gestational period (43), resulting in a net reduction in gestational heart rate reserve (HRR) (51). Resting blood pressure (BP) remains fairly consistent in uncomplicated pregnancies as the significant increase in blood volume is offset by systemic peripheral vascular dilation (5,51). Diastolic BP decreases approximately 15 mm Hg by mid-pregnancy, and systolic BP remains similar to or slightly decreases compared with the nonpregnant state (51). A reduction in mean arterial BP occurs by mid-second trimester, gradually returning to prepregnancy levels (5,43,51). The hemodynamic adaptations that occur during pregnancy often result in soft tissue edema most commonly observed during the third trimester and presenting as lower leg and ankle edema (27). Increased glomerular filtration rate accompanied by increased diuresis presents as renal adaptations during pregnancy (91). The respiratory/ventilatory adaptations include increased tidal volume, bronchiole dilation, an increase in minute ventilation by approximately 30%–50%, an increase in absolute oxygen consumption both at rest and with activity, and a reduced carbon dioxide threshold (43).

The most prevalent visible anatomical adaptation during pregnancy is gestational weight gain (13,25,55,56,75,90) ranging from 10 to 16 kg (22 to 35 lb) (5) primarily distributed at the breasts and the abdominal region (5,27,43). The distributional pattern of gestational weight gain results in an anterior translation of the center of gravity, which increases the risk for balance complications, most prevalent during the second and third trimesters (5,27). The adaptive pelvic posture that occurs during pregnancy often results in a functional imbalance between hip flexors and hip extensors, resulting in pseudo-hamstring tightness and positional instability of the hip abductors (27). Lumbar-pelvic postural alterations result in compensatory shoulder girdle postural accommodations, altering glenohumeral joint and cervical spine mechanics (27). A physiological and structural adaption that occurs during pregnancy is laxity of ligamentous structures derived from increased levels of estrogen, progesterone, and relaxin (41,91) primarily occurring at the pubic symphysis to accommodate childbirth; yet, joint laxity is demonstrated systemically (12,27,43). Bone density loss occurs during pregnancy and lactation yet rarely results in osteoporosis (27).

Metabolic and musculoskeletal anomalies frequently plague women during pregnancy including gestational hypertension (27), preeclampsia (6), gestational diabetes mellitus (GDM) (10,30,62,85), low back pain (LBP) (38,88), diastasis recti abdominis (27), lower extremity edema (27), carpal tunnel syndrome (27), and tarsal tunnel syndrome (27), to name a few.

Preparticipation Health Screening, Medical History, and Physical Examination

The ePARmed-X+ Physician Clearance Follow-Up Questionnaire (Fig. 9.1) is the recommended screening tool utilized by physicians and other obstetric health care providers to provide **medical clearance** for exercise initiation or continuation during pregnancy (18,93). The PARmed-X was designed to establish a line of communication between the woman during gestation, the health care provider, and the fitness specialist (18). The PARmed-X incorporates a gestational safety and care continuum including sections on Safety Considerations and Reasons to Consult a Physician, ensuring participant safety with exercise and when unscheduled medical consultation may be warranted (18).

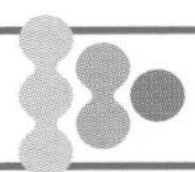

Exercise Testing Considerations

Maximal exercise testing is not indicated for women who are pregnant unless medically authorized and performed with medical supervision (1,3,5). The PARmed-X will assist the medical provider and the fitness professional in determining if exercise testing is required (93).

Exercise Prescription and Progression Considerations

Physical Activity and Exercise during Pregnancy

Because of its dynamically adaptive nature, pregnancy presents a challenge for fitness professionals regarding achievement of optimal gestational and postpartum outcomes for both mother and offspring. There is general consensus regarding **physical activity** during pregnancy among the American College of Obstetricians and Gynecologists (ACOG) (3), Society of Obstetricians and Gynaecologists of Canada (SOGC) (26), Canadian Society for Exercise Physiology (CSEP) (26), Royal College of Obstetricians and Gynaecologists (RCOG) (73), The Royal Australian and New Zealand College of Obstetricians and Gynaecologists (Sports Medicine Australia [SMA]) (78), and the American College of Sports Medicine (ACSM) (4,5,28). The available data strongly support and recommend physical activity prior to conception, during the gestational period, and through the postpartum period for healthy women with uncomplicated pregnancies not presenting with absolute and/or relative contraindications to exercise (Box 9.1). Initiation or continuation of an exercise program should be encouraged through the gestational period unless the woman presents with warning signs requiring exercise termination and medical consultation (see "Special Considerations for Exercise and Pregnancy" and Box 9.2). See Box 9.3 for the current committee opinion recommendations from ACOG regarding physical activity and exercise during pregnancy and through the postpartum period.

Regular participation in moderate-intensity physical activity during pregnancy has been demonstrated to be beneficial for both mother and fetus (5,55). See Box 9.4.

Women who continue with a healthy lifestyle and those who adopt a healthy lifestyle throughout pregnancy, inclusive of regular **aerobic** exercise, demonstrate specific activity-related adaptations, compared with sedentary peers, similar to the nonpregnant state such as reduced resting HR, increased stroke volume, enhanced glucose utilization, enhanced thermoregulation, and increased volume of oxygen consumed per unit time ($\dot{V}O_2$) response at a given HR (5,51).

Target HR ranges based on age and fitness level that correspond to moderate-intensity exercise have been validated and adopted for low-risk women who are pregnant (2,25,53,56) (Table 9.1).

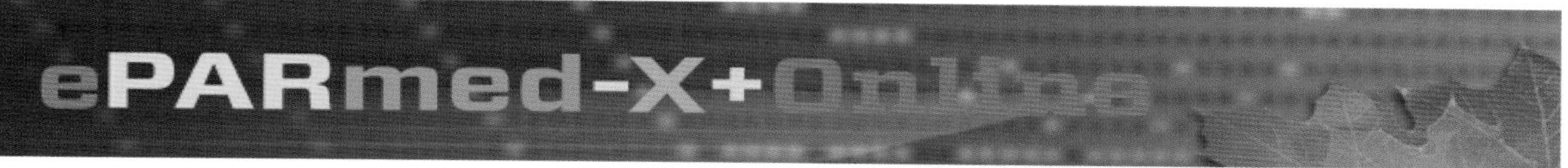

ePARmed-X+ Physician Clearance Follow-Up

This form is separated into three main sections:

A) Background information regarding the PAR-Q+ and ePARmed-X+ clearance process,
B) A brief history and demographic information regarding the participant, and
C) The physician's recommendations regarding the participant becoming more physically active.

At the end of this process, the participant is recommended to take this signed clearance form to a qualified exercise professional or other healthcare professional (as recommended in the ePARmed-X+) before becoming more physically active or engaging in a fitness appraisal.

A BACKGROUND INFORMATION REGARDING THE PAR-Q+ AND ePARMed-X+ CLEARANCE PROCESS

The ePARmed-X+ is an easy to follow interactive program (www.eparmedx.com) that can be used to determine an individual's readiness for increased physical activity participation or a fitness appraisal. The ePARmed-X+ supplements the paper and online versions of the new Physical Activity Readiness Questionnaire for Everyone (PAR-Q+).

Individuals who use the ePARmed-X+ have had a positive response to the PAR-Q+, or have been directed to the online program by a qualified exercise professional or another healthcare professional, owing to his/her current medical condition. At the end of the ePARmed-X+, it is possible that the participant is advised to consult a physician to discuss the various options regarding becoming more physically active. In this instance, the participant will be required to receive medical clearance for physical activity from a physician. Until this medical clearance is received, the participant is restricted to low intensity physical activity participation.

This document serves to assist both the participant and physician in the physical activity clearance process.

B PERSONAL INFORMATION

NAME: ____________________ SEX: ☐ M or ☐ F

ADDRESS: ____________________ BIRTHDATE (mm/dd/yy): __________
____
____

TELEPHONE: ____________________ HEALTH/MEDICAL NUMBER: __________

REASON FOR REFERRAL (SELECT ALL THAT APPLY):

☐ QUALIFIED EXERCISE PROFESSIONAL REFERRAL
☐ HEALTH CARE PROFESSIONAL REFERRAL
☐ ePARmed-X+ RECOMMENDATION

Version: September 7, 2014 Page 1 of 2

FIGURE 9.1. ePARmed-X+ Physician Clearance Follow-Up Questionnaire+. (Reprinted with permission from the PAR-Q+ Collaboration and the authors of the PAR-Q+ [Dr. Darren Warburton, Dr. Norman Gledhill, Dr. Veronica Jamnik, and Dr. Shannon Bredin].) *(continued)*

ePARmed-X+Online

C ePARmed-X+ PHYSICAL ACTIVITY READINESS PHYSICIAN REFERRAL FORM

Based on the current review of the health status of ________________________________(name)
I recommend the following course of action:

- ☐ The participant should avoid engaging in physical activity at this time.
- ☐ The participant should engage in only a medically supervised physical activity/exercise program involving the supervision of a qualified exercise professional (or other appropriately trained health care professional) and overseen by a physician.
- ☐ The participant is cleared for intensity and mode appropriate physical activity/exercise training under the supervision of a qualified exercise professional.
- ☐ The participant is cleared for intensity and mode appropriate physical activity/exercise training with limited supervision (i.e., unrestricted physical activity).

The following precautions should be taken when prescribing exercise for the aforementioned participant:

- ○ With the avoidance of: ____
____
____
____

- ○ With the inclusion of: ____
____
____
____

NAME OF PHYSICIAN: ________________________________

ADDRESS: ____

TELEPHONE: ________________________

Date of Medical Clearance (mm/dd/yy): ____________________

PHYSICIAN/CLINIC STAMP AND SIGNATURE

NOTE: This physical activity/exercise clearance is valid for a period of six months from the date it is completed and becomes invalid if the medical condition of the above named participant changes/worsens.

Version: September 7, 2014 Page 2 of 2

FIGURE 9.1. *(continued)*

Box 9.1 Contraindications for Exercising during Pregnancy

Absolute Contraindications

- Hemodynamically significant heart disease
- Restrictive lung disease
- Incompetent cervix or cerclage
- Multiple gestation at risk of premature labor
- Persistent second- or third-trimester bleeding
- Placenta previa after 26 weeks of gestation
- Premature labor during the current pregnancy
- Ruptured membranes
- Preeclampsia/pregnancy-induced hypertension

Relative Contraindications

- Severe anemia
- Unevaluated maternal cardiac dysrhythmia
- Chronic bronchitis
- Poorly controlled type 1 diabetes
- Extreme morbid obesity
- Extreme underweight (BMI less than 12)
- History of extremely sedentary lifestyle
- Intrauterine growth restriction in current pregnancy
- Poorly controlled hypertension
- Orthopedic limitations
- Poorly controlled seizure disorder
- Poorly controlled hyperthyroidism
- Heavy smoker

Reprinted with permission from American College of Obstetricians and Gynecologists. *Physical Activity and Exercise During Pregnancy and the Postpartum Period. Committee Opinion Number 650.* Washington (DC): American College of Obstetricians and Gynecologists; 2002. 8 p. From American College of Obstetricians and Gynecologists. *Physical Activity and Exercise During Pregnancy and the Postpartum Period. Committee Opinion Number 650. (Replaces Committee Opinion Number 267, January 2002).* Washington (DC): American College of Obstetricians and Gynecologists; 2015. 8 p.

Women who demonstrate at-risk pregnancies determined by the PARmed-X for Pregnancy, or determined through medical examination, characterized as high-risk women who are pregnant, should proceed with exercise planning only if cleared for exercise by their physician.

Types of Prescribed Exercises for Pregnancy

The prescribed resistance training session should contain a warm-up and cool-down component of approximately 8 minutes in duration each, and resistance exercises for 20–30 minutes with approximately 1 minute rest between sets and approximately 2 minutes rest between exercises (60). Greater rest time should be allotted for less fit women (69). Resistance can safely be derived from use of body weight resistance, resistance bands, resistance tubing, light dumbbells, water resistance, and appropriately positioned resistance machines (9,60,69).

Box 9.2 Warning Signs to Stop Exercise during Pregnancy

- Vaginal bleeding or (amniotic) fluid leakage
- Shortness of breath prior to exertion
- Dizziness, feeling faint, or headache
- Chest pain
- Muscle weakness
- Calf pain or swelling
- Decreased fetal movement
- Preterm labor

From American College of Obstetricians and Gynecologists. *Exercise During Pregnancy and the Postpartum Period. ACOG Committee Opinion Number 267.* Washington (DC): American College of Obstetricians and Gynecologists; 2002. 3 p.

Box 9.3 Current Committee Opinion Recommendations from the American College of Obstetricians and Gynecologists Regarding Physical Activity and Exercise during Pregnancy and the Postpartum Period

- Physical activity in pregnancy has minimal risks and has been shown to benefit most women, although some modification to exercise routines may be necessary because of normal anatomic and physiologic changes and fetal requirements.
- A thorough clinical evaluation should be conducted before recommending an exercise program to ensure that a patient does not have a medical reason to avoid exercise.
- Women with uncomplicated pregnancies should be encouraged to engage in aerobic and strength-conditioning exercises before, during, and after pregnancy.
- Obstetrician–gynecologists and other obstetric care providers should carefully evaluate women with medical or obstetric complications before making recommendations on physical activity participation during pregnancy. Although frequently prescribed, bed rest is only rarely indicated and, in most cases, allowing ambulation should be considered.
- Regular physical activity during pregnancy improves or maintains physical fitness.

From American College of Obstetricians and Gynecologists. *Physical Activity and Exercise During Pregnancy and the Postpartum Period. Committee Opinion Number 650. (Replaces Committee Opinion Number 267, January 2002).* Washington (DC): American College of Obstetricians and Gynecologists; 2015. 8 p.

Box 9.4 Benefits of Physical Activity before and during Pregnancy

Some benefits associated with regular physical activity before and during the gestational period include a reduced risk of the following:

- Preeclampsia (6)
- Gestational hypertension (HTN), GDM (85,86)
- Systemic inflammation (84)
- Excessive gestational weight gain (53)
- Gestational obesity (55)
- Gestational low BP (38,88)
- Generalized musculoskeletal discomfort (26)
- Urinary incontinence (65)
- Having a baby with macrosomia (86)
- Interventional delivery (9)
- Cesarean birth (9)
- Preterm birth (9)
- Low–birth-weight baby (11,17)
- Prevention/improvement of depressive symptoms
- Prevention of postpartum weight retention (55)

Table 9.1 Target Heart Rate Zones that Correspond to Moderate-Intensity Exercise for Healthy Low-Risk Women Who Are Pregnant and Lower Intensity Exercise Target Heart Rate Zones for Low-Risk Women Who Are Pregnant and Overweight or Obese

BMI 18.9–24.9 kg · m^{-2}		
Age (yr)	**Fitness Level**	**Heart Rate Range (bpm)**
<20	—	140–155
20–29	Low	129–144
	Active	135–150
	Fit	145–160
30–39	Low	128–144
	Active	130–145
	Fit	140–156
BMI ≥25 kg · m^{-2}		
Age (yr)		**Heart Rate Range (bpm)**
20–29		102–124
30–39		101–120

From Davenport MH, Charlesworth S, Vanderspank D, Sopper MM, Mottola MF. Development and validation of exercise target heart rate zones for overweight and obese pregnant women. *Appl Physiol Nutr Metab.* 2008;33:984–9. doi:10.1139/H08-086; Mottola MF. Exercise and pregnancy: Canadian guidelines for health care professionals. *Wellspring.* 2011;22(4):1–4; Mottola MF. Physical activity and maternal obesity: cardiovascular adaptations, exercise recommendations, and pregnancy outcomes. *Nutr Rev.* 2013;71(suppl 1):S31–6. doi:10.1111/nure.12064; and Mottola MF, Davenport MH, Brun CR, Inglis SD, Charlesworth S, Sopper MM. $\dot{V}O_{2peak}$ prediction and exercise prescription for pregnant women. *Med Sci Sports Exerc.* 2006;38(8):1389–95.

Exercises that promote lumbar-pelvic girdle and scapular-cervical postural stabilization, maintenance of muscle tone, **flexibility**, and general conditioning should be emphasized in order to minimize the deleterious effects of the postural adaptations common during pregnancy (34,51,60,69). Exercises performed in the supine position (lying on one's back) are contraindicated, and exercises performed in the prone position (lying on one's stomach) should be avoided beyond the first trimester (53). Resistance training can safely be performed in the seated position with lumbar support in order to avoid overloading posturally compromised joints (69). Exercises such as lunges, straight-legg deadlifts, and deep squats should be avoided during the gestational period (69). **Exercise prescription** should be individually designed based on specific needs and goals; therefore, the exercise specialist should be able to competently substitute a specific exercise for an exercise that has been contraindicated for the woman who is pregnant in order to avoid adverse outcomes.

The volume of exercise prescribed to the woman during pregnancy will be dependent on the woman's training status, musculoskeletal condition, and other individual factors that could vary day to day. Common exercise volume recommendations during pregnancy included one to two sets of 10–15 repetitions performed for six to eight exercises (9,34,60). The frequency, intensity, type, and time (FITT) table (Table 9.2) summarizes the frequency, intensity, time, type, volume, and progression (**FITT-VP**) recommended by the ACSM for pregnancy.

FITT

TABLE 9.2 FITT RECOMMENDATIONS ACROSS THE LIFESPAN

ACSM FITT Principle of the ExR_x

Chronic Medical Condition	Frequency (How often?)	Intensity (How hard?)	Time	Type (What kind?) Primary	Resistance	Flexibility	Special Considerations
Healthy Adult	$\geq$5 d · wk^{-1} of moderate exercise, or $\geq$3 d · wk^{-1} of vigorous exercise, or a combination of moderate and vigorous exercise on $\geq$3–5 d · wk^{-1} is recommended.	Moderate to vigorous. Light-to-moderate intensity exercise may be beneficial in deconditioned individuals.	If moderate intensity: $\geq$30 min · d^{-1} to total 150 min · wk^{-1}. If vigorous intensity: $\geq$20 min · d^{-1} to total 75 min · wk^{-1}.	Regular, purposeful exercise that involves major muscle groups and is continuous and rhythmic in nature is recommended.	2–3 d · wk^{-1} (nonconsecutive)	2–3 d · wk^{-1}; static stretch 10–30 s; 2–4 repetitions of each exercise	Sedentary behaviors can have adverse health effects, even among those who regularly exercise. Adding short physical activity breaks throughout the day may be considered as a part of the exercise.
Children and Adolescents	Daily	Most should be moderate (noticeable increase in HR and breathing) to vigorous intensity (substantial increases in HR and breathing). Include vigorous intensity at least 3 d · wk^{-1}.	As part of $\geq$60 min · d^{-1} of exercise	Enjoyable and developmentally appropriate activities, including running, brisk walking, swimming, dancing, bicycling, and sports such as soccer, basketball, or tennis	$\geq$3 d · wk^{-1}	N/A	Bone-strengthening activities include running, jump rope, basketball, tennis, resistance training, and hopscotch.
Older Adults	$\geq$5 d · wk^{-1} for moderate intensity; $\geq$3 d · wk^{-1} for vigorous intensity; 3–5 d · wk^{-1} for a combination of moderate and vigorous intensity	On a scale of 0–10 for level of physical exertion, 5–6 for moderate intensity and 7–8 for vigorous intensity	30–60 min · d^{-1} of moderate-intensity exercise; 20–30 min · d^{-1} of vigorous-intensity exercise; or an equivalent combination of moderate- and vigorous-intensity exercise; may be accumulated in bouts of at least 10 min each	Any modality that does not impose excessive orthopedic stress such as walking. Aquatic exercise and stationary cycle exercise may be advantageous for those with limited tolerance for weight-bearing activity.	$\geq$2 d · wk^{-1}	$\geq$2 d · wk^{-1}	
Women Who Are Pregnant	$\geq$3–5 d · wk^{-1}	Moderate intensity (3–5.9 METs; RPE of 12–13 on the 6–20 scale); vigorous-intensity exercise ($\geq$6 METs; RPE 14–17 on the 6–20 scale) for women who were highly active prior to pregnancy or for women who progress to higher fitness levels during pregnancy	~30 min · d^{-1} of accumulated moderate-intensity exercise to total at least 150 min · wk^{-1} or 75 min · wk^{-1} of vigorous-intensity aerobic exercise	A variety of weight- and non–weight-bearing activities are well tolerated during pregnancy (*e.g.*, hiking, group exercise, swimming).	2–3 d · wk^{-1} (nonconsecutive)	$\geq$2–3 d · wk^{-1} with daily being most effective	

ExR_x, exercise prescription.

Based on the FITT Recommendations present in *ACSM's Guidelines for Exercise Testing and Prescription.* 10th ed. Philadelphia (PA): Wolters Kluwer; 2018. 480 p.

Special Considerations for Exercise and Pregnancy

The following are special considerations to be used as guidelines relevant to pregnant women and exercise:

- Exercise should not be initiated, or should be immediately terminated, followed by immediate medical consultation if the pregnant woman presents with any of the following signs or symptoms: vaginal bleeding, dyspnea before exertion, dizziness, headache, chest pain, unexplained muscle weakness, calf pain or swelling, preterm labor, decreased fetal movement, uterine contractions lasting ≥30 minutes after exercise cessation, and/or amniotic fluid leakage (1). Women who are pregnant commonly present with lower extremity swelling/edema, but lower extremity swelling in combination with calf pain may be indicative of thrombophlebitis and/or deep vein thrombosis (DVT) and will require immediate medical examination for symptom resolution.
- A woman who is pregnant and sedentary or has a medical complication can initiate exercise at low intensity and progress with exercise **intensity** as appropriate based on the medical condition and the woman's tolerance to the exercise prescription in conjunction with medical clearance (53).
- Women who are obese, have GDM or gestational hypertension, and have been cleared by their physician to initiate or continue an exercise program require an adjusted exercise prescription based on the medical condition and the individual needs of the woman (3).
- Women who are pregnant need to avoid scuba diving, contact sports/activities, or those activities that pose a risk for loss of balance or falls that would result in trauma to the fetus such as gymnastics, vigorous racquet sports, soccer, basketball, softball, skiing/snowboarding, horseback riding, ice hockey, ice skating, and roller blading (3,26).
- Excessive heat exposure, especially during early pregnancy, can be teratogenic (resulting in neural tube defects) (51). Excessive heat exposure derived primarily from modalities such as hot tubs, saunas, and physiological manifestations such as fever appeared to demonstrate greater teratogenic effects than from exercise; however, exercise in hot and humid environments should be avoided (52). Exercise in a thermoneutral environment with air conditioning and loose fitting, breathable workout clothing is recommended.
- Women who are pregnant should avoid certain positions and avoid rapid positional changes (24). Women who are pregnant should avoid lying in the supine position after gestational week 16 as supine lying can result in inferior vena cava and abdominal aortic compression (24). Women who are pregnant should avoid quick changes of body position/posture when standing or in nonsupported positions because this can result in dizziness or syncope derived from orthostatic hypotension (24). Women who are pregnant should avoid exercises involved with prolonged, sustained standing positions which compromise venous return (24).
- Women who are pregnant should avoid performance of the Valsalva maneuver because this may result in moderate to severe BP spikes that could potentially harm the fetus (69) or limit venous return resulting in maternal reflex tachycardia and orthostasis.
- The estimated total energy cost of pregnancy is approximately 80,000 kcal, or an additional 300 kcal per day (43). The best measure of sufficient caloric intake is adequate weight gain throughout the gestational period (43). Additional caloric intake may be necessary to counteract the caloric expenditure derived from exercise.
- Stretching exercises (permanent lengthening of tissues that occurs only at end ranges of motion is not the equivalent of flexibility exercises that occur within the individual's available **range of motion**) should be avoided during pregnancy due to laxity of the support structures unless pathological adaptive shortenings are present (12,27,37). Stabilization structures will respond more readily to stretching with permanent joint instability resulting. Flexibility exercises performed within normal physiological range of motion are indicated during pregnancy (27).

- Weight-bearing exercise should be performed on level surfaces without quick directional changes to avoid joint damage including sprains, subluxations, and dislocations (27).
- Women who are pregnant should maintain proper hydration and are recommended to drink 6–8 oz of water for every 15 minutes of moderate-intensity exercise performed (2).
- Pregnancy is not the time for competitive training or to progress with training principles (FITT-VP) beyond that of prior training intensity in trained women (43).
- High-intensity, or prolonged, exercise ≥45 minutes can result in hypoglycemia; therefore, training session duration should be designed to minimize physiological risks, for example, through duration limitations and/or appropriate caloric intake before and during exercise (3).
- Physical activity can be resumed after pregnancy but should be incorporated gradually because of normal physiological **deconditioning** in the initial postpartum period. Generally, gradual exercise may begin approximately 4–6 weeks after a normal vaginal delivery or about 8–10 weeks (with medical clearance) after a cesarean section delivery (54). More fit women with more rigorous exercise routines prior to and during pregnancy may be able to resume exercise sooner (53). Light- to moderate-intensity exercise in the postpartum period is important for return to prepregnancy **body mass index** and does not interfere with breastfeeding (54).

CHILDREN AND YOUTH

Childhood and adolescence represent time periods where youth are in a state of growth and eventually go through the maturation process. Youth should not be viewed as miniature adults because their systems are immature and they do not have the same capabilities as adults. Most **children** and **adolescents** do not participate in adequate amounts of physical activity (20). Physical activity levels have a tendency to steadily decline from childhood to adolescence, with the majority of adolescents not meeting physical activity guidelines (21). Research has demonstrated that low levels of physical activity during childhood and adolescence tend to track into low physical activity levels in adulthood (47). Therefore, children who participate in a physically active lifestyle are more likely to be active as adults.

During early childhood, children begin to develop fundamental movement skills, which serve as building blocks for more complex motor skills essential for success in activities such as sport and dance (76). Proficiency of movement skills has been linked to higher physical activity levels and more favorable **body composition** (61,92). Evidence-based physical activity guidelines have been developed for school-age youth (6–17 yr old). The Physical Activity Guidelines for Americans recommend that children participate in at least 60 minutes of moderate- to vigorous-intensity activity daily that is enjoyable and developmentally appropriate. This activity should be accumulated over the course of the day (67). Meeting and exceeding these recommendations has been associated with more favorable cardiovascular disease risk profiles, improved mental health, and higher academic achievement (28,82).

This section focuses on physical activity recommendations for youth, exercise testing in the pediatric population, exercise prescription specific to the age level of the child, and special considerations for this population.

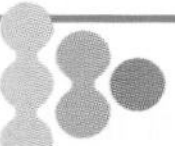

Exercise Testing Considerations

Clinical exercise testing in youth is usually safe with the exception of those with severe cardiopulmonary disease (63). Prior to assessment, it is important to choose the appropriate mode (treadmill or cycle) and protocol based on the purpose of the test and the functional aerobic capacity of the participant (72). There are advantages and disadvantages to both of these modes of testing.

Table 9.3 FITNESSGRAM Assessment Examples

Health-Related Fitness Components	Assessments
Aerobic capacity	PACER test 1-mile run Walk test
Muscular strength and endurance ▪ Abdominal ▪ Trunk extensor ▪ Upper body	Curl-ups Trunk extension Push-ups
Flexibility	Back-Saver sit-and-reach Shoulder stretch
Body composition	Body mass index Skinfold assessment Bioelectrical impedance analysis

The treadmill can be used by any age child and elicits a maximal HR and peak oxygen uptake ($\dot{V}O_{2peak}$). However, risk of injury is higher than that of the cycle, and a spotter should be readily available during the testing (72). The cycle has a lower risk of injury, results in lower maximal HR and $\dot{V}O_{2peak}$, and may not be the correct size for smaller children (72). There are a variety of testing protocols for the treadmill and cycle available (see *Pediatric Laboratory Exercise Testing: Clinical Guidelines* in "References" section). Procedures for exercise testing, as well as the variables that are assessed, generally follow the testing guidelines setup for adults (see Chapter 4). Familiarization with the mode of testing as well as the protocol is essential to achieving a true peak test. Pediatric exercise tests may require significant motivation and support during the assessment due to the maturity level of the child. The use of the OMNI Rating of Perceived Exertion (RPE) Scale may allow the technician to gain a subjective assessment of the participant's effort. This scale utilizes a 0–10 scale, text, and pictures to enable youth to be able to report their perceived exertion (87).

In addition to clinical exercise testing, field tests may also be used to assess health-related fitness. These types of assessments typically take place in schools and community centers (68). The FITNESSGRAM is a commonly used fitness testing battery that is used to assess aerobic capacity, **muscular strength** and **muscular endurance**, flexibility, and body composition. Specifics on the FITNESSGRAM testing protocols are located in the administration manual (83). Table 9.3 provides examples of the assessments that can be used for each of the health-related fitness components. Criterion-referenced standards have been developed for the FITNESSGRAM tests and can be used to classify youth who are considered fit (In Healthy Fitness Zone) and those who need to improve their fitness (Not in Healthy Fitness Zone). These classifications age- and sex-specific are available for all of the components of health-related fitness.

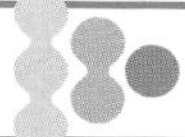

Exercise Prescription and Progression Considerations

The Physical Activity Guidelines for Americans recommend that children participate in at least 60 minutes of moderate- to vigorous-intensity activity daily that is enjoyable and developmentally appropriate (67). Vigorous-intensity activity should be included at least 3 days per week. Moderate-intensity activity includes walking briskly, whereas running would be considered a vigorous-intensity activity (67). Children tend to participate in activities that vary in tempo and are sporadic (7). Examples of appropriate activities for children include walking, running, and active games. Adolescents tend to participate in activity that is more structured and sustained. Typical activities for this age group include games that require object control skills (volleyball, baseball), endurance activities, and martial arts. With both groups, the activities should be fun and should be developmentally appropriate based on the youth's motor skill level, **physical literacy**, and health-related fitness status.

At least 3 days per week, youth should engage in physical activities that promote muscle and bone **strength**. These activities vary based on the age of the individual. Children's activities that strengthen muscle and bone include jumping, climbing, activities that use body weight as resistance, and possibly resistance training. Adolescents' activities consist of tug of war games, push-ups, and resistance training with weights or machines (67). Additionally, children and adolescents may safely participate in strength-training activities provided that they are adequately supervised, are properly trained to use equipment, and are emotionally mature (32). Recommendations for resistance training include a **moderate intensity** (60%–80% of estimated **one repetition maximum** [**1-RM**]), 8–15 repetitions for one to three sets, no more than 2–3 days per week on nonconsecutive days. Neuromuscular adaptations are primarily responsible for strength gains in prepubertal children, whereas the presence of higher levels of anabolic hormones contribute to muscle hypertrophy and strength gains in peri- and postpubertal youth. Although not specifically targeted in the Physical Activity Guidelines for Americans, youth should participate in activities that promote flexibility. Recommendations for a flexibility prescription should be similar to healthy adults (see FITT table, Table 9.2) and should emphasize the static stretching of each major muscle group. See FITT table (Table 9.2) for FITT-VP guidelines from the ACSM for youth and children.

Youth should gradually increase their physical activity levels until they are able to meet and eventually exceed federal recommendations. The high prevalence of overweight and obesity in the pediatric population in addition to low levels of regular physical activity may impede many children and adolescents' abilities to meet recommendations. A steady increase in the duration, frequency, and intensity of activity should be employed in order to facilitate the achievement of at least 60 minutes per day of physical activity that is of moderate-to-vigorous intensity. The gradual progression of the duration, frequency, and intensity of physical activity may reduce the risk of injury as well as improve adherence to a physically active lifestyle. Additionally, it is critical to reduce the amount of time youth spend in sedentary activities such as watching television, playing video games, and using electronic devices (12,28). Finally, youth should be introduced to activities that are enjoyable and promote lifelong activity and fitness (*i.e.*, walking, cycling, and tennis).

Special Considerations and Physical Activity Recommendations for Children and Youth

The following are physical activity recommendations and special considerations to be used as guidelines relevant to children and youth and exercise:

- Children and adolescents should participate in at least 60 minutes of moderate- to vigorous-intensity activity that is enjoyable and developmentally appropriate on a daily basis.
- Youth should engage in bone- and muscle-strengthening activities at least 3 days per week. Examples of activities include body weight resistance, calisthenics, and resistance training.
- Resistance training guidelines include moderate-intensity exercises (60%–80% of estimated 1-RM), 8–15 repetitions for one to three sets, 2–3 days per week on nonconsecutive days.
- Many common diseases and disorders (*e.g.*, asthma, diabetes mellitus, obesity, cystic fibrosis, and cerebral palsy) may impact a child or adolescent's ability to participate in regular physical activity.

- Several factors contribute to low activity levels in this population including symptoms, functional capacity, and the comfort level of parents and physicians allowing youth to be physically active. Youth with these conditions are likely to have a lower functional capacity compared with healthy youth.
- Most youth are capable of participating in regular physical activity, which usually results in decreased symptomology and improved fitness levels.

OLDER ADULTS

Older adults are defined as healthy individuals ≥65 years and/or individuals 50 years through 64 years with disabilities, chronic disease, and/or functional impairments (23,59). The older adult population is the fastest growing segment of society in the United States (94). Not all individuals reach older adulthood or progress through these years successfully (94). Individuals with the same chronological age often demonstrate significant differences in biological age as indicated by functional capacity and health status differences (59,64,66). Health status and functional capacity are often better indicators of exercise capacity than chronological age (58,66).

Aging has been associated with an increased risk of developing many chronic and degenerative diseases including cardiovascular disease, Type 2 diabetes mellitus, cancer, obesity, osteoporosis, and sarcopenia, all capable of limiting functional capacity, independence, and quality of life in the older adult (23). Most physiological and anatomical systems demonstrate functional and structural decline with advancing age (23).

A hallmark of the aging process is an alteration of body composition (23). Older adults tend to demonstrate a reduction in lean tissue and an increase in body fat with fat mass redistributed from subcutaneous to visceral regions (29,48). Visceral adipose has been positively associated with systemic inflammation, Type 2 diabetes mellitus, and cardiovascular disease (48).

A decrease in activity tends to be a hallmark of the aging process (89,94). Inactivity has been implicated as a modifiable risk factor for diabetes mellitus, cancer (colon and breast), obesity, hypertension, osteoporosis, osteoarthritis, and depression (89). The prevalence of **physical inactivity** is greater than that of all other associated modifiable disease risk factors for North Americans; therefore, distinguishing the effects of aging on physiological function/decline from the effects of inactivity, deconditioning, and/or disease is difficult (89).

Degenerative joint disease/osteoarthritis (DJD/OA) is a common condition that will vastly affect physical activity levels and exercise prescription for the older adult population (45). Exercise prescription for an individual with DJD/OA requires an individualized approach based on disease characteristics and joint abnormalities and whether the condition is acute and/or chronic in nature. Mild- to moderate-intensity joint loading on weight-bearing activities (aerobic and/or resistance training) results in enhanced proteoglycan synthesis (cartilage formation [extracellular matrix]) and reduction in markers of articular cartilage damage that are associated with high-intensity joint loading. High-intensity joint loading has been implicated in the development and progression of osteoarthritis in the older adult population (45).

Aging has been associated with a reduction in lean body mass, frequently referred to as **sarcopenia** (71). The measurable variables often associated with sarcopenia include reduced ambulatory capacity, functional mobility, energy intake, overall nutrient intake, independence, ventilation (71), chronic-systemic inflammation, oxidative stress, and insulin resistance (66). Rosenberg (71) suggested that proposing a name for the condition described earlier would bring recognition to the medical research community and the National Institutes of Health. He suggested that the name be derived from Greek origin and the condition be termed *sarcomalacia* or *sarcopenia*. *Sarx* in Greek is flesh and *penia* is loss, and thus, sarcopenia describes a critical change in body composition and physical function. These changes can be observed in magnetic resonance imaging (MRI) scans as a reduction in cross-sectional area of muscle, intramuscular adipose tissue deposition, and increased fat mass (71). Sarcopenia may lead to inactivity, and inactivity could hasten sarcopenia, a deleterious cyclical pattern (66).

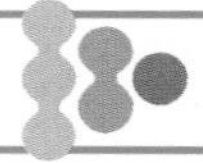

Exercise Prescription and Progression Considerations

The general principles of exercise prescription (FITT-VP) apply to adults of all ages. However, the exercise prescription becomes more complicated in the older adult population due to a high percentage of older adults who have chronic disease and require prescription medications. The relative adaptations to exercise and the percentage of improvement in the components of **physical fitness** among older adults are comparable with those reported in younger adults and are important for maintaining health and functional ability and attenuating many of the physiological changes that are associated with aging (Table 9.4). Low aerobic capacity, muscle weakness, and deconditioning are more common in older adults than in any other age group and contribute to loss of independence (23).

Overwhelming evidence supports the benefits of physical activity in (a) slowing physiological changes of aging that impair exercise and functional capacity, (b) optimizing age-related changes in body composition, (c) promoting psychological and cognitive well-being, (d) managing chronic diseases, (e) reducing the risks of physical impairment and disability, and (f) increasing quality-of-life years (23). Exercise prescription and adherence have been found to be beneficial for chronic disease management and prevention (89). Regular physical activity and enhanced fitness capacity have been associated with a >50% reduced risk of all-cause and cardiovascular mortality through both

Table 9.4 Effects of Aging on Selected Physiological and Health-Related Variables

Variable	Variable Change
Resting heart rate	Unchanged
Maximum heart rate	Lower
Maximum cardiac output	Lower
Resting and exercise blood pressure	Higher
Absolute and relative maximum oxygen uptake reserve ($\dot{V}O_2R_{max}$ $L \cdot min^{-1}$ and $mL \cdot kg^{-1} \cdot min^{-1}$)	Lower
Residual volume	Higher
Vital capacity	Lower
Reaction time	Slower
Muscular strength	Lower
Flexibility	Lower
Bone mass	Lower
Fat-free body mass	Lower
% Body fat	Higher
Glucose tolerance	Lower
Recovery time	Longer

From Skinner JS. Aging for exercise testing and exercise prescription. In: Skinner JS, editor. *Exercise Testing and Exercise Prescription for Special Cases: Theoretical Basis and Clinical Application.* 3rd ed. Baltimore: Lippincott Williams & Wilkins; 2005. pp. 85–99.

primary and secondary preventative mechanisms; decreased risk of Type 2 diabetes, certain forms of cancer, and osteoporosis; improved autonomic function; improved lipoprotein profiles; improved overall cardiovascular health (89,94); reduced medical costs (49); reduced prescription medication dependence (77); improvements in dimensions of sleep (44); improved global cognitive function (36,94); and improved psychological well-being (89).

Regular aerobic exercise negated age-related declines in vascular endothelial function and carotid compliance, attenuated age-related increases in arterial BP (48), and improved levels of cardiorespiratory and muscle fitness (89,94). Resistance training improved health and function in the older adult population via the following: improved fasting plasma insulin, improved insulin sensitivity, improved glucose tolerance, decreased percentage of body fat with associated increased lean body mass, increased energy metabolism, decreased sarcopenia, improved hormone regulation (48), improved bone mineral density (14), reduction in markers of oxidative stress, increased endogenous antioxidant enzyme synthesis, improved mitochondrial function (50), and maintained functional joint range of motion (79,80).

Despite these benefits, older adults are the least physically active of all age groups. Today, only 11% of individuals ≥65 years report engaging in aerobic and muscle-strengthening activities that complied with federal physical activity guidelines, and <5% of individuals age 85 years and older met these same guidelines; yet, a positive trend in physical activity participation by older adults has been identified (33). Only 6% of people ≥65 years met federal guidelines for physical activity in 1998 compared with 11% in 2010 (33).

One in 3 people 65 years and older will fall this year, and those who have demonstrated a fall are 2 to 3 times more likely to fall again within that same year (19). Half of the individuals 80 years and older will experience a fall each year in the United States (19). Falls are responsible for up to 75% of all emergency room visits in people 65 years and older in the United States (19). Falls are the leading contributor to financial burden associated with injury in the older adult population in the United States. One-third to one-half of older adults living at home will fall each year with an increased fall incidence in those who are more aged, institutionalized, female, single, divorced, widowed, demonstrate low walking speed, use assistive devices, demonstrate multiple comorbidities, and/or use multiple medications, to name the primary variables (81). The ACSM recommends that individuals who frequently fall or have mobility impairments partake in balance exercises (23).

The recommended exercises, if tolerated, include but should not be generalized to the older adult population and should be evaluated by a health care provider prior to administration by a certified exercise physiologist (23,35):

- Exercises with progressively challenging postures that serve to gradually reduce the individual's base of support from their position of limitation, seated or standing. Sample exercises include two-legged stand, semitandem stand, tandem stand, and one-legged stand (23).
- Exercises containing dynamic movements that serve to perturb the individual's center of gravity, making them less stable, such as tandem walking and circle turns (23)
- Exercises that stress postural muscle groups and target stability adaptations such as heel stands and toe stands (23)
- Exercises that reduce sensory input such as standing with eyes closed (23)

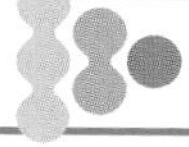

Special Considerations for Exercise and Older Adults

Physical activity has been found to be beneficial for a multitude of health-related variables in the older adult population with health-related outcomes optimized through individualized exercise prescription. Older adult individuals demonstrate similar adaptations to exercise as found in the young population; however, many variables must be considered and adjusted for prior to prescribing exercise, continually throughout the exercise session (HR, BP, RPE, dizziness, etc.), and over the course of the individual's exercise training period (months, years), such as changes in medications and health status. A thorough understanding of the confounding variables highly prevalent with aging and the impact of these variables on physiological and anatomical adaptations to exercise in the older adult population allows the fitness specialist to safely and effectively prescribe exercise.

The following special considerations must be taken into account to maximize the safe and effective development of an exercise program for an older adult:

- Intensity and duration of physical activity should be light (RPE 9–11 from original Borg 6–20 scale) at the beginning, in particular for older adults who are highly deconditioned, functionally limited, or have chronic conditions that affect their ability to perform physical tasks. This light intensity may be continued for 6 months until the participant is able to safely exercise for 30 minutes per session.
- Progression of physical activities should be individualized and tailored to tolerance and preference; a conservative approach is recommended for all older adults who are deconditioned and physically limited to reduce the risk of adverse events.
- Exercise should be terminated immediately with medical follow-up upon presentation of these signs/symptoms: dizziness, angina (chest pain), dyspnea before exertion, unexplained exertional dyspnea (shortness of breath not consistent with relative exercise intensity), retinal hemorrhage, onset of lower extremity edema, vasovagal response, preexercise or during exercise plasma glucose reading $<70\ \text{mL} \cdot \text{dL}^{-1}$, systolic BP >220 mm Hg, diastolic BP >105 mm Hg, syncope, and orthostasis. Medical clearance is required prior to exercise return.
- Small declines in **isometric** strength occur up until the sixth decade; however, decreases in isometric strength of 1.0%–1.5% per year from 50 to 70 years of age; and 3% per year after age 70 years (42). Upper extremity strength changes less with age than muscles of the lower extremity. Most older adults who are sedentary demonstrate a 1% decline in strength commencing in their 50s, with steeper muscular strength declines (3% per yr) after age 70 years. The muscular strength component of the exercise prescription is critical for maintaining independence in one's older years (23,35,59).
- The initial resistance training sessions must be supervised and monitored by personnel who are well versed in instructing the older adult on how to correctly execute a specific movement pattern whether using free weights or machines in order to optimize outcomes and minimize adverse events.
- In addition to training for strength (FITT table [see Table 9.2]), older adults may particularly benefit from power training because this element of muscle fitness declines most rapidly with aging, and insufficient power has been associated with a greater risk of accidental falls (15,22). Increasing muscle power in healthy older adults should include both single- and multiple-joint exercises (one to three sets) using light-to-moderate loading (30%–60% of 1-RM) for 6–10 repetitions with high velocity. Such power training decisions must be based on the older adults' current strength and weight-bearing stability status, experience with resistance training, and the potential for injury.
- Muscular strength is an imperative requirement for successful and independent aging; therefore, resistance training should be a component of the exercise prescription for all older adults, unless contraindicated. Increasing muscle strength in healthy older adults should include both single- and multiple-joint exercises (one to three sets) using moderate- to moderate-high loading (60%–75% of 1-RM) for 8–12 repetitions with high velocity. Such strength-training decisions must be based on the older adults' current strength and weight-bearing stability status, experience with resistance training, and the potential for injury.
- Individuals with sarcopenia, a marker of frailty, or those individuals who have been previously sedentary, need to increase muscular strength before they are physiologically capable of engaging in aerobic training.

- If chronic conditions preclude activity at the recommended minimum amount, older adults should perform physical activities as tolerated to avoid being sedentary.
- Older adults should gradually exceed the recommended minimum amounts of physical activity and attempt continued progression if they desire to improve and/or maintain their physical fitness if tolerated.
- Older adults should consider exceeding the recommended minimum amounts of physical activity to improve management of chronic diseases and health conditions when practical, for which a higher level of physical activity is known to confer a therapeutic benefit as tolerated by their condition.
- Moderate-intensity physical activity should be encouraged for individuals with cognitive decline given the known benefits of physical activity on cognition; safety is paramount (walking with a trained professional may be necessary in case of loss of balance). Individuals with significant cognitive impairment can engage in physical activity but may require individualized assistance.
- Structured physical activity sessions should end with an appropriate cool-down, particularly among individuals with cardiovascular disease. The cool-down should include a gradual reduction of effort and intensity, involving dynamic movements.
- Dehydration
  - Older adults are more susceptible to dehydration than other age group (8).
  - Fluid replacement for older adults can be complicated due to a multitude of variables but has been encouraged for the purpose of rehydration preexercise, during, and postexercise (46,74).
  - Older adults generally demonstrate reduced total body water by approximately 10%–15% with an altered extracellular to intracellular fluid balance compared with young individuals (31).
  - Reduced renal mass in conjunction with glomerular loss impairs older adults' capacity to retain water and concentrate urine based on an impaired sodium retention mechanism and may place them at greater risk for dysnatremia and hypovolemia (31).
  - Older adults demonstrate impaired water and electrolyte balance due to renal senescence, increasing the risk of dehydration in conjunction with electrolyte imbalances, enhanced during periods of physiological stress such as disease and exercise (31).
  - Older adults demonstrate increased atrial natriuretic peptide activity, antagonizing renin–angiotensin–aldosterone activity, increasing the likelihood of dehydration and electrolyte abnormalities (31,46).
  - Fluid intake in healthy older individuals primarily occurs through oral ingestion predicated upon each individual's thirst mechanism, which tends to be blunted in older adults (31,46).
  - Diuretics are a commonly prescribed form of medication for older adults, utilized as a mechanism for BP control, which could result in a multitude of adverse events including dehydration and electrolyte imbalance (31).
  - Fluid restriction in combination with a pharmacological regiment for the purpose of BP control are not uncommon for older adults.
  - A generalized older adult prescription for fluid replacement with exercise would not account for the many variables associated with water and electrolyte balance and could result in adverse events.
  - Fluid replacement for older adults who exercise should be individualized to prevent dehydration and hyperhydration and should be predicated on body weight and medical restrictions.
  - A commonly used equation used to determine fluid requirements with exercise based on fluid loss is as follows:
    1. (Preexercise body mass − postexercise body mass) = body weight difference (kg or g)
    2. If fluid consumed during exercise (drink volume [mL])
    3. (1 + 2) − urine volume (if produced before postexercise body mass) = sweat loss
    4. Sweat loss (mL) / exercise time (h or min) = sweat rate ($mL \cdot min^{-1}$ or $mL \cdot h^{-1}$) (57)
    5. Restoration of body fluids with exercise should be minimally based on sweat rate loss.

- Incorporation of behavioral strategies such as social support, self-efficacy, the ability to make healthy choices, and perceived safety, all may enhance participation in a regular exercise program.
- The exercise professional should provide regular feedback, positive reinforcement, and other behavioral/programmatic strategies to enhance adherence.
- Exercise prescription as an intervention for the mediation of balance issues in older adults falls outside of the scope of practice of the exercise physiologist (39). Generic exercise prescription for the mediation of balance issues and fall prevention in the older adult population was found to be ineffectual; yet, individualized programs based on a health care provider's assessment appeared more effective and with reduced injury rates (39).
- An exercise specialist must be familiar and competent with the indicated application and utilization of assisting and guarding (spotting) techniques when assisting a medical health care provider with expertise in fall prevention with balance exercises for the older adult population (39).
- An important distinction between older adults and their younger counterparts should be made relative to intensity when prescribing exercise. For apparently healthy adults, moderate- and vigorous-intensity physical activities are defined relative to **metabolic equivalents (METs)**, with moderate-intensity activities defined as 3–5.9 METs and vigorous-intensity activities as ≥6 METs. In contrast, for older adults, activities should be defined relative to an individual's physical fitness within the context of an RPE 6- to 20-point scale (16) with 6 indicating no exertion and 20 indicating maximal exertion. A moderate-intensity physical activity should produce a noticeable increase in HR and breathing, whereas a vigorous-intensity physical activity should produce a large increase in HR or breathing (59).
- A dose-response relationship for **cardiorespiratory fitness** was demonstrated in older adults who are sedentary with the largest maximal volume of oxygen consumed per unit time ($\dot{V}O_{2max}$) improvement derived from a mean intensity of 66% through 73% HRR (40). Higher intensity doses >75% through 80% HRR did not enhance $\dot{V}O_{2max}$ but resulted in declines (40).
- Approximately 81% of individuals between the ages of 57 and 85 years used at least one prescription medication, and 29% used ≥ five prescription medications concurrently, commonly taken with additional over-the-counter medications (70). Prescription medication use was most prevalent in the 65- to 74-year range and most commonly involved diuretics, statins, β-blockers, and angiotensin-converting enzyme (ACE) inhibitors (70). Prescription and over-the-counter medications may alter the expected physiological response to exercise and require a thorough understanding of the medication's pharmacokinetics, pharmacodynamics, and potential adverse reactions associated with exercise.
- Pain is a sensory-protective endogenous mechanism that, if present, requires the causative action be ceased or altered in order to avoid a deleterious inflammatory cascade and a potential exercise/functional setback.
- Monitor aerobic and resistance training form and plane of motion to reduce incidence of musculoskeletal injury.
- Older adults can demonstrate improvements in health status as a result of increased physical activity levels regardless of improvements in aerobic fitness (89). Many **activities of daily living** do not require a large aerobic capacity but do depend on other components of physical fitness, such as muscular strength and flexibility (89).
- As exercise professionals, we need to refocus attention on an older adult's functional, not performance, capacity. That is, instead of the usual "go for a walk to stay active," more emphasis on functional strength and mobility may be just as or more beneficial to an individual's quality of life. Exercise prescription for the older adult should be geared toward function, not performance with primary consideration given toward open and closed kinetic chain exercises.
- Working with the older adult must be a passion and a labor of love.

SUMMARY

The information provided in this chapter illustrates the special considerations that need to be undertaken when working with women who are pregnant, children and youth (*i.e.*, growth and maturation), and older adults. Information regarding exercise testing both in clinical and in field settings and physical activity guidelines for aerobic and bone and muscle strengthening activity have been provided.

REFERENCES

1. American College of Obstetricians and Gynecologists. *Exercise During Pregnancy and the Postpartum Period. ACOG Committee Opinion Number 267.* Washington (DC): American College of Obstetricians and Gynecologists; 2002. 3 p.
2. American College of Obstetricians and Gynecologists. *Physical Activity and Exercise During Pregnancy and the Postpartum Period. Committee Opinion Number 650.* Washington (DC): American College of Obstetricians and Gynecologists; 2002. 8 p.
3. American College of Obstetricians and Gynecologists. *Physical Activity and Exercise During Pregnancy and the Postpartum Period. Committee Opinion Number 650. (Replaces Committee Opinion Number 267, January 2002).* Washington (DC): American College of Obstetricians and Gynecologists; 2015. 8 p.
4. American College of Sports Medicine. *ACSM's Guidelines for Exercise Testing and Prescription.* 10th ed. Philadelphia (PA): Wolters Kluwer; 2018. 480 p.
5. Artal R, Clapp JF III, Vigil DV. *ACSM Current Comment: Exercise During Pregnancy.* Indianapolis (IN): American College of Sports Medicine.
6. Aune D, Saugstad OD, Henriksen T, Tonstad S. Physical activity and the risk of preeclampsia: a systematic review and meta-analysis. *Epidemiology.* 2014;25(3):331–43. doi:10.1097/EDE.0000000000000036.
7. Bailey RC, Olson J, Pepper SL, Porszasz J, Barstow TJ, Cooper DM. The level and tempo of children's physical activities: an observational study. *Med Sci Sports Exerc.* 1995;27(7):1033–41.
8. Baker LB, Munce TA, Kenney WL. Sex differences in voluntary fluid intake by older adults during exercise. *Med Sci Sports Exerc.* 2005;37(5):789–96. doi:10.1249/01.MSS.00000162622.78487.9C.
9. Barakat R, Lucia A, Ruiz JR. Resistance exercise training during pregnancy and newborn's birth size: a randomised control trial. *Int J Obes (Lond).* 2009;33:1048–57. doi:10.1038/ijo.2009.150.
10. Barakat R, Pelaez M, Lopez C, Lucia A, Ruiz JR. Exercise during pregnancy and gestational diabetes-related adverse effects: a randomized controlled trial. *Br J Sports Med.* 2013;47(10): 630–6. doi:10.1136/bjsports-2012-091788.
11. Barakat R, Ruiz JR, Stirling JR, Zakynthinaki M, Lucia A. Type of delivery is not affected by light resistance and toning exercise training during pregnancy: a randomized controlled trial. *Am J Obstet Gynecol.* 2009;201:590.
12. Blecher AM, Richmond JC. Transient laxity of an anterior cruciate ligament-reconstructed knee related to pregnancy. *Arthroscopy.* 1998;14:77–9.
13. Bodnar LM, Siega-Riz AM, Simhan HN, Himes KP, Abrams B. Severe obesity, gestational weight gain, and adverse birth outcomes. *Am J Clin Nutr.* 2010;91:1642–8.
14. Bolam KA, van Uffelen JG, Taaffe DR. The effect of physical exercise on bone density in middle aged and older men: a systematic review. *Osteoporosis Int.* 2013;24(11):2749–62. doi:10.1007/s00198-013-2346-1.
15. Bonnefoy M, Jauffret M, Jusot JF. Muscle power of lower extremities in relation to functional ability and nutritional status in very elderly people. *J Nutr Health Aging.* 2007;11(3):223–8.
16. Borg G. Psychophysical bases of perceived exertion. *Med Sci Sports Exerc.* 1982;14(5):377–81.
17. Campbell MK, Mottola MF. Recreational exercise and occupational activity during pregnancy and birth weight: a case-control study. *Am J Obstet Gynecol.* 2001;184(3):403–8.
18. Canadian Society for Exercise Physiology. *PARmed-X for Pregnancy.* Ottawa (Canada): Canadian Society for Exercise Physiology; 2015.
19. Centers for Disease Control and Prevention. *Important Facts About Falls* [Internet]. Atlanta (GA): Centers for Disease Control and Prevention; [cited 2017 Mar 22]. Available from: http://www.cdc.gov/homeandrecreationalsafety/falls/adultfalls.html
20. Centers for Disease Control and Prevention. Physical activity levels among children aged 9–13 years — United States, 2002. *MMWR Morb Mortal Wkly Rep.* 2003;52(33):785–8.
21. Centers for Disease Control and Prevention. Physical activity levels of high school students — United States, 2010. *MMWR Morb Mortal Wkly Rep.* 2011;60:773–7.
22. Chan BK, Marshall LM, Winters KM, Faulkner KA, Schwartz AV, Orwoll ES. Incident fall risk and physical activity and physical performance among older men: the osteoporotic fractures in men study. *Am J Epidemiol.* 2007;165(6):696–703.

23. Chodzko-Zajko WJ, Proctor DN, Fiatarone-Singh M, et al. American College of Sports Medicine position stand. Exercise and physical activity for older adults. *Med Sci Sports Exerc*. 2009;41(7):1510–30.
24. Clark SL, Cotton DB, Pivarnik JM, et al. Position change and central hemodynamic profile during normal third-trimester pregnancy and post-partum. *Am J Obstet Gynecol*. 1991;164(3):883–7.
25. Davenport MH, Charlesworth S, Vanderspank D, Sopper MM, Mottola MF. Development and validation of exercise target heart rate zones for overweight and obese pregnant women. *Appl Physiol Nutr Metab*. 2008;33:984–9. doi:10.1139/H08-086.
26. Davies GAL, Wolfe LA, Mottola MF, MacKinnon C. Joint SOGC/CSEP clinical practice guideline: exercise in pregnancy and the postpartum period. *Can J Appl Physiol*. 2003;28(3):330–41.
27. DeMaio M, Magann EF. Exercise and pregnancy. *J Am Acad Orthop Surg*. 2009;17:504–14.
28. Donnelly JE, Hillman CH, Castelli D, et al. Physical activity, fitness, cognitive function, and academic achievement in children: a systematic review. *Med Sci Sports Exerc*. 2016:48(6):1197–222.
29. Dunstan DW, Daly RM, Owen P, et al. High-intensity resistance training improves glycemic control in older patients with Type 2 diabetes. *Diabetes Care*. 2002;25(10):1729–36. doi:10.2337/diacare.25.10.1729.
30. Dye TD, Knox KL, Artal R, Aubry RH, Wojtowycz MA. Physical activity, obesity, and diabetes in pregnancy. *Am J Epidemiol*. 1997;146(11):961–5.
31. El-Sharkawy AM, Sahota O, Maughan RJ, Lobo DN. The pathophysiology of fluid and electrolyte balance in the older adult surgical patient. *Clin Nutr*. 2014;33:6–13.
32. Faigenbaum AD, Kraemer WJ, Blimkie CJ, et al. Youth resistance training: updated position statement paper from the National Strength and Conditioning Association. *J Strength Cond Res*. 2009;23(5 suppl):S60–79.
33. Federal Interagency Forum on Aging-Related Statistics. *Older Americans 2012: Key Indicators of Well-Being* [Internet]. Washington (DC): Federal Interagency Forum on Aging-Related Statistics. Available from: http://www.agingstats.gov
34. Fieril KP, Glantz A, Olsen MF. The efficacy of moderate-to-vigorous resistance exercise during pregnancy: a randomized controlled trial. *Acta Obstet Gynecol Scand*. 2015;94:35–42. doi:10.1111/aogs.12525.
35. Garber CE, Blissmer B, Deschenes MR, et al. American College of Sports Medicine position stand. Quantity and quality of exercise for developing and maintaining cardiorespiratory, musculoskeletal, and neuromotor fitness in apparently healthy adults: guidance for prescribing exercise. *Med Sci Sports Exerc*. 2011;43(7):1334–59.
36. Gill DP, Gregory MA, Zou G, et al. The healthy mind, healthy mobility trial: a novel exercise program for older adults. *Med Sci Sports Exerc*. 2016;48(2):297–306.
37. Giroux I, Inglis SD, Lander S, Gerrie S, Mottola MF. Dietary intake, weight gain, and birth outcomes of physically active pregnant women: a pilot study. *Appl Physiol Nutr Metab*. 2006;31:483–9. doi:10.1139/h06-024.
38. Gjestland K, Bø K, Owe KM, Eberhard-Gran H. Do pregnant women follow exercise guidelines? Prevalence data among 3482 women, and prediction of low-back pain, pelvic girdle pain and depression. *Br J Sports Med*. 2013;47:515–20.
39. Haas R, Maloney S, Pausenberger E, et al. Clinical decision making in exercise prescription for fall prevention. *Phys Ther*. 2012;92(5):666–79.
40. Huang G, Wang R, Chen P, Huang SC, Donnelly JE, Mehlferber JP. Dose-response relationship of cardiorespiratory fitness adaptation to controlled endurance training in sedentary older adults. *Eur J Prev Cardiol*. 2016;23(5):518–29. doi:10.1177/2047487315582322.
41. Kader M, Naim-Shuchana S. Physical activity and exercise during pregnancy. *Eur J Physiother*. 2014;16:2–9. doi:10.3109/21679169.2013.861509.
42. Kallman DA, Plato CC, Tobin JD. The role of muscle loss in the age-related decline of grip strength: cross-sectional and longitudinal perspectives. *J Gerontol*. 1990;45(3):M82–8.
43. Kawaguchi JK, Pickering RK. Population-specific concerns: the pregnant athlete, part 1: anatomy and physiology of pregnancy. *Athl Ther Today*. 2010;15(2):39–43.
44. King AC, Pruitt LA, Woo S, et al. Effects of moderate-intensity exercise on polysomnographic and subjective sleep quality in older adults with mild to moderate sleep complaints. *J Gerontol A Biol Sci Med Sci*. 2008;63(9):997–1004.
45. Leong DJ, Sun HB. Osteoarthritis — why exercise? *J Exerc Sports Orthop*. 2014;1(1):04.
46. Mack GW, Weseman CA, Langhans GW, Scherzer H, Gillen CM, Nadel ER. Body fluid balance in dehydrated healthy older men: thirst and renal osmoregulation. *J Appl Physiol*. 1994;76:1615–23.
47. Malina RM. Tracking of physical activity and physical fitness across the lifespan. *Res Q Exerc Sport*. 1996;67(3 suppl):S48–57.
48. Mazzeo RS, Tanaka H. Exercise prescription for the elderly: current recommendations. *Sports Med*. 2001;31(11):809–18.
49. McDermott AY, Mernitz H. Exercise and older patients: prescribing guidelines. *Am Fam Physician*. 2006;74:437–44.
50. Melov S, Tarnopolsky MA, Beckman K, Felkey K, Hubbard A. Resistance exercise reverses aging in human skeletal muscle. *PLos One*. 2007;2(5):e465. doi:10.1371/journal.pone.0000465.
51. Melzer K, Schultz Y, Boulvain M, Kayser B. Physical activity and pregnancy: cardiovascular adaptations, recommendations and pregnancy outcomes. *Sports Med*. 2010;40(6):493–507.
52. Milunsky A, Ulcickas M, Rothman KJ, Willet W, Jick SS, Jick H. Maternal heat exposure and neural tube defects. *JAMA*. 1992;268(7):882–5.
53. Mottola MF. Exercise and pregnancy: Canadian guidelines for health care professionals. *Wellspring*. 2011;22(4):1–4.
54. Mottola MF. Exercise prescription for overweight and obese women: pregnancy and postpartum. *Obstet Gynecol Clin North Am*. 2009;36:301–16. doi:10.1016/j.ogc.2009.03.005.

55. Mottola MF. Physical activity and maternal obesity: cardiovascular adaptations, exercise recommendations, and pregnancy outcomes. *Nutr Rev*. 2013;71(suppl 1):S31–6. doi:10.1111/nure.12064.
56. Mottola MF, Davenport MH, Brun CR, Inglis SD, Charlesworth S, Sopper MM. $\dot{V}O_{2peak}$ prediction and exercise prescription for pregnant women. *Med Sci Sports Exerc*. 2006;38(8):1389–95.
57. Murray R. Exercise and Fluid Replacement: The American College of Sports Medicine Position Stand. *Gatorade Sports Science Institute. Med Sci Sports Exercise*. 1996;9(4).
58. Myers J, Kaykha A, George S, et al. Fitness versus physical activity patterns in predicting mortality in men. *Am J Med*. 2004;117(12):912–8.
59. Nelson ME, Rejeski WJ, Blair SN, et al. Physical activity and public health in older adults: recommendation from the American College of Sports Medicine and the American Heart Association. *Circulation*. 2007;116(9):1094–105.
60. O'Connor PJ, Poudevigne MS, Cress ME, Motl RW, Clapp JF III. Safety and efficacy of supervised strength training adopted in pregnancy. *J Phys Act Health*. 2011;8(3):309–20.
61. Okely AD, Booth ML, Chey T. Relationships between body composition and fundamental movement skills among children and adolescents. *Res Q Exerc Sport*. 2004;75(3):238–47.
62. Padayachee C, Coombes JS. Exercise guidelines for gestational diabetes mellitus. *World J Diabetes*. 2015;6(8):1033–44. doi:10.4239/wjd.v6.i8.1033.
63. Paridon SM, Alpert BS, Boas SR, et al. Clinical stress testing in the pediatric age group: a statement from the American Heart Association Council on Cardiovascular Disease in the Young, Committee on Atherosclerosis, Hypertension, and Obesity in Youth. *Circulation*. 2006;113(15):1905–20.
64. Paterson DH, Jones GR, Rice CL. Ageing and physical therapy activity: evidence to develop exercise recommendations for older adults. *Appl Physiol Nutr Metab*. 2007;32:589–5108. doi:10.1139/1107-111.
65. Pelaez M, Gonzalez-Cerron S, Montejo R, Barakat R. Pelvic floor muscle training included in a pregnancy exercise program is effective in primary prevention of urinary incontinence: a randomized controlled trial. *Neurourol Urodyn*. 2014;33(1):67–71.
66. Peterson MD, Gordon PM. Resistance exercise for the aging adult: clinical implications and prescription guidelines. *Am J Med*. 2011;124:194–8.
67. Physical activity guidelines for Americans. *Okla Nurse*. 2008;53(4):25.
68. Plowman SA, Meredith MD, editors. *Fitnessgram/Activitygram Reference Guide*. 4th ed. Dallas (TX): The Cooper Institute; 2013.
69. Pujol TJ, Barnes JT, Elder CL. Resistance training during pregnancy. *Strength Cond J*. 2007;29(2):44–6.
70. Qato DM, Alexander GC, Conti RM, Johnson M, Schumm P, Lindau ST. Use of prescription and over-the-counter medications and dietary supplements among older adults in the United States. *JAMA*. 2008;300(24):2867–78. doi:10.1001/jama.2008.892.
71. Rosenberg IH. Sarcopenia: origins and clinical relevance. *J Nutr*. 1997;127(5 suppl):990S–1S.
72. Rowland TW. *Pediatric Laboratory Exercise Testing: Clinical Guidelines*. Champaign (IL): Human Kinetics; 1993.
73. Royal College of Obstetricians and Gynaecologists. *RCOG Statement No. 4: Exercise in Pregnancy* [Internet]. [cited 2016 Feb 1]. London (United Kingdom): Royal College of Obstetricians and Gynaecologists. Available from: http://www.rcog.org.uk/womens-health/clinical-guidance/exercise-pregnancy
74. Sawka MN, Burke LM, Eichner ER, Maughan RJ, Montain SJ, Stachenfeld NS. American College of Sports Medicine position stand. Exercise and fluid replacement. *Med Sci Sports Exerc*. 2007;39(2):377–90.
75. Shankar K, Harrell A, Liu X, Gilchrist JM, Ronis MJ, Badger TM. Maternal obesity at conception programs obesity in the offspring. *Am J Physiol Regul Integr Comp Physiol*. 2008;294:R528–38. doi:10.1152/ajpregu.00316.2007.
76. SHAPE America. *Active Start: A Statement of Physical Activity Guidelines for Children From Birth to Age 5*. 2nd ed. Reston (VA): SHAPE; 2009.
77. Simmonds B, Fox K, Davis M, et al. Objectively assessed physical activity and subsequent health service use of UK adults aged 70 and over: a four to five year follow up study. *PLoS One*. 2014;9(5):e97676. doi:10.1371/journal.pone.0097676.
78. Sports Medicine Australia. SMA statement the benefits and risks of exercise during pregnancy. *J Sci Med Sport*. 2002;5;11–9.
79. Stathokostas L, Little RMD, Vandervoot AA, Paterson DH. Flexibility training and functional ability in older adults: a systematic review. *J Aging Res*. 2012;2012:306818. doi:10.1155/2012/306818.
80. Stathokostas H, McDonald MW, Little RMD, Paterson DH. Flexibility of older adults aged 55–86 years and the influence of physical activity. *J Aging Res*. 2013;2013:743843. doi:10.1155/2013/743843.
81. Stenhagen M, Ekström H, Nordell E, Elmståhl S. Falls in the general elderly population: a 3- and 6-year prospective study of risk factors using data from the longitudinal population study "Good ageing in Skane." *BMC Geriatr*. 2013;13:81.
82. Strong WB, Malina RM, Blimkie CJ, et al. Evidence based physical activity for school-age youth. *J Pediatr*. 2005;146(6):732–7.
83. The Cooper Institute. *Fitnessgram & Activitygram Test Administration Manual*. 4th ed. Chicago (IL): Human Kinetics; 2007. 152 p.
84. Tinius RA, Cahill AG, Strand EA, Cade WT. Maternal inflammation during late pregnancy is lower in physically active compared with inactive obese women. *Appl Physiol Nutr Metab*. 2016;41(2):191–8. doi:10.1139/apnm-2015-0316.
85. Tobias DK, Zhang C, van Dam RM, Bowers K, Hu FB. Physical activity before and during pregnancy and risk of gestational diabetes mellitus: a meta-analysis. *Diabetes Care*. 2011;34:223–9. doi:10.2337/dc10-1368.
86. Tomić V, Sporiš G, Tomić J, Milanović Z, Zigmundovac-Klaić D, Pantelić S. The effect of maternal exercise during pregnancy on abnormal fetal growth. *Croat Med J*. 2013;54:362–8. doi:10.3325/cmj.2013.54.362.
87. Utter AC, Robertson RJ, Nieman DC, Kang J. Children's OMNI Scale of Perceived Exertion: walking/running evaluation. *Med Sci Sports Exerc*. 2002;34(1):139–44.

88. Wang SM. Dezinno P, Maranets I, Berman MR, Caldwell-Andrews AA, Kain ZN. Low back pain during pregnancy: prevalence, risk factors, and outcomes. *Obstet Gynecol.* 2004;104(1):65–70.
89. Warburton DER, Nicol CW, Bredin SS. Health benefits of physical activity: the evidence. *CMAJ.* 2006;174(6):801–9.
90. Wasinski F, Bacurau RF, Estrela GR, et al. Exercise during pregnancy protects adult mouse offspring from diet-induced obesity. *Nutr Metab.* 2015;12:56. doi:10.1186/s12986-015-0052-z.
91. Weissgerber TL, Wolfe LA. Physiological adaptation in early human pregnancy: adaptation to balance maternal-fetal demands. *Appl Physiol Nutr Metab.* 2006;31:1–11. doi:10.1139/h05-003.
92. Williams HG, Pfeiffer KA, O'Neill JR, et al. Motor skill performance and physical activity in preschool children. *Obesity (Silver Spring).* 2008;16(6):1421–6.
93. Wolfe LA, Davies GLA. Canadian guidelines for exercise in pregnancy. *Clin Obstet Gynecol.* 2003;46(2):488–95.
94. World Health Organization. *Global Strategy on Diet, Physical Activity and Health, WHO Information Fact Sheet* [Internet]. Geneva (Switzerland): World Health Organization; 2016.

PART IV

Exercise Testing and Prescription for Special Populations

CHAPTER 10

Special Considerations for Cardiovascular Disease: Chronic Stable Angina and Coronary Artery Bypass Graft Surgery

INTRODUCTION

For patients with cardiovascular disease, **exercise** is a critically important intervention and should be prioritized to slow the progression of disease and prevent or reverse physical **deconditioning**. Along with other therapeutics prescribed to patients with cardiovascular disease, exercise training should be viewed as medicinal. As is the case with all medicines, it is critically important that the optimal "dose" of exercise is recommended to patients. This chapter presents background and special considerations related to exercise testing, prescription, and progression for individuals with chronic stable angina and for postsurgical patients following coronary revascularization. Although there are issues and concerns that specifically pertain to individuals who have been revascularized versus those with chronic angina, many of the benefits and limitations of exercise training apply to both types of patients.

Case Study 10-1

Ms. Case Study-Angina

Ms. Case Study-Angina is a 64-year-old female that recently retired from providing pastoral care at a local college. She has a past history of endometriosis, Ménière disease, gastroesophageal reflux disease (GERD), asthma, hyperlipidemia, osteoporosis, and metabolic syndrome. For many months, she has been experiencing exertional subscapular pain. Additionally, she frequently experiences chest pain which, at a minimum, is partially related to GERD. Unlike the subscapular pain, the chest pain is more random, occurring both while at rest and with exertion. She underwent nuclear imaging testing that was positive for electrocardiogram (ECG) changes that occurred with chest and subscapular pain. Ms. Case Study-Angina had a heart catheterization which revealed a 50% obstruction of the left anterior descending artery and a 90% obstruction of a small right coronary artery, neither of which was amenable to intervention. Thus, she is being treated for her GERD, cardiovascular disease, and angina pectoris medically with the following regimen: aspirin, isosorbide mononitrate, 30 mg; extended-release metoprolol, 25 mg; atorvastatin, 40 mg; and omeprazole, 40 mg.

Ms. Case Study-Angina reports to cardiac rehabilitation (CR) for her baseline exercise tolerance test and consult with a preventive cardiologist 28 days after her catheterization. Her cardiac risk factor history includes a positive family history for premature coronary artery disease, hypertension, hyperlipidemia, and insulin resistance. She reports that she continues to have moderate threshold exertional angina which always resolved with rest. In particular, she reported experiencing subscapular pain when exerting in the cold weather. She claims that her symptoms are slightly but not substantially better since starting with isosorbide mononitrate and β-blocker therapy.

An exercise tolerance test was performed, and she exercised for 6.5 minutes of a standard Bruce protocol. Ms. Case Study-Angina first reported subscapular pain at about 5 minutes into the test and at a heart rate (HR) of 114 bpm. At peak exercise, she reported 2 out of 4 angina pain with ECG changes of 1- to 2-mm ST depression. Her peak HR and volume of oxygen consumed per unit time ($\dot{V}O_2$) were 124 bpm and 17.5 mL $O_2 \cdot kg^{-1} \cdot min^{-1}$, respectively. Her respiratory exchange ratio was 1.02, which would suggest that the test was physiologically not **maximal**. Her peak $\dot{V}O_2$ measures would place her at about 20% above age- and gender-matched females entering CR with a similar diagnosis (1). On the other hand, her fitness measures would place her at about the 25th percentile of otherwise healthy women of a similar age (11). Currently, her **body mass index (BMI)** is 27, which would categorize her as overweight. Other baseline values include the following:

- Waist circumference = 94 cm (37 in)
- Resting ECG: HR is normal sinus rhythm = 68 bpm
- Resting blood pressure (BP): 144/80 mm Hg
- Blood test
  - Total cholesterol = 124 mg $\cdot$ dL^{-1}
  - Triglyceride = 59 mg $\cdot$ dL^{-1}
  - High-density lipoprotein (HDL) cholesterol = 54 mg $\cdot$ dL^{-1}
  - Low-density lipoprotein (LDL) cholesterol = 58 mg $\cdot$ dL^{-1}
  - Glycolated hemoglobin (HbA1C) = 5.9

Based on the results of the stress test, a short-term goal for CR was established that the exercise program would include treadmill walking, rowing and cycle ergometry, and **strength** training (Table 10.1). Additionally, given that her recent HbA1C level was elevated at 5.9, the importance of weight loss was emphasized. A mutually agreed on goal of 2.5–5 kg (5.5–11 lb) weight loss was established.

A target HR of 104 bpm for aerobic training was established based on the guidelines that recommend that patients with angina exercise at an HR of at least 10 bpm below their angina threshold (3). At the first session of CR, Ms. Case Study-Angina walked on the treadmill for 15 minutes at a speed of 2.0 mph, 1% grade.

(continues)

Case Study 10-1 (continued)

Table 10.1 Cardiac Rehabilitation Exercise Training Summary for Ms. Case Study-Angina

			Treadmill					
Session	HR (bpm)	BP (mm Hg)	Time	Speed/G	HR/RPE	Rower Time/HR	Cycle Time/HR	Angina Scale
1	73	130/80	:15	2.0/1.0	98/12	:05/94	:05/92	1/4
3	72	120/84	:19	2.0/0.5	90/11	:06/88	:06/87	0/4
6	66	140/90	:22	2.0/1.0	97/12	:07/93	:09/93	1/4
9	73	130/80	:26	2.0/1.0	102/12	:08/90	:08/92	0/4
12	72	120/84	:30	2.1/0.5	98/12	:08/88	:08/87	2/4
15	66	140/90	:30	2.0/1.0	97/11	:08/93	:08/93	1/4
18	78	144/94	:30	2.3/2.5	98/12	:08/94	:08/99	1/4
19	77	132/84	:30	2.1/1.0	96/13	:08/93	:08/96	2/4
20	76	130/78	:30	2.1/1.0	94/13	:08/97	:08/91	2/4
21	73	130/80	:30	2.3/2.0	96/12	:08/94	:08/92	1/4
24	72	120/84	:30	2.3/2.0	94/13	:10/88	:10/87	1/4
27	66	124/80	:30	2.3/2.5	95/13	:10/93	:10/95	1/4
30	84	128/72	:30	2.3/2.5	97/13	:10/96	:10/94	1/4
33	66	150/84	:30	2.4/2.5	93/13	:10/98	:10/88	1/4
36	76	160/80	:30	2.5/2.5	95/13	:10/93	:10/95	1/4

G, grade.

The speed and grade was selected based on the patient reporting that it was "moderate" (rating of perceived exertion [RPE] = 12) intensity. At the end of the 15 minutes, her HR was 98, and she reported 2 out of 4 subscapular pain and 2 out of 4 chest angina pain, both of which subsided with the cessation of walking. She also exercised for 5 minutes each on the rower and cycle ergometer, experiencing no discomfort. By session 6, she had increased the duration on the treadmill, cycle, and rower to 22, 7, and 9 minutes, respectively. She continued to experience angina each time she walked on the treadmill.

At session 6, the following resistance training exercises were introduced: arm curl, overhead press, triceps extension, bench press, lateral pull-down, leg extension and press, and hamstring curl. The weight for each of the exercises was selected using a conservative approach and done so while directly observing the patient performing the exercise. Proper technique was emphasized, and the initial weight for the various exercises was determined by selecting a resistance that patient perceived to be "light." The patient was instructed to exhale during the **concentric** phase of the exercise and to inhale during the **eccentric** phase. The goal is to gradually titrate the weight upward so that, eventually, the 10th repetition of a particular set is considered to be "heavy" or "hard" (10).

At session 7, an extended warm-up on the treadmill was attempted. Ms. Case Study-Angina started at 1.5 mph for 5 minutes, and then the speed was increased to 2 mph and the grade was elevated to 1% gradually over the next 5 minutes. She denied any angina despite walking on the treadmill for a total of 25 minutes. By session 12, she had increased the total duration of exercise to 46 minutes, with 30 minutes spent on the treadmill and 8 minutes on both the cycle and rowing ergometers. At session 12, however, she reported 2 out of 4 angina on the treadmill despite the extended warm-up. Starting with session 13, she began to take nitroglycerin about 15

Case Study 10-1 (continued)

minutes before commencing with her exercise session. Ms. Case Study-Angina took sublingual nitroglycerin while resting in a chair in an attempt to cause vasodilatation of the coronary arteries before beginning exercise. Prior to getting on the treadmill, her BP was rechecked to make sure that it was not too low. Her BP decreased from an entry value of 120/84 to 108/74 mm Hg. She denied any significant symptoms, but she experienced a low-level headache for a few minutes after taking the nitroglycerin. She was able to complete her exercise session without experiencing any angina.

By session 18, she was able to walk for 30 minutes at a speed and grade of 2.3 mph at a 2.5% grade. However, Ms. Case Study-Angina had complaints of experiencing frequent subscapular pain while doing **activities of daily living (ADL)**, in particular walking in the cold and carrying laundry upstairs. Entry BP readings upon arrival at CR have been normal to slightly elevated. In an attempt to remedy her predictably occurring angina, her cardiologist increased her dose of isosorbide mononitrate from 30 to 60 mg.

The first 2 sessions (sessions 19 and 20) after the increase in isosorbide mononitrate, the practice of taking the sublingual nitroglycerin prior to the exercise session was discontinued. In both of these sessions, angina came on at a much lower speed and grade. At session 21, the practice of administering the nitroglycerin 15 minutes prior to beginning the exercise session was reestablished. By session 27, she was able to exercise for a total of 50 minutes of exercise. Her speed and grade on the treadmill was increased to 2.3 mph and 2.5%, respectively.

Prior to session 28, Ms. Case Study-Angina consulted with her cardiologist. Persistent angina pain while doing everyday activities and exercise precipitated a change from isosorbide mononitrate to ranolazine 500 mg, another type of antianginal medication. As was the case when the dose of isosorbide mononitrate was increased, the practice of administering the sublingual nitroglycerin prior to exercise was eventually discontinued. She was able to exercise at her previous intensity with only minimal symptoms. After completing 36 sessions of CR, Ms. Case Study-Angina went through a post-program evaluation that included an exercise tolerance test and blood work. Her pre- and post-program values are included in Table 10.2.

On her exit stress test, she was able to increase the exercise duration from 6:30 to 8:45 minutes. Her stress test was stopped due to dyspnea. She experience no scapular angina pain but did have 1/10 chest pressure. Her aerobic fitness improved by 7%. Her peak HR on the exit test was 133 bpm with 1-mm ST-segment depression in leads V_2 through V_4. Consequently, she was able to work to a higher peak HR on her exit test than at entry (133 vs. 114 bpm) while experiencing fewer anginal symptoms.

Table 10.2 Cardiac Rehabilitation Pre/Post-Program Values for Ms. Case Study-Angina

	CR Entry	CR Exit	% Change
Weight (kg)	64.5	63	−2.3
Waist circumference (cm)	94	91	−3.1
Peak $\dot{V}O_2$ (mL $O_2 \cdot kg^{-1} \cdot min^{-1}$)	17.5	18.8	+7.5
Stress test treadmill time (min) (Bruce protocol)	6:30	8:45	+18.2
Estimated METs	7	10	+42.9
Total cholesterol (mg/dL)	124	129	+4.0
Triglyceride (mg/dL)	59	64	+8.5
HDL cholesterol (mg/dL)	54	57	+5.6
LDL cholesterol (mg/dL)	58	59	No change
HbA1C (%)	5.9	5.7	−3.4

METs, metabolic equivalents.

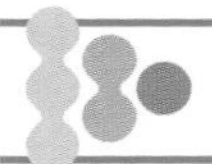

Description, Prevalence, and Etiology of Angina Pectoris

Ischemic heart disease is a major public health problem. It is estimated that 1 in 3 adults (about 81 million people) in the United States has some form of ischemic heart disease, including nearly 10 million people with angina pectoris (9). Common symptoms associated with heart disease are angina, dyspnea at rest or at low levels of exertion, orthopnea, peripheral edema, palpitations, dizziness, and syncope. Angina is defined as chest pain, pressure, discomfort, or fullness that is the manifestation of diminished blood flow resulting in inadequate oxygen delivery to the myocardium. Angina is not a disease but rather the symptom of an underlying heart problem. Typically, angina is brought on by exertion or psychological stress and will resolve with rest or medications that induce vasodilatation. Angina-related symptoms may occur in isolation or in combination. Management of symptoms is of paramount importance in the treatment of patients with heart disease and is important reason for referral to CR.

Angina can be a recurring problem or a sudden, acute health concern. Worsening ("crescendo") angina, sudden-onset angina at rest, and angina lasting more than 15 minutes are symptoms of "unstable" angina. Chronic "stable" angina is usually related to myocardial ischemia. A typical presentation of stable angina occurs following the initiation of **physical activity**. Generally, symptoms at rest are nonexistent. The anginal symptoms generally resolve with a cessation of activity, a decrease in physical activity intensity, or administration of vasodilator medication.

Education and counseling are important when developing an exercise training program for an individual who experiences chronic, stable angina (9). Patients need to understand and be able to recognize their symptoms. Specifically, patients need to be able to identify the nature of their angina (*e.g.*, location, precipitating factors, associated symptoms, and radiation patterns) and understand that activity patterns need to be adjusted according to the severity of symptoms. It should be clearly communicated to the patient that although experiencing lesser levels of anginal discomfort is acceptable and safe, highly intense pain is to be avoided. Also, reinforcing adherence to medical therapy is of paramount importance. Medications such as β-blockers, nitrates, and calcium channel blockers may influence an individual's ischemic threshold and should be taken at the prescribed intervals and dose. In addition to the daily prescribed medication, using nitroglycerin prophylactically can be an effective means for an individual to avoid experiencing exercise-induced angina. Taking nitroglycerin about 15 minutes before starting an exercise session may allow a patient to exercise symptom-free at higher workloads than would be possible otherwise.

Case Study 10-2

Mr. Case Study-CABGS

Mr. Case Study-CABGS is a 62-year-old male optometrist. He has a past medical history of asthma, hypertension, and hyperlipidemia. He describes being physically active throughout his typical day but participates in no regular exercise. He presents to his primary care physician with complaints of classic angina symptoms of exertional, substernal chest pain that radiates to the left arm. He was referred for an exercise tolerance test, which was markedly positive with 3- to 4-mm ST-segment depression occurring at 6 minutes on the Bruce protocol. He was immediately put on antianginal medication, lipid-lowering (statin) therapy, and aspirin and was referred for a cardiac catheterization. The catheterization revealed diffuse disease in left main, left anterior descending, left circumflex, and right coronary arteries. His ejection fraction was preserved at 65%. Coronary artery bypass graft surgery (CABGS) was recommended. Surgery included a full sternotomy, a bypass of the left anterior descending artery with the left anterior mammary artery, and saphenous vein grafts to the second obtuse and right coronary arteries. Mr. Case Study-CABGS was in and out of atrial fibrillation during surgery but experienced no serious complications. He did experience atrial fibrillation on post-op day 1. Consequently, metoprolol and warfarin were initiated. By post-op day 5, normal sinus rhythm had been restored, and he was discharged to home.

Case Study 10-2 (continued)

As an outpatient, his recovery proceeded without complications and he arrived at CR 28 days post-surgery for his baseline consultation and cardiopulmonary exercise tolerance test. He reports that he has been walking for approximately 10 minutes per day. He denies any symptoms other than moderate sternal and saphenous vein-related soreness. His height and weight were 175 cm and 89 kg, respectively. He has lost about 2.5 kg since his surgery, claiming that he does not have much of an appetite. Currently, his BMI is 28, which would categorize him as overweight.

- Waist circumference = 104 cm (41 in)
- Resting ECG: HR is normal sinus rhythm = 64 bpm
- Resting BP: 140/70 mm Hg
- Blood test (preoperative)
  - Total cholesterol = 176 $mg \cdot dL^{-1}$
  - Triglyceride = 198 $mg \cdot dL^{-1}$
  - HDL cholesterol = 39 $mg \cdot dL^{-1}$
  - LDL cholesterol = 97 $mg \cdot dL^{-1}$
  - HbA1C = 5.8

Mr. Case Study-CABGS's medications were reviewed, and his statin therapy was increased from 5 to 20 mg of rosuvastatin to comply with statin therapy treatment guidelines for individuals with a diagnosis of coronary heart disease (17). Otherwise, his medications were held constant and included warfarin, 10 mg of amlodipine, 81 mg of aspirin, and 25 mg of metoprolol.

A cardiopulmonary exercise tolerance test utilizing the Bruce protocol was performed as part of his baseline assessment. He was able to exercise for 3 minutes. His peak HR, $\dot{V}O_2$, and respiratory exchange ratio were 107 bpm, 17.2 $mL\ O_2 \cdot kg^{-1} \cdot min^{-1}$, and 1.38, respectively. The exercise ECG revealed no abnormalities, and he denied experiencing any angina-related symptoms. Therefore, he was cleared to begin CR and was instructed to start increasing the duration of his daily walks on non-CR days.

A goal was established for Mr. Case Study-CABGS to increase his daily walking time by 5 minutes each week until he is walking for 30 minutes on nearly all his non-CR days. It was also recommended that he log his activity daily so that it can be reviewed periodically with the CR staff to assess adherence to exercise.

The first session of CR is intended to familiarize the participant with the program, identify goals and objectives, and initiate an individualized exercise training regimen. In consultation with the CR case manager, the following goals for CR were identified for Mr. Case Study-CABGS:

- Improve aerobic fitness and strength.
- Lose weight.
- Lower HbA1C value.
- Lower triglycerides and raise HDL-cholesterol.

A primary goal of the **exercise prescription**, along with improve aerobic fitness, is to maximize caloric expenditure to promote weight loss (2). Consequently, non–weight-supported exercise is prioritized. Additionally, a dual-action cycle ergometer is selected as an exercise modality because it allows for an upper body activity as he continues to recover from his sternotomy. Table 10.3 has specific information for exercise sessions 1, 3, and 6. Additionally, we tracked his caloric expenditure utilizing the "on-board" displays for the exercise equipment. Caloric expenditure estimates for sessions 1, 3, and 6 were 160, 205, and 230 calories, respectively.

Prior to every CR exercise session, the general health status of the patient is evaluated. Additionally, adherence to medication home exercise and dietary recommendation are assessed. At session 6, Mr. Case Study-CABGS arrives to CR with an elevated HR but denied any symptoms. Telemetry monitory revealed that he was in atrial fibrillation. He confirmed that he was continuing to taking warfarin. The medical director was consulted and he, in turn, conferred with the patient's cardiologist. The patient was instructed to make a follow-up appointment with his cardiologist but was allowed to exercise given the lack of symptoms.

(continues)

Case Study 10-2 (continued)

Table 10.3 Cardiac Rehabilitation Exercise Training Summary for Mr. Case Study-CABGS

			Treadmill						
Session	Weight (kg)	HR (bpm)	BP (mm Hg)	Time	Speed/G	HR/RPE	Combined Arm/Leg Cycle Time/HR	Elliptical Time/HR	Calories Expended
1	85	72	140/70	:25	2.8/2	84/12	N/A	:05/88	160
3	84	57	118/84	:25	2.8/3	74/11+	:06/79	:05/84	205
6	84	98	140/80	:25	3.0/3	120/11+	:08/110	:06/120	230
9	83	84	148/88	:14 :16	3.1/2.5 3.8/2.5	84/12 108/15	:12/108	:08/112	320
18	82.5	107	138/80	:14 :16	3.1/2.5 3.8/3.0	102/12 108/15	:14/108	:12/104	365
21	82.5	72	148/88	:14 :16	3.3/3.0 3.8/3.0	90/12 96/15	:15/96	:13/94	397
29	81	102	138/80	:14 :16	3.3/4.0 3.9/4.0	102/12 108/15	:14/108	:12/104	425
36	80	98	134/80	:14 :16	3.3/4.0 4.0/4.0	96/12 102/15	:15/108	:15/106	435

G, grade.

Instead of relying on target HR as a primary gauge for assessing exercise intensity, the atrial fibrillation required the utilization of RPE. Despite significantly higher HRs, the patient tolerated the exercise session without any adverse effects. After conferring with his cardiologist, the plan for Mr. Case Study-CABGS was for him to have an electrical cardioversion in 4 weeks. He was subtherapeutic on warfarin, which necessitated a switch to apixaban. Meanwhile, he continued to come to CR, adjusting exercise training intensity by perceived exertion.

At exercise session 7 (about 7 weeks post-surgery), resistance training was started. A week prior, Mr. Case Study-CABGS had a routine, post-surgery chest x-ray and consult with his cardiothoracic surgeon. The chest x-ray confirmed that the sternum was healing as expected. Surgery-related weight restrictions limit upper extremity lifting to less than 4.5 kg for 12 weeks from the date of surgery. Specifically, he was instructed to do one set each of bicep curls and lateral raises with 2.5 kg (5 lb) dumbbells in each hand for 10 repetitions. Also, he was instructed to do one set each of the leg press, extension, and curl. Even though there are no absolute weight limits for lower body weight resistance exercise, weight selection was based on the individual's ability to complete 10 repetitions while maintaining proper form and through the fullest **range of motion** possible with minimal strain.

Baseline aerobic fitness at entry to CR for Mr. Case Study-CABGS was very low (1). He was about 10% below age-matched men with a similar diagnosis who were entering CR. Further highlighting just how unfit he was, his fitness level would put him in just the 5th percentile for age-matched, otherwise healthy males (11). Consequently, to specifically target Mr. Case Study-CABGS's low level of aerobic fitness, interval training was introduced at session 9. For Mr. Case Study-CABGS, a 2-minute interval was selected with the higher intensity interval subjectively rated as hard, whereas the lower intensity interval was rated as moderate.

At session 18 (12 weeks post-surgery), bench press, lateral pull-downs, and triceps extension exercises were added to his resistance training regimen. He continued to do leg press, bicep curls, and lateral raises. Relatively light weight was used for the first session. Gradually, thereafter, he was instructed to increase the weight until he found the weight

Case Study 10-2 (continued)

that caused fatigue with 10 repetitions but allowed for proper form through the fullest range of motion as possible. RPE was used to gauge exercise intensity while performing resistance training exercise. Mr. Case Study-CABGS was instructed to aim for an RPE of 15 (hard) when completing the 10th repetition of a particular exercise.

Prior to session 21, Mr. Case study-CABGS underwent successful cardioversion of atrial fibrillation to normal sinus rhythm with a 100 J biphasic shock. He was released from the hospital and returned to CR. Given that he was on the same amount of rate control medication as when he underwent his entry exercise tolerance test, target HR was used again to guide exercise intensity.

At session 29, Mr. Case Study-CABGS reported to CR with a regular but rapid HR. A 12-lead ECG revealed atrial flutter with 2:1 conduction. As was the case when he experienced atrial fibrillation, he denied symptoms and was allowed to continue with his exercise training.

After completing 36 sessions of CR, Mr. Case Study-CABGS went through a post-program evaluation that included an exercise tolerance tests and blood work. His pre- and post-program values are included in Table 10.4.

At baseline, he had all five of the components of metabolic syndrome: (history of) hypertension, insulin resistance, abdominal obesity, low HDL cholesterol, and high triglycerides. At exit, lipids and hypertension were well maintained on the combination of medical therapy and lifestyle. Weight loss and exercise also resulted in a decrease in abdominal obesity as measured by waist circumference and improved insulin sensitivity as reflected by a decline in HbA1C values. His weight loss achievement is even more impressive when one considers that he had lost 2.5 kg (5.5 lb) prior to starting CR. Therefore, through dietary change and exercise, he was able to not only sustain his initial, postsurgical weight loss but also go beyond that to achieve a weight loss total of 7.5 kg (16.5 lb).

Table 10.4 Cardiac Rehabilitation Pre/Post-Program Values for Mr. Case Study-CABGS

	CR Entry	CR Exit	Percentage Change
Weight (lb)	187	176	−5.9
Waist circumference (in)	41	38	−6.5
Peak $\dot{V}O_2$ (mL $O_2 \cdot kg^{-1} \cdot min^{-1}$)	17	22.7	+33.5
Estimated METs	7	10	+42.9
Total cholesterol (mg/dL)	176	115	−34.7
Triglyceride (mg/dL)	198	81	−59.1
HDL cholesterol (mg/dL)	39	51	+30.8
LDL cholesterol (mg/dL)	97	48	−50.5
HbA1C (%)	5.8	5.5	−5.2

METs, metabolic equivalents.

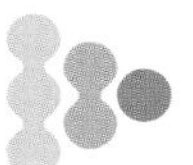

Description, Prevalence, and Etiology of Coronary Artery Bypass Graft Surgery

There are different methods of coronary revascularization that vary significantly regarding the level of invasiveness and the time required for convalescence. The least invasive method for revascularization is a catheter-based, percutaneous intervention. CABGS is the most durable and complete treatment for coronary heart disease. Nearly 400,000 CABGSs are performed each year in the United States (12).

Although CABGS results in revascularization, it should not be viewed as a permanent fix. Patients who have undergone CABGS remain at risk for the progression of coronary artery disease of the native arteries or the development of vein graft atherosclerosis. Exercise is a critically important component of the secondary prevention strategy for patients after CABGS.

CABGS is an invasive method to achieve revascularization and involves surgically grafting a harvested blood vessel (*i.e.*, saphenous vein, internal mammary artery, and radial artery) to a coronary artery. Essentially, the CABG procedure bypasses an area of the coronary artery that has restricted blood flow as a result of atherosclerosis. Typically, the conventional CABG procedure involves accessing the heart by way of a sternum-splitting incision. Surgical advances have led to techniques that allow for minimally invasive surgeries that do not require separating the sternum. In theory, minimally invasive surgeries allow for a more speeding recovery than surgery involving a sternotomy. Recovery times after minimally invasive operations are from 2 to 4 weeks. For a patient undergoing sternotomy, significant activity restrictions are put in place, particularly for upper body activities. Upper body weight restrictions are often put in place for up to 8–12 weeks from the date of surgery. A patient needs not to wait until 12 weeks to start with an exercise program, however. Patients undergoing CABGS can start with lower intensity exercise as early as 2 weeks post-surgery with an initial focus on lower body, aerobic activity.

Preparticipation Health Screening, Medical History, and Physical Examination

After experiencing a cardiac event and prior to starting an exercise training program, **medical clearance** is recommended (10). It is recommended that patients undergo a baseline evaluation where medical and surgical history — including the most recent cardiovascular event, comorbidities, and other pertinent medical history — are reviewed (3). The baseline assessment should include a physical examination with an emphasis on the cardiopulmonary and musculoskeletal systems. Current medications including dose, means by which the drug is administered, and frequency need to be confirmed, and cardiovascular risk factors should be identified. The baseline physical examination should be performed by a physician or other appropriate health care provider under the direction of a physician who is actively involved in the care of patients with coronary artery disease. Identification of contraindications for exercise training have been developed and should be considered prior to having an individual with coronary artery disease initiate an exercise training program.

Case Study Quiz:

Preparticipation Health Screening, Medical History, and Physical Examination

Case Study 10-1

1. Ms. Case Study-Angina had a positive stress test with angina. Is it appropriate for her to start CR?
2. What are your concerns and what precautions are advised when a patient takes a nitroglycerin?

Case Study 10-2

1. Regarding targeting coronary artery risk factors, what are the goals of the exercise prescription for Mr. Case Study-CABGS?
2. Metabolic syndrome is linked to development of coronary artery disease. Does this man meet the criteria that would classify him as having metabolic syndrome?

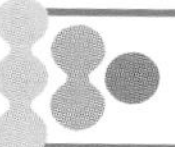

Exercise Testing Considerations

As part of the baseline evaluation, it is highly preferred for a patient to perform a symptom-limited exercise tolerance test (*e.g.*, exercise stress test). Information obtained from an exercise test is necessary for developing an *individualized*, safe, and appropriate exercise prescription and is useful for guiding a patient's return to work or home/leisure activities. Because some medications affect HR, BP, and exercise tolerance, a patient should be instructed to take medications as prescribed on the day of the stress test.

Unfortunately, many individuals do not perform an exercise test prior to initiating an exercise training program. For these individuals, the exercise prescription should be implemented conservatively with close surveillance. For all patients, regardless of whether an exercise tolerance test is administered, RPE should be used as a tool to guide and adjust exercise intensity while maintaining patients within their physical limitations and below their symptomatic threshold.

Case Study Quiz:

Exercise Testing Considerations

Case Study 10-1

3. Explain how administering nitroglycerin prophylactically can help decrease angina symptoms.

Case Study 10-2

3. Mr. Case Study-CABGS was able to exercise for only 3 minutes. Would this be considered a submaximal test?

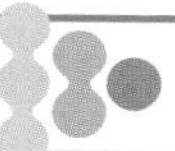

Exercise Prescription and Progression Considerations

Prescriptive techniques for determining exercise dosage or the frequency, intensity, time, and type (FITT) of an exercise prescription for chronic stable angina and coronary artery bypass surgery patients are detailed in the FITT table (Table 10.5) (4).

Typically, an exercise session consists of a 5- to 10-minute warm-up and cool-down period in addition to the aerobic training phase (3). The warm-up and cool-down phases should include range of motion, stretching, and low-intensity aerobic activities. For patients with chronic stable angina, a lower intensity and prolonged warm-up might help avoid the development of symptoms, ECG changes, arrhythmias, and cardiac dysfunction (3). Conversely, an extended exercise cool-down phase facilitates the gradual return of HR and BP to resting values. Irrespective of an individual's qualifying diagnosis or whether an exercise tolerance test was performed, it is generally recommended that patients initially exercise at the lower end of the recommended training intensity (40%–60% heart rate reserve [HRR] or 11–13 on the RPE scale) (4). Exercise training intensity should be progressively increased as tolerated, up to 80% of HRR or 14–17 on the RPE scale.

The deleterious consequences of low fitness have been well documented (13). Evidence suggests that fitness level is an important, independent predictor of long-term health outcomes. Exercise training programs for individuals with coronary artery disease have traditionally targeted a light-to-moderate intensity for exercise training (3). The vast majority of studies reporting outcomes in cardiac patients have used a training regimen of moderate-intensity exercise.

FITT

TABLE 10.5 FITT RECOMMENDATIONS FOR INDIVIDUALS IN OUTPATIENT CARDIAC REHABILITATION

ACSM FITT Principle of the ExR_x

Chronic Medical Condition	Frequency (How often?)	Intensity (How hard?)	Time	Type (What kind?) Primary	Resistance	Flexibility	Special Considerations
Healthy Adult	$\geq$5 d · wk^{-1} of moderate exercise, or $\geq$3 d · wk^{-1} of vigorous exercise, or a combination of moderate and vigorous exercise on $\geq$3–5 d · wk^{-1} is recommended.	Moderate to vigorous. Light-to-moderate intensity exercise may be beneficial in deconditioned individuals.	If moderate intensity: $\geq$30 min · d^{-1} to total 150 min · wk^{-1}. If vigorous intensity: $\geq$20 min · d^{-1} to total 75 min · wk^{-1}.	Regular, purposeful exercise that involves major muscle groups and is continuous and rhythmic in nature is recommended.	2–3 d · wk^{-1} (nonconsecutive)	2–3 d · wk^{-1}; static stretch 10–30 s; 2–4 repetitions of each exercise	Sedentary behaviors can have adverse health effects, even among those who regularly exercise. Adding short physical activity breaks throughout the day may be considered as a part of the exercise.
CVD in Outpatient CR	Minimal 3 d · wk^{-1}; preferably 5 d · wk^{-1}	With an exercise test, use 40%–80% of exercise capacity, using HRR, $\dot{V}O_2R$, or $\dot{V}O_{2peak}$. Without an exercise test, use seated or standing HR_{rest} + 20–30 bpm or an RPE of 12–16 on a 6–20 scale.	20–60 min	Arm ergometer, upper and lower (dual action) extremity ergometer, upright and recumbent cycles, recumbent stepper, rower, elliptical, stair climber, or treadmill	2–3 d · wk^{-1} (nonconsecutive) at 40%–60% 1-RM or RPE ~11–13 (6–20 scale) 10–15 repetitions. Without fatigue, 1–3 sets per exercise. 8–10 different muscle groups. Select equipment that is safe for the patient to use.	2–3 d · wk^{-1}; with daily being most effective. Stretch to the point of feeling tightness or slight discomfort. 15 s hold for static stretching; >4 repetitions of each exercise. Static and dynamic stretching focused on major muscle groups of the limbs and lower back; consider PNF stretching.	Special considerations for those with angina to stay below the ischemic threshold; medications such as β-blockers, nitrates, and calcium channel blockers may influence the ischemic threshold. Patients with CABGS with sternotomy need to ensure that the sternum is fully healed and stable. Significant restrictions for upper body activities for up to 8–12 wk from the date of surgery. Encourage patients with CABGS to start to exercise prior to 12 wk.

ExR_x, exercise prescription; CVD, cardiovascular disease; $\dot{V}O_2R$, oxygen uptake reserve; $\dot{V}O_{2peak}$, peak oxygen uptake; HR_{rest}, resting heart rate; 1-RM, one repetition maximum; PNF, proprioceptive neuromuscular facilitation.

Based on the FITT Recommendations present in *ACSM's Guidelines for Exercise Testing and Prescription*. 10th ed. Philadelphia (PA): Wolters Kluwer; 2018. 480 p.

These studies have provided overwhelming evidence that moderate-intensity exercise is both beneficial and safe (5). More recently, however, a number of studies utilizing higher intensity interval training have demonstrated significantly greater improvements in **cardiorespiratory fitness** (8) and selected cardiovascular risk factors (13,14). Additionally, there is reasonable evidence that high intensity is safe (15), even in "relatively" higher risk cardiac patients. Studies employing interval training have used high-intensity intervals of as short as 30 seconds to as long as 4 minutes. Generally, the recovery interval is at least equivalent in duration as the higher intensity interval.

Aerobic exercise training for patients with coronary artery disease should include activities that employ large muscle groups through rhythmic activities such as walking, jogging, cycling, elliptical, stair climbing, and rowing. The duration should be individually titrated upward from an amount that can be performed without adverse events to as much as 60 minutes per session.

Eventually, for most individuals with coronary artery disease, some type of physical activity should be undertaken nearly every day of the week. Physical activity guidelines (16) for secondary prevention of coronary heart disease recommend 30 minutes of moderate-intensity aerobic activity at least 5 days and preferably 7 days per week. Moreover, the goal for patients with coronary artery disease is the long-term habituation of physical activity. In addition to accruing the health benefits that come from near daily exercise, developing a regimen that includes frequently repeated exercise sessions helps to establish the behavior as a habit (6).

In addition to aerobic activity, resistance training is important for patients with cardiovascular disease. Resistance training results in improved muscle strength and endurance, both of which are important for the safe return to ADL along with occupational and avocational pursuits. Resistance training has been shown to be well tolerated and effective in increasing strength and physical function in **older adults** (7). A commonly recommended resistance training program consists of performing one set of 8–12 repetitions of 8–10 different exercises targeting major muscle groups (18). As is the case with aerobic exercise, resistance training programs should start at a relatively low weight and progressed upward. Utilizing RPE is a useful means by which to select the resistance for a particular exercise. After a period of acclimatization, the final repetition of a particular set should be described, effort-wise, as "hard" to complete. Proper form should be maintained through the entirety of the range of motion and individuals should be counseled to refrain from holding their breath during resistance training. Patients should be instructed to exhale during the concentric phase of the exercise and to inhale during the eccentric contraction. Patients undergoing a catheterization with or without percutaneous intervention and those who experienced an uncomplicated myocardial infarction may begin resistance training program as early as 3 and 5 weeks from the date of the event, respectively. It is generally recommended that for patients undergoing CABGS involving sternotomy, upper body resistance training should be avoided for 8–12 weeks from the date of surgery or until sternal healing has fully occurred. Initiating lightweight resistance training prior to when the weight restrictions are removed, however, is useful to promote range of motion and to minimize muscle atrophy.

CR is the ideal location to care for a patient recovering from a recent cardiovascular event. CR participation is associated with improved long-term outcomes including decreased mortality and morbidity, less disability, and improved fitness. Although the benefits to patients are enormous, participation in CR is suboptimal. Evidence suggests that only 20%–30% of patients who are eligible for CR actually participate. Obviously, the majority of eligible do not participate in CR. Just some of the reasons for poor participation include lack of interest, socioeconomic factors, family and work obligations, lack of program availability, inadequate insurance coverage, and cost. Given the low rates of participation in CR, alternative methods of getting individuals with coronary heart disease to exercise regularly need to be considered. As such, health care providers outside of the practice of CR should develop the knowledge base required to provide counsel about exercise to patients with coronary heart disease.

Case Study Quiz:

Exercise Prescription and Progression Considerations

Case Study 10-1

4. Why is it not unexpected that Mrs. Case Study-Angina experiences angina when exerting herself in the cold or carrying laundry upstairs? What advice would you give to help mitigate these symptoms?

Case Study 10-2

4. Calculate an exercise target heart zone for Mr. Case Study-CABGS.
5. Is it safe and appropriate for this patient to exercise with new-onset atrial fibrillation?
6. What would you do to guide exercise intensity now that he is in atrial fibrillation?

SUMMARY

A summary of exercise training and prescription considerations for individuals with stable angina and CABGS is presented as follows:

- Exercise is a critical component of the long-term strategy of secondary prevention of coronary artery disease. Chronic exercise has a positive impact on most of the risk factors linked to the development and progression of coronary artery disease.
- Given the breadth and strength of its effects, exercise needs to be prioritized for managing cardiovascular risk factors, preventing disability, and improving an individual's general well-being.
- Health care providers need to work closely with the individual with heart disease to develop a safe and appropriate exercise training program.
- Many of these patients do not perform an exercise test prior to initiating an exercise training program. As a result, the exercise professional may need to rely on other measures of intensity and symptomatology to guide initial exercise prescription and programming.
- Appropriate and often extended warm-up and cool-down are very important in this population of patients.
- Although initial moderate-intensity exercise is most often appropriate for patients with coronary artery disease, utilizing higher intensity interval training provides greater improvements in cardiorespiratory fitness and selected cardiovascular risk factors.
- Resistance training should be encouraged in this population for muscle strength and endurance, both of which are important for the safe return to ADL along with occupational and avocational pursuits.

REFERENCES

1. Ades PA, Savage PD, Brawner CA, et al. Aerobic capacity in patients entering cardiac rehabilitation. *Circulation*. 2006;113(23):2706–12.
2. Ades PA, Savage PD, Toth MJ, et al. High-calorie-expenditure exercise: a new approach to cardiac rehabilitation for overweight coronary patients. *Circulation*. 2009;119(20):2671–8.
3. American Association of Cardiovascular and Pulmonary Rehabilitation. The continuum of care: from inpatient and outpatient cardiac rehabilitation to long-term secondary prevention. In: *Guidelines for Cardiac Rehabilitation and Secondary Prevention Programs*. 5th ed. Champaign (IL): Human Kinetics; 2013. p. 5–18.

4. American College of Sports Medicine. *ACSM's Guidelines for Exercise Testing and Prescription.* 10th ed. Philadelphia (PA): Wolters Kluwer; 2018. 480 p.
5. Anderson L, Oldridge N, Thompson DR, et al. Exercise-based cardiac rehabilitation for coronary heart disease: Cochrane systematic review and meta-analysis. *J Am Coll Cardiol.* 2016;67(1):1–12. doi:10.1016/j.jacc.2015.10.044.
6. Artinian NT, Fletcher GF, Mozaffarian D, et al. Interventions to promote physical activity and dietary lifestyle changes for cardiovascular risk factor reduction in adults: a scientific statement from the American Heart Association. *Circulation.* 2010;122(4):406–41. doi:10.1161/CIR.0b013e3181e8edf1.
7. Brochu M, Savage P, Lee M, et al. Effects of resistance training on physical function in older disabled women with coronary heart disease. *J Appl Physiol (1985).* 2002;92(2):672–8.
8. Elliott AD, Rajopadhyaya K, Bentley DJ, Beltrame JF, Aromataris EC. Interval training versus continuous exercise in patients with coronary artery disease: a meta-analysis. *Heart Lung Circ.* 2015;24(2):149–57. doi:10.1016/j.hlc.2014.09.001.
9. Fihn SD, Gardin JM, Abrams J, et al. 2012 ACCF/AHA/ACP/AATS/PCNA/SCAI/STS guideline for the diagnosis and management of patients with stable ischemic heart disease: a report of the American College of Cardiology Foundation/American Heart Association Task Force on Practice Guidelines, and the American College of Physicians, American Association for Thoracic Surgery, Preventive Cardiovascular Nurses Association, Society for Cardiovascular Angiography and Interventions, and Society of Thoracic Surgeons. *J Am Coll Cardiol.* 2012;60(24):e44–164. doi:10.1016/j.jacc.2012.07.013.
10. Fragnoli-Munn K, Savage PD, Ades PA. Combined resistive-aerobic training in older patients with coronary artery disease early after myocardial infarction. *J Cardiopulm Rehabil.* 1998;18(6):416–20.
11. Kaminsky LA, Arena R, Myers J. Reference standards for cardiorespiratory fitness measured with cardiopulmonary exercise testing: data from the Fitness Registry and the Importance of Exercise National Database. *Mayo Clin Proc.* 2015;90(11):1515–23.
12. Kulik A, Ruel M, Jneid H, et al. Secondary prevention after coronary artery bypass graft surgery: a scientific statement from the American Heart Association. *Circulation.* 2015;131(10):927–64. doi:10.1161/CIR.0000000000000182.
13. Munk PS, Breland UM, Aukrust P, Ueland T, Kvaløy JT, Larsen AI. High intensity interval training reduces systemic inflammation in post-PCI patients. *Eur J Cardiovasc Prev Rehabil.* 2011;18(6):850–7. doi:10.1177/1741826710397600.
14. Ramos JS, Dalleck LC, Tjonna AE, Beetham KS, Coombes JS. The impact of high-intensity interval training versus moderate-intensity continuous training on vascular function: a systematic review and meta-analysis. *Sports Med.* 2015;45(5):679–92. doi:10.1007/s40279-015-0321-z.
15. Rognmo Ø, Moholdt T, Bakken H, et al. Cardiovascular risk of high- versus moderate-intensity aerobic exercise in coronary heart disease patients. *Circulation.* 2012;126(12):1436–40. doi:10.1161/CIRCULATIONAHA.112.123117.
16. Smith SC Jr, Benjamin EJ, Bonow RO, et al. AHA/ACCF secondary prevention and risk reduction therapy for patients with coronary and other atherosclerotic vascular disease: 2011 update: a guideline from the American Heart Association and American College of Cardiology Foundation. *Circulation.* 2011;124(22):2458–73. doi:10.1161/CIR.0b013e318235eb4d.
17. Stone NJ, Robinson JG, Lichtenstein AH, et al. Treatment of blood cholesterol to reduce atherosclerotic cardiovascular disease risk in adults: synopsis of the 2013 American College of Cardiology/American Heart Association cholesterol guideline. *Ann Intern Med.* 2014;160(5):339–43. doi:10.7326/M14-0126.
18. Williams MA, Haskell WL, Ades PA, et al. Resistance exercise in individuals with and without cardiovascular disease: 2007 update: a scientific statement from the American Heart Association Council on Clinical Cardiology and Council on Nutrition, Physical Activity, and Metabolism. *Circulation.* 2007;116(5):572–84.

CHAPTER 11

Special Considerations for Cardiovascular Diseases: Ventricular Assist Devices and Heart Transplantation

INTRODUCTION

Patients with advanced chronic heart failure (stage D, end stage) treated with **maximal** medical therapy, optimal lifestyle including regular **exercise** and healthy eating habits, and implantable cardiac defibrillator (ICD)/pacemaker therapy (cardiac resynchronization therapy) when indicated often have refractory symptoms, very limited exercise tolerance, and poor quality of life. One-year survival is ≤25% and is particularly dismal for patients with a peak volume of oxygen consumed per unit time ($\dot{V}O_2$) of ≤12 mL · kg^{-1} · min^{-1} (3,35). The purpose of this chapter is to describe two treatment options that allow patients with advanced chronic heart failure to function outside of the hospital: mechanical circulatory support with a left ventricular assist device (LVAD) and heart transplantation. In addition, responses to acute and chronic exercise for each treatment option for these patients are described.

Case Study 11-1

Mr. Case Study-HtTxp

The patient is a 46-year-old man with a 17-year history of familial nonischemic dilated cardiomyopathy that is managed medically. An ICD was inserted in 2011. Other pertinent medical history includes severe obesity with bariatric surgery in 2010, which resulted in a 100-lb (45 kg) weight loss, obstructive sleep apnea, cerebrovascular accident with complete resolution of symptoms, and left lower extremity deep vein thrombosis.

He recently became progressively more symptomatic with minimal **physical activity** (New York Heart Association class IV) and was hospitalized in his hometown and found to be in severe congestive heart failure (CHF) with frequent episodes of nonsustained ventricular tachycardia. Subsequently, he was transferred to the Mayo Clinic for a 42-day inpatient stay. The echocardiogram revealed severe left ventricular enlargement with an ejection fraction of 14%, generalized hypokinesis and increased filling pressure, moderate right ventricular enlargement, moderate-to-severe reduction in systolic function, and an elevated right ventricular systolic pressure of 51 mm Hg.

Aggressive diuresis was successful in improving symptoms to the point that he was able to perform a cardiopulmonary exercise test a week later with a peak $\dot{V}O_2$ of 7 $mL \cdot kg^{-1} \cdot min^{-1}$, 19% of predicted for his age (Table 11.1). His heart catheterization revealed normal coronary arteries with evidence of moderate pulmonary hypertension with a mean pulmonary artery pressure of 42 mm Hg. An intra-aortic balloon pump was inserted to support cardiac output.

He was considered to be a candidate for heart transplantation, but because of concern for his immediate survival, he underwent surgery to remove the intra-aortic balloon pump and to install a continuous-flow LVAD as a bridge to transplant. Approximately 2 weeks after the operation, the patient developed abdominal pain and was found to have necrotic cholecystitis. A laparoscopic cholecystectomy was performed. A week later, he underwent separate catheter ablations for both symptomatic atrial fibrillation and symptomatic nonsustained ventricular tachycardia.

The patient returned to his hometown after discharge from the hospital and gradually increased walking duration to 30 minutes at a moderate pace most days of the week. He returned to the Mayo Clinic 2 months later for treatment of a LVAD drive-line infection. An echocardiogram at the time demonstrated partial recovery of left ventricular

Table 11.1 Cardiopulmonary Exercise Test Data

	Sequence of Cardiopulmonary Exercise Tests			
	Pre-LVAD	85 Days after LVAD	105 Days after Transplant	363 Days after Transplant
Body weight (kg)	101.2	92.0	91.1	95.8
Rest HR (bpm)	88	83	107	111
Peak HR (bpm)	100	115	131	196
HR 1 min (bpm)	95	104	142	184
Rest SBP (mm Hg)	80	—	134	140
Peak SBP (mm Hg)	80	—	158	164
Peak $\dot{V}O_2$ ($mL \cdot min^{-1}$)	710	1160	1561	1821
Peak $\dot{V}O_2$ ($mL \cdot kg^{-1} \cdot min^{-1}$)	7.0	12.6	17.2	18.9
% Predicted	19	34	47	53
Peak RER	1.16	1.12	1.27	1.39
$\dot{V}E/\dot{V}CO_2$ slope	38	30	37	31

HR 1 min, heart rate at 1 minute after peak exercise; SBP, systolic blood pressure; RER, respiratory exchange ratio; $\dot{V}E/\dot{V}CO_2$, minute volume/carbon dioxide production.

(continues)

Case Study 11-1 (continued)

function with an ejection fraction to 37%. Peak $\dot{V}O_2$ measured with cardiopulmonary exercise testing had improved to 12.6 mL · kg^{-1} · min^{-1}, 34% of predicted (see Table 11.1).

Five months after implantation of the LVAD, a suitable donor organ became available, and the patient underwent orthotopic heart transplantation as well as removal of the LVAD and ICD. Postoperative course was uncomplicated, and the physical medicine and rehabilitation health care providers worked with the patient to increase physical activity, beginning ambulation 24 hours postoperative when intubation was discontinued. The patient was discharged from the hospital 10 days after surgery. The transplant team consulted with the patient on a frequent basis after hospital discharge, and periodic right ventricular biopsies were performed with only two episodes of very mild acute rejection diagnosed in the first several months after the transplant. The patient was required to reside close to the hospital for the first 3 months after surgery to facilitate close monitoring by the transplant team. Selected prescribed medications included the following:

- Immunosuppressants: mycophenolate mofetil, prednisone (with a gradual taper over time), and tacrolimus, which was transitioned to sirolimus a few months after transplantation
- Cardiovascular medications: furosemide, amlodipine, pravastatin, sildenafil, and aspirin

The patient began outpatient cardiac rehabilitation (CR) 14 days after transplantation. Initial 6-minute walk distance was 338 m (1108 ft), 53% of his predicted. The initial estimated **one repetition maximum (1-RM)** for the leg press was 221 lb. He completed questionnaires for both depression and neuromuscular deficits, and both were negative. For the first 6 weeks of CR, the patient participated in seven supervised exercise sessions using the treadmill for **aerobic** exercise (gradual increase in duration to 30 min per session), free weights (biceps curl, triceps extension, shoulder press), and weight machines (leg press, leg curl, upright row), one to two sets of 8–15 slow repetitions per exercise, keeping the resistance for upper extremity exercises at ≤10 lb for the first 8 weeks after surgery to allow for sternal healing. The intensity for both aerobic and **strength** exercise was prescribed using ratings of perceived exertion (RPEs) of 12–14 on the 6–20 scale. Over the next 7 weeks, he performed more frequent exercise sessions, with a total of 23 supervised exercise sessions at completion of 3 months of outpatient CR.

At the end of outpatient CR, the estimated 1-RM for the leg press was 466 lb, and his cardiopulmonary exercise test demonstrated a peak $\dot{V}O_2$ of 17.2 mL · kg^{-1} · min^{-1}, 47% of predicted (see Table 11.1). Repeat 6-minute walk distance was 541 m (1774 ft), 84% of his predicted distance. The patient was discharged to home by the transplant team and an exercise prescription was provided by CR staff: treadmill or outdoor walking, RPE 12–14, 30–45 minutes 5–6 days per week and strength training exercises as performed in rehabilitation, 2–3 days per week.

A year after transplantation, Mr. Case Study-HtTxp reported a favorable quality of life and was walking >30 minutes, three times weekly. A repeat cardiopulmonary exercise test demonstrated a peak $\dot{V}O_2$ of 18.9 mL · kg^{-1} · min^{-1}, 53% of predicted (see Table 11.1).

Description, Prevalence, and Etiology

For patients with advanced heart failure, heart transplantation remains the gold standard therapy. However, there exists a substantial donor-organ shortage, and many patients are not candidates for transplantation due to comorbid conditions (37). LVAD therapy is an attractive option for maintaining patient viability while awaiting transplantation (LVAD as a bridge to transplant) or as permanent use for a patient not deemed suitable for transplantation (LVAD as destination therapy). LVAD therapy may also be used as a bridge to recovery in patients with the possibility of improvement in cardiac function or as a bridge to decision of treatment options in rapidly deteriorating patients (20). Approximately 2,400 LVADs were implanted in the United States in 2014 (20).

Left Ventricular Assist Devices

An LVAD is a battery-powered (external battery pack) pump surgically implanted in the upper abdomen (Fig. 11.1). Circulatory support is provided by pulling blood from the left ventricle and pumping it into the aorta. The current LVAD technology provides continuous blood flow and results in lower mortality than the previous pulsatile flow devices (37). There may be no palpable pulse due to absent pulsatile flow, and blood pressure (BP) may be difficult or impossible to measure using standard auscultatory techniques. BP can be measured using a Doppler probe but may represent the pressure at any point in the cardiac cycle and should not be considered the actual systolic, diastolic, or mean pressure (38). During exercise, for some patients with LVAD, it is difficult or impossible to detect BP even with Doppler. Continuous-flow LVADs unload the left ventricle and operate at a fixed speed which may be adjusted to optimize left ventricular unloading. Cardiac output is relatively fixed and changes little during exercise.

Cardiac output is normal at rest and is provided primarily by the LVAD; the aortic valve remains closed throughout the cardiac cycle in most patients. During exercise, there is variable contribution

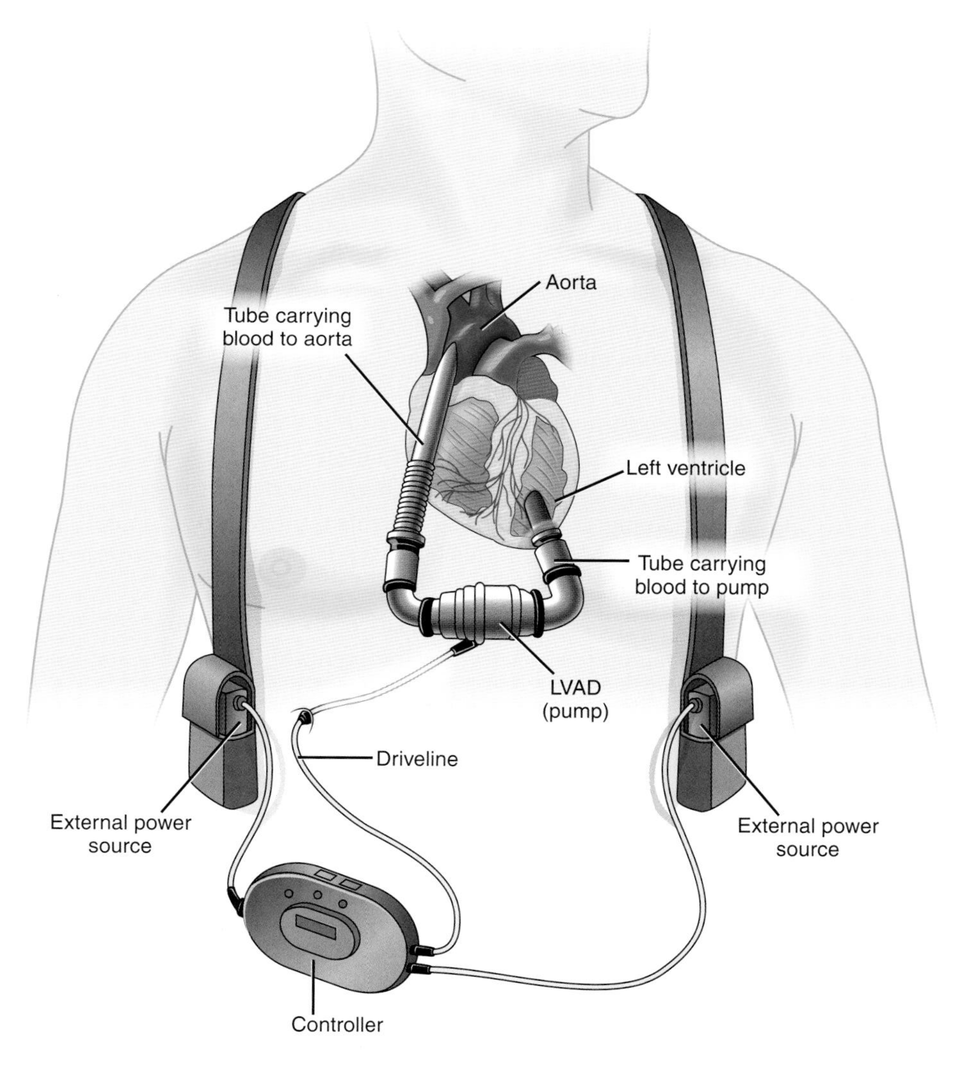

FIGURE 11.1. Left ventricular assist device. (Used with permission of Mayo Foundation for Medical Education and research, all rights reserved.)

of the native left ventricle, and in the majority of patients, the aortic valve remains open during exercise (27). LVADs typically provide 66%–93% of the total cardiac output during exercise with the remaining portion of the cardiac output provided by the stroke volume of the native heart (1). The cardiac output is adequate for many usual physical activities. However, exercise cardiac output is subnormal, and exercise capacity is limited with peak $\dot{V}O_2$ averaging 12–18 mL · kg^{-1} · min^{-1} (27). Additional reasons for below normal exercise capacity include the persistent CHF-related abnormalities, such as chronotropic incompetence, skeletal myopathy, endothelial dysfunction, right ventricular dysfunction, and anemia.

One-year survival for patients using an LVAD as a bridge to transplant is 68% (41). One- and 2-year survivals for destination therapy are 75% and 62%, respectively (3). After implantation, there may be spontaneous improvement in exercise capacity, reduced symptoms, improved end-organ function, and improved appetite, but full benefit is not achieved for 12–26 weeks. In some patients, reverse left ventricle remodeling may occur resulting in partial normalization of left ventricle systolic function with a concomitant reduction in pulmonary congestion and dead space ventilation (recovery) (1,11,27). **Older adult** patients appear to derive less benefit than younger patients.

After implantation, patients continue to receive complicated medical care related to their CHF and multisystem dysfunction as well as LVAD-specific issues. Patients with LVAD require anticoagulant therapy with an attendant increased bleeding risk. These patients are also at increased risk for fluid imbalance, stroke, hemolysis, infection, arrhythmias, and right ventricular and multiorgan failure (1,37). CR programs are well positioned to assist these patients with their complex care and to provide medical surveillance (1). CR staff should work with the LVAD team at the institution that performed the implant regarding the specific device characteristics, such as proper driveline immobilization and care, device alarm settings, etc. An important consideration in a medical emergency involving a patient with LVAD is that cardiopulmonary resuscitation (CPR) should not be performed due to risk of dislodgement of the device.

Patients with LVAD may be challenging candidates for exercise training due to profound **deconditioning**, low cardiac output state, fatigue, and skeletal muscle weakness. After LVAD implantation, most patients have persistent functional limitations. Kerrigan et al. (16) reported an average peak $\dot{V}O_2$ 90 days postimplantation of only 12.9 ± 3.1 mL · kg^{-1} · min^{-1}. The limited numbers of exercise training studies performed thus far have demonstrated that exercise training is safe; no major exercise-related adverse events have been reported. Some patients demonstrate an improved peak $\dot{V}O_2$ after training. Essentially, all patients improve **submaximal** exercise endurance (longer exercise time to fatigue at a fixed workload) (1). However, the long-term effects of exercise training have not been investigated.

Two recent randomized, controlled trials of exercise training after LVAD implantation merit discussion. Kerrigan and associates (15) randomized 27 patients, an average of 2.8 months after implantation, to either CR-supervised exercise training or usual care. Exercise training consisted of 18 sessions over 6 weeks and included treadmill or cycle exercise for 30 minutes initially at 60% of heart rate reserve (HRR), increasing to 80% of HRR. There were no significant changes in peak $\dot{V}O_2$ for the usual care group. The exercise group increased peak $\dot{V}O_2$ from 13.6 to 15.3 mL · kg^{-1} · min^{-1}. Although strength training was not a component of the CR program, knee extension strength increased by 17% in the exercise group and did not change with usual care. Quality of life score and 6-minute walk distance increased more for the exercise group than for the usual care group. In 313 supervised exercise sessions, one syncopal episode occurred, although a cardiovascular etiology was not determined.

Laoutaris and associates (25) randomized 15 LVAD or biventricular assist device (LVAD + right ventricular assist device [RVAD]) recipients to either home-based exercise training and inspiratory muscle training or usual care. Both groups were encouraged to walk 30–45 minutes daily. The home exercise training took place on either cycle ergometers or treadmills with a goal of 45 minutes, three to five times per week, at RPE levels of 12–14 on the Borg 6–20 scale. Inspiratory muscle training took place twice weekly at the hospital at an intensity of 60% of maximal inspiratory strength to exhaustion. Peak $\dot{V}O_2$ did not change for the usual care group but did increase from 16.8 to 19.3 $mL \cdot kg^{-1} \cdot min^{-1}$ in the exercise group. Improvements in the quality of life score, 6-minute walk distance (65 m vs. 18 m), and the minute volume/carbon dioxide production ($\dot{V}E/\dot{V}CO_2$) slope were greater for the exercise group than the usual care group.

Early mobilization, including walking with and without supervision, may begin within 1 week of surgery. Patients may begin outpatient exercise training 2–4 weeks after implantation (1). Some patients with LVAD will require physical medicine and rehabilitation assessment and treatment to prepare them for outpatient CR due to profound deconditioning, frailty, and cachexia (wasting syndrome). Exercise prescription for patients with LVAD follows the same format as for other patients with heart failure. For patients with continuous-flow devices, exercise intensity should be prescribed on the basis of RPE of 11–14 (2).

Based on the results of the exercise test, an **exercise prescription** may be developed for the patient with the goal of maintaining or even improving **cardiorespiratory fitness** (to better tolerate surgery and early recuperation) while waiting for a donor organ. Ideally, the exercise program should be carried out under medical supervision, although many patients have performed home-based, independent exercise successfully. The exercise prescription follows the same guidelines used for other patients with chronic heart failure, as described in Chapter 12.

Heart Transplantation

Heart transplantation is the treatment of choice for eligible patients with advanced chronic heart failure resulting in markedly improved survival, functional status, and quality of life compared with alternative treatments (29). The Registry of the International Society for Heart and Lung Transplantation's 2015 report (29) contained 112,521 heart transplantations performed worldwide between 1982 and 2013 with 1- and 5-year survival of 82% and 69%, respectively. Survival for 1 year was better for transplants performed between 2009 and 2013 (86%) than for earlier years. Survival is similar for both patients with and without circulatory support with an LVAD before transplantation. Causes of death include graft failure (primary graft dysfunction and acute rejection), infection, and multi-organ failure in the early years after surgery. Late mortality is due primarily to malignancy, cardiac allograft vasculopathy (CAV), and renal failure.

In 2013, there were 3,817 adult and 577 pediatric (≤18 yr) patients reported to the Registry worldwide (7,29). The age range of heart transplant recipients is from newborn to the eighth decade of life. For adults, the average age at transplant is approximately 54 years and 75% are men. Approximately 50% of children who receive a transplant are ≤5 years of age. The average age of the donors is approximately 35 years. Combined organ transplant (heart + liver, kidney or both, or heart-lung) accounts for 3% of transplants. Almost 70% of transplant candidates require pretransplant hospitalization, and mechanical circulatory support before transplant is common with 40% of patients with LVAD, 1% with a total artificial heart (TAH), and 1% with RVAD. Retransplantation accounts for 2.5% of cases.

The waiting time for an organ is dependent on blood type and the degree of medical urgency. Unfortunately, the number of potential candidates for heart transplantation greatly exceeds the available supply of donor organs. For example, for 2012, in the United States, 6,700 patients were eligible and listed for transplantation, but only 2,400 transplants were performed (49).

Approximately 90% of adult patients who require transplantation suffer from either coronary heart disease (ischemic left ventricular dysfunction, 45%) or idiopathic dilated cardiomyopathy (46%) (29). Additional diseases resulting in terminal heart failure include hypertension, valvular heart disease, myocarditis, alcohol abuse, chemotherapy, AIDS, complex congenital heart disease, infiltrative diseases of the myocardium (amyloidosis, hemochromatosis), and peripartum (19). For children, the most common indications for transplantation are complex congenital heart disease and cardiomyopathy (7).

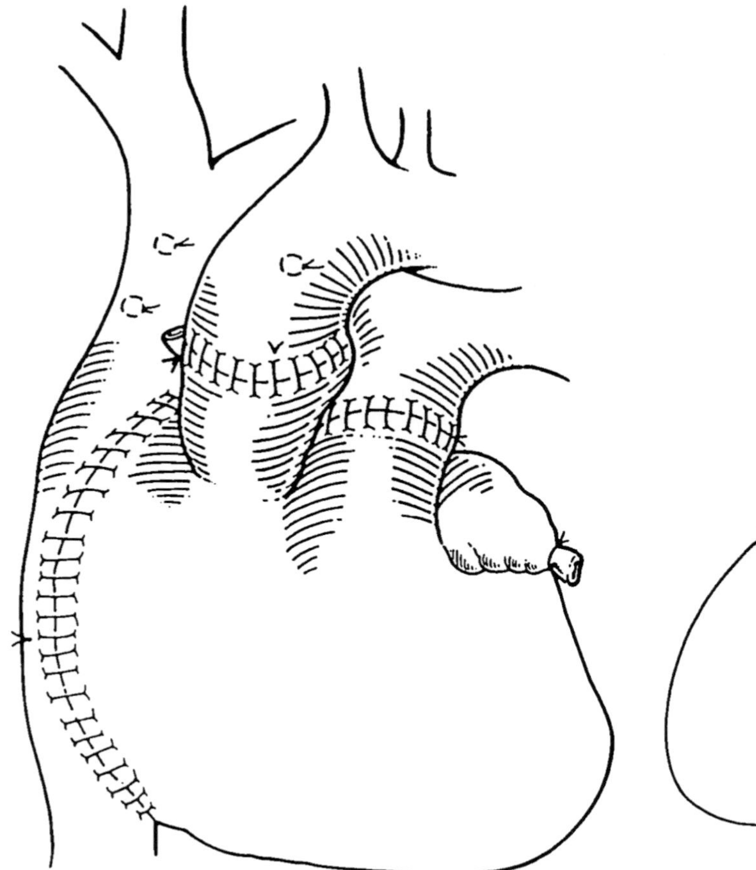

FIGURE 11.2. Orthotopic cardiac transplant technique. (From Squires RW. Exercise training after cardiac transplantation. *Med Sci Sports Exerc.* 1991;23:686–94.)

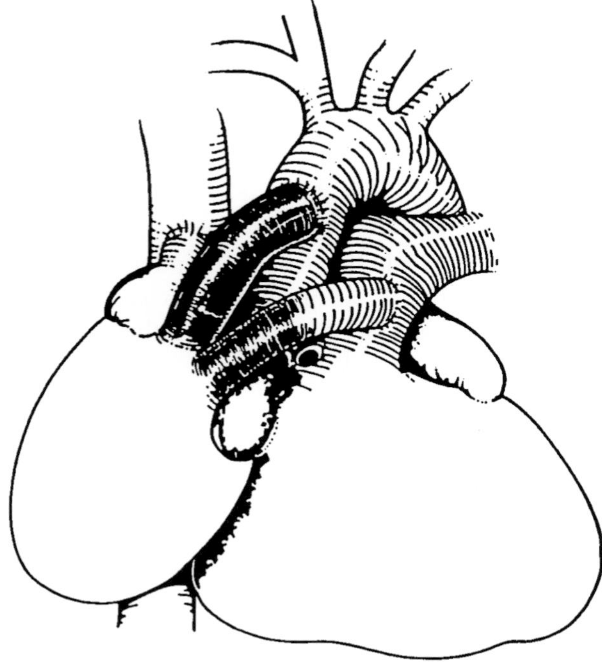

FIGURE 11.3. Heterotopic cardiac transplantation technique. (From Squires RW. Exercise training after cardiac transplantation. *Med Sci Sports Exerc.* 1991;23:686–94.)

Orthotopic transplantation, depicted in Figure 11.2, is the usual surgical technique with excision of the recipient's diseased heart and anastomosis of the donor heart to the great vessels and atria of the recipient (42). Rarely, in the circumstances of excessive pulmonary vascular resistance with severe pulmonary hypertension, or a marked donor–recipient body weight mismatch, a heterotopic or "piggyback" transplant, shown in Figure 11.3, may be used. With this procedure, the recipient's diseased heart is left intact and the donor heart is sewn in parallel to the existing heart. This procedure results in the unique electrocardiographic appearance of two separate QRS complexes on the electrocardiogram (ECG).

Case Study 11-1 Quiz:

Description, Prevalence, and Etiology

1. What were the diagnosis and clinical findings that resulted in implantation of the LVAD?
2. What clinical factors and test factors (echocardiograms, cardiopulmonary exercise tests pre-LVAD vs. 85 days after LVAD) provide evidence that the LVAD improved the cardiovascular health of the patient?

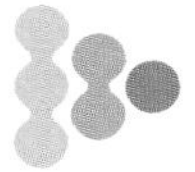

Preparticipation Health Screening, Medical History, and Physical Examination

The goals of cardiac transplantation are improved survival, reduced symptoms, improved quality of life, and an increased exercise capacity. After recovery from surgery, most patients report an improved functional capacity (40). Many patients return to work, school, or their usual avocational activities, although exercise capacity generally remains below average as will be discussed later in the chapter. Employment for patients aged 25–60 years is approximately 50% (29). However, due to the immunosuppressant medications and other transplant-related factors, patients are prone to develop complications and comorbidities. Table 11.2 lists the prevalence of common medical problems observed in cardiac transplant recipients. In terms of medical screening for cardiac transplant patients, it is similar to methods used with patients who have undergone coronary bypass, coronary valve, or other cardiothoracic surgery.

Graft Dysfunction

The transplanted heart may fail soon after surgery due to primary graft dysfunction, pulmonary hypertension, or hyperacute rejection. Primary graft dysfunction is caused by ischemia and reperfusion injury related to the transplant procedure and results in the majority of early mortality (19). Contributing factors include brain death of the donor, ischemic time, and hypothermia of the donor heart. The incidence is variable but occurs in at least 5% of patients. The pathophysiology includes both increased pulmonary vascular resistance and systemic inflammation (22).

Rejection

Rejection of the transplanted heart is a major cause of hospitalization and death in the first year after surgery (51). There are four types of rejection: hyperacute, acute cellular, acute humoral (vascular), and chronic (CAV).

Hyperacute Rejection

Hyperacute rejection occurs shortly after surgery and is caused by preformed antibodies to the donor heart (51). This type of rejection results in acute inflammatory infiltration with vessel necrosis

Table 11.2 Cumulative Prevalence of Medical Problems in Survivors within Seven Years of Cardiac Transplantation

Condition	Prevalence
Hypertension	97%
Hyperlipidemia	89%
Cardiac allograft vasculopathy	43%
Renal dysfunction	36%
Diabetes mellitus	35%
Malignancy	24%

From Taylor DO, Edwards LB, Boucek MM, Trulock EP, Keck BM, Hertz MI. The Registry of the International Society for Heart and Lung Transplantation: twenty-first official adult heart transplant report — 2004. *J Heart Lung Transplant.* 2004;23:796–803.

of the transplanted organ and patient death. Fortunately, with immunologic matching of donor and recipient, hyperacute rejection is rare.

Acute Cellular Rejection

Acute cellular rejection is most common during the first 6 months after transplantation, affecting approximately 50% of patients, and is due to T lymphocyte and macrophage infiltration of the myocardium (18). The diagnosis is made using routine, periodic transvenous endomyocardial biopsy of the right ventricle. If not treated promptly, myocardial injury and necrosis may occur, although mild acute cellular rejection may not require acute treatment (29). Based on tissue sample analysis, acute cellular rejection is graded from mild to severe. The treatment of acute cellular rejection involves additional immunosuppressants and may require hospitalization. Severe acute rejection, resulting in substantial myocyte necrosis and fibrosis, may produce left ventricular dysfunction and heart failure (42).

Acute Humoral Rejection

Acute humoral (vascular) rejection occurs within days to weeks of transplantation and is a relatively rare phenomenon (51). Initiated by antibodies, the process may impair coronary vasodilatory reserve resulting in ventricular dysfunction. Diagnosis is made by identifying immunoglobulins or complement in the vessels of the graft using biopsy material.

Chronic (Cardiac Allograft Vasculopathy) Rejection

CAV, also called *chronic rejection* or *accelerated graft coronary artery disease*, occurs months to years after transplantation (51). CAV is the major limiting factor in long-term survival after cardiac transplantation, affecting 43% of patients within 7 years of transplantation (see Table 11.2). The disease is an unusually accelerated form of coronary disease affecting epicardial and intramyocardial coronary arteries and veins (41). The pathophysiology is incompletely understood but is thought to be associated with repetitive immunological endothelial injury, ischemia-perfusion injury, viral infection, immunosuppressant medications, and traditional coronary risk factors such as dyslipidemia, insulin resistance, and hypertension. The lesions usually diffusely involve the entire vessel, although focal obstructive lesions are sometimes seen. This disease process occurs in pediatric and adult recipients with equal regularity. Annual coronary angiography or imaging stress testing may be performed to detect the disease. Because of the diffuse nature of the typical lesions, retransplantation is the most common treatment. In patients with discrete, focal lesions, revascularization, either catheter-based or coronary bypass graft surgery, may be effective.

Medications

Immunosuppressants

Immunosuppressant medications are given to prevent acute rejection of the donor heart (42). Maintenance drugs generally include combination therapy with a calcineurin inhibitor (sirolimus, tacrolimus, or cyclosporine), an antiproliferative agent (mycophenolate mofetil or azathioprine), and a corticosteroid (prednisone) (28,51). These powerful drugs enable the patient to tolerate the donor heart but are associated with several common side effects as listed in Table 11.3. Prednisone, in the dose range used in transplantation, is particularly bothersome. It alters body fat distribution with resultant truncal obesity and a moonfaced appearance for many patients. Prednisone may also cause mood swings as well as skeletal muscle atrophy and weakness, osteoporosis, and dyslipidemia. During the first 1–2 years after transplantation, an attempt is usually made to taper and stop prednisone.

Table 11.3 Common Immunosuppressant Drugs and Associated Side Effects

Drug (Brand Name)	Potential Common Side Effects
Tacrolimus (Prograf)	Tremor, headache, diarrhea, hypertension, nausea, renal dysfunction
Sirolimus (Rapamune)	Skin irritation, tremor, light-headedness, weight gain, abdominal pain, diarrhea
Mycophenolate mofetil (CellCept)	Diarrhea, leukopenia, sepsis, vomiting, infection, edema
Prednisone	Muscle atrophy/weakness, hypertension, fluid retention, osteoporosis, aseptic necrosis of bone, "moon" face appearance, truncal obesity, increased insulin resistance, cataracts, glaucoma, mood swings, personality change, insomnia, peptic ulcer disease
Cyclosporine (Gengraf, Neoral, Sandimmune)	Renal dysfunction, tremor, hypertension, hirsutism, gum hyperplasia, muscle cramps, acne
Azathioprine (Imuran)	Nausea/vomiting, leukopenia, thrombocytopenia, anemia

HMG-CoA Reductase Inhibitors (Statins)

Statin medications may slow progression of accelerated graft coronary disease and improve survival (12,48,53). In addition, statins have been shown to reduce the incidence of acute rejection and to improve left ventricular function (23,31). These benefits appear to be independent of these drugs' effects in improving the blood lipid profile.

Common Nonrejection Medical Problems

Infection and Malignancy

Immunosuppressed transplant recipients are at a higher risk for opportunistic infections and malignancy than the general population of patients with cardiovascular diseases. During the first several weeks after surgery, pulmonary bacterial infections are common (26). Late after transplantation, viral, bacterial, and fungal infections pose a threat. Special precautions should be taken to minimize the chances of exposure to persons with active infections. Patients are encouraged to wear a surgical mask and gloves as an infection barrier in public places particularly during the first 3 months after surgery. Malignancy risk is substantial for transplant patients. At 7 years after surgery, the incidence of malignancy (primarily skin cancers) is 24% (48).

Hypertension

Hypertension is common after transplantation, affecting >95% of patients at 7 years (50). The extremely high prevalence is thought to be due to the use of calcineurin inhibitors and their adverse effects on renal function (41). Use of combination antihypertensive drug therapy is often required. BP after transplantation is usually sensitive to the dietary sodium load.

Obesity

Weight gain and obesity after cardiac transplantation are commonly observed. In a cohort of 95 patients at our institution, **body mass index (BMI)** averaged 28 ± 1 kg · m^{-2} at the time of surgery (52). The average increase in BMI and body weight by the first anniversary after transplantation was 2.1 ± 3.6 kg · m^{-2} and 6.3 ± 8.7 kg (13.86 ± 19 lb), respectively. Corticosteroid use plays a major role in posttransplant weight gain.

Dyslipidemia

Blood lipid abnormalities after cardiac transplantation are almost as universal as is hypertension (52). Immunosuppressants, diuretics prescribed for the treatment of hypertension, and renal insufficiency contribute to the problem. Statin medications are effective in treating dyslipidemia in these patients, although the risk of rhabdomyolysis is increased with concurrent statin and calcineurin inhibitor use.

Diabetes

Diabetes is common after transplant and is present in 35% of patients at 7 years (3). Pretransplant diabetes, glucocorticoid and calcineurin inhibitor use, and obesity contribute to the high prevalence of the disease (26). Diabetes is associated with a poorer long-term survival in cardiac transplant recipients.

Chronic Renal Insufficiency

Renal insufficiency, defined as creatinine levels >2 mg · dL^{-1}, is a common side effect of calcineurin inhibitors (26). Fortunately, less than 10% of transplant recipients develop end-stage renal disease.

Osteoporosis

Advanced heart failure is associated with osteopenia and osteoporosis before transplantation. Glucocorticoid use after transplantation results in additional loss of bone mineral. Osteoporosis resulting in vertebral fractures is common in heart transplant recipients, affecting up to 30% of patients (26).

Depression

Depression has been reported in approximately 25% of heart transplant recipients at 1–3 years after surgery (26). Therefore, many of these patients take antidepressant medications.

Psychological Factors

The psychological response to the transplant process is understandably intense for most patients (44). During the period of waiting for the operation after acceptance as a transplant candidate, emotions range from relief and happiness to anxiety (indefinite waiting time, lack of absolute assurance that the transplant will occur) and thoughts of death. Patients who require continuous hospitalization while waiting for an organ may find the environment supportive or merely tedious and boring. Immediately after transplantation, patients are usually relieved at the prospects for a longer, higher quality life.

As the period of convalescence continues, patients must adjust to the tedium of medical appointments and procedures. As previously discussed, the immunosuppressant prednisone may cause mood swings and personality change. The first episode of acute rejection may result in heightened feelings of anxiety and transient depression. As the recovery from surgery progresses and the degree of medical surveillance decreases, patients generally shift their attention from transplant-related activities to becoming more independent, resuming family roles, and occupational and avocational pursuits. The readjustment to life after transplantation requires months, and the 1-year anniversary is an important milestone in this process. Most patients are able to return to productive and meaningful lives.

Nonadherence to treatment as evidenced by inconsistent taking of medications, poor attendance at clinic appointments, smoking, lack of regular exercise or poor attendance at CR classes, and dietary lapses are unfortunately common in transplant patients (17). Predictors of that include young age at transplant, lower educational level, depression, anxiety, hostility, substance abuse, and poor social support.

Case Study 11-1 Quiz:

Preparticipation Health Screening, Medical History, and Physical Examination

3. How was the patient screened for acute rejection?
4. Did the patient experience episodes of acute rejection?

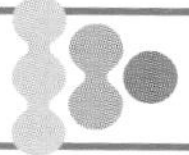

Graded Exercise Testing Considerations: Pretransplant

As part of the evaluation process for transplantation, ambulatory patients usually undergo cardiopulmonary exercise testing. Peak $\dot{V}O_2$ is a powerful prognostic indicator: Patients with an aerobic capacity of 14 $mL \cdot kg^{-1} \cdot min^{-1}$ (4 METs) or below experience a markedly reduced 1-year survival, independent of left ventricular ejection fraction (30).

Based on the results of the exercise test, an exercise prescription may be developed for the patient with the goal of maintaining or even improving cardiorespiratory fitness while waiting for a donor organ. Ideally, the exercise program should be carried out under medical supervision, although many patients have performed home-based, independent exercise successfully. The exercise prescription follows the same guidelines used for other patients with chronic heart failure, as described in Chapter 12.

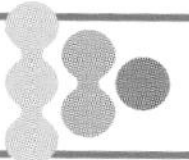

Graded Exercise Testing Considerations: Posttransplant

Exercise testing after cardiac transplantation is helpful in determining the exercise capacity, prescribing exercise training, and in counseling patients regarding the timing of return to work or school or resumption of avocational pursuits. The ECG of transplant recipients commonly demonstrates right bundle-branch block and nonspecific repolarization abnormalities. The sensitivity of the exercise ECG in detecting the presence of CAV is poor (<25%) unless combined with myocardial imaging (8).

Due to the healing and recovery process after surgery and the usual deconditioned state prior to surgery, it is best to wait 6–8 weeks after surgery before performing graded exercise testing to maximal effort. For patients with more complicated postoperative courses, an even longer period of recovery is recommended before performance of an exercise test.

Treadmill or cycle ergometer protocols with continuous exercise (2- or 3-min stages) or ramp tests may be used. Arm cranking protocols may also be employed after adequate sternal healing, for a specific upper extremity fitness evaluation, or an arm cranking exercise prescription (18). The initial exercise intensity should be approximately 2 METs, with 1–2 MET increments in intensity per stage (14,18). Continuous multilead ECG monitoring with BP measurement and Borg RPE for each stage is recommended. For precise determination of aerobic capacity and the ventilatory anaerobic threshold, direct measurement of $\dot{V}O_2$ and associated variables is highly desirable. The endpoints of the **graded exercise test** should be maximal effort (symptom-limited maximum) or standard signs of exertional intolerance (9).

The responses of heart transplant recipients to acute exercise are unique and related, in part, to the following factors (13,34,42):

1. With harvesting of the donor organ, the transplanted heart is surgically denervated and receives no direct efferent input from the autonomic nervous system and provides no direct afferent signals to the central nervous system. Months after transplantation, some patients demonstrate signs of partial cardiac reinnervation. This will be discussed later in this chapter.
2. During organ harvesting and with transplantation, the donor heart has experienced ischemic time and reperfusion.
3. There is no intact pericardium.
4. Diastolic dysfunction (elevated filling pressures at rest and with exercise) is common. Reasons for abnormal diastolic function include hypertension (common after transplant), acute rejection episodes resulting in myocardial scarring and fibrosis, and CAV.
5. Abnormal skeletal muscle histology and energy metabolism, developed during the course of chronic heart failure, may continue after transplantation.
6. Peripheral and coronary vasodilatory capacity may be impaired, in part, due to endothelial dysfunction.

Heart Rate and Exercise

As a result of the loss of parasympathetic innervation of the donor heart with transplantation, heart rate (HR) at rest is elevated at approximately 95–115 bpm and represents the inherent rate of depolarization of the sinoatrial node (29). With graded exercise, for the majority of patients, the HR typically does not increase during the first several minutes (delayed increase), followed by a gradual rise with peak HR slightly lower than normal (approximately 150 bpm) due to sympathetic nervous system denervation. Many patients achieve their highest exercise HR during the first few minutes of recovery from exercise rather than at the point of maximal exercise intensity. HR may remain near peak values for several minutes during recovery before gradually returning to resting levels (delayed decrease). The chronotropic reserve (the difference between the maximal and resting HRs) is less than normal. Regulation of HR during exercise is dependent on circulating catecholamines. Figure 11.4 shows the HR response to graded exercise of the same patient 1 year before and 3 months after orthotopic transplantation. Note the delayed increase in

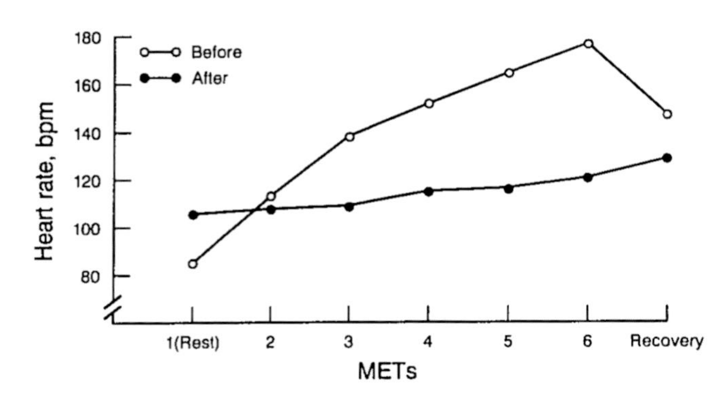

FIGURE 11.4. Heart rates measured during graded exercise in the same patient 1 year before and 3 months after orthotopic cardiac transplantation. Note the elevated resting heart rate and the delayed increase in heart rate during exercise after transplantation consistent with complete denervation. (From Squires RW. Cardiac rehabilitation issues for heart transplantation patients. *J Cardiopulm Rehabil.* 1990;10:159–68.)

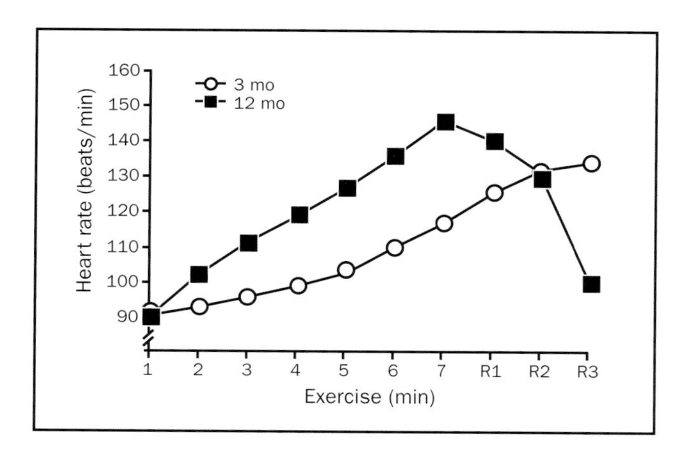

FIGURE 11.5. Heart rate responses to graded exercise in the same patient at 3 months and 12 months after cardiac transplantation demonstrating both denervation (at 3 months) and partial reinnervation (at 24 months). (From Squires RW, Leung TC, Cyr NS, et al. Partial normalization of the heart rate response to exercise after cardiac transplantation: frequency and relationship to exercise capacity. *Mayo Clin Proc.* 2002;77:1295–300.)

HR during the first few minutes of exercise and the highest rate during recovery after transplantation. At 1 year after transplantation, approximately one-third of patients exhibit partial cardiac reinnervation with a more normal increase in HR during graded exercise and decrease in HR during recovery (47) (Fig. 11.5).

Blood, Intracardiac, and Vascular Pressures

BP at rest is mildly elevated in heart transplant patients, even though most patients receive antihypertensive medications. During exercise, BP generally increases appropriately, although peak exercise BP is slightly lower than expected for normal persons (24). Vascular resistance is elevated, and intracardiac and pulmonary vascular pressures (particularly right-sided pressures) are elevated (5).

Left Ventricular Function

For most heart transplant patients, left ventricular ejection fraction is normal at rest and during exercise (5). However, as mentioned previously, left ventricular diastolic function is often impaired, as evidenced by an elevated filling pressure for a given end-diastolic volume. This impairment results in a below normal increase in stroke volume during exercise. The impaired rise in stroke volume, coupled with the below normal HRR, results in an impaired exercise cardiac output.

Exercise Cardiac Output

With the onset of exercise, cardiac output in transplant recipients with complete cardiac denervation increases due to augmentation of stroke volume via the Frank-Starling mechanism. Later, increased HR also contributes to augmentation of cardiac output (42). Table 11.4 demonstrates the greater increase, relative to controls, in left ventricular end-diastolic volume index during exercise in transplant patients that results in an enhanced Frank-Starling effect. However, at rest and during exercise, the cardiac index is lower for transplant recipients than for normal persons (Fig. 11.6) (42).

Pulmonary Function and Arterial Oxygenation

The efficiency of pulmonary ventilation during exercise is below normal during at least the first several months after transplantation, illustrated by an elevation in the ratio of minute ventilation to carbon dioxide production (the ventilatory equivalent for CO_2, $\dot{V}E/\dot{V}CO_2$) (5). This excess ventilation results in a heightened sense of shortness of breath during exercise. The normal increase in tidal volume during exercise is blunted, probably as a result of respiratory muscle weakness,

Table 11.4 Exercise Responses in Normal and Transplant Subjects

	Exercise Stage				
	Rest	EX1	EX2	Peak	Post
Heart rate (beats/min)					
Normal	67 ± 3	90 ± 3	100 ± 2	132 ± 5	91 ± 4
Transplant	88 ± 3	91 ± 3	98 ± 3	117 ± 5	112 ± 4
p Value	0.001	NS	NS	0.05	0.001
Blood pressure (S/D) (mm Hg)					
Normal	130 ± 3/82 ± 3	146 ± 4/87 ± 2	163 ± 5/90 ± 3	209 ± 7/96 ± 4	151 ± 6/76 ± 2
Transplant	137 ± 3/83 ± 2	141 ± 4/84 ± 2	148 ± 4/86 ± 3	174 ± 5/84 ± 3	157 ± 4/80 ± 4
p Value	NS NS	NS NS	0.02 NS	0.001 0.05	NS NS
Ejection fraction (%)					
Normal	61 ± 2	65 ± 2	66 ± 2	68 ± 2	71 ± 1
Transplant	61 ± 2	64 ± 2	65 ± 2	67 ± 2	66 ± 2
p Value	NS	NS	NS	NS	NS
End-diastolic index (ml/m^2)					
Normal	83 ± 5	81 ± 4	87 ± 5	84 ± 5	80 ± 4
Transplant	67 ± 4	76 ± 4‡	76 ± 4‡	75 ± 5‡	59 ± 3‡
p Value	0.02	NS	0.02	NS	0.001
End-systolic index (ml/m^2)					
Normal	32 ± 2	29 ± 2*	29 ± 2*	27 ± 3†	23 ± 2‡
Transplant	26 ± 2	27 ± 2	26 ± 2	24 ± 2	19 ± 2‡
p Value	0.05	NS	NS	NS	NS
Stroke index (ml/m^2)					
Normal	51 ± 3	52 ± 2	58 ± 3†	56 ± 3	57 ± 3
Transplant	41 ± 3	49 ± 3‡	49 ± 3‡	50 ± 3‡	40 ± 3
p Value	0.05	NS	NS	NS	0.001
Cardiac index (liters/min per m^2)					
Normal	3.3 ± 0.2	4.6 ± 0.2	5.7 ± 0.3	7.4 ± 0.4	5.3 ± 0.3
Transplant	3.6 ± 0.3	4.4 ± 0.2	4.8 ± 0.3	5.8 ± 0.4	4.5 ± 0.3
p Value	NS	NS	0.05	0.01	NS

For cardiac volumes; *$p < 0.05$, †$p < 0.01$, ‡$p < 0.001$ versus rest. Data are presented as mean values ± 1 SEM. D = diastolic; EX = exercise; S = systolic.

The change in left ventricular end-diastolic volume index (LVEDVI) during graded, supine exercise in cardiac transplant recipients compared with healthy persons.

Reprinted from Pflugfelder PW, Purves PD, McKenzie FN, Kostuk WJ. Cardiac dynamics during supine exercise in cyclosporine-treated orthotopic heart transplant recipients: assessment by radionuclide angiography. *J Am Coll Cardiol.* 1987;10:336–41.

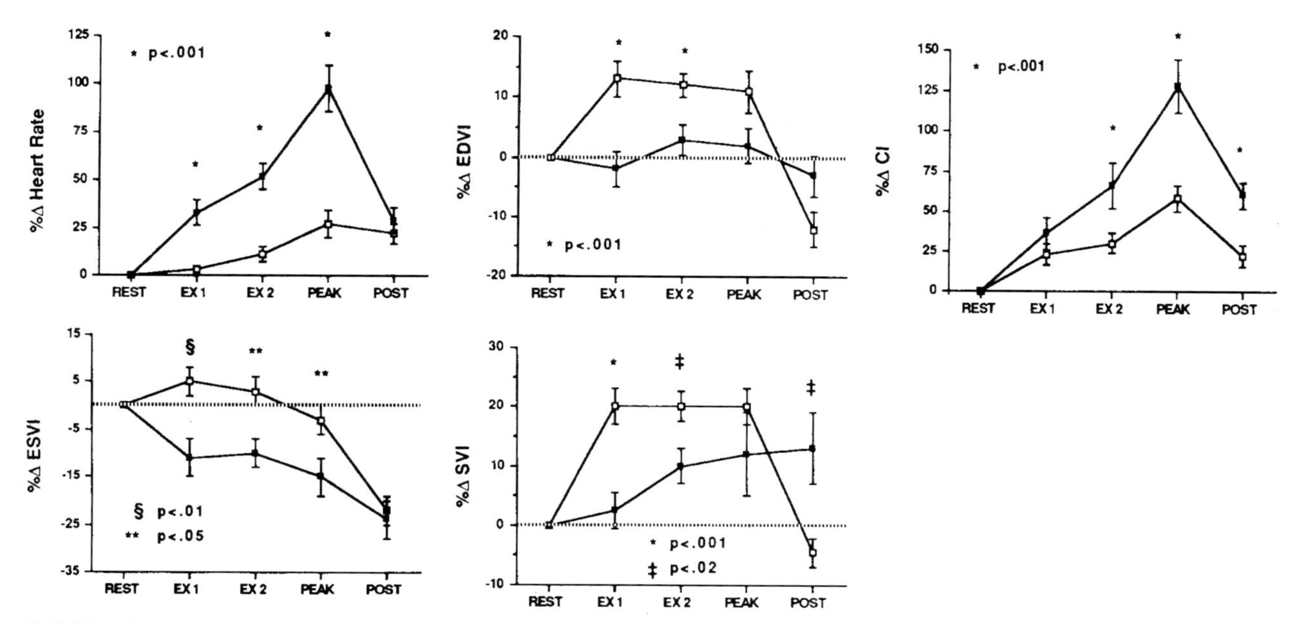

FIGURE 11.6. The change in cardiac index (CI) during graded, supine exercise in cardiac transplant recipients compared with healthy persons. (From Pflugfelder PW, Purves PD, McKenzie FN, Kostuk WJ. Cardiac dynamics during supine exercise in cyclosporine-treated orthotopic heart transplant recipients: assessment by radionuclide angiography. *J Am Coll Cardiol.* 1987;10:336–41.)

deconditioning, and the effects of corticosteroid medications (5). Alveolar gas diffusion impairment is present in approximately 40% of patients. However, arterial oxygen saturation at rest and during exercise is normal for most patients (46). A minority of patients with pretransplant diffusion abnormalities experience mild arterial desaturation (to approximately 90%) with exercise (8). Azathioprine may cause anemia in some patients, resulting in reduced arterial oxygen content (42).

Oxygen Extraction by Exercising Skeletal Muscle

Extraction of oxygen from the arterial blood by metabolically active body tissues, as indicated by the arterial-mixed venous oxygen difference, is normal at rest after transplantation. However, during exercise, the arterial-mixed venous oxygen difference does not increase in a normal manner and reflects abnormalities with both the delivery of capillary blood to the exercising skeletal muscle and impairment of the oxidative capacity of the muscle (13).

Oxygen Uptake Kinetics, Peak Exercise $\dot{V}O_2$

With the onset of exercise, the rate of increase in $\dot{V}O_2$ (oxygen uptake kinetics) is slower than normal as a result of both an impaired rise in cardiac output and a diminished oxidative capacity of the skeletal muscle (reduced arterial-mixed venous oxygen difference) (33). Figure 11.7 shows oxygen uptake versus cycle ergometer power output during graded exercise for the same patient measured 1 year before and 3 months after cardiac transplantation. Although peak $\dot{V}O_2$ was 18% higher after transplantation, for any given submaximal power output, oxygen uptake was consistently lower than before the transplant, consistent with slower $\dot{V}O_2$ kinetics.

Because of the dual abnormalities of an impaired exercise cardiac output and a reduced arterial-mixed venous oxygen difference described earlier, peak exercise $\dot{V}O_2$ is usually below normal for transplant patients (average of 62% of age- and gender-predicted peak exercise $\dot{V}O_2$) (47). There are additional interesting abnormal exercise physiology findings in cardiac transplant recipients. Box 11.1 lists the most common abnormalities.

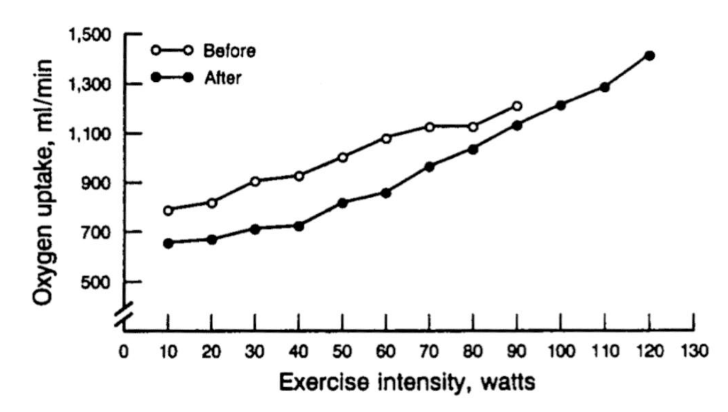

FIGURE 11.7. Oxygen uptake versus cycle ergometer power output for the same patient measured 1 year before and 3 months after orthotopic cardiac transplantation. (From Squires RW. Cardiac rehabilitation issues for heart transplantation patients. *J Cardiopulm Rehabil.* 1990;10:159–68.)

Case Study 11-1 Quiz:

Graded Exercise Testing Considerations

5. For the cardiopulmonary exercise test performed 105 days after transplantation, the HR response was markedly different than for the test performed 85 days after LVAD implantation. What were the differences? What is an explanation for each difference?
6. Was the peak $\dot{V}O_2$ (as a percentage of age- and gender-predicted) measured 105 days after transplantation typical?
7. For the exercise tests performed 105 days and 363 days after transplantation, the resting HRs were similar, but the peak exercise HRs were very different. Why?

Box 11.1 Abnormal Exercise Physiology Findings in Cardiac Transplant Patients

- Increased resting HR
- Delayed HR increase at onset of exercise
- Blunted maximal HR
- Delayed return of HR to resting level after cessation of exercise
- Reduced HRR
- Increased exercise left ventricular end-diastolic pressure (diastolic dysfunction)
- Increased exercise pulmonary artery pressure, pulmonary capillary wedge pressure, right atrial pressure
- Increased left ventricular end-systolic and end-diastolic volume indices
- Impaired increase in stroke volume during exercise
- Reduced exercise cardiac output
- Decreased exercise arterial-mixed venous oxygen difference
- Slowed oxygen uptake kinetics during exercise
- Decreased maximal oxygen uptake
- Reduced maximal power output during exercise testing
- Decreased ventilatory anaerobic threshold
- Increased exercise ventilatory equivalents for oxygen and carbon dioxide

The first report of exercise training after heart transplant was published in 1983 (45). However, there have been relatively few reports on the subject. Investigators have employed various approaches to exercise training with differences in intensity, session duration, frequency, and length of the training program. The time between transplant and starting exercise training has varied widely between studies.

Cardiac transplant recipients are excellent candidates for progressive exercise training for several reasons:

- Pretransplant syndrome of chronic heart failure with poor exercise capacity due to central and peripheral circulatory abnormalities as well as skeletal muscle pathology
- Deconditioning and the healing process with open-heart surgery similar to that observed with coronary or valvular surgery
- Posttransplant use of corticosteroid medications with resultant skeletal muscle atrophy and weakness

Potential additional benefits of regular exercise for transplant recipients include the following (43):

- Improved submaximal exercise endurance
- Increased peak treadmill exercise workload or peak cycle power output
- Increased maximal HR
- Decreased exercise HR at the same absolute submaximal workload
- Increased ventilatory (anaerobic) threshold
- Decreased submaximal exercise minute ventilation
- Reduced exercise ventilatory equivalent for CO_2
- Lessened symptoms of fatigue and/or dyspnea
- Reduced rest and submaximal exercise systolic and diastolic BP
- Decreased peak exercise diastolic BP
- Reduced submaximal exercise RPEs
- Improved psychosocial function
- Increased lean body mass
- Reduced body fat mass
- Increased bone mineral content

Resistance Exercise

Most cardiac transplant patients require prednisone, at least during the first several months after surgery, for immunosuppression. Skeletal muscle atrophy and weakness are common side effects related to prednisone use. Resistance exercise training partially reverses corticosteroid-related myopathy and improves skeletal muscle strength. Horber and associates (10) found definite evidence of skeletal muscle wasting and weakness in the lower extremities of renal transplant patients who received prednisone. Fifty days of isokinetic strength training substantially increased muscle mass and strength in these patients. In addition, strength training has been shown to improve bone density and to reduce the potential development of osteoporosis (also caused by prednisone) in cardiac transplant recipients (4).

Effect of Exercise Training on Immune Function and Longevity

An obvious and important question concerning exercise training in immunosuppressed cardiac transplant recipients is the effects of training on immune function. Traditional, moderate-intensity training does not increase or decrease the number or severity of episodes of acute rejection (22). In addition, training does not require changes in immunosuppressant dosage or treatment. Infection risk is not changed by exercise training (21).

A recent report from the Mayo Clinic, the only study to date that addresses exercise training and longevity, included 201 heart transplant recipients in the modern era of transplantation: 2000–2013 (36).

Table 11.5 Mayo Clinic Cardiopulmonary Treadmill Exercise Test Protocol

Stage	Duration (min)	Speed (mph)	Grade (%)
1	2.0	2.0	0
2	2.0	2.0	7.0
3	2.0	2.0	14.0
4	2.0	3.0	12.5
5	2.0	3.0	17.5
6	2.0	3.4	18.0
7	2.0	3.8	20.0
8	2.0	5.0	18.0
9	2.0	5.5	20.0
10	2.0	6.0	22.0
Cool-down	3.0	1.7	0

From Daida H, Squires RW, Allison TG, Johnson BD, Gau GT. Sequential assessment of exercise tolerance in heart transplantation compared with coronary artery bypass surgery after phase II cardiac rehabilitation. *Am J Cardiol.* 1996;77:696–700.

All transplant patients discharged from the Mayo Clinic are enrolled in outpatient CR and remain in town for 3 months for close follow-up by the transplant team. The number of CR exercise sessions attended predicted survival to 10 years (82% survival overall) with a hazard ratio of 0.31 (69% reduction) for mortality if patients participated in eight or more sessions (Table 11.5).

Early Mobilization and Inpatient Exercise Training

After surgery, patients are extubated expeditiously, usually within 24 hours. Passive range-of-motion exercises for both the upper and lower extremities, sitting up in a chair, and slow ambulation may begin and progress gradually after extubation (32). Walking or cycle ergometry may be increased in duration to 20–30 minutes as tolerated. Exercise intensity is guided using the Borg RPE scale ratings of 11–13 ("fairly light" to "somewhat hard"), keeping the respiratory rate below 30 breaths per minute and arterial oxygen saturation above 90%. Exercise frequency is two to three sessions per day (42). Patients whose postoperative courses are uncomplicated typically remain hospitalized for 7–10 days.

During inpatient rehabilitation, as well as during the outpatient phases, episodes of acute rejection of a moderate or greater severity may require alteration of the exercise plan depending on the preferences of the transplant team. In general, if the rejection episode is graded as moderate, activity may be continued at the current level but should not progress until after the rejection has been adequately treated. Severe acute rejection necessitates suspension of all physical activity with the exception of passive range-of-motion exercises.

Outpatient Exercise Training

Cardiac transplant recipients may enter an outpatient CR program as soon as they are dismissed from the hospital (42). Patients are generally required by the transplant team to remain near the transplant center for close follow-up for approximately 3 months. Ideally, they should exercise in both a supervised environment (three sessions per week) and independently (an additional three sessions per week).

Continuous monitoring of the ECG during the first few supervised exercise sessions is standard practice, although many weeks of ECG-monitored exercise are seldom useful because target HRs are not used for monitoring as well as the rarity of clinically important dysrhythmia. It is not necessary to perform graded exercise testing before beginning the outpatient exercise program.

Performance of a 6-minute walk is helpful in assessing functional capacity, however. Graded exercise testing may be performed 6–8 weeks after surgery for patients without complicated recoveries, when the patient has recovered sufficiently from surgery to assess the cardiopulmonary responses to exercise and to refine the exercise prescription.

Exercise prescription for cardiac transplant patients is similar to methods used with patients who have undergone coronary bypass, coronary valve, or other cardiothoracic surgery. The one exception is that a target HR is not used, unless the patient exhibits a partially normalized HR response to exercise as discussed previously. The typical denervated heart increases in rate slowly during submaximal exercise, and the HR may either drift gradually higher during steady-state exercise or plateau after several minutes (44). Borg RPE scale ratings of 12–14 ("somewhat hard") may be used to prescribe exercise intensity (42).

The HRR (also called *chronotropic response*), defined as the difference between the HR at rest and the highest value during maximal exercise, increases during the first 6 weeks after transplantation in many patients. In a subset of patients, the HRR increases further over the next 6–12 months (6). A more rapid decline in HR from peak exercise to baseline is observed in some patients at 1–2 years after transplantation (39).

Recently, high-intensity interval training (HIIT) has been used in exercise programs for transplant recipients and is well tolerated with favorable effects on fitness (38). The exercise prescription should include standard warm-up and cool-down activities, a gradual increase in aerobic exercise duration to 30–60 minutes, and a frequency of four to six sessions per week. Typical modes of aerobic exercise used during the early outpatient recovery period include walking outdoors (or in shopping centers, schools), treadmill walking, cycle ergometry, and stair climbing.

Because of the sternal incision, special emphasis on upper extremity active range-of-motion exercises is required. At approximately 6 weeks after surgery, when sternal healing is nearly completed, rowing, arm cranking, combination arm/leg ergometry, outdoor cycling, hiking, and jogging become additional options, depending on a patient's fitness levels. Sports such as tennis and golf may be performed as early as 6 weeks after surgery if patient fitness is adequate (5 METs or greater) and sternal healing is nearly complete.

Skeletal muscle weakness in cardiac transplant recipients is very common and is related to the following factors:

- Skeletal muscle atrophy due to advanced heart failure
- Pretransplant deconditioning
- Corticosteroid use posttransplant as part of the immunosuppressant regimen

Muscle strengthening exercises should be incorporated into the exercise program to counteract these factors. For the first 6 weeks after surgery, bilateral arm lifting is restricted to less than 10 lb to avoid sternal nonunion. During this early stage of rehabilitation, light hand weights are an excellent method of introducing resistance exercise. After at least 6 weeks of healing, patients may be started on standard weight machines, emphasizing moderate resistance, 10–20 slow repetitions per set, one to three sets of exercises for the major muscle groups, with a frequency of two or three sessions per week (17,42). Elastic band exercises are also another excellent mode of resistance training for these patients. We recommend Borg RPE scale of 12–14 to gauge the intensity of lifting. Strength gains of 25%–50% or greater commonly occur after 8 weeks of strength training in these patients. Performance of the strengthening exercises immediately following the aerobic portion of the exercise prescription (after the cool-down) is recommended. Because cardiac transplant recipients are likely to require antihypertensive medications, periodic BP measurement during both aerobic and strengthening exercise is recommended.

Encouragement to continue a lifelong exercise program should be a consistent message from the transplant team and the primary health care provider. Patients should continue either in a supervised exercise program indefinitely, exercise independently, or use a combination of supervised and unsupervised exercise. We recommend annual graded exercise tests with revision of the exercise prescription, as necessary, see frequency, intensity, time, and type (FITT) table (Table 11.6).

FITT

TABLE 11.6 FITT RECOMMENDATIONS FOR INDIVIDUALS WITH HEART TRANSPLANTATION AND LEFT VENTRICULAR ASSIST DEVICE

ACSM FITT Principle of the ExR_x

Chronic Medical Condition	Frequency (How often?)	Intensity (How hard?)	Time	Type (What kind?) Primary	Resistance	Flexibility	Special Considerations
Healthy Adult	$\geq$5 d · wk^{-1} of moderate exercise, or $\geq$3 d · wk^{-1} of vigorous exercise, or a combination of moderate and vigorous exercise on $\geq$3–5 d · wk^{-1} is recommended.	Moderate to vigorous. Light-to-moderate intensity exercise may be beneficial in deconditioned individuals.	If moderate intensity: $\geq$30 min · d^{-1} to total 150 min · wk^{-1}. If vigorous intensity: $\geq$20 min · d^{-1} to total 75 min · wk^{-1}.	Regular, purposeful exercise that involves major muscle groups and is continuous and rhythmic in nature is recommended.	Muscle strengthening 2–3 d · wk^{-1} (nonconsecutive) Moderate-to-vigorous intensity; 2–4 sets of 8–12 repetitions	2–3 d · wk^{-1}; static stretch 10–30 s; 2–4 repetitions of each exercise	Sedentary behaviors can have adverse health effects, even among those who regularly exercise. Adding short physical activity breaks throughout the day may be considered as a part of the exercise.
Heart Transplantation	3–5 d · wk^{-1}	Use RPE of 11–14 on a 6–20 scale.	Progressively increase from 15–20 min · d^{-1} up to 30–60 min · d^{-1}	Treadmill or free walking, stationary cycling, and dual-action stationary bike	Slowly increase upper body activities over several weeks to months from 40% of 1-RM to 70% of 1-RM. Lower body excises should begin at 50% of 1-RM. 1–2 sets of 10–15 repetitions for each exercise Weight machines are best, but dumbbells, elastic bands, and body weight can be used.	2–3 d · wk^{-1} with daily being most effective Stretch to the point of feeling tightness or slight discomfort. 10–30 s hold for static stretching 2–4 repetitions of each exercise Static, dynamic, and/or PNF stretching	Pretransplant patients make excellent candidates for reconditioning with significant potential posttransplant benefits. Posttransplant patients can expect similar benefits from aerobic and resistance exercise compared to apparently healthy with additional benefits to reverse corticosteroid-related myopathy.
LVAD	3–5 d · wk^{-1}	If HR data is available from a recent GXT, set intensity between 60% and 80% of HRR. In the absence of data from a GXT or if atrial fibrillation is present, use RPE of 11–14 on a 6–20 scale.	Progressively increase to 30 min · d^{-1} and then up to 60 min · d^{-1}.	Early mobilization such as walking may begin within 1 week of surgery. Progress to treadmill, free walking, and cycling.	1–2 nonconsecutive d · wk^{-1} Begin at 40% 1-RM for upper body and 50% 1-RM for lower body exercises. Gradually increase to 70% 1-RM over several weeks to months. 2 sets of 10–15 reps focusing on major muscle groups Machines may be best due to loss of strength and balance.	$\geq$2–3 d · wk^{-1} with daily being most effective Stretch to the point of tightness or slight discomfort. 10–30 s hold for static stretching; 2–4 repetitions of each exercise Static, dynamic, and/or PNF stretching	Exercise conditioning important to better outcomes and recuperation postsurgery. Using RPE key for this very deconditioned population.

ExR_x, exercise prescription; PNF, proprioceptive neuromuscular facilitation; GXT, graded exercise test.

Based on the FITT Recommendations present in *ACSM's Guidelines for Exercise Testing and Prescription.* 10th ed. Philadelphia (PA): Wolters Kluwer; 2018. 480 p.

Case Study 11-1 Quiz:

Graded Exercise Testing Considerations

8. How long after transplantation did the patient begin supervised outpatient exercise in the CR program?

SUMMARY

A summary of exercise training and prescription considerations for patients with advanced chronic heart failure who are treated with either LVAD or heart transplantation follows:

- Patients with LVAD and heart transplant receive similar benefits of exercise training as patients with other forms of heart disease.
- These patients are ideal candidates for outpatient CR programs and are encouraged to adopt and maintain long-term active lifestyles.

REFERENCES

1. Alsara O, Perez-Terzic C, Squires RW, et al. Is exercise training safe and beneficial in patients receiving left ventricular assist device therapy? *J Cardiopulm Rehabil Prev*. 2014;34:233–40.
2. American College of Sports Medicine. Exercise prescription for patients with cardiovascular disease. In: *ACSM's Resource Manual for Guidelines for Exercise Testing and Prescription*. 7th ed. Philadelphia (PA): Lippincott Williams & Wilkins; 2014. p. 619–34.
3. Balady GJ, Arena R, Sietsema K, et al. Clinician's guide to cardiopulmonary exercise testing in adults: a scientific statement from the American Heart Association. *Circulation*. 2010;122:191–225.
4. Braith RW, Mills RM, Welsch MA, Keller JW, Pollock ML. Resistance exercise training restores bone mineral density in heart transplant recipients. *J Am Coll Cardiol*. 1996;28:1471–7.
5. Brubaker PH, Brozena SC, Morley DL, Walter JD, Berry MJ. Exercise-induced ventilatory abnormalities in orthotopic heart transplant patients. *J Heart Lung Transplant*. 1997;16:1011–7.
6. Daida H, Squires RW, Allison TG, Johnson BD, Gau GT. Sequential assessment of exercise tolerance in heart transplantation compared with coronary artery bypass surgery after phase II cardiac rehabilitation. *Am J Cardiol*. 1996;77:696–700.
7. Dipchand AI, Rossano JW, Edwards LB, et al. The Registry of the International Society for Heart and Lung Transplantation: eighteenth official pediatric heart transplantation report — 2015; focus theme: early graft failure. *J Heart Lung Transplant*. 2015;34:1233–43.
8. Ehrman JK, Keteyian SJ, Levine AB, et al. Exercise stress tests after cardiac transplantation. *Am J Cardiol*. 1993;71:1372–3.
9. Gibbons RJ, Balady GJ, Beasley JW, et al. ACC/AHA guidelines for exercise testing: a report of the American College of Cardiology/American Heart Association Task Force on Practice Guidelines (Committee on Exercise Testing). *J Am Coll Cardiol*. 1997;30:260–311.
10. Horber FF, Scheidegger JR, Grünig BE, Frey FJ. Evidence that prednisone-induced myopathy is reversed by physical training. *J Clin Endocrinol Metab*. 1985;61:83–8.
11. Jaski BE, Lingle RJ, Reardon LC, Dembitsky WP. Left ventricular assist device as a bridge to patient and myocardial recovery. *Prog Cardiovasc Dis*. 2000;43:5–18.
12. Jenkins GH, Grieve LA, Yacoub MH, Singer DRJ. Effect of simvastatin on ejection fraction in cardiac transplant recipients. *Am J Cardiol*. 1996;78:1453–6.
13. Kao AC, Van Trigt P III, Shaeffer-McCall GS, et al. Central and peripheral limitations to upright exercise in untrained cardiac transplant recipients. *Circulation*. 1994;89:2605–15.
14. Kavanagh T. Physical training in heart transplant recipients. *J Cardiovasc Risk*. 1996;3:154–9.
15. Kerrigan DJ, Williams CT, Ehrman JK, et al. Cardiac rehabilitation improves functional capacity and patient-reported health status in patients with continuous-flow left ventricular assist devices: the Rehab-VAD randomized controlled trial. *JACC Heart Fail*. 2014;2:653–9.

16. Kerrigan DJ, Williams CT, Ehrman JK, et al. Muscular strength and cardiorespiratory fitness are associated with health status in patients with recently implanted continuous-flow LVADs. *J Cardiopulm Rehabil Prev*. 2013;33:396–400.
17. Keteyian SJ, Brawner C. Cardiac transplant. In: Durstine JL, editor. *ACSM's Exercise Management for Persons With Chronic Diseases and Disabilities*. Champaign (IL): Human Kinetics; 1997. p. 54–8.
18. Keteyian SJ, Brawner C. Cardiac transplant. In: Durstine JL, Moore GE, editors. *ACSM's Exercise Management for Persons With Chronic Diseases and Disabilities*. 2nd ed. Champaign (IL): Human Kinetics; 2003. p. 70–5.
19. Kirklin JK, Naftel DC, Pagani FD, et al. Long-term mechanical circulatory support (destination therapy): on track to compete with heart transplantation? *J Thorac Cardiovasc Surg*. 2012;144:584–603.
20. Kirklin JK, Naftel DC, Pagani FD, et al. Seventh INTERMACS annual report: 15,000 patients and counting. *J Heart Lung Transplant*. 2015;34:1495–504.
21. Kobashigawa JA, Leaf DA, Lee N, et al. A controlled trial of exercise rehabilitation after heart transplantation. *N Engl J Med*. 1999;340:272–7.
22. Kobashigawa JA, Zuckermann A, Macdonald P, et al. Report from a consensus conference on primary graft dysfunction after cardiac transplantation. *J Heart Lung Transplant*. 2014;33:327–40.
23. Kuhn WF, Davis MH, Lippmann SB. Emotional adjustment to cardiac transplantation. *Gen Hosp Psychiatry*. 1988;10:108–13.
24. Lampert E, Mettauer B, Hoppeler H, Charloux A, Charpentier A, Lonsdorfer J. Structure of skeletal muscle in heart transplant recipients. *J Am Coll Cardiol*. 1996;28:980–4.
25. Laoutaris ID, Dritsas A, Adamopoulos S, et al. Benefits of physical training on exercise capacity, inspiratory muscle function, and quality of life in patients with ventricular assist devices long-term postimplantation. *Eur J Cardiovasc Prev Rehabil*. 2011;18:33–40.
26. Lindenfeld J, Page RL II, Zolty R, et al. Drug therapy in the heart transplant recipient: part III: common medical problems. *Circulation*. 2005;111:113–7.
27. Loyaga-Rendon RY, Plaisance EP, Arena R, Shah K. Exercise physiology, testing, and training in patients supported by a left ventricular assist device. *J Heart Lung Transplant*. 2015;34:1005–16.
28. Lund LH, Edwards LB, Kucheryavaya AY, et al. The Registry of the International Society for Heart and Lung Transplantation: thirty-first official adult heart transplant report — 2014; focus theme: retransplantation. *J Heart Lung Transplant*. 2014;33:996–1008.
29. Lund LH, Edwards LB, Kucheryavaya AY, et al. The Registry of the International Society for Heart and Lung Transplantation: thirty-second official adult heart transplantion report — 2015; focus theme: early graft failure. *J Heart Lung Transplant*. 2015;34:1244–54.
30. Mancini DM, Eisen H, Kussmaul W, Mull R, Edmunds LH Jr, Wilson JR. Value of peak exercise oxygen consumption for optimal timing of cardiac transplantation in ambulatory patients with heart failure. *Circulation*. 1991;83:778–86.
31. Marconi C, Marzorati M. Exercise after heart transplantation. *Eur J Appl Physiol*. 2003;90:250–9.
32. McGregor CG. Cardiac transplantation: surgical considerations and early postoperative management. *Mayo Clin Proc*. 1992;67:577–85.
33. Mettauer B, Zhao QM, Epailly E, et al. $\dot{V}O_2$ kinetics reveal a central limitation at the onset of subthreshold exercise in heart transplant recipients. *J Appl Physiol*. 2000;88:1228–38.
34. Pope SE, Stinson EB, Daughters GT II, Schroeder JS, Ingels NB Jr, Alderman EL. Exercise response of the denervated heart in long-term cardiac transplant recipients. *Am J Cardiol*. 1980;46:213–8.
35. Rogers JG, Butler J, Lansman SL, et al. Chronic mechanical circulatory support for inotrope-dependent heart failure patients who are not transplant candidates: results of the INTrEPID trial. *J Am Coll Cardiol*. 2007;50:741–7.
36. Rosenbaum AN, Kremers WK, Schirger JA, et al. Association between early cardiac rehabilitation and long-term survival in cardiac transplant recipients. *Mayo Clin Proc*. 2016;91:149–56.
37. Roussel JC, Baron O, Périgaud C, et al. Outcome of heart transplants 15 to 20 years ago: graft survival, post-transplant morbidity, and risk factors for mortality. *J Heart Lung Transplant*. 2008;27:486–93.
38. Rustad LA, Nytrøen K, Amundsen BH, Gullestad L, Aakhus S. One year of high-intensity interval training improves exercise capacity, but not left ventricular function in stable heart transplant recipients: a randomised controlled trial. *Eur J Prev Cardiol*. 2014;21:181–91.
39. Scott CD, Dark JH, McComb JM. Evolution of the chronotropic response to exercise after cardiac transplantation. *Am J Cardiol*. 1995;76:1292–6.
40. Slaughter MS, Pagani FD, Rogers JG, et al. Clinical management of continuous-flow left ventricular assist devices in advanced heart failure. *J Heart Lung Transplant*. 2010;29(4 suppl):S1–39.
41. Slaughter MS, Rogers JG, Milano CA, et al. Advanced heart failure treated with continuous-flow left ventricular assist device. *N Engl J Med*. 2009;361:2241–51.
42. Squires RW. Cardiac rehabilitation issues for heart transplantation patients. *J Cardiopulm Rehabil*. 1990;10:159–68.
43. Squires RW. Exercise therapy for cardiac transplant recipients. *Prog Cardiovasc Dis*. 2011;53:429–36.
44. Squires RW. Transplant. In: Pashkow FJ, Dafoe WA, editors. *Clinical Cardiac Rehabilitation: A Cardiologist's Guide*. 2nd ed. Baltimore (MD): Lippincott Williams & Wilkins; 1999. p. 175–191.
45. Squires RW, Arthur PA, Gau GT, Muri A, Lambert WB. Exercise after cardiac transplantation: a report of two cases. *J Cardiac Rehabil*. 1983;3:570–4.

46. Squires RW, Hoffman CJ, James GA, et al. Arterial oxygen saturation during graded exercise testing after cardiac transplantation. *J Cardiopulm Rehabil.* 1998;18:348.
47. Squires RW, Leung TC, Cyr NS, et al. Partial normalization of the heart rate response to exercise after cardiac transplantation: frequency and relationship to exercise capacity. *Mayo Clin Proc.* 2002;77:1295–300.
48. Stapleton DD, Mehra MR, Dumas D, et al. Lipid-lowering therapy and long-term survival in heart transplantation. *Am J Cardiol.* 1997;80:802–5.
49. Stehlik J, Stevenson LW, Edwards LB, et al. Organ allocation around the world: insights from the ISHLT International Registry for Heart and Lung Transplantation. *J Heart Lung Transplant.* 2014;33:975–84.
50. Taylor DO, Edwards LB, Boucek MM, Trulock EP, Keck BM, Hertz MI. The Registry of the International Society for Heart and Lung Transplantation: twenty-first official adult heart transplant report — 2004. *J Heart Lung Transplant.* 2004;23:796–803.
51. Weis M, von Scheidt W. Cardiac allograft vasculopathy: a review. *Circulation.* 1997;96:2069–77.
52. Wenke K, Meiser B, Thiery J, et al. Simvastatin reduces graft vessel disease and mortality after heart transplantation: a four-year randomized trial. *Circulation.* 1997;96:1398–402.
53. Wu AH, Ballantyne CM, Short BC, et al. Statin use and risks of death or fatal rejection in the heart transplant lipid registry. *Am J Cardiol.* 2005;95:367–72.

CHAPTER 12

Special Considerations for Cardiovascular Disease: Heart Failure

INTRODUCTION

This chapter presents background, special considerations related to **exercise** testing, prescription, and progression for individuals with chronic heart failure (HF). The case study that follows outlines the results for a middle-aged woman with HF who participated in a combined 24-week exercise regimen at both her cardiac rehabilitation facility (12 wk) and her fitness club (12 wk). This case study presents guidance for the design of a progressive resistance training program and **aerobic** conditioning with a primary goal of return to work for an individual with stable systolic HF.

Case Study 12-1

Mrs. Case Study-HF

Mrs. Case Study-HF is a 54-year-old woman weighing 67.7 kg (149 lb) with a height of 163 cm (64 in). She has a history of anteroseptal myocardial infarction (MI) treated with a percutaneous transluminal coronary angioplasty (PTCA) and stent placement. Risk factors for the subject included a family history of heart disease as both her mother and father died of MIs. She works as a United Parcel Service package handler at a large midwestern airport, and her primary goal for an exercise program is to facilitate her return to work. She is married and attributes high stress to both her job and marriage. She had been a smoker for most of her life; however, on the night of her MI, she quit cold turkey and has been smoke-free ever since. Her medications at discharge from her MI included metoprolol (a β-blocker), 25 mg; lisinopril (angiotensin-converting enzyme [ACE] inhibitor), 10 mg; baby aspirin, 81 mg; and simvastatin (anti-lipidemic), 10 mg. Her blood pressure (BP) levels have been below 120/80 mm Hg since medical management. She then performed 24 weeks of exercise: 12 weeks in cardiac rehabilitation and 12 weeks at her neighborhood fitness facility.

She was asymptomatic for 4 years and at that time began to notice episodes of chest discomfort and dyspnea during walking and cutting the grass. Chest pains were random, with pain present during an activity on one occasion but not the next. She scheduled an appointment with her cardiologist and informed him of her symptoms. He suggested she either have a treadmill test or undergo a cardiac catheterization to evaluate possible progression of disease. She opted for the cardiac catheterization procedure. Results of the catheterization procedure showed akinesis of anterolateral, anteroapical, and inferoapical walls, with anterobasal hypokinesis and an ejection fraction of 30%. Coronary artery analysis demonstrated 10% ostial left main coronary artery disease and 60%–70% in-stent restenosis of the mid-left anterior descending artery. Because of these findings, she was admitted to the hospital for a myocardial viability study that was negative. Because of the negative myocardial viability study, medical management was continued and her dosage of lisinopril was increased to 20 mg. Since then, she has not complained of any chest discomfort. Two years later, her physician again increased her lisinopril to 40 mg daily to achieve maximum benefit with ACE-inhibitor therapy. She continues to do well with medical management. Recently, a **graded exercise test** was performed to evaluate the patient's appropriateness for a supervised exercise program (Table 12.1).

During the graded exercise test, the patient stopped at the end of the second minute of stage IV due to fatigue and mild dyspnea. Muscle strength was measured by the **one repetition maximum (1-RM)** method according to

Table 12.1 Treadmill Graded Exercise Test Results for Mrs. Case Study-HF

Protocol: Naughton protocol was performed while patient was on medications.
Control blood pressure: 128/80 mm Hg
Resting heart rate: 76 bpm

3 min Stages	Speed (mph)	Grade (%) and Estimated METs		Blood Pressure (mm Hg)	Heart Rate (bpm)
I	2.0	0	1.6	140/80	118
II	2.0	3.5	3	150/80	134
III	2.0	7	4	160/80	156
IV	2.0	10.5	5	180/80	166

Recovery Phase	Blood Pressure	Heart Rate
Immediately	—	—
2 min	140/76	126
5 min	—	78

(continues)

Case Study 12-1 (continued)

Table 12.2 Progressive Resistance Training Program for Weeks 1–12 for Mrs. Case Study-HF

Week	Monday (% RM, Sets × Repetitions)	Friday (% RM, Sets × Repetitions)
1	Baseline 1-RM testing	50, 2 × 12
2	60, 2 × 10	1-RM testing
3	70, 2 × 8	80, 2 × 8
4	80, 2 × 8	80, 2 × 8
5	80, 1 × 8	1-RM testing
6–8	60, 2 × 8	70, 2 × 8
9	80, 1 × 8	80, 2 × 8
10–11	60, 2 × 8	70, 3 × 8
12	80, 1 × 8	1-RM testing

accepted standards for leg press, horizontal squat, shoulder press, leg extension, latissimus dorsi pull-down, and biceps curl exercises.

Mrs. Case Study-HF performed the following exercise prescription/progression for 12 weeks at cardiac rehabilitation and then for an additional 12 weeks at her fitness club in her neighborhood. Her exercise training program consisted of cardiovascular training 3 days a week and resistance training 2 days a week for 24 weeks (12 wk in cardiac rehabilitation and 12 wk at her fitness club). She trained 15 minutes on both the treadmill and Schwinn Airdyne bike at 60%–80% of her heart rate reserve (HRR) following a 5-minute warm-up at 50% of HRR. Exercise intensity was increased 0.5 **metabolic equivalents (METs)** per week consistent with patient tolerance. During the first 12 weeks of training at cardiac rehabilitation, heart rate (HR) and rhythm were monitored continuously using a Nihon-Kohden WEP-9430 Cardiac Telemetry System. The following exercises were used for resistance training: leg press, shoulder press, leg extension, lateral pull-down, cable biceps curl, and horizontal squat starting at 50% of her 1-RM and progressing to 80%. During weeks 1 and 2, she worked at 50% and 60% of her 1-RM, respectively. During week 3, she worked at 70% of her 1-RM. For weeks 4–12, she trained at 80% of her 1-RM as outlined in Table 12.2.

Table 12.3 presents the exercise program recommended for Mrs. Case Study-HF that transitioned her from cardiac rehabilitation to her fitness center and was accomplished with the help of a personal trainer with experience in

Table 12.3 Progressive Resistance Training Program for Weeks 13–24 for Mrs. Case Study-HF

Week	Monday (% RM, Sets × Repetitions)	Friday (% RM, Sets × Repetitions)
13	60, 2 × 8	70, 3 × 8
14–15	80, 3 × 8	80, 3 × 8
16	80, 1 × 8	1-RM testing
17	60, 2 × 8	70, 3 × 8
18–19	80, 3 × 8	80, 3 × 8
20	80, 1 × 8	1-RM testing
21	70, 2 × 8	70, 3 × 8
22–23	70, 3 × 8	80, 3 × 8
24	80, 1 × 8	1-RM testing

Case Study 12-1 (continued)

resistance training for individuals with HF. At week 13, dumbbell lunges, dumbbell shoulder press, and dumbbell curl were substituted for the leg extension, the machine shoulder press, and cable biceps curl, respectively. The addition of the dynamic free weight program at week 13 is beneficial for several reasons:

- First, the neuromuscular system will likely be optimally challenged by activities that affect **activities of daily living (ADL)** so crucial to the quality of life for individuals with HF.
- Second, the free weight program is reproducible outside of the clinic and thus provides the subjects with resistance training techniques that can be performed independently after completion of supervised exercise.
- Lastly, the dynamic free weight program mimics the balance and **strength** requirements of activities such as walking and climbing stairs, facilitating the transfer of **muscular strength** gains to activities of daily life. This aggressive resistance training program was designed to facilitate return to work and was accomplished safely and effectively.

Description, Prevalence, and Etiology

HF is an abnormality of myocardial function in which the heart is not able to pump blood at a rate commensurate with the requirements of the metabolizing tissues or to do so only from an elevated filling pressure. There are two types of HF: systolic HF, in which the individual has a reduced ejection fraction (<35%) (HFrEf), and diastolic HF, in which the individual has a normal ejection fraction with elevated filling pressure (HFpEF). HF may also exist as a combination of the two types. HF affects about 5 million individuals in the United States, and more than 550,000 patients are diagnosed each year (17). Nearly, 1 in 100 individuals older than the age of 65 years have chronic HF, which is the most common cause of hospitalization for this age group. The total direct cost of treating patients with HF is estimated to be approximately $300 billion annually, an amount that constitutes more than what is spent on any other diagnosis (17). Etiologic factors for HF include ischemic, hypertensive, and valvular heart disease as well as a variety of metabolic, infectious, and toxic agents (11).

Exercise intolerance is a hallmark finding with chronic HF. These individuals often have a poor quality of life related to this factor as well as frequent rehospitalizations for their condition (1). As the disease progresses, patients become more incapacitated and deconditioned, unable to perform simple daily tasks without limiting dyspnea or fatigue. Muscle atrophy and loss of muscle strength and endurance are also exhibited in individuals with HF and partly explain the exercise intolerance and decreased ability to perform ADL. A comprehensive program of aerobic conditioning and resistance training has been found to improve muscle strength, muscular endurance, and **cardiorespiratory fitness** as well as function and quality of life (4,11,15–17). Furthermore, the landmark Heart Failure: A Controlled Trial to Investigate Outcomes of Exercise Training (HF-ACTION) clinical trial (12) found that morbidity and mortality were modestly affected by aerobic training when added to usual care versus usual care alone.

Reduced cardiopulmonary factors in patients with HF were believed to be the primary contributor to the exercise intolerance demonstrated. Ejection fraction does not correlate well with exercise intolerance or dyspnea. This lack of correlation has led investigators to search for other explanations for muscle fatigue observed with HF. Results have found that peripheral factors such as blood flow, intrinsic skeletal muscle abnormalities, and neurohormonal alterations are primarily responsible for the poor exercise tolerance. The *muscle hypothesis* provides a connection between left ventricular dysfunction and peripheral abnormalities that include skeletal muscle myopathy and dyspnea. The peripheral abnormalities have been associated with reduced ability to perform ADL leading to a reduced quality of life in patients with HF (Fig. 12.1). The muscle hypothesis states that reduced left

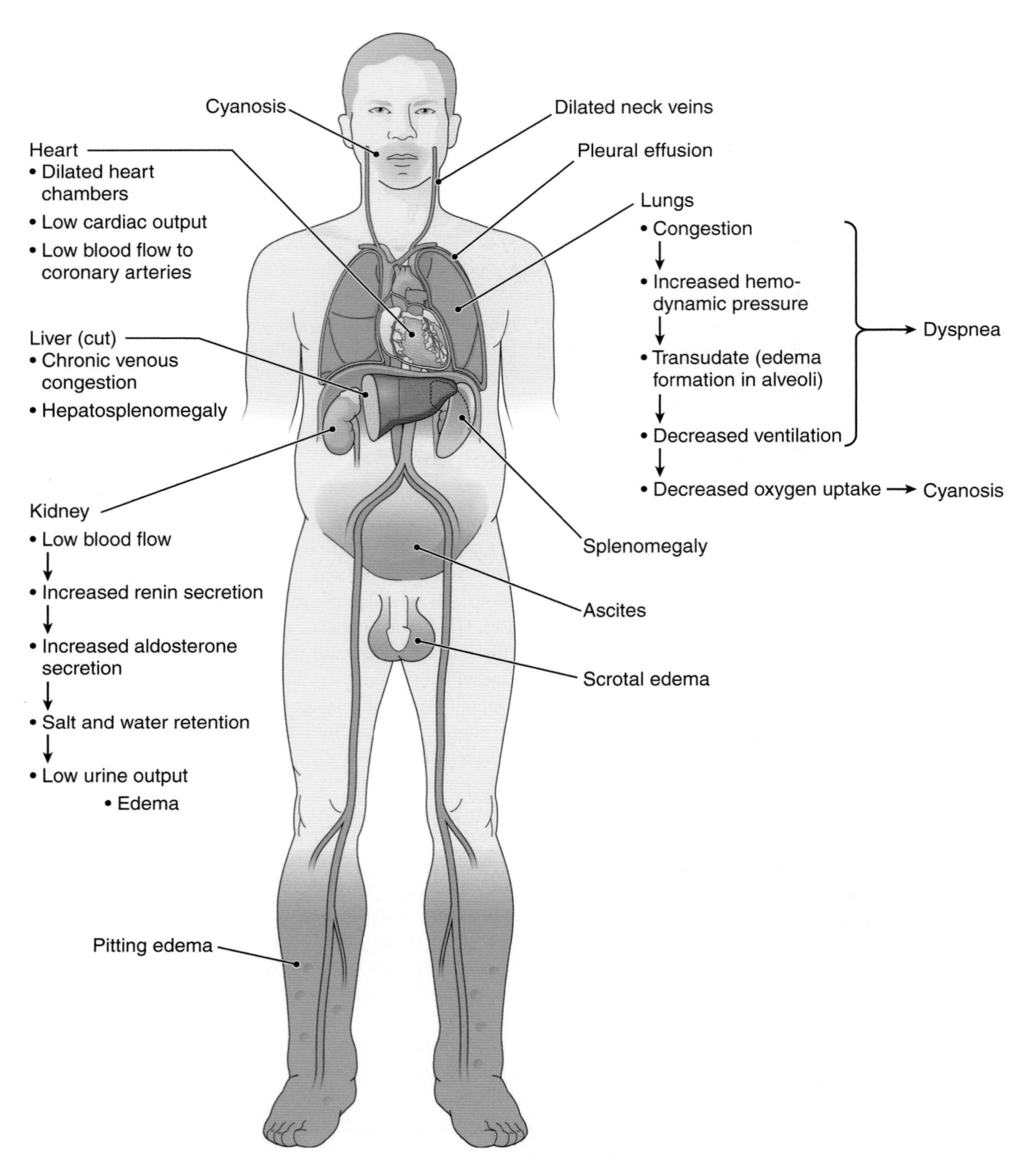

FIGURE 12.1. Cycle by which long-term left ventricular (LV) dysfunction leads to reduced exercise capacity and muscle fatigue. The cycle begins at the LV dysfunction and continues with exacerbating conditions. (From McConnell TH. *The Nature of Disease: Pathology for the Health Professions*. 2nd ed. Philadelphia [PA]: Wolters Kluwer; 2014. 800 p.)

ventricular function results in low perfusion to the skeletal muscle. The low muscle perfusion leads to a reduced metabolic state in the skeletal muscle, causing skeletal muscle myopathy. The skeletal muscle myopathy results in an accumulation of metabolic by-products, causing muscle fatigue and activating ergoreceptors in the skeletal muscle. Ergoreceptors are afferent nerve endings that transmit signals to the central nervous system. These signals result in increased ventilation and sympathetic nervous system (SNS) stimulation, causing increased dyspnea and peripheral resistance, respectively. The long-term negative consequences of the increase in SNS activity is an increase in vasoconstriction and afterload, both of which perpetuate the HF cycle. Both aerobic exercise and resistance training positively affect the muscle, vasculature, and autonomic system, thus effectively altering this cycle (14).

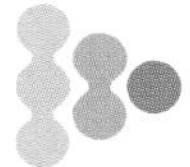

Preparticipation Health Screening, Medical History, and Physical Examination

An extensive medical history, including presence of comorbidities such as diabetes (which affects nearly 35% of patients with HF) or age (most patients with HF are **older adults**), and **physical activity** history should be performed prior to initiating exercise for the individual with HF (2). In addition, a medical screening examination consisting of a physical examination and an echocardiogram to determine ejection fraction should be performed. The drug regimen is extensive and should be assessed and side effects should be considered before implementing any exercise program. Standard medical therapy includes diuretics (loop, thiazide, potassium sparing) to reduce blood volume and edema, vasodilators (*e.g.*, ACE inhibitors or angiotensin receptor blockers) to reduce afterload and restore neurohumoral balance and systemic vascular resistance, and β-adrenergic receptor blockers to interrupt the "toxic effects" of the overactive SNS (9,10,13). Combination drugs such as sacubitril/valsartan (angiotensin receptor blocker plus a medication to reduce BP) are increasingly popular because of their effectiveness and lower patient burden. The use of digoxin in patients with HF and atrial fibrillation may be appropriate in patients who cannot tolerate β-blockers for rate control because of intractable HF. Other agents that may be used with this population include antiplatelet and anticoagulation therapies and an aldosterone antagonist. Biventricular pacing is a technique to enhance the stroke volume for patients with HF who experience left bundle-branch block and a very prolonged QRS duration. Heart transplantation and ventricular assist devices are end-stage treatments for HF. Use of implantable cardioverter defibrillators (ICDs) and wearable defibrillator devices is also becoming more common in this population of patients. The exercise professional should be aware of the upper limits in terms of HRs for these individuals that could potentially precipitate the delivery of an electrical shock.

Case Study 12-1 Quiz:

Preparticipation Health Screening, Medical History, and Physical Examination

1. Why was medical management the recommendation for this patient?
2. What are the guidelines for this patient in terms of preparticipation medical clearance?

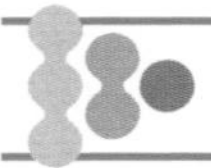

Exercise Testing Considerations

A symptom-limited cardiopulmonary exercise test using a low-intensity protocol with small, 1 MET increments in work requirements/stage such as a modified Naughton may be performed prior to exercise prescription. The Bruce protocol is never appropriate for patients with HF unless the patient clearly already has a more normalized exercise capacity. Other modes of testing include 6-minute walk and pharmacological stress testing (1). Absolute contraindications to exercise testing and exercise training for HF are presented in *ACSM's Guidelines for Exercise Testing and Prescription, 10th edition* (*GETP10*) (2). The most common concerns related to exercise testing and specific to HF include postexercise hypotension, arrhythmias, and worsening HF symptoms. A summary of exercise testing considerations follows:

- Postexercise symptoms including hypotension, arrhythmias, and disproportionate dyspnea need to be monitored closely.
- Symptoms for patients with HF will occur at lower workloads, and thus, exercise tests need to be low level with modest MET increments between stages; ramped protocols are appropriate.
- Six-minute walk tests may be used in this population.
- Gas exchange measurements including **maximal oxygen consumption** and ventilatory measures, although not available to all patients with HF, can provide valuable data for clinicians regarding patient status and prognosis.
- Test termination criteria should be more focused on symptoms rather than target HRs.

Case Study 12-1 Quiz:

Exercise Testing Considerations

3. What are the intended actions and their potential impact on exercise testing of the three medications prescribed for Mrs. Case Study-HF?
4. Was the Naughton protocol appropriate for this patient? Why or why not? Is there another protocol you would select for this patient? Justify your answer.
5. What precaution(s) need to be taken for a patient with HF for safe 1-RM testing?

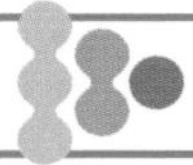

Exercise Prescription and Progression Considerations

General guidelines for exercise prescription and progression for individuals with HF are presented in frequency, intensity, time, and type (FITT) table (Table 12.4). Important considerations when designing a comprehensive exercise program for individuals with HF include individualization of program and goal setting. Aerobic conditioning recommendations for individuals with HF include the following (13): The mode should be large muscle group activities, most likely walking, treadmill, or cycling performed at an intensity of 40%–70% volume of oxygen consumed per unit time ($\dot{V}O_2$) or HRR, 4–7 days per week accumulating 20–60 minutes per day. **Intensity** can also be gauged by rating of perceived exertion (RPE) of 11–14/20 or 5–7/10 on the CR-10 scale. High-intensity interval training (HIIT), although popular, is appropriate for only a selected subsection of the HF population. Training intensities of up to 90% of the HRR

TABLE 12.4 FITT RECOMMENDATIONS FOR INDIVIDUALS WITH CHRONIC HEART FAILURE

ACSM FITT Principle of the ExR_x

Chronic Medical Condition	Frequency (How often?)	Intensity (How hard?)	Time	Type (What kind?) Primary	Resistance	Flexibility	Special Considerations
Healthy Adult	$\geq$5 d · wk^{-1} of moderate exercise, or $\geq$3 d · wk^{-1} of vigorous exercise, or a combination of moderate and vigorous exercise on $\geq$3–5 d · wk^{-1} is recommended.	Moderate to vigorous. Light-to-moderate intensity exercise may be beneficial in deconditioned individuals.	If moderate intensity: $\geq$30 min · d^{-1} to total 150 min · wk^{-1}. If vigorous intensity: $\geq$20 min · d^{-1} to total 75 min · wk^{-1}.	Regular, purposeful exercise that involves major muscle groups and is continuous and rhythmic in nature is recommended.	Muscle strengthening 2–3 d · wk^{-1} (nonconsecutive) Moderate to vigorous intensity; 2–4 sets of 8–12 repetitions	2–3 d · wk^{-1}; static stretch 10–30 s; 2–4 repetitions of each exercise	Sedentary behaviors can have adverse health effects, even among those who regularly exercise. Adding short physical activity breaks throughout the day may be considered as a part of the exercise.
Heart Failure	3–5 d · wk^{-1}	If HR data is available from a recent GXT, set intensity between 60% and 80% of HRR. In the absence of data from a GXT or if atrial fibrillation is present, use RPE of 11–14 on a 6–20 scale.	Progressively increase to 30 min · d^{-1} and then up to 60 min · d^{-1}	Treadmill or free walking and stationary cycling	1–2 d · wk^{-1} (nonconsecutive) Begin at 40% 1-RM for upper body and 50% for lower body exercises. Two sets of 10–15 repetitions focusing on major muscle groups. Machines may be best due to loss of strength and balance.	2–3 d · wk^{-1} with daily being most effective; 10–30 s for static stretching; 2–4 repetitions of each exercise Static, dynamic, and/or PNF	Exercise is especially important for patients with HF who may exhibit exercise intolerance due to skeletal muscle myopathy. Resistance training is needed to assist with ADL. HIIT, although popular, is only appropriate for a selected subsection of this population.

ExR_x, exercise prescription; GXT, graded exercise test; PNF, proprioceptive neuromuscular facilitation.

Based on the FITT Recommendations present in *ACSM's Guidelines for Exercise Testing and Prescription*. 10th ed. Philadelphia (PA): Wolters Kluwer; 2018. 480 p.

may be appropriate for stable individuals. Significant improvement was seen as a result of HITT with peak oxygen uptake ($\dot{V}O_{2peak}$) improving by 46% (2).

In terms of resistance training, design of a program should include **maximal** strength testing (1-RM) for evaluating baseline strength levels, establishing weight loads for training, and tracking changes in strength over time (2,7). Circuit weight training protocols are currently used in cardiac rehabilitation because they are safe, efficient, and effective (2,4,5,6). Circuit weight training programs consist of a series of resistance training exercises performed in sequence with minimal rest (30–60 s) between exercises. Approximately 8–12 repetitions of each exercise are performed per circuit at a relative intensity of 60%–80% of 1-RM. Individuals may gradually progress to two sets of 12 repetitions at 80% of 1-RM. Examples of exercises that could be included for the individual with HF are the leg press, squat, shoulder press, leg extension, latissimus dorsi (lat) pull-down, and cable biceps curl exercises for weeks 1 through 12. These exercises, among others (Table 12.5), have the potential to contribute to the ability to perform

Table 12.5 Exercises that Assist with Functional Activities for the Patient with Heart Failure

Exercise	Muscle Groups Involved	ADL Affected by Exercise
Leg press	Quadriceps, hamstrings, glutes	Pushing off to move from a seated to a standing position
Deadlift	Spinal erectors, quadriceps, hamstrings, glutes	Proper technique for picking up something from the floor
Step up	Quadriceps, hamstrings, glutes	Walking up and down stairs
Squat	Quadriceps, hamstrings, glutes, spinal erectors	Getting out of a chair
Shoulder press	Deltoids, triceps	Putting something on a top shelf, such as dishes
One arm row with dumbbell	Latissimus dorsi, brachialis, biceps	Pull something toward the body, such as a grandchild, to hug them
Lateral pull-down	Latissimus dorsi, brachialis, biceps	Pulling oneself to a seated position using shower safety bars in case of a fall
Chest press	Pectorals, deltoids, triceps	Pushing a lawnmower up a hill or around obstacles
Biceps curl	Brachialis, biceps	Picking up a jug of milk and putting it in a cart

ADLs so crucial to quality of life for the individual with chronic HF as well as add variety to prevent plateaus in fitness gains (3). Individuals should be properly oriented to each exercise procedure and piece of equipment. Intermittent monitoring of HR and BP should take place to ensure patient's safety. Signs or symptoms of worsening HF include weight gain of 1.5–2.0 kg over previous 3–5 days, increased HR, increased dyspnea including orthopnea, and paroxysmal nocturnal dyspnea. Visual inspection for increasing peripheral edema and auscultatory findings of pulmonary edema are important for the exercise professional to evaluate. If telemetry monitoring is available, increasing arrhythmia may also be present. Any of these findings would require cessation of exercise testing or training and may require additional evaluation and treatment (8,9). Alterations in autonomic nervous system function and medications may affect reflex response to positional changes, so the clinician needs to be careful during lifting exercises that involve postural changes.

Case Study 12-1 Quiz:

Exercise Prescription and Progression Considerations

6. Compare and contrast the application of the FITT principle in this case study with the recommendations as presented in the *GETP10* (see FITT table, Table 12.5). Identify any significant differences and discuss whether you agree or disagree with these different applications of the FITT recommendations. Justify your answer.
7. Can you suggest other exercises that would be beneficial for this patient given the strong desire to return to work as a package handler at United Parcel Service?

SUMMARY

This chapter presents relevant information regarding exercise testing, prescription, and progression recommendations for individuals with HF. A case study is presented as a means to clarify the concepts discussed. It should be noted that HF often exists with other comorbidities such as diabetes (see Chapter 14) and pulmonary disease (see Chapter 16) and is more common in older individuals (see Chapter 9), so the clinician working with this population should be familiar with the exercise testing, prescription, and progressions for these special populations.

A summary of exercise training and prescription considerations for individuals with HF follows:

- Preexercise assessment of the patient should include a visual inspection for ankle edema, routine monitoring of body weight, and unusual dyspnea or fatigue with usual activity.
- Warm-up and cool-down aspects of exercise programming may need to be extended.
- Alteration of the relationship between HR and exercise intensity with the use of β-blockers or other pharmacological therapies may require the use of RPE 11–14.
- There should be emphasis on exercise duration and frequency before intensity
- When appropriate, inclusion resistance training usually after a period of adjustment to aerobic exercise conditioning

REFERENCES

1. ACC/AHA 2005 Guidelines update for the diagnosis and management of chronic heart failure in the adult: a report of the American College of Cardiology/American Heart Association task force on practice guidelines (writing committee to update the 2001 guidelines for the evaluation and management of heart failure) [Internet]. Washington (DC): American College of Cardiology; [cited 2005]. Available from: http://www.acc.org/clinical/guidelines/failure/index.pdf
2. American College of Sports Medicine. *ACSM's Guidelines for Exercise Testing and Prescription*. 10th ed. Philadelphia (PA): Wolters Kluwer; 2018. 480 p.
3. Barnard K. Exercise testing and training strategies for coronary heart disease. In: Swank AM, Hagerman P, editors. *Resistance Training for Special Populations*. Clifton Park (NY): Delmar Cengage; 2009. p. 261–70.
4. Barnard KL, Adams KJ, Swank AM, Kaelin M, Kushnik MR, Denny DM. Combined high-intensity strength and aerobic training in patients with congestive heart failure. *J Strength Cond Res*. 2000;14(4):383–88.
5. Braith RW, Beck DT. Resistance exercises: training adaptations and developing a safe exercise prescription. *Heart Fail Rev*. 2008;13:69–79.
6. Delagardelle C, Feiereisen P, Krecké R, Essamri B, Beissel J. Objective effects of a 6 months' endurance and strength training program in outpatients with congestive heart failure. *Med Sci Sport Exerc*. 1999;31:1102–7.
7. Fleck SJ, Kraemer WJ. *Designing Resistance Training Programs*. 2nd ed. Champaign (IL): Human Kinetics; 1997. p. 1–32.
8. Hanson P. Exercise testing and training in patients with chronic heart failure. *Med Sci Sports Exerc*. 1994;26:527–37.
9. Keteyian SJ, Brawner CA, Schairer JR. Exercise testing and training of patients with heart failure due to left ventricular dysfunction. *J Cardiopulm Rehabil*. 1997;17:19–28.
10. Maiorana A, O'Driscoll G, Cheetham C, et al. Combined aerobic and resistance exercise training improves functional capacity and strength in CHF. *J Appl Physiol (1985)*. 2000;88:1565–70.
11. Myers JN, Brubaker PH. Chronic heart failure. In: Durstine JL, Moore GE, Painter PL, Roberts SO, editors. *ACSM's Exercise Management for Persons With Chronic Diseases and Disabilities*. Champaign (IL): Human Kinetics; 2009. p. 92–8.
12. O'Connor CM, Whellan DJ, Lee KL, et al. Efficacy and safety of exercise training in patients with chronic heart failure: HF-ACTION randomized controlled trial. *JAMA*. 2009;301(14):1439–50. doi:10.1001/jama.2009.454.
13. Oka RK, DeMarco T, Haskell WL, et al. Impact of a home-based walking and resistance training program on quality of life in patients with heart failure. *Am J Cardiol*. 2000;85:365–9.
14. Pu CT, Johnson MT, Forman DE, et al. Randomized trial of progressive resistance training to counteract the myopathy of chronic heart failure. *J Appl Physiol (1985)*. 2001;90:2341–50.

15. Santoro C, Cosmas A, Forman D, et al. Exercise training alters skeletal muscle mitochondrial morphometry in heart failure patients. *J Cardiovasc Risk.* 2002;9:377–81.
16. Selig SE, Carey MF, Menzies DG, et al. Moderate-intensity resistance exercise training in patients with chronic heart failure improves strength, endurance, heart rate variability and forearm blood flow. *J Card Fail.* 2004;10(1):21–30.
17. Thom T, Haase N, Rosamond W, et al. Heart disease and stroke statistics — 2006 update: a report from the American Heart Association Statistics Committee and Stroke Statistics Subcommittee. *Circulation.* 2006;113:e85–151.

CHAPTER 13

Special Considerations for Cardiovascular Disease: Valvular Heart Disease and Peripheral Artery Disease

INTRODUCTION

This chapter presents background and special considerations related to **exercise** testing, prescription, and progression for individuals with valvular heart disease (VHD) and for individuals with peripheral artery disease (PAD). The first section of this chapter addresses VHD. The case study presented outlines the diagnosis of an older woman with aortic stenosis and follows her through her recovery during 12 weeks of cardiac rehabilitation. This case study provides guidance for the design of a progressive aerobic conditioning and eventual resistance training program with a primary goal of return to **activities of daily living** for an individual with VHD.

VALVULAR HEART DISEASE

Case Study 13-1

Mrs. Case Study-Valve

Mrs. Case Study-Valve is a 73-year-old woman weighing 65 kg (143 lb) with a height of 1.6764 m (5 ft 6 in) tall. She has a 2-month history of feeling light-headed while carrying laundry up one flight of stairs at home. This occurs less often when not carrying anything upstairs. She has not lost consciousness during any of these episodes, nor has she had chest pain or unusual shortness of breath. However, she is not physically active outside of her activities of daily living around her home. She has no history of high cholesterol, smoking, or significant family history for coronary artery disease (CAD). Her blood glucose is slightly elevated with a glycolated hemoglobin (HbA1c) of 5.9 and a long history of hypertension that currently is well controlled with a diuretic and angiotensin-converting enzyme (ACE) inhibitor.

She saw her primary care physician (PCP), who noted a 3/6 systolic murmur. She was asked to follow up with an echocardiogram and routine treadmill testing to better evaluate her symptoms.

She underwent exercise stress testing on a treadmill using a Cornell protocol. Her resting electrocardiogram (ECG) demonstrated normal sinus rhythm, normal heart rate, normal axis, and no concerning acute ST changes. She was able to complete 8 minutes and 40 seconds (speed of 2.5 mph with 12% grade). Her heart rate increased from 67 bpm at rest to 127 bpm (86% of predicted maximal capacity) at the peak workload. Her blood pressure (BP) initially increased from 132/80 mm Hg at rest to 140/78 mm Hg at 3 minutes and then fell to 136/74 at 6 minutes and 118/68 at the peak workload. Her ECG had no concerning changes, but between 6 minutes and peak effort, she began having frequent, unifocal premature ventricular contractions (PVCs), which resolved within 2 minutes of recovery. She denied chest pain or palpitations but complained of light-headedness that correlated with her falls in systolic BP during testing. This also resolved within a couple minutes of exercise (Table 13.1).

Table 13.1 Treadmill Graded Exercise Test Results for Mrs. Case Study-Valve

Pretest Data
Protocol: Cornell
Resting HR: 67 bpm
BP: 132/80 mm Hg

2 min Stages	Speed (mph)	Grade (%) and Estimated METs		HR (bpm)	BP (mm Hg)
0	1.7	0	2	81	
0.5	1.7	5	3	95	140/78
1.0	1.7	10	5	109	136/74
1.5	2.1	11	6	121	
2.0	2.5	12	7	127	118/68

Recovery Phase
Immediately: HR —; BP —
2 min: HR: 85; BP: 132/78 mm Hg
5 min: HR: 70; BP: 130/82 mm Hg

HR, heart rate; BP; blood pressure.

Case Study 13-1 (continued)

Table 13.2 Progressive Aerobic Training Program for Mrs. Case Study-Valve during Cardiac Rehabilitation

Week	Treadmill Workload (METs)	Treadmill Time (min)
1	2.0	5–10
2	2.3	15
3–4	2.6	20–25
5–6	3.2	25–30
7–8	3.5	30
9–10	3.8	30–35
11–12	4.0	30–40

The patient stopped at 8 minutes and 40 seconds (stage 2.0) due to light-headedness. She had a follow-up echocardiogram 2 days later which revealed normal biventricular, systolic function (left ventricular ejection fraction [LVEF] about 55%–60%), mild-to-moderate left ventricular hypertrophy (LVH), moderate-to-severe aortic stenosis, and no other issues noted. Due to a symptomatic stress test and significant valvular disease, she was referred for aortic valve replacement surgery.

After a successful surgery and discharge from the hospital 5 days later, Mrs. Case Study-Valve was referred to a traditional cardiac rehabilitation program. She attended monitor exercise sessions three times a week for 12 weeks and was given a weekly home **exercise prescription** to follow on the off days from cardiac rehabilitation. Her exercise program began with building her endurance and incorporating gentle stretching exercises. For the first week, she walked on the treadmill at a pace she could comfortably sustain for 10 minutes without symptoms. The workload was 1.5 mph or 2.0 **metabolic equivalents (METs)**. Each successive week, she was progressed by no more than 5 minutes and 0.5 METs each week (Table 13.2). She also performed a total body, gentle stretching routine without pain and was encouraged to stretch daily after her aerobic exercise sessions.

To gain upper body conditioning, 1 month after surgery she began using a recumbent stepper for 5–10 minutes in addition to the treadmill exercise. Her heart rate and MET level were matched to heart rate and MET level on the treadmill. For upper body strength, 2 months after surgery she began a strength training routine for the major muscles of the arms and trunk, including biceps curls, lateral shoulder raises, standing triceps kickback extensions, and standing dumbbell rows (Table 13.3). Muscle strength was assessed for each exercise using the 10-repetition maximum method. She continued to progress in her **aerobic**, **flexibility**, and **strength** training routine through the end of cardiac rehabilitation. At that point, she graduated and maintained her exercise routine at home.

Table 13.3 Progressive Resistance Training Program for Weeks 13–24 for Mrs. Case Study-Valve

Week	Day 1 (% RM, Sets × Repetitions)	Day 2 (% RM, Sets × Repetitions)
8	60, 1 × 12	60, 1 × 15
9	70, 2 × 10	70, 2 × 12
10	80, 2 × 10	80, 2 × 12
11	70, 3 × 10	1-RM testing
12	60, 2 × 12	60, 2 × 15

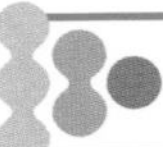

Description, Prevalence, and Etiology

VHD is any disease or abnormality of a single heart valve or any combination of the four valves. The most prevalent valvular diseases are those of the aortic and mitral valves due to the higher pressure on the left side of the heart. Tricuspid and pulmonary valve diseases are much less common (4). Over 5 million Americans are diagnosed with VHD each year (15), and approximately 10% of people older than 75 years of age have some form of VHD (15). VHD can be congenital or acquired later in life; however, most cases of VHD are the result of aging (15).

Heart murmurs (the sound of valve dysfunction) can be detected with a stethoscope, but an echocardiogram is the primary imaging tool used to diagnose VHD. Valvular diseases are typically classified as a leaky valve (regurgitation) or the inability of a valve to completely open (stenosis). Over time, both regurgitation and stenosis can reduce cardiac output and lead to cardiac hypertrophy and, eventually, myocardial dysfunction or heart failure (6). Exercise training has not been shown to improve valve function but can improve peripheral adaptations and functional capacity in patients with VHD (6).

Preparticipation Health Screening, Medical History, and Physical Examination

Evaluation of VHD will usually happen before the patient is referred to cardiac rehabilitation or a supervised exercise program. However, the exercise professional should be familiar with the most common symptoms of VHD. Symptoms originating from VHD can vary dependent on several factors: the specific valve(s) involved, the condition and severity of the valve(s), and the presence of other comorbidities.

Symptoms of VHD may be more subtle at the onset and can be difficult to discern through an initial patient interview, which can lead to multiple differential diagnoses and a "shotgun" approach to testing. Gradually, if not diagnosed correctly in the early stages, symptoms can worsen considerably and lead to more debilitating conditions such as heart failure.

During exercise, many of the symptoms listed in Box 13.1 may be present. The specific symptoms will vary depending on which valve is involved and the degree of impairment. Normal mild-to-moderate valve disease may not impair the ability to exercise, but progression toward more severe VHD can result in multiple abnormal conditions during exercise (Table 13.4).

Box 13.1 Common Symptoms of Valvular Heart Disease

- Shortness of breath
- Dyspnea on exertion
- Fatigue
- Palpitations
- Chest discomforts
- Near syncope
- Syncope
- Unexplained coughing
- Swelling in lower extremities

Table 13.4 Signs and Conditions Related to the Dysfunction of Specific Valves

Conditions	Mitral Stenosis	Mitral Regurgitation	Aortic Stenosis	Aortic Regurgitation
Reduced CO	X		X	
Exertional hypotension	X		X	
Exertional syncope	X		X	
Inadequate $M\dot{V}O_2$	X		X	
Chest discomfort	X		X	
ECG changes		X	X	X
LVH/false positive result		X	X	X
Diastolic dysfunction			X	?
Systolic dysfunction		X		X
Ventricular ectopy		X	X	X

CO, cardiac output; $M\dot{V}O_2$, myocardial oxygen consumption.

Although this chapter does not go into detail on the different heart sounds (heart murmurs) related to significant VHD, it is in the best interest of the clinical exercise professional to be able to distinguish between a normal and abnormal heart sound and to be able to communicate findings to a qualified medical professional.

In many cases, if a heart murmur is detected and if symptoms are suggestive of a possible heart valve disorder, an ultrasound (echocardiogram) of the heart may be ordered. The echocardiogram will look at the structure and function of the heart muscle and valves and provide valuable information to the physician about the best plan of care for the patient.

Case Study 13-1 Quiz:

Preparticipation Health Screening, Medical History, and Physical Examination

1. What intensity for cardiovascular exercise would you suggest for this patient if medical management is decided on?
2. Assuming this patient continues with medical management for aortic stenosis, would you perform regular, nonimaging, exercise stress testing to evaluate for detection of CAD? If so, why?

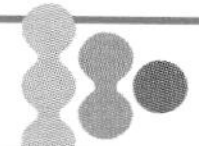

Exercise Testing Considerations

Exercise testing is often a valuable tool to evaluate overall prognosis of individuals with VHD. Specifically, it can measure the degree of physical impairment from symptoms, the thresholds of abnormal hemodynamic responses, the thresholds for arrhythmias, the efficacy of medical management, and the need for surgeries and interventions.

Table 13.5 Types of Exercise Testing and Quantifiable Data

Type of Testing	Prognosis/ Capacity	Hemodynamic Response	Arrhythmia	Symptom Threshold	$\dot{V}O_2$	Ischemia
Routine exercise ECG only	X	X	X	X		
Stress nuclear imaging	X	X	X	X		X
Stress echocardiogram	X	X	X	X		X
Cardiopulmonary	X	X	X	X	X	

$\dot{V}O_2$, volume of oxygen consumed per unit time.

The type of exercise stress testing must be carefully selected and specific to medical needs. Issues such as LVH and false positive ECG changes suggestive of ischemia can result from VHD when performing exercise testing (Table 13.5).

Endpoints for exercise testing with those suffering from VHD are generally the same as noted in *ACSM's Guidelines for Exercise Testing and Prescription, 10th edition* (3). Specifically for this population, look for the onset of serious arrhythmias, excessive ST depression on ECG, plateau or drop in systolic BP with increased work rate (especially in presence of symptoms or ECG changes), slowing of heart rate with increased work rate, or excessive increase in systolic/diastolic BP (11).

Case Study 13-1 Quiz:

Exercise Testing Considerations

3. The patient's systolic BP fell during exercise testing, from 132/80 to 118/68 mm Hg at peak exercise. Would this be considered a *relative* or *absolute* indication for terminating exercise testing?
4. Would the Bruce protocol have been appropriate for this patient? Why or why not? Name another protocol you could select for this patient and justify your answer.
5. What precaution(s) need to be taken for a patient post–valve-replacement surgery for one repetition maximum (1-RM) testing to be safe?

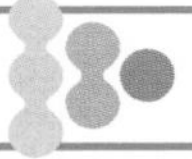

Exercise Prescription and Progression

The exercise prescription and progression for patients with VHD will largely depend on the severity of the disease, the presence of symptoms, and the type of treatment. Most patients with VHD are encouraged to exercise. Asymptomatic patients with mild VHD, normal left ventricular function, and normal pulmonary artery pressures may participate in vigorous exercise and competitive sports without restrictions (5,16). Exercise prescription and progression guidelines for these patients would be the same as the general population (see Chapter 6).

Patients with more than mild VHD or with ventricular dysfunction in addition to VHD should avoid competitive sports. Also, patients with moderate-to-severe aortic stenosis should avoid both vigorous exercise and competitive sports due to the risk of sudden cardiac death (5). However, most dysfunctional valves can be replaced or repaired with surgical or catheter-based techniques.

Exercise training after valve replacement or repair is encouraged to increase functional capacity and prevent other cardiac problems (20). Patients who receive valve replacements, both bioprosthetic and mechanical, should limit the intensity of exercise to a moderate level. Patients on anticoagulation therapy such as warfarin for either a mechanical valve or atrial fibrillation should avoid contact sports or activities due to the risk of bleeding (6). Exercise prescription and progression guidelines for postsurgical patients would be the same as for patients post-surgery for coronary artery bypass grafting (see Chapter 9).

Case Study 13-1 Quiz:

Exercise Prescription and Progression

6. Shorter, less intense intervals of cardiovascular exercise were prescribed, along with low volume and intensity strength training between cardiovascular exercise intervals. Please explain why this particular approach was taken.
7. What could the cardiac rehabilitation team do to help with long-term adherence to an exercise program?

PERIPHERAL ARTERY DISEASE

Case Study 13-2

Mr. Case Study-PAD

Mr. Case Study-PAD is a 57-year-old man weighing 94.5 kg (208 lb) and is 1.8 m (5 ft 10 in) tall. He has a 30-pack-year history of smoking but quit 2 years ago. He has no known history of heart disease but has mildly elevated cholesterol, an HbA1c of 6.3, hypertension controlled with ACE inhibitor and diuretic, and no family history of cardiovascular disease. He works as a machine shop supervisor but does not participate in recreational activities or structured exercise.

Mr. Case Study-PAD complains of a 2-year history of bilateral thigh numbness and fatigue, greater on the left than on the right, brought on only with exertion, but inconsistently. His symptoms are not brought on by long periods of sitting, standing, or repetitive lifting.

An initial workup included lower back x-ray and magnetic resonance imaging (MRI), which were negative for any significant findings. He was referred for physical therapy which seemed initially to provide moderate relief from symptoms. The exercise prescription from physical therapy at the time included a series of daily mobility and strengthening movements as well as suggestion of some moderate effort exercise on a home stationary bike 3 days a week for 20 minutes.

He was consistent with this program for about 3 months and then returned to his normal lifestyle and symptoms returned about 2 months later. He did not seek follow-up consultation with his physician or with physical therapist. Over the next 6 months, the symptoms worsened and started to include left buttock tightness and cramping and some worsening bilateral thigh numbness and fatigue.

Only when his ambulation was limited to less than three blocks did he seek consultation with his physician, where he described the left buttock cramping and bilateral leg fatigue with ambulation of short distances, which was not brought on by long-term sitting, standing, or repetitive lifting. His physician then ordered bedside ankle/brachial systolic pressure index (ABI) testing, which revealed normal results of 1.12 on the right and

(continues)

Case Study 13-2 (continued)

1.06 on the left. His physician, still concerned about possible PAD, then consulted with the vascular surgery department, which subsequently ordered pre- and postexercise ABI testing.

Preexercise his resting ABIs were measured at 1.09 on the right and 1.03 on the left. He was able to exercise to maximal tolerated claudication pain of 7/10 on a typical PAD testing protocol (constant speed of 2.0 mph starting at 0% grade with increase of 3.5% grade every 3 min). The onset of bilateral thigh fatigue occurred at 3 minutes and 45 seconds and the onset of left buttock cramping by 5 minutes. His resting ECG was normal sinus rhythm, regular rate and rhythm, normal axis, and no acute ST changes at a rate of 78 bpm. His resting BP was 120/64 mm Hg, and he had no resting cardiovascular symptoms. His heart rate increased to 125 bpm at peak (77% of predicted maximal heart rate), BP increased normally to 164/62 mm Hg, and he only had a few isolated PVCs during the entirety of the test. There were some mild up sloping ST-segment depression noted in inferior and lateral leads that did not meet criteria for ischemia. He did not complain of anginal symptoms.

The postexercise recovery period was unremarkable for concerning cardiac findings. His ABIs postexercise was measured at 0.34 on the right and 0.29 on the left, suggesting moderate disease with absolute drop of 35 mm Hg on the right and 41 mm Hg on the left helping to confirm presence of PAD.

The vascular surgeon decided to go directly to lower extremity computed tomography angiography (CTA) to delineate the anatomy of disease so he could better discuss treatment and possible revascularization options. CTA revealed distal abdominal aorta disease that did not appear to be obstructive of less than 50%; however, of note was more proximal bilateral common iliac disease of about 65%–70% on the right and 80%–85% on the left. It appeared that some collateral circulation had developed.

After discussions with the patient, he was referred for exercise counseling and prescription in a supervised exercise program. The program was case management style with an initial consultation and testing (as needed) with individualized follow-up to include exercise sessions, test follow-ups, phone calls, and e-mails. The patient attended an initial exercise consultation and evaluation with a clinical exercise physiologist. After review of medical chart, medications, exercise history, current exercise, and goals, it was decided to undergo a session of interval walking on the treadmill because there was a recent monitored exercise test to screen for any concerning cardiovascular conditions. During the exercise test, he had onset of symptoms at stage 3 of a typical PAD protocol (2.0 mph with 3.5% grade), so it was decided to start with that particular exercise intensity. He performed three walking intervals at 2.0%–3.5% grade with the results shown in Box 13.2.

Following the exercise session, the patient and the clinical exercise physiologist collaborated on the exercise regimen. It was decided that the patient could perform the interval walking program for 3 days a week, and 1–2 days a week would include higher intensity exercise bike session and four strengthening exercises that could be done easily at the clubhouse near where the patient lived. Box 13.3 provides details of Mr. Case Study-PAD home exercise program.

A 4-week follow-up was conducted over the phone. The patient reported good adherence to the walking intervals, starting with 2 days a week on a treadmill and progressing to 30 minutes, with only 1:30 for each rest period, and a speed up to 3.0 mph with 2% grade. He stopped at about 8–9 minutes into each interval due to claudication pain. He was not as consistent with the exercise bike and reported about one session every other week. He had been

Box 13.2 Exercise Test Results for Mr. Case Study-PAD

Interval 1 — onset symptoms 3:23, total walking time of 5:30
  Rest — 2:00 to total symptom resolution
Interval 2 — onset of symptoms 3:50, total walking time of 6:15
  Rest — 1:50 to total resolution
Interval 3 — onset of symptoms 4:00, total walking time of 6:25
Total walking time of 18:10, resting time of 3:50 — total time of 22:00

Case Study 13-2 (continued)

Box 13.3 Mr. Case Study-PAD's Home Exercise Program

Walking

- 3 or more days a week
- Treadmill
- 2.0–2.5 mph with 0%–5% grade
- Adjust speed so will stop due to claudication pain between 5 and 10 min. Indication to stop was decided to be right before patient would start to limp to help avoid development of orthopedic issues.
- If the patient is able to walk longer than 10 min, then either increase speed by 0.2–0.3 mph or increase grade 1%–2% or a combination of the two.
- Minimum of 30 min total, including rest periods

Exercise Bike

- 1–2 days a week
- Will have to experiment a little. Ideally will want to adjust resistance at a comfortable cadence (revolutions per minute) where will only have to stop to rest once during a 20-min session.
- Keep any rest periods to 2 min or less.
- If he finds that has to stop more often due to claudication pain, then he should perform three higher intensity intervals at 5 or more min each.

Strength Training

- Chest press
- Lateral pull-down
- Seated leg press
- Body weight calf raise
- Adjust chest press, lateral pull-down and leg press to a weight where patient can perform 12–15 repetitions without struggling to complete, holding breath, or bearing down.
- 2–3 days a week

regular with strength training as prescribed and had not increased the weight with any of the exercises despite the exercises feeling easier. He also reported that his claudication pain was less intense overall and he was able to walk further and faster before the onset and stopping less often due to pain. There were no concerning cardiac symptoms at this time.

At 6 weeks from the initial exercise consultation, the patient called to report the onset of exertional chest tightness. These new symptoms only occurred during exercise and usually resolved within a minute or so. He felt his exercise sessions were the most exertion he performed during the week.

A note was sent to his PCP who requested a pharmacological stress testing due to fact that he may not be able to get an adequate heart rate and BP response with exercise. The patient was asked to refrain from exercise until his symptoms could be evaluated. He completed the test about 1 week later and tolerated the procedure well. The imaging report came back suggesting reversible ischemia in the left anterior coronary artery heart function. He was referred to cardiology, which scheduled an outpatient cardiac catheterization for the next week and advised him to continue with only normal daily activities.

Cardiac catheterization revealed an 85%–90% occlusion of his mid-distal left anterior descending coronary artery. Two overlapping drug-eluding stents were deployed with zero residual occlusion. His diuretic medication was discontinued and ACE dosage lowered with the addition of a β-blocker taken twice daily as well as clopidogrel and aspirin.

(continues)

Case Study 13-2 (continued)

A referral for outpatient cardiac rehabilitation was made, and he had his first visit 1 week later. The clinical exercise physiologist who was following him in the supervised exercise program contacted the cardiac rehabilitation program, and they agreed to work together with him. He continued his walking interval program with them for the next 3 months as well as a slightly expanded strengthening regimen.

By the end of the 3 months with cardiac rehabilitation, he was walking on a treadmill 3 days a week for 40 minutes at a speed of 3.6 mph with 5% grade with no stops. However, two to three times during the session, he would have to take the grade down to 0% due to onset of claudication symptoms. He was performing strength training 3 days a week, using eight different upper and lower body exercises for two sets of 12–15 repetitions. He discontinued use of the exercise bike at home during this time.

The patient denied any symptoms of claudication with normal daily activities and general walking. Only during higher intensity would his claudication appear, which would quickly resolve by simply lowering the grade on the treadmill.

Description, Prevalence, and Etiology

PAD is atherosclerosis of the systemic arteries outside of the heart and most often affects the lower extremities. Approximately 8.5 million Americans in the United States and 202 million people worldwide have PAD, which is associated with significant morbidity and mortality (14). The major risk factors for PAD include hypertension, smoking, diabetes, and chronic kidney disease (14).

PAD accelerates functional decline, leading to physical disability (12). Hamburg and Balady (10) cited multiple studies that both symptomatic and asymptomatic patients demonstrate significant declines in physical functioning. This suggests that there may be something in the progression of the disease that has an impact on the periphery and decreasing the ability of an individual to be active, or creates a situation where exercise tolerance gradually declines, and the person just attributes it to aging. It may be the case that the individual is purposely avoiding activities that produce the pain or discomfort, so he or she may appear asymptomatic. Either way, PAD contributes to functional decline and increased risk of adverse events (9).

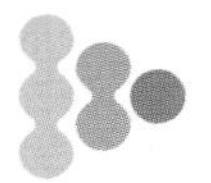

Preparticipation Health Screening, Medical History, and Physical Examination

Claudication originating from PAD is typically a cramping or tightness sensation in the lower extremities caused by reduced arterial blood flow that predictably waxes and wanes with exercise and rest. Claudication most often presents itself in one or both calves but can also occur in buttocks and thighs. This discomfort can also present itself in various other forms such as aching, muscular fatigue, weakness, burning, and numbness. Other signs and symptoms can include sores (ulcers) on the lower extremities that will not heal, color change in the legs, hair loss on the legs, and toenail color change.

When taking a symptom history, it is important to establish a pattern of exertional symptoms that do not have another potential cause that could be neuromuscular or musculoskeletal in origin. These can include spinal canal stenosis, peripheral neuropathy, peripheral nerve pain, herniated disc, osteoarthritis of the hip or knee, venous claudication, Baker cyst, chronic compartment syndrome, muscle spasms, cramps, or restless leg syndrome (1). Symptoms can vary greatly depending on the location, number and length of the occlusions, prior exercise training history, current exercise levels, and comorbidities. Box 13.4 outlines tips for conducting a patient history.

Box 13.4 Suggestions for Conducting a Patient History of Peripheral Artery Disease

It is very important to make the most of your initial symptom interview; some tips to remember are the following:

- Remember that you will likely have limited visits and ability to interact personally.
- Discuss other potential symptoms and limitations to the ability to walk and exercise.
- Make sure you take your time to understand what is most limiting and take into consideration that the claudication may not really be the most limiting factor.
- Conducting a detailed, thorough history will help you build a better exercise prescription but also gain their trust and increase the likelihood of the patient listening and adhering to your advice.

In a paper by Gardner et al. (8), they suggest that despite our best efforts during an interview, and using a well-established questionnaire such as the San Diego Claudication Questionnaire, providers still miss identifying claudication from PAD. Some of the suggested reasons included varying interpretations of pain, different walking speeds accounting for differences in definition of onset of pain, participants adjusting walking speeds and habits to accommodate pain over time, and those who unknowingly slow down walking to alleviate pain.

McDermott et al. (13) suggest that older age, diabetes, and being male may increase the likelihood of absence of exertional leg symptoms. With older age, a lack of typical symptoms could be related to a decline in daily activity and a lack of activity intense enough to produce symptoms. Diabetic neuropathy was also discussed as having role in altering the sensation of claudication symptoms (atypical), making it more difficult to diagnose from history alone.

After claudication due to PAD is suspected, there are multiple evaluations that may be performed. The ABI test can be performed in a primary care office if there are appropriate equipment and trained personnel. It is simply a measurement of ankle versus brachial pressures. Ideally, the ratio between the readings should be around 1.0. Box 13.5 describes the ABI evaluation criteria. A noninvasive vascular assessment is sometimes a first-line evaluation. A combination of various pressures in the lower extremity (thigh, calf, ankle, toes) are compared with brachial pressures as well as ultrasound pictures of the lower vasculature. This is helpful in detecting location and possible severity of arterial occlusions and ultimately how much blood flow is reaching the foot.

A CTA may be performed if a physician is considering possible intervention such as balloon angioplasty, stenting, or bypass surgery. This is useful in mapping the precise location of occlusions and if interventions are likely to succeed. An invasive angiogram is usually done if there is an intention to intervene on a specific occlusion, or if CTA is inconclusive or not available.

Box 13.5 Resting Ankle/Brachial Systolic Pressure Index Values

≥1.30: Noncompressible
1.0–1.29: Normal
0.91–0.99: Borderline (equivocal)
0.41–0.90: Mild-to-moderate disease
≤0.40: Severe disease

Case Study 13-2 Quiz:

Preparticipation Health Screening, Medical History, and Physical Examination

1. What made this person's symptoms of claudication atypical?
2. Which risk factor was most likely the reason for developing PAD in this individual?

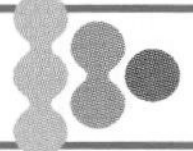

Exercise Testing Considerations

Exercise testing can be performed in patients with PAD to determine functional capacity, to assess exercise limitations, to determine time to onset of claudication pain, to determine total walking time, and to diagnose the presence of cardiovascular disease (11).

It is well known that individuals with PAD are high risk for developing significant CAD. The choice to screen for possible significant CAD has to be considered carefully by the clinical exercise physiologist. If the patient already has known CAD and has been followed closely by a cardiologist and is symptoms-free, then exercise testing may be performed to assist in the development of an exercise prescription. The clinical exercise physiologist should consider a variety of issues, however, including ability of the patient to attain an adequate double-product, alternative modalities for testing and referral for pharmacological test. When performing exercise testing, the *ACSM's Exercise Management for Persons with Chronic Diseases and Disabilities* (2) suggests the following:

1. Obtain reliable measures of claudication pain times.
2. Obtain reliable measures of ankle pressure following exercise (exercise Postexercise Ankle/Brachial Systolic Pressure Index).
3. Assess whether CAD is present.
4. Obtain information for exercise prescription.

Additionally, when testing, consider selecting a protocol that utilizes a constant speed (2 mph) and an increase in grade of 2% every 2 minutes, starting with an initial grade of 0%. Variations may include using a protocol that is similar with a constant speed (1.5, 2.0, or 2.5 mph) that starts at 0% grade and increases 3.5% every 2–3 minutes. Selections of speed and stage time can be chosen depending on pretest interviews and observations of normal walking speed of the patient as he or she is escorted to the testing lab.

Box 13.6 Postexercise Ankle/Brachial Systolic Pressure Index

No Change or Increase — Within Normal Limits

>0.5: Mild disease
>0.2: Moderate disease
<0.2: Severe disease

Change in Ankle Systolic Pressure

Increase or <20 mm Hg drop: Normal
>20 mm Hg drop: Abnormal

There are occasions when an exercise ABI test is needed. This test should be conducted with a treadmill and includes taking resting ABIs prior to exercise and then immediately postexercise taking another set of ABIs to compare with the resting values. Box 13.6 shows a set of normal and abnormal postexercise values to be considered.

Case Study 13-2 Quiz:

Exercise Testing Considerations

3. Why do you think that his CAD was not detected on the initial exercise test?
4. What are some alternative types of testing that may have better demonstrated that the patient had significant CAD?
5. Elaborate on why the physician still had concerns for PAD despite somewhat atypical leg symptoms and completely normal resting ABIs.

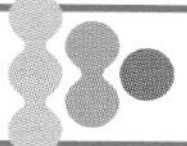

Exercise Prescription and Progression Considerations

Frequency, intensity, time, and type (FITT) recommendations for exercise prescription and progression for individuals with PAD are presented in the FITT table (Table 13.6) (3). An important consideration when designing an exercise program for patients with PAD is the use of weight-bearing exercise. As mentioned previously, the hallmark symptom of PAD is claudication, which often presents only with walking. Non–weight-bearing exercises can have many beneficial effects for patients with PAD but show less improvement in walking distance or less of a decrease in symptoms with walking. Evidence from multiple randomized controlled trials demonstrates that repeated bouts of walking, either on a treadmill or ambulating freely, to the point of claudication has a greater impact on pain-free walking distance than alternative modes of exercise (17).

Other evidence suggests higher intensity arm ergometry done in shorter intervals compares favorably with improvements in maximal walking distance with treadmill exercise (19,20,22). Still, others have shown that higher intensity cycle training has improved walking distance and claudication symptoms (18,21). It is suggested that the lack of claudication pain during arm and cycle ergometry allows individuals with PAD to exercise at much higher intensities, thus potentially gaining greater contributions from systemic cardiovascular improvements. Arm and cycle ergometry, in conjunction with walking, can be part of a well-rounded program for individuals with PAD to lower the risk of CAD in this population.

Exercise that elicits claudication should take place at least 3 days a week, but more days a week are not necessarily better. This is possibly because adherence rates to programs that required significant pain to perform can have a negative effect on overall adherence and patients may not work as hard if they know they will have to endure significant pain most, if not all, days of the week (7). To optimize adherence to PAD training protocols, it is recommended that patients begin an exercise routine under supervision. Supervised exercise programs appear to increase functional ability to a greater extent than unsupervised training (5). This increase may be related to greater patient adherence and greater intensity of exercise with supervision than during independent walking.

Individuals with PAD are also encouraged to include resistance and flexibility exercises for total body **muscular strength** and conditioning. Strength training and flexibility guidelines for individuals with PAD, as seen in FITT table (see Table 13.6), are similar to the guidelines for the general population (also see Chapter 9).

FITT

TABLE 13.6 FITT RECOMMENDATIONS FOR INDIVIDUALS WITH LOWER EXTREMITY, SYMPTOMATIC PERIPHERAL ARTERY DISEASE AND FOR INDIVIDUALS WITH CARDIOVASCULAR DISEASE PARTICIPATING IN OUTPATIENT CARDIAC REHABILITATION

ACSM FITT Principle of the ExR_x

Chronic Medical Condition	Frequency (How often?)	Intensity (How hard?)	Time	Type (What kind?) Primary	Resistance	Flexibility	Special Considerations
Healthy Adult	≥5 d · wk^{-1} of moderate exercise, or ≥3 d · wk^{-1} of vigorous exercise, or a combination of moderate and vigorous exercise on ≥3–5 d · wk^{-1} is recommended.	Moderate to vigorous. Light-to-moderate intensity exercise may be beneficial in deconditioned individuals.	If moderate intensity: ≥30 min · d^{-1} to total 150 min · wk^{-1}. If vigorous intensity: ≥20 min · d^{-1} to total 75 min · wk^{-1}.	Regular, purposeful exercise that involves major muscle groups and is continuous and rhythmic in nature is recommended.	2–3 d · wk^{-1} (nonconsecutive)	2–3 d · wk^{-1}; static stretch 10–30 s; 2–4 repetitions of each exercise	Sedentary behaviors can have adverse health effects, even among those who regularly exercise. Adding short physical activity breaks throughout the day may be considered as a part of the exercise.
Valvular Heart Disease	Minimally 3 d · wk^{-1}, preferably 5 d · wk^{-1}	With an exercise test, use 40%–80% of exercise capacity using HRR, $\dot{V}O_2R$, or $\dot{V}O_{2peak}$. Without a test, use seated or standing HR_{rest} +20 to +30 bpm or an RPE of 12–16 on a 6–20 scale.	20–60 min	Arm ergometer Upper and lower extremity ergometer, upright and recumbent cycles, recumbent stepper, elliptical, stair climber, treadmill	2–3 d · wk^{-1} (nonconsecutive) 10–15 repetitions without significant fatigue, RPE 11–13 or 40%–60% of a 1-RM. 1–3 sets: 8–10 different exercises of major muscle groups. Select equipment that is both safe and comfortable.	2–3 d · wk^{-1} with daily being most effective Stretch to the point of feeling tightness or slight discomfort. 15 s hold for static stretching. >4 repetitions of each exercise. Static, dynamic, and/or PNF stretching of the major joints of the limbs and lower back.	The specific symptoms of valvular heart disease as well as modification to exercise prescription will vary depending on which valve is involved and the degree of impairment. These patients may also follow guidelines for healthy adults.
Peripheral Artery Disease	3–5 d · wk^{-1}	Moderate intensity (*i.e.*, 40%–59% $\dot{V}O_2R$) to the point of moderate pain (*i.e.*, 4 out of 5 on the claudication pain scale)	30–45 min · d^{-1} (excluding rest periods) for up to 12 weeks. May progress to 60 min · d^{-1}.	Weight bearing (*i.e.*, free or treadmill walking)	60%–80% 1-RM 3 sets of 8–12 repetitions; 6–8 exercises targeting major muscle groups	≥2–3 d · wk^{-1} with daily being most effective Stretch to the point of tightness or slight discomfort 10–30 s hold for static stretching; 2–4 repetitions of each exercise Static, dynamic, and or PNF stretching	An important consideration is the use of weight-bearing exercise that elicit pain.

ExR_x, exercise prescription; HRR, heart rate reserve; $\dot{V}O_2R$, oxygen uptake reserve; $\dot{V}O_{2peak}$, peak oxygen uptake; HR_{rest}, resting heart rate; RPE, rating of perceived exertion; PNF, proprioceptive neuromuscular facilitation.

Based on the FITT Recommendations present in *ACSM's Guidelines for Exercise Testing and Prescription*. 10th ed. Philadelphia (PA): Wolters Kluwer; 2018. 480 p.

Case Study 13-2 Quiz:

Prescription and Progression Considerations

6. After increasing volume and intensity of exercise, why did his symptoms of significant CAD finally appear?
7. What alternative exercise modes may also be effective for this individual and why?

SUMMARY

This chapter presents relevant information regarding exercise testing and prescription and progression recommendations for individuals with VHD and for individuals with PAD. It should be noted that VHD as well as PAD often exist with comorbidities such as diabetes (see Chapter 10), chronic obstructive pulmonary disease (see Chapter 9), and aging (see Chapter 7), so the clinician working with these populations should be familiar with the exercise testing, prescription, and progressions for these special populations. The following points should be considered when working with these populations:

- The specific symptoms of VHD as well as modification to exercise prescription will vary depending on which valve is involved and the degree of impairment.
- Exercise prescription and progression guidelines for patients with VHD would be the same as the general population.
- Patients on anticoagulation therapy such as warfarin for either a mechanical valve or for atrial fibrillation should avoid contact sports or activities due to the risk of bleeding.
- In terms of PAD, atherosclerosis of the peripheral arteries contributes to significant functional decline and increased risk of adverse events.
- Claudication, the most common symptom of PAD, most often presents itself in one or both calves but can also occur in buttocks and thighs. This discomfort can also present itself in various other forms such as aching, muscular fatigue, weakness, burning, and numbness.
- An important consideration for exercise prescription is the use of weight-bearing exercises that elicits pain.

REFERENCES

1. American Association of Cardiovascular and Pulmonary Rehabilitation/Vascular Disease Foundation. *PAD Toolkit — PAD Coalition*; 2010. Available from: www.vdf.org or www.aacvpr.org
2. American College of Sports Medicine. *ACSM's Exercise Management for Persons With Chronic Diseases and Disabilities*. 4th ed. Champaign (IL): Human Kinetics; 2016. 416 p.
3. American College of Sports Medicine. *ACSM's Guidelines for Exercise Testing and Prescription*. 10th ed. Philadelphia (PA): Wolters Kluwer; 2018. 480 p.
4. Baliga RR, Eagle KA. *Practical Cardiology: Evaluation and Treatment of Common Cardiovascular Disorders*. 2nd ed. Philadelphia (PA): Lippincott Williams & Wilkins; 2008. 720 p.
5. Bendermacher BL, Willigendael EM, Teijink JA, Prins MH. Supervised exercise therapy versus non-supervised exercise therapy for intermittent claudication. *Cochrane Database Syst Rev*. 2006;(2):CD005263.
6. Bonow RO, Cheitlin MD, Crawford MH, Douglas PS. Task force 3: valvular heart disease. *J Am Coll Cardiol*. 2005;45(8):1334–40.
7. Bulmer AC, Coombes JS. Optimising exercise training in peripheral arterial disease. *Sports Med*. 2004;34(14):983–1003.
8. Gardner AW, Montgomery PS, Afaq A. Exercise performance in patients with peripheral arterial disease who have different types of exertional leg pain. *J Vasc Surg*. 2007;46:79–86.

9. Gardner AW, Montgomery PS, Parker DE. Physical activity is a predictor of all-cause mortality in patients with intermittent claudication. *J Vasc Surg.* 2008;47:117–22.
10. Hamburg NM, Balady GJ. Exercise rehabilitation in peripheral artery disease: functional impact and mechanisms of benefits. *Circulation.* 2011;123:87–97.
11. Hirsch AT, Haskal ZJ, Hertzer NR, et al. ACC/AHA 2005 practice guidelines for the management of patients with peripheral arterial disease (lower extremity, renal, mesenteric, and abdominal aortic): a collaborative report from the American Association for Vascular Surgery/Society for Vascular Surgery, Society for Cardiovascular Angiography and Interventions, Society for Vascular Medicine and Biology, Society of Interventional Radiology, and the ACC/AHA Task Force on Practice Guidelines (Writing Committee to Develop Guidelines for the Management of Patients with Peripheral Arterial Disease): endorsed by the American Association of Cardiovascular and Pulmonary Rehabilitation; National Heart, Lung, and Blood Institute; Society for Vascular Nursing; TransAtlantic Inter-Society Consensus; and Vascular Disease Foundation. *Circulation.* 2006;113(11):e463–654.
12. McDermott MM, Liu K, Greenland P, et al. Functional decline in peripheral arterial disease: associations with the ankle brachial index and leg symptoms. *JAMA.* 2004;292:453–61.
13. McDermott MM, Mehta S, Greenland P. Exertional leg symptoms other than intermittent claudication are common in peripheral arterial disease. *Arch Intern Med.* 1999;159:387–92.
14. Mozaffarian D, Benjamin EJ, Go AS, et al. Heart disease and stroke statistics — 2015 update: a report from the American Heart Association. *Circulation.* 2015;131:e29–322.
15. Nishimura RA, Otto CM, Bonow RO, et al. 2014 AHA/ACC guideline for the management of patients with valvular heart disease: a report of the American College of Cardiology/American Heart Association Task Force on Practice Guidelines. *J Am Coll Cardiol.* 2014;63(22):2438–88.
16. Nkomo VT, Gardin JM, Skelton TN, et al. Burden of valvular heart disease: a population-based study. *Lancet.* 2006;368:1005–11.
17. Parmenter BJ, Raymond J, Dinnen P, Singh MA. A systematic review of randomized controlled trials: walking versus alternative exercise prescription as treatment for intermittent claudication. *Atherosclerosis.* 2011;218(1):1–12.
18. Sanderson B, Askew C, Stewart I, Walker P, Gibbs H, Green S. Short-term effects of cycle and treadmill training on exercise tolerance in peripheral arterial disease. *J Vasc Surg.* 2006;44:119–27.
19. Tew G, Nawaz S, Zwierska I, Saxton J. Limb-specific and cross-transfer effects of arm-crank exercise training in patients with symptomatic peripheral artery disease. *Clin Sci.* 2009;117:405–13.
20. Treat-Jacobson D, Bronas UG, Leon AS. Efficacy of arm-ergometry versus treadmill exercise training to improve walking distance in patients with claudication. *Vasc Med.* 2009;14(3):203–13.
21. Tuner SL, Easton C, Wilson J, et al. Cardiopulmonary responses to treadmill and cycle ergometry exercise in patients with peripheral vascular disease. *J Vasc Surg.* 2008;47:123–30.
22. Walker RD, Nawaz S, Wilkinson CH, Saxton JM, Pockley AG, Wood RF. Influence of upper- and lower-limb exercise training on cardiovascular function and walking distances in patients with intermittent claudication. *J Vasc Surg.* 2000;31:662–9.

CHAPTER 14

Special Considerations for Type 1 and Type 2 Diabetes Mellitus

INTRODUCTION

Diabetes mellitus is characterized by abnormal glucose metabolism resulting from defects in insulin release, action, or both (5). According to the Centers for Disease Control and Prevention (CDC) (17), 29 million people or 9.3% of the U.S. population have diabetes, with 28% of those undiagnosed. This complex metabolic disease requires rigorous self-management combined with an appropriate balance of nutritional intake, medication(s), and regular exercise for blood glucose control. This chapter focuses on the most common forms of diabetes: Type 1 diabetes (T1D) and Type 2 diabetes (T2D). Safe and effective exercise recommendations are presented to assist in diabetes management and the associated diabetes-related health complications.

Case Study 14-1

Mrs. Case Study-DM

Mrs. Case Study-DM, a 52-year-old woman diagnosed with T2D 7 years earlier, was having trouble controlling her weight and blood pressure (BP). She is 1.63 m (64 in) tall and weighs 86 kg (190 lb), classifying her as obese based on a **body mass index** of 33 kg · m^{-2}. Her resting heart rate is 85 bpm, and her resting BP is 138/86 mm Hg (medicated). Her lab work showed her to be in suboptimal control of her diabetes, with a fasting plasma glucose of 158 mg · dL^{-1} and a glycolated hemoglobin (HbA1C) of 7.2% (indicating an average blood glucose level of around 160 mg · dL^{-1} over the prior 2–3 months). Her lipid profile revealed a total cholesterol of 190 mg · dL^{-1}, high-density lipoprotein cholesterol (HDL-C) at 38 mg · dL^{-1} with elevated low-density lipoprotein cholesterol (LDL-C) and fasting triglycerides (132 mg · dL^{-1} and 200 mg · dL^{-1}, respectively). She reported testing her blood glucose fairly regularly (*i.e.*, at least once a day).

Her medications included DiaBeta (sulfonylurea) and an antihypertensive agent. She was not currently participating in any structured exercise and had not regularly participated in the past. She stated that she was motivated to be more active mainly because of her physician's recommendation and her unhappiness with her weight gain. She received medical clearance from her doctor to start increasing her activity level with no specific restrictions. Her physician referred her to a certified fitness professional to discuss safe and appropriate ways to be more physically active and improve her overall health and blood glucose management.

The fitness professional working with Mrs. Case Study-DM interviewed her to discuss her personal beliefs, past experiences, preferences, and concerns regarding exercise. The fitness professional reminded Mrs. Case Study-DM of the importance of monitoring her blood glucose before and after exercise and carrying a form of carbohydrate during activity. She was also told that in her case, it would be best to start with exercise at a low intensity and progress slowly with structured activities to avoid the development of activity-related injuries, exercise nonadherence, or lack of motivation, with a goal of increasing her amount of exercise gradually over a period of weeks to months.

The initial focus of her exercise program was on lifestyle exercise using low- to moderate-intensity types of exercise, particularly focusing on ones that she enjoys doing. Because Mrs. Case Study-DM was sedentary, the fitness professional encouraged inclusion of short activity bouts that could be incorporated into her daily routine. She was advised to start with a walking program consisting of 5–10 minutes of slow walking several times each day, 5–6 days a week. The exercise duration was to be gradually increased to 10 minutes per session, 3 times a day, and walking speed increased slowly as tolerated. Mrs. Case Study-DM was encouraged to engage in more daily movement and to use strategies to break up her sedentary time whenever possible. Her long-term exercise goals focused on progressively increasing amounts and frequency of activity to minimum recommended levels (150 min of moderate-to-vigorous exercise spread throughout the week, with no more than 24 h of inactivity between exercise sessions) (3).

In addition to helping Mrs. Case Study-DM identify activities that she might be interested in trying to incorporate into her daily lifestyle, the fitness professional suggested that she try using a simple pedometer (step counter) to obtain feedback about her activity levels, with a goal of increasing her number of baseline steps over a period of weeks to months. Behavior change strategies appropriate for the contemplation and preparation stages were used, including offering information on the benefits of exercise, discussing the pros and cons of increasing exercise, helping Mrs. Case Study-DM identify and build a support system, and identifying barriers to exercise and brainstorming possible solutions. Self-efficacy was enhanced by helping her set goals that were likely to be reached, such as making a list of five ways to be more active throughout the day. Finally, Mrs. Case Study-DM was encouraged to ask questions and come up with ideas for becoming more active to promote autonomy and build confidence to promote adherence to her new fitness-promoting lifestyle choices.

Description, Prevalence, and Etiology

T2D accounts for 90% of all diabetes, with T1D making up the remaining 5%–10% (5). Although T1D is one of the most common chronic diseases diagnosed in children, it also occurs in adults, usually with a slower onset than typically seen in youth (5). Likewise, although T2D was formerly seen mostly among **older adults**, the diagnosis in youth has risen dramatically over the past two decades (9). The burden of diabetes disproportionately affects minorities. It is now estimated that 1 in 3 Americans born in 2000 or later will develop diabetes during their lifetimes, with rates closer to 50% in high-risk, ethnic populations (57,58).

Diabetes-related complications exacerbate morbidity and increase the likelihood of physical limitation or disability (34). Hyperglycemia for an extended period of time is linked with chronic diabetes-related complications that worsen macrovascular, microvascular, and neural processes. Because of daily fluctuations in blood glucose occurring in diabetes, therapeutic interventions focus on blood glucose control, management of heart disease risk factors, and prevention of diabetes-related complications (30,32).

The diagnosis of diabetes is based on established criteria (5). Table 14.1 provides the major characteristics of T1D and T2D. Effective management involves use of self-monitoring of blood

Table 14.1 Major Characteristics of Type 1 and Type 2 Diabetes

Factor	Type 1	Type 2
Age at onset	More often early in life but may occur at any age	Usually older than age 30 yr but may occur at any age
Type of onset	Rapid, with short duration of symptoms in children; slower progression when onset occurs during adulthood	Slow progression (*e.g.*, years)
Genetic susceptibility	HLA-related DR3 and DR4, ICAs, IAAs; limited family history	Frequent genetic background; not HLA-related
Environmental factors	Virus, toxins, autoimmune stimulation	Obesity, poor nutrition, physical inactivity, POP exposure
ICA	Present at onset	Usually not observed
Endogenous insulin	Minimal or absent	Stimulated response either adequate with delayed secretion or reduced but not absent; insulin resistance present
Nutritional status	Thin or overweight; catabolic state (recent weight loss)	Obese, overweight, or normal; little or no recent weight loss
Symptoms	Thirst, polyuria, polyphagia, fatigue	Mild or frequently none; acanthosis nigricans; PCOS in females
Ketosis	Common at onset or during insulin deficiency	Unusual (resistant to ketosis except during infection or stress)
Control of diabetes	Often difficult, with wide glucose fluctuation	Variable; helped by dietary adherence, weight loss, exercise
Dietary management	Essential but must be balanced with insulin dosage	Essential; may suffice for glycemic control
Insulin	Required for all	Used by ~40%
Oral or injected antihyperglycemic medications	Usually minimally effective (unless insulin resistant as well)	Effective

HLA, human leukocyte antigen; DR, D-related antigen; ICA, islet cell antibody; IAA, insulin autoantibodies; POP, persistent organic pollutants; PCOS, polycystic ovary syndrome.

glucose, use of appropriate medications to regulate blood glucose levels, regular participation in **physical activity** (PA)/**exercise**, and body weight management as well as good dietary habits (5,68). Exercise interventions for individuals with diabetes should ideally involve a multidisciplinary team of specialists to facilitate individual education and lifestyle changes to manage this disease. Self-management skills are essential to success, and diabetes education is an important tool to improve glycemic control (56).

Precise hormonal and metabolic events that normally regulate glucose homeostasis are frequently disrupted in diabetes because of defects in insulin release, action, or both (5). Glucose control requires near-normal balance between hepatic glucose production and peripheral glucose uptake, combined with effective insulin responses (76). With diabetes, a reduced ability to precisely match glucose production and utilization results in daily glucose fluctuations and requires adjustments in dosages of exogenous insulin and/or antihyperglycemic medications (Table 14.2). These adjustments should be combined with adequate changes in dietary intake, particularly when anticipating exercise (85).

After diagnosis, clinical emphasis is placed on self-monitoring of blood glucose, which benefits glycemic control regardless of the type of diabetes. Adjustments to insulin dose, oral medications, and/or carbohydrate intake can be fine-tuned using the detailed information provided by continuous glucose monitoring (62).

Concomitant lifestyle improvements (*i.e.*, dietary changes and exercise) assist in the control of blood glucose levels and reduce the risk of acute and long-term diabetes-related complications (6).

Table 14.2 Risk of Hypoglycemia with Use of Diabetes Medications

No or Minimal Risk		Higher Risk
Acarbose:	Liraglutide:	Glimepiride:
Precose®	Victoza®	Amaryl®
Metformin and combinations with metformin:	Alogliptin:	Glipizide and combinations with glipizide:
	Nesina/Galvus	Glucotrol®, Glucotrol XL®
Glucophage®	Linagliptin:	MetaGlip (glipizide/metformin)
Avandamet® (metformin/rosiglitizone)	Tradjenta	Glyburide and combinations with glyburide:
Miglitol:	Linagliptin and empagliflozin:	DiaBeta
Glyset®	Glyxambi	Glynase® PresTab®
Pioglitazone:	Sitagliptin:	Micronase®
Actos®	Januvia®	Glucovance® (glyburide/metformin)
Rosiglitizone:	Saxagliptin:	Nateglinide:
Avandia®	Onglyza®	Starlix®
Bromocriptine:	Pramlintide:	Repaglinide:
Cycloset®	Symlin®	Prandin®
Albiglutide:	Canagliflozin:	Insulin:
Tanzeum	Invokana®	All types and delivery methods
Dulaglutide:	Dapagliflozin:	
Trulicity	Farxiga®	
Exenatide:	Empagliflozin:	
Byetta® (daily)	Jardiance	
Bydureon™ (weekly)		

Well-known brand names are listed following the generic names. Always consider new diabetes medications that may not be listed and medications prescribed for diabetes complications or other conditions.

Reprinted with permission from Colberg S. Chapter 17: Exercise prescription. In: Mensing C, editor. *The Art & Science of Diabetes Self-Management Education Desk Reference*. 4th ed. Chicago (IL): American Association of Diabetes Educators; 2017. p. 888.

Overall glycemic control is assessed by measuring HbA1C, which reflects a time-averaged blood glucose concentration over the previous 2–3 months. The recommended HbA1C goal is <7.0% (7). Using the estimated average glucose conversion, this goal equates to <154 mg · dL^{-1} (or 8.6 mmol · L^{-1}). HbA1C levels should ideally be assessed every 3–4 months (7).

Regular exercise facilitates improved blood glucose control in T2D (39,52,55,64,74). Although regular exercise does not uniformly provide glycemic management in those with T1D unless appropriate regimen changes are made, exercise is still considered a safe and effective adjunct therapy for the management of T1D (79). Exercise, in combination with dietary improvements and weight loss, has been demonstrated to favorably modify lipids and lipoproteins, thereby lowering cardiovascular disease (CVD) risk in diabetes (64). Also, reductions in BP have been demonstrated through exercise and weight loss and may be partially explained by improved insulin sensitivity and loss of visceral fat (67). Glucose control is improved through exercise in individuals with T2D. A lower HbA1C generally reduces the risk for diabetes-related complications, including CVD (14,66,86). Table 14.3 summarizes benefits of chronic exercise for individuals with T1D and T2D.

Table 14.3 Effects of Exercise in Diabetes

Parameter	Type 1	Type 2
Cardiovascular		
Aerobic capacity or fitness level	↑	↑/↔
Resting pulse rate and rate–pressure product	↓	↓
Resting systolic BP (in mild-to-moderate hypertension)	↓	↓
HR at submaximal loads (aerobic only)	↓	↓
Lipid and lipoprotein alterations		
HDL-C	↑	↑
LDL-C	↓/↔	↓/↔
VLDL-C	↓	↓
Total cholesterol	↔	↔
Cardiovascular risk ratio (total cholesterol/HDL)	↓	↓
Anthropometric measures		
Body mass (aerobic exercise in particular)	↓/↔	↓
Fat mass (including visceral fat)	↓	↓
Fat-free mass (resistance exercise mainly)	↑	↑/↔
Metabolic parameters		
Insulin sensitivity and glucose/fat metabolism	↑	↑
HbA1C (overall glycemic control)	↓/↔	↓
Postprandial thermogenesis or thermic effect of food	↑	↑
Presumed psychological outcomes		
Self-concept and self-esteem	↑	↑
Depression and anxiety	↓	↓
Stress response to psychological stimuli	↑	↑

HR, heart rate; VLDL-C, very low density lipoprotein cholesterol; ↑, increase; ↓, decrease; ↔, no change.

Acutely uncontrolled diabetes is a relative contraindication to exercise participation. Self-monitoring of blood glucose before and after exercise is essential, especially in insulin users, to allow individuals to make appropriate adjustments in insulin or other medications and food intake (29,68). Although light-intensity exercise will expend calories and assist with weight maintenance, it will likely lower blood glucose levels less than moderate-intensity workouts. Conversely, vigorous exercise may result in transient hyperglycemia because glucose production tends to increase more than glucose use (65,71). Thus, two common risks associated with exercise in individuals with diabetes are hypoglycemia and hyperglycemia; however, practical precautions can be taken to reduce the risk or avoid their onset.

Case Study 14-1 Quiz:

Description, Prevalence, and Etiology

1. What health benefits is Mrs. Case Study-DM likely to experience from becoming and staying regularly physically active? Are the benefits different for people with T2D versus T1D?

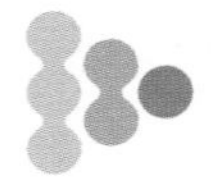

Preparticipation Health Screening, Medical History, and Physical Examination

The *ACSM's Guidelines for Exercise Testing and Prescription* (*GETP*) (3) evidence-based model for **preparticipation health screening** for those with T1D and T2D is based, in part, on the individual's current level of exercise. **Medical clearance** rather than medical exams/graded exercise testing is only recommended, and the decision to include these tests is left to the health care provider. For exercise more vigorous than brisk walking or exceeding the demands of everyday living, sedentary and older individuals with diabetes may benefit from being more thoroughly assessed for conditions that are associated with a higher risk of CVD (including uncontrolled hypertension), contraindications to exercise, or diabetes-related factors that may predispose them to injury (*e.g.*, autonomic neuropathy, peripheral neuropathy, a history of foot lesions, and untreated proliferative retinopathy) (6,22). Preexercise assessments may include a symptom-limited exercise test depending on the age of the person, diabetes duration, and the presence of additional CVD risk factors (22).

The best protocol for screening asymptomatic individuals with diabetes for coronary artery disease remains unclear, and routine screening is not recommended (6). Although a symptom-limited exercise test may be done, it may not be necessary in young individuals with diabetes and those with a low risk of CVD. Specific indications for a symptom-limited exercise test are shown in Box 14.1. Following these criteria will avoid automatic inclusion of lower risk individuals with diabetes and advise such testing primarily for previously sedentary individuals who plan to engage in exercise more intense than normally undertaken during **activities of daily living**. Although a symptom-limited exercise test may be used for **exercise prescription** and risk stratification, its comprehensive use to diagnose myocardial ischemia in asymptomatic individuals is not recommended. A recent meta-analysis suggested that systematic detection of silent ischemia in high-risk, asymptomatic patients with diabetes is unlikely to provide any major benefit in individuals whose cardiovascular risk is controlled by an optimal medical treatment (51).

Box 14.1 Indications for Symptom-Limited Exercise Testing Prior to Vigorous Exercise Participation

Individuals with diabetes and at least one of the following:

- Age >35 years
- T1D for >10-year duration or T2D for >15-year duration
- Any additional cardiovascular risk factor (see *GETP*, Table 3.1)
- Microvascular disease evidenced by proliferative retinopathy or nephropathy including microalbuminuria
- Autonomic dysfunction

Any of the following, regardless of age:

- Diagnosed cardiovascular disease including prior coronary and peripheral vascular atherosclerotic disease
- New or changing symptoms suggestive of cardiovascular disease as detected by Physical Activity Readiness Questionnaire for Everyone (PAR-Q+)
- End-stage renal disease
- Patients with symptomatic or diagnosed pulmonary disease

Brown RJ, Wijewickrama RC, Harlan DM, Rother KI. Uncoupling intensive insulin therapy from weight gain and hypoglycemia in Type 1 diabetes. *Diabetes Technol Ther.* 2001;13:457–60; and Brown SJ, Handsaker JC, Bowling FL, Boulton AJ, Reeves ND. Diabetic peripheral neuropathy compromises balance during daily activities. *Diabetes Care.* 2015;38:1116–22.

Case Study 14-1 Quiz:

Preparticipation Health Screening, Medical Screening, and Physical Examination

2. Mrs. Case Study-DM obtained medical clearance from her doctor prior to starting an exercise program. What are recommendations for preparticipation screening of Mrs. Case Study-DM prior to the initiation of her exercise program?

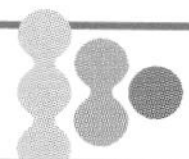

Exercise Prescription and Progression Considerations

In general, **aerobic** exercise programming for individuals without complications follows the FITT guidelines (frequency, intensity, time [duration], and type or mode of activities) presented in Table 14.4. Appropriate exercise prescription is critical for preventing compliance issues related to the development of overuse injuries and motivational factors, particularly in people with diabetes who are more prone overall to developing tendinopathy (61).

For individuals with T1D, exercise recommendations are closely aligned with those for apparently healthy persons (31,36), whereas recommendations for individuals with T2D are more closely aligned with guidelines for individuals with obesity, hypertension, and sedentary lifestyles and who are older (59). Most individuals with T2D are obese (5) and have low **cardiorespiratory fitness** levels (12,21,69).

FITT

TABLE 14.4 FITT RECOMMENDATIONS FOR INDIVIDUALS WITH TYPE 1 AND TYPE 2 DIABETES

ACSM FITT Principle of the ExR_x

Chronic Medical Condition	Frequency (How often?)	Intensity (How hard?)	Time	Type (What kind?) Primary	Resistance	Flexibility	Special Considerations
Healthy Adult	≥5 d · wk^{-1} of moderate exercise, or ≥3 d · wk^{-1} of vigorous exercise, or a combination of moderate and vigorous exercise on ≥3–5 d · wk^{-1} is recommended.	Moderate to vigorous. Light-to-moderate intensity exercise may be beneficial in deconditioned individuals.	If moderate intensity: ≥30 min · d^{-1} to total 150 min · wk^{-1}. If vigorous intensity: ≥20 min · d^{-1} to total 75 min · wk^{-1}.	Regular, purposeful exercise that involves major muscle groups and is continuous and rhythmic in nature is recommended.	2–3 d · wk^{-1} (nonconsecutive)	2–3 d · wk^{-1}; static stretch 10–30 s; 2–4 repetitions of each exercise	Sedentary behaviors can have adverse health effects, even among those who regularly exercise. Adding short physical activity breaks throughout the day may be considered as a part of the exercise.
T1D	3 d vigorous or 5 d moderate Greater regularity may benefit diabetic management.	Moderate (40%–59% $\dot{V}O_2R$ or 11–12 RPE) to vigorous (60%–89% $\dot{V}O_2R$ or 14–17 RPE)	At least 150 min · wk^{-1} of moderate intensity, 60 min · wk^{-1} at vigorous intensity, or a combination	Walk, jog, cycle, row, swim, aquatic activities, seated exercises, team sports	2–3 d · wk^{-1} at 60%–80% 1-RM (lower intensity to start) RPE ~11–15 (6–20 scale) 8–12 repetitions/exercise (10–15 to start) 1–3 sets per exercise All major muscle groups Upper body: 4–5 exercises Lower body/core: 4–5 exercises	Static, dynamic, and/or PNF stretching Stretch to the point of feeling tightness or slight discomfort Hold static stretch for 10–30 s; 2–4 repetitions of each exercise	Clinical emphasis is based on monitoring of blood glucose before and after exercise. Adjustments to insulin dose and/or carbohydrate intake can be fine-tuned using that information from the continuous glucose monitoring.
T2D	7 d · wk^{-1} (no more than 2 consecutive days without PA/exercise)	Moderate (40%–59% $\dot{V}O_2R$ or 11–12 RPE) to vigorous (60%–89% $\dot{V}O_2R$ or 14–17 RPE); individuals who are severely deconditioned may start out lower (30%–59% $\dot{V}O_2R$).	At least 150 min · wk^{-1} of moderate-to-vigorous (3.0 METs and higher) intensity	Walk, jog, cycle, row, swim, aquatic activities, seated exercises, team sports	2–3 d · wk^{-1} at 60%–80% 1-RM (lower intensity to start) RPE ~11–15 (6–20 scale) 8–12 repetitions/exercise (10–15 to start) 1–3 sets per exercise All major muscle groups Upper body: 4–5 exercises Lower body/core: 4–5 exercises	Static, dynamic, and/or PNF stretching Stretch to the point of feeling tightness or slight discomfort. Hold static stretch for 10–30 s; 2–4 repetitions of each exercise	Regular exercise facilitates improved blood glucose control in T2D. Clinical emphasis is based on monitoring of blood glucose before and after exercise.

ExR_x, exercise prescription; $\dot{V}O_2R$, oxygen uptake reserve; RPE, rating of perceived exertion; MET, metabolic equivalent; PNF, proprioceptive neuromuscular facilitation.

Based on the FITT Recommendations present in *ACSM's Guidelines for Exercise Testing and Prescription*. 10th ed. Philadelphia (PA): Wolters Kluwer; 2018. 480 p.

A minimum of 3 days of exercise per week is recommended for all individuals with diabetes, and ideally no more than 2 days should lapse between bouts of activity in order to maintain a heightened insulin action (22,31,60). For people with T1D, engaging in daily exercise may improve the balance between insulin dose and caloric needs and make blood glucose management easier (19). For long-term weight loss and maintenance, larger amounts of exercise ($7 \text{ h} \cdot \text{wk}^{-1}$ of moderate or vigorous activity) for individuals who are overweight with T1D or T2D are recommended (26,50).

Both high-intensity interval training and continuous resistance training are recommended forms of vigorous-intensity exercise for individuals with diabetes mellitus (42). Training with alternating intensity improves whole-body glucose disposal in adults with T2D (43), although when matched for energy expenditure, prolonged continuous low- to moderate-intensity aerobic training is equally effective as continuous moderate- to high-intensity training in lowering HbA1C levels and increasing aerobic capacity in adults who are obese with T2D (35).

Recent guidelines from Exercise & Sports Science Australia organization recommend that adults with T2D or prediabetes undertake even more exercise: at least 210 minutes per week of moderate-intensity exercise or 125 minutes per week of vigorous exercise, with no more than 2 consecutive days without training (66). In support of both sets of these recommendations, a recent meta-analysis showed that structured exercise training that consists of aerobic exercise, resistance training, or both is associated with HbA1C reductions in adults with T2D, and total training (of all types) of more than 150 minutes per week is associated with greater improvements in glycemic control than that of 150 minutes or less per week (73).

Doing interspersed, faster intervals during an aerobic training session may increase fitness gains in T2D (44) as well as lower risk for nocturnal hypoglycemia in T1D (38). Whereas general mode recommendations for individuals with uncomplicated T1D are similar to advice for adults without diabetes (31), walking is a preferred low-impact exercise that lessens joint loading (compared with jogging or running) for those with T2D (22,40). Non–weight-bearing or low-impact activities (*e.g.*, cycle ergometer, aquatic exercise classes, elastic bands, yoga, tai chi) may be healthful alternatives to lessen joint stress (2).

Poorly controlled diabetes increases the likelihood of dehydration (72). Ensuring proper hydration in any environmental condition is important. Exercising in a thermally challenging environment (*e.g.*, hot and/or humid) can pose difficulties for those with diabetes because of hydration issues and heightened glucose metabolism. Exercise professionals should offer precautionary measures and prevention strategies to avoid dehydration and/or hypoglycemia in those with diabetes. In some instances, outdoor exercise should be postponed to ensure a safe environment in which to participate. A complete list of diabetes-related complications, neuropathological, microvascular, and macrovascular, can be found in Table 14.5.

Resistance training is recommended for persons with diabetes and follows guidelines for apparently healthy individuals, with age and experience as prime considerations in program development (see FITT table, Table 14.4). Such training has been shown to improve musculoskeletal health, maintain independence in performing daily activities, and reduce the possibility of injury (4). Properly designed resistance programs may improve cardiovascular function, glycemic control, **strength**, and **body composition** in individuals with diabetes (9,16,22,25,78,79).

Typically, lower intensity training is suggested for persons with T1D or T2D and requires 15 seconds to 1 minute of rest, whereas higher intensity training may necessitate up to 2–3 minutes of rest between sets. In terms of intensity, using a **one repetition maximum (1-RM)** to define the amount of weight that an individual can successfully lift one time, resistance training should be moderate (50% of 1-RM) or vigorous (75%–80% of 1-RM) in intensity to optimize gains in strength and insulin action (27,28,33). Higher intensity resistance exercise is safe and effective in lowering HbA1C (27,77).

For safe and effective exercise participation, it is imperative that glucose levels are carefully managed particularly because resistance exercise may cause elevations in blood glucose (71).

Table 14.5 Special Precautions for Diabetes-Related Complications

Complication	Precaution
Autonomic neuropathy[a]	Likelihood of hypoglycemia, abnormal BP (↑/↓), and impaired thermoregulation; abnormal resting HR (↑) and maximal HR (↓); impaired SNS or PNS nerves yield abnormal exercise HR, BP, and SV; use of RPE is suggested; prone to dehydration and hyperthermia/hypothermia.
Peripheral neuropathy	Check feet daily and minimize participation in exercise that may cause trauma to the feet (*e.g.*, prolonged hiking, jogging, or walking on uneven surfaces). Non–weight-bearing exercises (*e.g.*, cycling, chair exercises, swimming) may be more appropriate in some cases, although risk of reulceration is not increased by walking if ulcers are fully healed. Aquatic exercises are not recommended if active ulcers are present. Regular assessment of the feet is recommended. Keep feet clean and dry. Choose shoes carefully for proper fit. Avoid activities requiring a great deal of balance.
Nephropathy	Avoid exercise that increases BP (*e.g.*, weightlifting, high-intensity aerobic exercise) excessively and refrain from breath holding. High BP is common. Lower intensity exercise is recommended.
Retinopathy[a,b]	With proliferative and severe stages of retinopathy, avoid vigorous, high-intensity activities that involve breath holding (*e.g.*, weightlifting and isometrics) or overhead lifting. Avoid activities that lower the head (*e.g.*, yoga, gymnastics) or that risk jarring the head. Consult an ophthalmologist for specific restrictions and limitations. In the absence of peak HR identified through a maximal exercise test, use of RPE is recommended (10–12 on 6–20 scale).
Hypertension	Avoid heavy weightlifting or breath holding. Perform dynamic exercises using large muscle groups, such as walking and cycling at a low-to-moderate intensity. Follow BP guidelines. In the absence of peak HR identified through a maximal exercise test, use of RPE is recommended (10–12 on 6–20 scale).
All individuals	Carry identification with diabetes information. Maintain hydration (drink fluids before, during, and after exercise). Avoid exercise in the heat of the day and in direct sunlight (wear hat and sunscreen when in the sun). Carry rapid-acting carbohydrate sources with you during all exercise and consider packing a glucagon kit in your workout bag to treat severe hypoglycemia.

HR, heart rate; SNS, sympathetic nervous system; PNS, parasympathetic nervous system; SV, stroke volume; RPE, rating of perceived exertion; ↑, increase; ↓, decrease.

[a]Submaximal exercise testing is recommended for individuals with proliferative retinopathy and autonomic neuropathy.

[b]If individual has proliferative retinopathy and has recently undergone photocoagulation or surgical treatment or is not properly treated, exercise is contraindicated.

Appropriate attention to modifying the intensity of the lifting session may reduce the risk for increases in BP, glucose, and musculoskeletal injuries. Individuals with joint limitations or other health complications should complete one set of exercises for all major muscle groups, starting with 10–15 repetitions and progressing to 15–20 repetitions before additional sets are added (4). Although studies have found that moderate- to high-intensity resistance training provoked no evidence of ischemia, resistance exercises should be dynamic and undertaken at a moderate intensity to ensure a safe and effective program. Individuals should avoid the Valsalva maneuver and breathe on effort to avoid untoward outcomes of resistance training, particularly with respect to increased

BP that may contribute to retinal damage. In cases of untreated, severe diabetic retinopathy, intense resistance training may be contraindicated (23).

Prescribing both aerobic and resistance exercise training is recommended for individuals with T1D and T2D. A recent **systematic review and meta-analysis** found no evidence that resistance exercise differs from aerobic exercise in impact on cardiovascular risk markers or safety in individuals with T2D; therefore, selecting one modality of exercise over another may be less important than engaging in any form of exercise (78). Combined training three times weekly in individuals with T2D may be of greater benefit to glycemic control than either aerobic or resistance exercise alone (20,25,53,78), even when caloric expenditure is held constant for the combination (43). Similar training in individuals with T1D results in significantly lower insulin requirements, with unchanged HbA1C values (25). At present, it is unknown whether daily, but alternating, training is more effective than both types undertaken on the same day. Alternate types of physical, such as yoga and tai chi, may bestow some benefits with regard to short- and long-term control of blood glucose levels, **flexibility**, and balance, but more research is needed (2,9,18,49).

Individuals with diabetes should be encouraged to engage in other types of exercise outside of scheduled exercise sessions (*i.e.*, more daily movement). Prolonged sedentary time has been found to be independently associated with deleterious health outcomes, such as T2D and all-cause mortality; however, the deleterious outcome effects associated with sedentary time generally decrease with higher levels of exercise (11). All individuals are recommended to reduce the amount of time spent being sedentary (*e.g.*, working at a computer, watching television) particularly by breaking up extended amounts of time (>90 min) spent sitting by briefly standing or walking (45,46). Individuals with diabetes who are physically deconditioned and sedentary may incorporate more unstructured exercise into daily living to initially increase their daily activity levels and build a fitness base (50,75).

Case Study 14-1 Quiz:

Exercise Prescription and Programming

3. What recommendations would you give to this individual for increasing her aerobic activity level? Do you agree or disagree with the ones that she was given?
4. What aerobic exercise precautions would you suggest that she take?
5. Mrs. Case Study-DM was not given a resistance exercise training prescription. What might be the benefits of a resistance training program and how should she begin?
6. What recommendations would you give to this individual for increasing her activity level outside any programmed exercise sessions she may perform?

Hypoglycemia and Exercise

In individuals managing T2D with diet and exercise alone, the risk of developing hypoglycemia during or after exercise is minimal, even though undertaking longer duration and lower intensity exercise generally reduces glycemic levels (52). More intense activities can cause transient blood glucose elevations in individuals with diabetes (65,71). As a precaution, though, glucose monitoring can be performed before and after exercise to assess its individualized effect.

Declines in blood glucose frequently occur during exercise and cause symptoms even when blood glucose is well above 70 mg · dL^{-1}, or they may occur without generating noticeable symptoms. Hypoglycemia is less common in patients with diabetes who are not treated with insulin or insulin-secreting agents, and no preventive measures for hypoglycemia are usually advised in these cases. If controlled with diet or other oral medications, or if insulin levels can be decreased during exercise, most individuals will not need supplemental carbohydrate for exercise lasting less than an hour or for short, intense workouts because of the release of glucose-raising hormones (48). In insulin users, changing the order of different types of exercise, such as undertaking resistance training before aerobic, may help prevent hypoglycemia during exercise (81,82), as can engaging in short sprints or intermittent high-intensity work (15,38,83).

Importantly, hypoglycemia may be delayed and can occur up to 12 hours (or more) postexercise, even with reductions in insulin doses (1,80). Blood glucose uptake into muscles appears to be elevated during and shortly following 45 minutes of moderate aerobic exercise and again 7–11 hours afterward, suggesting a biphasic glycemic response to exercise in some individuals (54). Consumption of either whole milk and sports drinks before, during, and after 1 hour of moderate exercise may lower the risk of later onset hypoglycemia in T1D (37). Similarly, the risk of nocturnal hypoglycemia following exercise may be lowered with ingestion of a bedtime snack and/or reduced basal rates of insulin overnight (24,41,70).

Common symptoms associated with hypoglycemia include shakiness, weakness, abnormal sweating, nervousness, anxiety, tingling of the mouth and fingers, and hunger. Neuroglycopenic symptoms may include headache, visual disturbances, mental dullness, confusion, amnesia, seizures, and coma. Any incidences of hypoglycemia should be treated with ingestion of rapidly absorbed carbohydrate sources, such as glucose tablets or gels, hard candy, regular soda, skim milk, or juice (8). Severe hypoglycemia resulting in an inability to self-treat or unconsciousness may require the use of a glucagon injection (8).

Hyperglycemia and Exercise

In the presence of low insulin levels, insulin-stimulated glucose uptake in skeletal muscle is reduced and exercise-induced hepatic glucose output is increased, frequently resulting in hyperglycemia, sometimes after exercise (47,63,84). In T1D and other very insulin deficient states, after glucose levels exceed 250–300 mg · dL^{-1}, urinary ketones begin to form as a result of ineffective fat metabolism and contribute to diabetic ketoacidosis if hyperglycemia persists (72). This scenario requires insulin to be administered to lower the glucose level and reestablish euglycemia prior to the initiation of exercise. If blood glucose is elevated (*e.g.*, >250–300 mg · dL^{-1}) before exercise, an acute bout may cause further elevation in blood glucose (hyperglycemia) if moderate or higher levels of ketones are evident. Poor glycemic control may negatively affect exercise training adaptations, such as **maximal oxygen consumption**, workload, heart rate, stroke volume, and cardiac output (10,13).

Case Study 14-1 Quiz:

Exercise Prescription and Progression

7. Does Mrs. Case Study-DM have any known complications that would complicate exercise or make it less safe for her to do? If so, what exercise precautions would you suggest?
8. Many individuals with diabetes have some degree of peripheral neuropathy (nerve damage and loss of sensation) in their feet. What precautions would they need to take to ensure that their exercise training is safe for them?

Box 14.2 Exercise Training and Prescription Considerations for Type 1 Diabetes and Type 2 Diabetes

Perform SMBG.	Check before and after each exercise session. Allow the individual to understand glucose response to PA. It is important to ensure that glucose is in relatively good control before beginning exercise. If blood glucose is >250–300 mg · dL^{-1} plus ketones, exercise should be postponed; if >250–300 mg · dL^{-1} without ketones, exercise is okay but use caution; if <100 mg · dL^{-1}, some individuals using insulin may need to consume a carbohydrate-based snack based on insulin regimen and circulating insulin levels during PA; and if 100–250 mg · dL^{-1}, exercise is recommended without limitations.
Keep a daily log.	Record the time of day the SMBG values are obtained and the amount of any pharmacological agent (*e.g.*, oral drugs, insulin). Also, approximate the duration (minutes), intensity (HR or rating of perceived exertion), and distance (miles or meters) of exercise session. Over time, this aids the individual in understanding the type of glucose response to anticipate from an exercise bout.
Plan for exercise sessions.	How much (*e.g.*, duration and intensity) exercise is anticipated allows adjusting insulin or oral drugs. If needed, carry extra carbohydrate feedings (~10–15 g · 30 min · $^{-1}$) to limit hypoglycemia. Hydrate before and rehydrate after each exercise session to prevent dehydration.
Modify caloric intake accordingly.	Through frequent SMBG, caloric intake can be regulated more carefully on days of and after exercise.
Adjust insulin accordingly.	If using insulin, reduce rapid- or short-acting insulin dosage by 50% to limit hypoglycemia episodes.
Exercise with a partner.	This affords a support system for the exercise habit. Initially, individuals with diabetes should exercise with a partner until their glucose response is known.
Wear a diabetes identification tag.	A diabetes necklace or shoe tag with relevant medical information should always be worn. Hypoglycemia and other problems can arise that require immediate attention.
Wear good shoes.	Always wear proper-fitting and comfortable footwear with socks to minimize foot irritations and limit orthopedic injury to the feet and lower legs.
Practice good hygiene.	Always take extra care to inspect feet for any irritation spots to prevent possible infection. Tend to all sores immediately and limit any irritations.

HR, heart rate.

SUMMARY

Regular exercise is an essential part of the therapeutic regimen in diabetes management and care. Diabetes presents challenges for the individual and for the exercise professional that require comprehensive evaluation of individual status, assessment of individual ability, and individualization of the exercise prescription to meet the needs and goals of those with any type of diabetes. Careful attention to individuals and their diabetes-related comorbidities is required for safe and effective exercise training. Summary of exercise training and prescription considerations for individuals with T1D and T2D are provided in Box 14.2.

RECOMMENDED RESOURCES

American College of Sports Medicine: http://www.acsm.org
American Diabetes Association: http://www.diabetes.org
American Association of Diabetes Educators: http://www.diabeteseducators.org
Centers for Disease Control and Prevention, National Center for Chronic Disease Prevention and Health Promotion (Diabetes Public Health Resource): http://www.cdc.gov/diabetes/index.htm
National Institute of Diabetes and Digestive and Kidney Diseases: http://www2.niddk.nih.gov

REFERENCES

1. Admon G, Weinstein Y, Falk B, et al. Exercise with and without an insulin pump among children and adolescents with type 1 diabetes mellitus. *Pediatrics*. 2005;116:e348–55.
2. Ahn S, Song R. Effects of Tai Chi exercise on glucose control, neuropathy scores, balance, and quality of life in patients with type 2 diabetes and neuropathy. *J Altern Complement Med*. 2012;18:1172–8.
3. American College of Sports Medicine. *ACSM's Guidelines for Exercise Testing and Prescription*. 10th ed. Philadelphia (PA): Wolters Kluwer; 2018. 480 p.
4. American College of Sports Medicine. American College of Sports Medicine position stand. Progression models in resistance training for healthy adults. *Med Sci Sports Exerc*. 2009;41:687–708.
5. American Diabetes Association. 2. Classification and diagnosis of diabetes. *Diabetes Care*. 2016;39(suppl 1):S13–22.
6. American Diabetes Association. 3. Foundations of care and comprehensive medical evaluation. *Diabetes Care*. 2016;39(suppl 1): S23–35.
7. American Diabetes Association. 5. Glycemic targets. *Diabetes Care*. 2016;39(suppl 1):S39–46.
8. American Diabetes Association. 6. Glycemic targets. *Diabetes Care*. 2015;38(suppl 1):S33–40.
9. American Diabetes Association. 11. Children and adolescents. *Diabetes Care*. 2016;39(suppl 1):S86–93.
10. Baldi JC, Cassuto NA, Foxx-Lupo WT, Wheatley CM, Snyder EM. Glycemic status affects cardiopulmonary exercise response in athletes with type I diabetes. *Med Sci Sports Exerc*. 2010;42:1454–9.
11. Biswas A, Oh PI, Faulkner GE, et al. Sedentary time and its association with risk for disease incidence, mortality, and hospitalization in adults: a systematic review and meta-analysis. *Ann Intern Med*. 2015;162:123–32.
12. Boulé NG, Kenny GP, Haddad E, Wells GA, Sigal RJ. Meta-analysis of the effect of structured exercise training on cardiorespiratory fitness in Type 2 diabetes mellitus. *Diabetologia*. 2003;46:1071–81.
13. Brassard P, Ferland A, Bogaty P, Desmeules M, Jobin J, Poirier P. Influence of glycemic control on pulmonary function and heart rate in response to exercise in subjects with type 2 diabetes mellitus. *Metabolism*. 2006;55:1532–7.
14. Buse JB, Ginsberg HN, Bakris GL, et al. Primary prevention of cardiovascular diseases in people with diabetes mellitus: a scientific statement from the American Heart Association and the American Diabetes Association. *Circulation*. 2007;115: 114–26.
15. Bussau VA, Ferreira LD, Jones TW, Fournier PA. The 10-s maximal sprint: a novel approach to counter an exercise-mediated fall in glycemia in individuals with type 1 diabetes. *Diabetes Care*. 2006;29:601–6.
16. Bweir S, Al-Jarrah M, Almalty AM, et al. Resistance exercise training lowers HbA1c more than aerobic training in adults with type 2 diabetes. *Diabetol Metab Syndr*. 2009;1:27.
17. Centers for Disease Control and Prevention. *National Diabetes Statistics Report, 2014: Estimates of Diabetes and Its Burden in the United States*. Atlanta (GA): Centers for Disease Control and Prevention; 2014. 12 p.
18. Chimkode SM, Kumaran SD, Kanhere VV, Shivanna R. Effect of yoga on blood glucose levels in patients with type 2 diabetes mellitus. *J Clin Diagn Res*. 2015;9:CC01–3.
19. Chu L, Hamilton J, Riddell MC. Clinical management of the physically active patient with type 1 diabetes. *Phys Sportsmed*. 2011;39:64–77.
20. Church TS, Blair SN, Cocreham S, et al. Effects of aerobic and resistance training on hemoglobin A1c levels in patients with type 2 diabetes: a randomized controlled trial. *JAMA*. 2010;304:2253–62.
21. Church TS, LaMonte MJ, Barlow CE, Blair SN. Cardiorespiratory fitness and body mass index as predictors of cardiovascular disease mortality among men with diabetes. *Arch Intern Med*. 2005;165:2114–20.
22. Colberg SR, Albright AL, Blissmer BJ, et al. Exercise and type 2 diabetes: American College of Sports Medicine and the American Diabetes Association: joint position statement. Exercise and type 2 diabetes. *Med Sci Sports Exerc*. 2010;42:2282–303.
23. Colberg SR, Sigal RJ. Prescribing exercise for individuals with type 2 diabetes: recommendations and precautions. *Phys Sportsmed*. 2011;39:13–26.
24. Delvecchio M, Zecchino C, Salzano G, et al. Effects of moderate-severe exercise on blood glucose in Type 1 diabetic adolescents treated with insulin pump or glargine insulin. *J Endocrinol Invest*. 2009;32:519–24.
25. D'hooge R, Hellinckx T, Van Laethem C, et al. Influence of combined aerobic and resistance training on metabolic control, cardiovascular fitness and quality of life in adolescents with type 1 diabetes: a randomized controlled trial. *Clin Rehabil*. 2011;25:349–59.

26. Donnelly JE, Blair SN, Jakicic JM, et al. American College of Sports Medicine position stand. Appropriate physical activity intervention strategies for weight loss and prevention of weight regain for adults. *Med Sci Sports Exerc.* 2009;41(2):459–71.
27. Dunstan DW, Daly RM, Owen N, et al. High-intensity resistance training improves glycemic control in older patients with type 2 diabetes. *Diabetes Care.* 2002;25:1729–36.
28. Dunstan DW, Daly RM, Owen N, et al. Home-based resistance training is not sufficient to maintain improved glycemic control following supervised training in older individuals with type 2 diabetes. *Diabetes Care.* 2005;28:3–9.
29. Farmer A, Balman E, Gadsby R, et al. Frequency of self-monitoring of blood glucose in patients with type 2 diabetes: association with hypoglycaemic events. *Curr Med Res Opin.* 2008;24:3097–104.
30. Fox CS, Pencina MJ, Wilson PW, et al. Lifetime risk of cardiovascular disease among individuals with and without diabetes stratified by obesity status in the Framingham heart study. *Diabetes Care.* 2008;31:1582–4.
31. Garber CE, Blissmer B, Deschenes MR, et al. American College of Sports Medicine position stand. Quantity and quality of exercise for developing and maintaining cardiorespiratory, musculoskeletal, and neuromotor fitness in apparently healthy adults: guidance for prescribing exercise. *Med Sci Sports Exerc.* 2011;43:1334–59.
32. Gimeno Orna JA, Boned Juliani B, Lou Arnal LM, Castro Alonso FJ. Microalbuminuria and clinical proteinuria as the main predictive factors of cardiovascular morbidity and mortality in patients with type 2 diabetes. *Rev Clin Esp.* 2003;203:526–31.
33. Gordon BA, Benson AC, Bird SR, Fraser SF. Resistance training improves metabolic health in type 2 diabetes: a systematic review. *Diabetes Res Clin Pract.* 2009;83:157–75.
34. Gregg EW, Gu Q, Cheng YJ, Narayan KM, Cowie CC. Mortality trends in men and women with diabetes, 1971 to 2000. *Ann Intern Med.* 2007;147:149–55.
35. Hansen D, Dendale P, Jonkers RA, et al. Continuous low- to moderate-intensity exercise training is as effective as moderate- to high-intensity exercise training at lowering blood HbA(1c) in obese type 2 diabetes patients. *Diabetologia.* 2009;52:1789–97.
36. Haskell WL, Lee IM, Pate RR, et al. Physical activity and public health: updated recommendation for adults from the American College of Sports Medicine and the American Heart Association. *Med Sci Sports Exerc.* 2007;39:1423–34.
37. Hernandez JM, Moccia T, Fluckey JD, Ulbrecht JS, Farrell PA. Fluid snacks to help persons with type 1 diabetes avoid late onset postexercise hypoglycemia. *Med Sci Sports Exerc.* 2000;32:904–10.
38. Iscoe KE, Riddell MC. Continuous moderate-intensity exercise with or without intermittent high-intensity work: effects on acute and late glycaemia in athletes with Type 1 diabetes mellitus. *Diabet Med.* 2011;28:824–32.
39. Ishiguro H, Kodama S, Horikawa C, et al. In search of the ideal resistance training program to improve glycemic control and its indication for patients with type 2 diabetes mellitus: a systematic review and meta-analysis. *Sports Med.* 2016;46:67–77.
40. Johnson ST, Boulé NG, Bell GJ, Bell RC. Walking: a matter of quantity and quality physical activity for type 2 diabetes management. *Appl Physiol Nutr Metab.* 2008;33:797–801.
41. Kalergis M, Schiffrin A, Gougeon R, Jones PJ, Yale JF. Impact of bedtime snack composition on prevention of nocturnal hypoglycemia in adults with type 1 diabetes undergoing intensive insulin management using lispro insulin before meals: a randomized, placebo-controlled, crossover trial. *Diabetes Care.* 2003;26:9–15.
42. Karstoft K, Christensen CS, Pedersen BK, Solomon TP. The acute effects of interval- vs continuous-walking exercise on glycemic control in subjects with type 2 diabetes: a crossover, controlled study. *J Clin Endocrinol Metab.* 2014;99:3334–42.
43. Karstoft K, Winding K, Knudsen SH, et al. Mechanisms behind the superior effects of interval vs continuous training on glycaemic control in individuals with type 2 diabetes: a randomised controlled trial. *Diabetologia.* 2014;57:2081–93.
44. Karstoft K, Winding K, Knudsen SH, et al. The effects of free-living interval-walking training on glycemic control, body composition, and physical fitness in type 2 diabetic patients: a randomized, controlled trial. *Diabetes Care.* 2013;36:228–36.
45. Katzmarzyk PT. Standing and mortality in a prospective cohort of Canadian adults. *Med Sci Sports Exerc.* 2014;46:940–6.
46. Katzmarzyk PT, Church TS, Craig CL, Bouchard C. Sitting time and mortality from all causes, cardiovascular disease, and cancer. *Med Sci Sports Exerc.* 2009;41:998–1005.
47. Kitabchi AE, Umpierrez GE, Miles JM, Fisher JN. Hyperglycemic crises in adult patients with diabetes. *Diabetes Care.* 2009;32:1335–43.
48. Kreisman SH, Halter JB, Vranic M, Marliss EB. Combined infusion of epinephrine and norepinephrine during moderate exercise reproduces the glucoregulatory response of intense exercise. *Diabetes.* 2003;52:1347–54.
49. Lee MS, Choi TY, Lim HJ, Ernst E. Tai chi for management of type 2 diabetes mellitus: a systematic review. *Chin J Integr Med.* 2011;17:789–93.
50. Levine JA, McCrady SK, Lanningham-Foster LM, Kane PH, Foster RC, Manohar CU. The role of free-living daily walking in human weight gain and obesity. *Diabetes.* 2008;57:548–54.
51. Lièvre MM, Moulin P, Thivolet C, et al. Detection of silent myocardial ischemia in asymptomatic patients with diabetes: results of a randomized trial and meta-analysis assessing the effectiveness of systematic screening. *Trials.* 2011;12:23.
52. MacLeod SF, Terada T, Chahal BS, Boulé NG. Exercise lowers postprandial glucose but not fasting glucose in type 2 diabetes: a meta-analysis of studies using continuous glucose monitoring. *Diabetes Metab Res Rev.* 2013;29:593–603.
53. Marcus RL, Smith S, Morrell G, et al. Comparison of combined aerobic and high-force eccentric resistance exercise with aerobic exercise only for people with type 2 diabetes mellitus. *Phys Ther.* 2008;88:1345–54.
54. McMahon SK, Ferreira LD, Ratnam N, et al. Glucose requirements to maintain euglycemia after moderate-intensity afternoon exercise in adolescents with type 1 diabetes are increased in a biphasic manner. *J Clin Endocrinol Metab.* 2007;92(3):963–8.

55. Moreira SR, Simões GC, Moraes JV, Motta DF, Campbell CS, Simões HG. Blood glucose control for individuals with type-2 diabetes: acute effects of resistance exercise of lower cardiovascular-metabolic stress. *J Strength Cond Res.* 2012;26:2806–11.
56. Naik AD, Palmer N, Petersen NJ, et al. Comparative effectiveness of goal setting in diabetes mellitus group clinics: randomized clinical trial. *Arch Intern Med.* 2011;171:453–9.
57. Narayan KM, Boyle JP, Geiss LS, Saaddine JB, Thompson TJ. Impact of recent increase in incidence on future diabetes burden: U.S., 2005-2050. *Diabetes Care.* 2006;29:2114–6.
58. Narayan KM, Boyle JP, Thompson TJ, Sorensen SW, Williamson DF. Lifetime risk for diabetes mellitus in the United States. *JAMA.* 2003;290:1884–90.
59. Nelson ME, Rejeski WJ, Blair SN, et al. Physical activity and public health in older adults: recommendation from the American College of Sports Medicine and the American Heart Association. *Med Sci Sports Exerc.* 2007;39:1435–45.
60. O'Gorman DJ, Karlsson HK, McQuaid S, et al. Exercise training increases insulin-stimulated glucose disposal and GLUT4 (SLC2A4) protein content in patients with type 2 diabetes. *Diabetologia.* 2006;49:2983–92.
61. Ranger TA, Wong AM, Cook JL, Gaida JE. Is there an association between tendinopathy and diabetes mellitus? A systematic review with meta-analysis. *Br J Sports Med.* 2016;50:982–9.
62. Riddell MC, Milliken J. Preventing exercise-induced hypoglycemia in type 1 diabetes using real-time continuous glucose monitoring and a new carbohydrate intake algorithm: an observational field study. *Diabetes Technol Ther.* 2011;13:819–25.
63. Rosenbloom AL. Hyperglycemic crises and their complications in children. *J Pediatr Endocrinol Metab.* 2007;20:5–18.
64. Schwingshackl L, Missbach B, Dias S, König J, Hoffmann G. Impact of different training modalities on glycaemic control and blood lipids in patients with type 2 diabetes: a systematic review and network meta-analysis. *Diabetologia.* 2014;57:1789–97.
65. Sigal RJ, Fisher SJ, Manzon A, et al. Glucoregulation during and after intense exercise: effects of alpha-adrenergic blockade. *Metabolism.* 2000;49:386–94.
66. Snowling NJ, Hopkins WG. Effects of different modes of exercise training on glucose control and risk factors for complications in type 2 diabetic patients: a meta-analysis. *Diabetes Care.* 2006;29:2518–27.
67. Stewart KJ. Exercise training and the cardiovascular consequences of type 2 diabetes and hypertension: plausible mechanisms for improving cardiovascular health. *JAMA.* 2002;288:1622–31.
68. St John A, Davis WA, Price CP, Davis TM. The value of self-monitoring of blood glucose: a review of recent evidence. *J Diabetes Complications.* 2010;24:129–41.
69. Sui X, Hooker SP, Lee IM, et al. A prospective study of cardiorespiratory fitness and risk of type 2 diabetes in women. *Diabetes Care.* 2008;31:550–5.
70. Taplin CE, Cobry E, Messer L, McFann K, Chase HP, Fiallo-Scharer R. Preventing post-exercise nocturnal hypoglycemia in children with type 1 diabetes. *J Pediatr.* 2010;157:784–8.e1.
71. Turner D, Gray BJ, Luzio S, et al. Similar magnitude of post-exercise hyperglycemia despite manipulating resistance exercise intensity in type 1 diabetes individuals. *Scand J Med Sci Sports.* 2016;26:404–12.
72. Ugale J, Mata A, Meert KL, Sarnaik AP. Measured degree of dehydration in children and adolescents with type 1 diabetic ketoacidosis. *Pediatr Crit Care Med.* 2012;13(2):e103–7.
73. Umpierre D, Ribeiro PA, Kramer CK, et al. Physical activity advice only or structured exercise training and association with HbA1c levels in type 2 diabetes: a systematic review and meta-analysis. *JAMA.* 2011;305:1790–9.
74. Van Dijk JW, Manders RJ, Canfora EE, et al. Exercise and 24-h glycemic control: equal effects for all type 2 diabetes patients? *Med Sci Sports Exerc.* 2013;45:628–35.
75. Vanhecke TE, Franklin BA, Miller WM, deJong AT, Coleman CJ, McCullough PA. Cardiorespiratory fitness and sedentary lifestyle in the morbidly obese. *Clin Cardiol.* 2009;32:121–4.
76. Wahren J, Ekberg K. Splanchnic regulation of glucose production. *Annu Rev Nutr.* 2007;27:329–45.
77. Willey KA, Singh MA. Battling insulin resistance in elderly obese people with type 2 diabetes: bring on the heavy weights. *Diabetes Care.* 2003;26:1580–8.
78. Yang Z, Scott CA, Mao C, Tang J, Farmer AJ. Resistance exercise versus aerobic exercise for type 2 diabetes: a systematic review and meta-analysis. *Sports Med.* 2014;44:487–99.
79. Yardley JE, Hay J, Abou-Setta AM, Marks SD, McGavock J. A systematic review and meta-analysis of exercise interventions in adults with type 1 diabetes. *Diabetes Res Clin Pract.* 2014;106:393–400.
80. Yardley JE, Iscoe KE, Sigal RJ, Kenny GP, Perkins BA, Riddell MC. Insulin pump therapy is associated with less post-exercise hyperglycemia than multiple daily injections: an observational study of physically active type 1 diabetes patients. *Diabetes Technol Ther.* 2013;15:84–8.
81. Yardley JE, Kenny GP, Perkins BA, et al. Effects of performing resistance exercise before versus after aerobic exercise on glycemia in type 1 diabetes. *Diabetes Care.* 2012;35:669–75.
82. Yardley JE, Kenny GP, Perkins BA, et al. Resistance versus aerobic exercise: acute effects on glycemia in type 1 diabetes. *Diabetes Care.* 2013;36:537–42.
83. Yardley JE, Mollard R, MacIntosh A, et al. Vigorous intensity exercise for glycemic control in patients with type 1 diabetes. *Can J Diabetes.* 2013;37(6):427–32.

84. Yardley JE, Zaharieva DP, Jarvis C, Riddell MC. The "ups" and "downs" of a bike race in people with type 1 diabetes: dramatic differences in strategies and blood glucose responses in the Paris-to-Ancaster Spring Classic. *Can J Diabetes*. 2015;39(2):105–10.
85. Zaharieva DP, Riddell MC. Prevention of exercise-associated dysglycemia: a case study-based approach. *Diabetes Spectr*. 2015;28:55–62.
86. Zoungas S, Chalmers J, Ninomiya T, et al. Association of HbA1c levels with vascular complications and death in patients with type 2 diabetes: evidence of glycaemic thresholds. *Diabetologia*. 2012;55: 636–43.

SELECTED REFERENCES FOR FURTHER READING

American Diabetes Association. Physical activity/exercise and diabetes. *Diabetes Care*. 2004;27:S58–62.

Colberg SR. *Diabetic Athlete's Handbook: Your Guide to Peak Performance*. Champaign (IL): Human Kinetics; 2009. 284 p.

Colberg SR. *The 7 Step Diabetes Fitness Plan: Living Well and Being Fit With Diabetes, No Matter Your Weight*. New York (NY): Marlowe; 2006. 272 p.

Colberg SR, Sigal RJ, Fernhall B, et al. Exercise and Type 2 diabetes: the American College of Sports Medicine and the American Diabetes Association: joint position statement. *Diabetes Care*. 2010;33:e147–67.

CHAPTER 15

Special Considerations for Metabolic Syndrome, Hypertension, and Dyslipidemia

INTRODUCTION

Lifestyle therapy (*i.e.*, beneficial modifications in diet and **physical activity**) is prescribed in the prevention and treatment of many cardiometabolic diseases, including high blood pressure (BP) (hypertension), abnormal blood lipids (dyslipidemia), or the clustering of cardiovascular and metabolic risk factors known as the *metabolic syndrome*. **Exercise** training may be just as effective, if not more, than certain pharmacological monotherapies for preventing mortality from cardiovascular disease (CVD) (22). This finding requires clinicians to understand the unique considerations for prescribing exercise training to ameliorate cardiovascular and metabolic risk factors. This chapter presents disease etiology and special considerations related to exercise testing, prescription, and progression for individuals with three cardiovascular or **metabolic disorders**: metabolic syndrome, hypertension, and dyslipidemia. The accompanying case study details a patient with hypertension and elevated low-density lipoprotein cholesterol (LDL-C) who wishes to increase his physical activity in order to alleviate side effects associated with several of the prescription medications he has been taking.

Case Study 15-1

Mr. Case Study-BP

Mr. Case Study-BP is a 48-year-old male contractor who has recently been faced with some health concerns. He is self-employed and has only carried catastrophic health insurance for most of his adult life. When he became eligible to purchase insurance through a health insurance exchange in his state, he found a primary care physician and went for his first routine physical in over 20 years. At that time, Mr. Case Study-BP was diagnosed with stage 1 hypertension as his BP was 145/84 mm Hg. His doctor immediately prescribed a low-dose diuretic to bring his BP down. Mr. Case Study-BP was also diagnosed with an LDL-C of 185 mg · dL^{-1} and, as a result, was started on 5 mg of a statin medication to be taken once daily. His doctor was very direct when she weighed Mr. Case Study-BP, stating that he was 9 kg (20 lb) overweight and was at risk for metabolic syndrome, diabetes, stroke, and heart disease. He was anxious and overwhelmed by the visit but felt thankful that his hypertension and elevated LDL-C were going to be treated immediately. Six months later, however, Mr. Case Study-BP has been frustrated by his inability to lose weight. Although his BP is now 136/82 mm Hg, he hates taking three daily medications (he also takes an over-the-counter baby aspirin at his physician's recommendation) and is worried that he will need increasing amounts of medication to control his cardiovascular risk. The adult education catalog in his town advertises a 4-week health and wellness class for adults, so Mr. Case Study-BP signs up. The second class focuses on exercise with each participant receiving an individualized exercise prescription using an online program. His prescription is as follows:

Weeks 0–4: Exercise 20 minutes per day, three times per week, alternating 4 minutes walking with 1 minute running.
Weeks 5–8: Exercise 30 minutes per day, three to five times per week, alternating 2 minutes walking with 3 minutes running.
Weeks 9 onward: Run 30 minutes per day, 4–5 days per week.

He is also instructed not to perform heavy resistance exercise due to his hypertension; instead, he is instructed to do low-intensity body weight exercises such as push-ups and sit-ups twice a week.

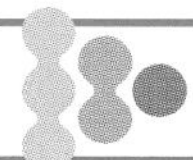

Description, Prevalence, and Etiology

Metabolic Syndrome

Metabolic syndrome is defined as the clustering of individual cardiovascular and metabolic risk factors that are related to obesity, insulin resistance, hypertension, and dyslipidemia. This clustering of abnormal risk increases an individual's disease predisposition for both Type 2 diabetes and CVD. By definition, an individual is classified as having metabolic syndrome if he or she is diagnosed with any three of five risk factors: fasting plasma glucose ≥100 mg · dL^{-1} (or being treated pharmacologically for elevated glucose), high-density lipoprotein cholesterol (HDL-C) <40 mg · dL^{-1} in men or <50 mg · dL^{-1} in women (or being treated for reduced HDL-C), triglycerides (TG) ≥150 mg · dL^{-1} (or being treated for high TG), waist circumference >102 cm in men or >88 cm in women, and systolic blood pressure (SBP) ≥130 mm Hg or diastolic blood pressure (DBP) ≥85 mm Hg (or being treated for hypertension) (1). Recent statistics indicate that the prevalence of metabolic syndrome has dropped slightly overall in the United States from approximately 26% in 2000 to 23% in 2010 (21). However, disproportionately higher rates are observed in ethnic groups such as Hispanic/Latinos, American Indians, and Alaska natives such that prevalence rates in these groups may be almost twice as high as overall rates. The burden of metabolic syndrome is substantial because, in addition to the health risks associated with each individual cardiometabolic component, overall risk of CVD morbidity and mortality is two- to threefold higher in patients with metabolic syndrome (14).

Metabolic syndrome is considered largely a disease of unhealthy lifestyle practices, with many of the underlying risk factors for development of the syndrome involving poor diet and exercise, such as low levels of physical activity and fitness; high intake of soft drinks, diet soda, carbohydrates, meat, and fried foods; and unhealthy behaviors such as skipping breakfast and heavy alcohol consumption. Moreover, public awareness of the metabolic syndrome and its cardiovascular and metabolic risk is low. Consequently, treatment guidelines from the American Heart Association (AHA)/National Heart, Lung, and Blood Institute emphasize that the primary aim of treatment for metabolic syndrome is to treat the modifiable, underlying risk factors (obesity, **physical inactivity**, and atherogenic diet) through lifestyle changes (15). Guidelines include reducing body weight by 7%–10% over the first year of therapy with the goal to achieve a **body mass index (BMI)** <25 kg · m^{-2}; following a diet low in fat, trans fat, cholesterol, and simple sugars; and participating in 30 minutes per day of moderate-intensity exercise at least 5 days per week (but preferably achieving 60 min daily).

The primary goal of treatment in individuals with the metabolic syndrome is to reduce risk for clinical atherosclerotic disease, so treatment is designed to improve the major cardiovascular risk factors: elevated LDL-C, hypertension, and diabetes (blood glucose) (15). If absolute risk is sufficiently high to warrant drug therapy above and beyond lifestyle changes, then clinical guidelines for metabolic syndrome suggest following treatment guidelines for each individual risk factor. As pharmacological treatment for hypertension and dyslipidemia are discussed in the following sections, medications for treating elevated blood glucose alone will be presented in this section.

The American Diabetes Association (ADA) guidelines (3) suggest biguanides (metformin) as first-line therapy. These drugs reduce the amount of glucose released by the liver and moderately increase peripheral insulin sensitivity. Other classes of drugs include sulfonylureas and meglitinides (which stimulate the pancreas to release more insulin), thiazolidinediones (insulin sensitizers), and α-glucosidase inhibitors (which slow the absorption of carbohydrates into the bloodstream). Second-line polypharmacy often involves one or more of these drugs in addition to insulin supplementation. Of note is that, especially in patients who use insulin and/or insulin secretagogues (drugs that stimulate pancreatic release of insulin), acute exercise can evoke hypoglycemia (low blood sugar). Thus, the American College of Sports Medicine (ACSM)/ADA joint position statement on exercise and Type 2 diabetes recommends that individuals using these medications consider ingesting carbohydrates prior to and possibly after exercise and/or consider reducing oral medications or insulin dosing before and possibly after exercise (8). However, this recommendation is specific to the duration and intensity of exercise, the patient's glucose level at the time of exercise, and the type and dose of medication(s) being used and should be interpreted on an individual clinical basis. Readers are encouraged to refer to a more comprehensive coverage of **exercise prescription** for individuals with Type 2 diabetes (see Chapter 14).

Hypertension

BP is defined as the force exerted by the blood against artery walls during the heart's contraction and relaxation, with high BP or hypertension representing a pathological condition which contributes to CVD risk. A patient is classified as having hypertension if he or she has an SBP $\geq$140 mm Hg and/or DBP $\geq$90 mm Hg, or is taking antihypertensive medicine, or has been told at least twice by a physician or other health care provider that he or she has high BP (9). Even small elevations in BP over time increase the future risk of hypertension and cardiovascular events, and thus, the category of prehypertension is defined as untreated SBP of 120–139 mm Hg or untreated DBP of 80–89 mm Hg. Classification of BP categories according to the frequently used Seventh Report of the Joint National Committee on Prevention, Detection, Evaluation, and Treatment of High Blood Pressure (JNC 7) (7) as well as the updated guidelines by the Eighth Report of the Joint National Committee on Prevention, Detection, Evaluation, and Treatment of High Blood Pressure (JNC 8) (16) are described in Table 15.1.

Table 15.1 Quantitative Differences between JNC 7 and JNC 8 Guidelines

JNC 7 Guidelines (SBP and DBP)	JNC 8 Guidelines (SBP and DBP)
Blood pressure classification system	Blood pressure goals
Normal	<60 yr or with diabetes or CKD
<120 and <80 mm Hg	<140 and 90 mm Hg
Prehypertension	≥60 yr
120–139 or 80–89 mm Hg	<150 and 90 mm Hg
Stage 1 hypertension	
140–159 or 90–99 mm Hg	
Stage 2 hypertension	
≥160 or ≥100 mm Hg	

CKD, chronic kidney disease.

From National High Blood Pressure Education Program. *The Seventh Report of the Joint National Committee on Prevention, Detection, Evaluation, and Treatment of High Blood Pressure.* Bethesda (MD): National Heart, Lung, and Blood Institute (US); 2004 Aug. Available from: https://www.ncbi.nlm.nih.gov/books/NBK9630/; and James PA, Oparil S, Carter BL, et al. 2014 Evidence-based guideline for the management of high blood pressure in adults: report from the panel members appointed to the Eighth Joint National Committee (JNC 8). *JAMA.* 2014;311(5):507–20.

Other important categories of BP classification routinely assessed by the National Health and Nutrition Examination Survey (NHANES) include being aware of one's hypertension, being treated for hypertension, and having controlled hypertension (see Table 15.2 for specific definitions) (9). Hypertension is the most important CVD risk factor, accounting for 40% of all CVD deaths (23). Approximately one-third (32.6%) of U.S. adults ≥20 years of age have hypertension, and 17.2% of these individuals are unaware of their elevated BP (21). Even individuals who reach the age of 50 years with normal BP still have a 90% risk of developing hypertension within their lifetime (6).

As the estimated medical cost for treatment of hypertension is $46.4 billion annually (21), the impact of hypertension on the U.S. health care system has made it a critical public health concern. Hypertension is a multifaceted disease with risk factors including age, race/ethnicity, family history of hypertension and genetic factors, lower education and socioeconomic status, greater weight,

Table 15.2 Definitions of Hypertension According to the National Health and Nutrition Examination Survey

Awareness: IF the patient with hypertension answers yes to the following question: "Have you ever been told by a doctor or health care provider that you had hypertension, also called high blood pressure?" THEN he or she is AWARE of his or her hypertension.
Treatment: IF the patient with hypertension answers yes to the following questions: "Because of your high blood pressure/hypertension, have you ever been told to take prescribed medicine?" and "Are you now following this advice to take prescribed medicine?" THEN he or she is being TREATED for his or her hypertension.
Control: IF the patient with hypertension has an SBP below 140 mm Hg and DBP below 90 mm Hg THEN he or she has CONTROLLED hypertension.

From Crim MT, Yoon SS, Ortiz E, et al. National surveillance definitions for hypertension prevalence and control among adults. *Circ Cardiovasc Qual Outcomes.* 2012;5(3):343–51.

lower physical activity, tobacco use, psychosocial stressors, sleep apnea, and dietary factors (including dietary fats, higher sodium intake, lower potassium intake, and excessive alcohol intake) (21). Evidence suggests that despite the various mechanisms and etiologies underlying hypertension, modifiable factors such as diet and exercise comprise a large proportion of an individual's overall risk for hypertension (25).

According to JNC 7 (7), patients with hypertension should be treated with medically supervised diet and lifestyle modifications first (*i.e.*, reduced-sodium diets, increased physical activity, and recommendations for weight loss). Patients not at goal after these initial modifications should then be started on pharmacological therapy of one or more drugs depending on stage of hypertension (stage 1 or 2) and existent underlying disease such as chronic kidney disease or diabetes. In JNC 8 (16), these guidelines were revised to relax BP treatment goals by 10 mm Hg for **older adults** >60 years of age as well as patients with chronic kidney disease or diabetes. JNC 8 guidelines, however, were not wholly embraced by the medical community, many of whom continue to utilize JNC 7 treatment paradigms for patients. Qualitative differences between the guidelines are summarized in Table 15.3.

Table 15.3 Major Qualitative Differences between JNC 7 and JNC 8 Guidelines

JNC 7 Guidelines	JNC 8 Guidelines
Standardized definitions ▪ Numerical quantification of ranges and thresholds for prehypertension and hypertension	No definitions for diagnosis ▪ No definitions of prehypertension and hypertension ▪ Quantifies numerical thresholds for pharmacological treatment
Treatment regimen depends on other diseases. ▪ Defines different treatment approaches for singular/uncomplicated hypertension than hypertension with comorbidities such as chronic kidney disease and diabetes	Treatment regimen is more uniform independent of disease. ▪ Treatment of hypertension with and without comorbid disease is uniform except in certain disease pathologies where evidence supports specific treatments.
Comprehensive description of lifestyle therapy ▪ Recommended lifestyle modifications were based on literature review and expert opinion.	References guidelines for lifestyle therapy ▪ Endorsed previously published guideline of the Lifestyle Work Group
Five classes of drugs ▪ Recommended five classes of drugs with diuretics as first-line option if no other compelling indication	Four classes of drugs ▪ Recommends a choice between four classes of drugs for initial therapy
Comprehensive topic coverage ▪ Addressed multiple issues including blood pressure measurement	Limited topic coverage ▪ Addressed a limited number of high priority questions

From Chobanian AV, Bakris GL, Black HR, et al. The Seventh Report of the Joint National Committee on Prevention, Detection, Evaluation, and Treatment of High Blood Pressure: the JNC 7 report. *JAMA.* 2003;289(19):2560–72; and James PA, Oparil S, Carter BL, et al. 2014 Evidence-based guideline for the management of high blood pressure in adults: report from the panel members appointed to the Eighth Joint National Committee (JNC 8). *JAMA.* 2014;311(5):507–20.

There are many classes of antihypertensive medications that influence peripheral vascular resistance or cardiac output (or both). These include medications that target rate-limiting enzymes of the renin-angiotensin-aldosterone system, β-adrenergic receptors in the heart, vasodilation, or fluid balance, among others. JNC 8 recommends any drug from one of the four following classes to be a good choice as initial therapy: thiazide-type diuretics, calcium channel blockers, angiotensin-converting enzyme inhibitors, or angiotensin II receptor antagonists (16). Drug monotherapy typically results in a reduction in SBP or DBP of 5–10 mm Hg, but these reductions are dependent on factors such as the patient's baseline BP and the mechanism underlying hypertension. In addition, combining doses of multiple classes of BP-lowering drugs is preferred because this treatment is more effective than doubling the dose of one BP drug (34). Multiple other factors contribute to the choice to utilize one or more antihypertensive drugs from the various classes (*e.g.*, race, disease, age) (16), and thus pharmacological management of hypertension requires adjustment of doses and classes of medications over time.

Dyslipidemia

Dyslipidemia is defined as abnormal levels of blood lipids. There are three atherogenic lipoproteins: very low density lipoprotein (VLDL), intermediate-density lipoprotein (IDL), and LDL-C. LDL-C is the major atherogenic protein and lipid risk marker; a 10% increase in LDL-C leads to an approximate 20% increase in coronary heart disease (CHD) risk (35). TG are also associated with an increase in CHD events, although their link to CHD is complex and may be related to the other risk factors such as LDL-C and HDL-C subfractions, abdominal obesity, insulin resistance, and hypertension (13). HDL-C, by contrast, reduces the risk of atherosclerosis and CHD. The four major blood lipid measurements (total cholesterol [TC], with components of HDL-C, LDL-C, TG) and their ratios in relationship to each other are the primary targets used to diagnose and treat CVD risk.

Dyslipidemia is a major public health problem. Approximately 13% of U.S. adults have elevated TC (21), and 30% elevated LDL-C, the latter which doubles their heart disease risk (23). Because CVD (heart disease and stroke) accounts for about 1 of every 3 deaths in the United States, treating abnormal blood lipids is vital to reduce heart disease deaths in the United States.

Treatment guidelines based primarily on serum LDL-C levels were established by the National Cholesterol Education Program Adult Treatment Panel III (ATP III) in May 2001 (13). These guidelines suggest an LDL-C treatment goal, based on current and estimated cardiovascular risk and risk factors, ranging from 100 to 160 $mg \cdot dL^{-1}$ for patients. Recently released 2013 guidelines (32) by the American College of Cardiology (ACC) and the AHA dramatically revised the treatment guidelines for hyperlipidemia, focusing on risk of stroke and coronary disease rather than strictly defined target LDL-C levels as a rationale to treat an individual. These ACC/AHA guidelines emphasized a benefit of pharmacological treatment for individuals with LDL-C $>$190 $mg \cdot dL^{-1}$ and/or diabetes, established CVD, or high risk of CVD. For both sets of guidelines, lifestyle modification such as routine **aerobic** and resistance exercise and heart-healthy diet adherence are recommended as initial therapy and in addition to pharmacology. Quantitative and qualitative differences between the two guidelines are summarized in Table 15.4 and Table 15.5, respectively.

There are five major classes of drugs to treat dyslipidemia. These include hydroxy-methyl-glutaryl (HMG) coenzyme A reductase inhibitors (statins), niacin, fibric acid derivatives, bile acid binding resins, and cholesterol absorption inhibitors. With the exception of niacin, which increases HDL-C, the major target associated with these drugs is a reduction in LDL-C. Statins are the most effective of the cholesterol-lowering drugs; the average reduction in LDL-C with routine statin monotherapy ranges from 25% to 50% even at low doses (13). Consequently, statins reduce cardiac events by 20%–44% in both patients with coronary artery

Table 15.4 Quantitative Differences between ATP III and ACC/AHA Guidelines

ATP III Guidelines		ACC/AHA Guidelines
LDL goal		LDL goal
<100 mg · dL^{-1}	CHD, 10-yr risk >20%	No recommendation
<130 mg · dL^{-1}	2+ risk factors	
<160 mg · dL^{-1}	0–1 risk factors	
Threshold of LDL of which to initiate drug therapy		Threshold of LDL of which to initiate statin therapy
≥130 mg · dL^{-1}	CHD, 10-yr risk >20%	■ ≥190 mg · dL^{-1}
≥130 mg · dL^{-1}	2+ risk factors, 10-yr risk 10%–20%	■ 70–189 mg · dL^{-1}, 40–75 yr, with diabetes ■ 70–189 mg · dL^{-1}, 40–75 yr, and estimated 10-yr ASCVD risk ≥7.5%
≥160 mg · dL^{-1}	2+ risk factors, 10-yr risk <10%	■ Any level, but with clinical ASCVD
≥190 mg · dL^{-1}	0–1 risk factors	
Classification of LDL (mg · dL^{-1})		Classification of LDL (mg · dL^{-1})
<100	Optimal	No recommendation
100–129	Near optimal	
130–159	Borderline high	
160–189	High	
≥190	Very high	
Classification of HDL (mg · dL^{-1})		Classification of HDL (mg · dL^{-1})
<40	Low	No recommendation
≥60	High	
Classification of TC (mg · dL^{-1})		Classification of TC (mg · dL^{-1})
<200	Desirable	No recommendation
200–239	Borderline high	
≥240	High	

ASCVD, atherosclerotic cardiovascular disease.

From Expert Panel on Detection, Evaluation, and Treatment of High Blood Cholesterol in Adults. Executive summary of the third report of the National Cholesterol Education Program (NCEP) Expert Panel on Detection, Evaluation, and Treatment of High Blood Cholesterol in Adults (Adult Treatment Panel III). *JAMA*. 2001;285(19):2486–97; and Stone NJ, Robinson JG, Lichtenstein AH, et al. 2013 ACC/AHA guideline on the treatment of blood cholesterol to reduce atherosclerotic cardiovascular risk in adults: a report of the American College of Cardiology/American Heart Association Task Force on Practice Guidelines. *Circulation*. 2014;129(25 suppl 2):S1–45.

disease (CAD) (31) and in previously healthy subjects (10). Statins are so effective that they are among the most prescribed drugs in the United States and the world; most recent data indicate that use of these drugs explains the statistically significant decline in TC over the last 5 years in the United States (21). The recent release of the 2013 ACC/AHA guidelines (32) for the treatment of cholesterol is likely to expand the use of statins. Comparing the new 2013 ACC/AHA guidelines with the prior ATP III guidelines suggest that the number of U.S. adults eligible right now for statin therapy will increase from 43.2 million (37.5% of U.S. adults) to 56.0 million (48.6%) (28).

Table 15.5 Qualitative Differences between ATP III Guidelines and ACC/AHA Guidelines

ATP III Guidelines	ACC/AHA Guidelines
Treat to target approach ■ Quantitative guidelines for LDL-C, HDL-C, and TG based on number of CV risk factors	Not enough evidence for targets ■ Randomized control trials do not support evidence for numerical targets. ■ Suggests treating four groups who may benefit from statin therapy
No distinction between cholesterol-lowering drugs ■ Emphasizes treatment with cholesterol-lowering drugs to achieve targets	Recommends statin therapy to reduce blood lipids ■ Identifies high- and moderate-intensity statins for use in secondary and primary prevention ■ Non-statin therapies do not provide substantial risk reduction relative to potential adverse effects.
Cardiovascular disease risk calculated from Framingham score ■ Does not include stroke in calculation, only heart attacks	Uses a new equation to estimate 10-yr ASCVD risk ■ Includes stroke and heart attack in calculation of risk
Treatment decisions based on guidelines ■ Clinicians base treatment decisions on guidelines.	Clinician flexibility in treatment decisions ■ Treatment decisions for patients who fall outside of the four predefined groups involve physician discretion.

ASCVD, atherosclerotic cardiovascular disease.

From Expert Panel on Detection, Evaluation, and Treatment of High Blood Cholesterol in Adults. Executive summary of the third report of the National Cholesterol Education Program (NCEP) Expert Panel on Detection, Evaluation, and Treatment of High Blood Cholesterol in Adults (Adult Treatment Panel III). *JAMA.* 2001;285(19):2486–97; and Stone NJ, Robinson JG, Lichtenstein AH, et al. 2013 ACC/AHA guideline on the treatment of blood cholesterol to reduce atherosclerotic cardiovascular risk in adults: a report of the American College of Cardiology/American Heart Association Task Force on Practice Guidelines. *Circulation.* 2014;129(25 suppl 2):S1–45.

Case Study 15-1 Quiz:

Description, Prevalence, and Etiology

1. How would you classify Mr. Case Study-BP's BP (according to JNC 7 guidelines) after 3 months on the diuretic?
2. Mr. Case Study-BP's doctor used his body weight as an indication that he was overweight and at risk for metabolic syndrome. Is body weight the best predictor of obesity as it relates to metabolic risk?
3. What lifestyle recommendations could the doctor have given Mr. Case Study-BP in addition to prescribing regular medication use?

Preparticipation Health Screening, Medical History, and Physical Examination

ACSM's new guidelines for preparticipation screening state that "insufficient evidence is available to suggest that the presence of CVD risk factors *without underlying disease* confers substantial risk of adverse exercise-related cardiovascular events." Consequently, exercise professionals are encouraged to "complete a CVD risk factor assessment with their patients as part of the preexercise evaluation" to rely on **medical clearance** rather than exercise testing (which poorly predicts the likelihood of an acute cardiac event) to guide the development of exercise prescription (30). For metabolic syndrome, hypertension, and dyslipidemia, Figure 2.2 of the *ACSM's Guidelines for Exercise Testing and Prescription, 10th edition* (*GETP10*) indicates that the majority of asymptomatic individuals not participating in regular exercise do not need medical clearance prior to initiating a light- to moderate-intensity exercise training program (2). Indeed, these individuals may also progress to more **vigorous intensity** exercise provided they follow ACSM's basic exercise prescription guidelines for progression. However, clinicians should be aware of the following considerations, as outlined in *GETP10* (2), that may require additional supervision and/or clinical oversight:

- Individuals with metabolic syndrome, hypertension, and dyslipidemia may have other health conditions, including undetected CVD, and thus, a detailed medical evaluation and screening for factors such as blood glucose control, other CVD risk factors, symptoms, and concurrent medications by a physician may be helpful prior to initiating and exercise program. This process will better personalize and tailor the exercise prescription and desired goals.
- Individuals with hypertension typically also do not require medical clearance prior to initiating low- to moderate-intensity exercise, according to the updated **preparticipation health screening** guidelines (30). However, the degree to which hypertension is existent, treated, and controlled may influence the need for and recommended types of medical clearance.

As noted in the previous sections, lifestyle therapy, notably modifications of diet and patterns of physical activity, is a cornerstone of therapy for all of these health conditions. The *GETP10* notes that increasing physical activity, alone and in conjunction with diet modification and/or weight loss, exerts beneficial effects (ranging in magnitude) on BP, insulin sensitivity, blood glucose levels, HDL-C, LDL-C, and TG. Therefore, even an increase in physical activity in these populations from low- to moderate-intensity exercise will incur some benefit.

Case Study 15-1 Quiz:

Preparticipation Screening Considerations

4. Is an exercise test indicated for Mr. Case Study-BP prior to beginning his exercise program? Why or why not?

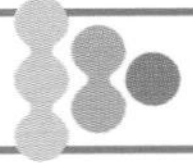

Exercise Testing Considerations

In general, exercise testing is not required for asymptomatic patients with metabolic syndrome, hypertension, or dyslipidemia prior to beginning a low-intensity exercise training program such as walking. Standard exercise testing protocols may be used for an individual with dyslipidemia and metabolic syndrome unless that individual presents with other health risk factors described in this chapter or others. According to updated preparticipation health screening guidelines (30), exercise testing is not required prior to initiating a low- to moderate-intensity exercise training program but may be useful for establishing baseline performance or individualizing an exercise prescription.

In hypertension cases where exercise testing is needed, special considerations for exercise testing include the magnitude of hypertension present (*i.e.*, stage 1 vs. stage 2), whether the hypertension is controlled (<140/90 mm Hg) or uncontrolled (≥140/90 mm Hg) with medication use, whether BP responses are being used to guide exercise prescription, and whether the individual usually takes antihypertensive medications at night or in the morning (before or after exercise) (2,29). In addition, individuals with hypertension who plan to engage in higher intensity exercise programs may be screened for an exaggerated BP response to exercise, which can occur even if BP is controlled. Standardized BP monitoring before and after exercise testing should also be emphasized. Table 15.6 documents common questions a clinician may ask an individual with hypertension to guide decision-making processes for exercise testing in a hypertensive individual.

Medication is frequently prescribed for the management of metabolic syndrome, hypertension, and dyslipidemia. An additional consideration for exercise testing and prescription in these conditions is the use of concomitant medications that may influence physical activity and alter exercise tolerance. Consequently, clinicians encouraging patients to exercise should be aware of medications the patient is taking as well as their potential interactions with exercise. An obvious example is the risk of hypotension following a bout of aerobic exercise in older adults who are prescribed multiple BP-lowering drugs to treat chronic hypertension. Adults on several antihypertensive medications may experience such a substantial drop in BP with postexercise hypotension that they experience transient orthostatic intolerance that translates into balance disturbance and increased fall risk. By contrast, however, recent evidence finds that certain medications, in conjunction with exercise, facilitate greater improvements in health outcomes and risk factors above those that are achieved with exercise alone.

As has been previously noted, cholesterol-lowering drugs — particularly statins — are extremely efficacious for lowering LDL-C. Therefore, clinicians may emphasize cholesterol-lowering drugs over exercise for treating hypercholesterolemia. Data suggest, however, that the combination of exercise training and cholesterol-lowering drugs may be most efficacious for patients with elevated LDL-C. For example, after 12 weeks of resistance training in older adults, LDL-C was reduced by an average 18 $mg \cdot dL^{-1}$, and reductions were greater with concurrent use of cholesterol-lowering drugs (4). Similarly, an analysis of over 10,000 adults in the Veteran's Affairs medical system (18) found that although both high fitness and statin drug use decreased mortality risk, individuals who were both highly fit and taking a statin had the lowest mortality risk of any study participants. Therefore, routine exercise may interact with, potentiate, and/or be influenced by common medications used to treat hypercholesterolemia.

Table 15.6 Helpful Questions to Ask When Considering Exercise Testing for the Individual with Hypertension

- Is this individual going to perform moderate- to vigorous-intensity exercise? Would exercise testing be valuable to determine if he or she has an exaggerated blood pressure response to exercise?
- Does this individual have controlled hypertension? IF NOT, has he or she consulted with his or her physician prior to initiating exercise?
- Does this individual have stage 2 hypertension (SBP 160 mm Hg and/or DBP >100 mm Hg) or target organ disease? If so, a medically supervised symptom-limited exercise test is recommend, in addition to a medical evaluation and adequate BP control, prior to initiating an exercise program.
- What medications is this individual taking? Will they affect exercise responses by influencing heart rate, electrolyte balance, fluid balance, or postexercise hypotension?

Case Study 15-1 Quiz:

Exercise Testing Considerations

5. What are the daily medications Mr. Case Study-BP is taking, and how might they have an impact on his response to daily exercise training?

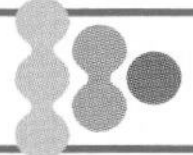

Exercise Prescription and Progression Considerations

Frequency, intensity, time, and type (FITT) table (Table 15.7) documents exercise prescription and special considerations for a healthy adult as well as an adult with chronic conditions of hypertension, dyslipidemia, and overweight/obesity from *GETP10* (2). The premise of this table is to guide the reader in comparing and contrasting between the exercise prescriptions. In general, these exercise prescriptions, based on FITT principles, are largely similar with several considerations for each chronic condition as detailed in the following sections.

Metabolic Syndrome

Individuals with metabolic syndrome are encouraged to engage in physical activity and/or diet modification sufficient to evoke weight loss and reduce cardiovascular and metabolic risk. Therefore, an adequate exercise prescription such as that prescribed to adults with overweight/obesity will optimize the potential for caloric expenditure. This prescription involves a gradual progression of aerobic exercise (starting at low-to-moderate intensity) until the individual progresses from 30 to 60 minutes per day to total 300 minutes or more each week.

Resistance exercise training increases metabolically active muscle tissue and is critical to the exercise prescription. Resistance training is known to attenuate the hypoglycemic effects of aerobic exercise alone and additionally can moderate risk factors such as obesity, waist girth, and prehypertension that all contribute to the metabolic syndrome. The exercise prescription considerations listed in the following sections may also be applicable. Individuals with the metabolic syndrome are not classified as diabetic; however, patients with metabolic syndrome may exhibit hyperglycemia, and thus, an exercise prescription based on considerations for hyperglycemia and/or use of medications influencing glucose and insulin levels should be followed as discussed in other sections of this book (see Chapter 14). A general rule of thumb for the individual with metabolic syndrome is to tailor the exercise prescription on individual risk factors, fitting it to the most conservative approach warranted.

Hypertension

The most visible difference between the FITT principles for exercise in healthy adults and in adults with hypertension is the frequency of exercise, which is increased in adults with hypertension to 5–7 days per week (see Table 15.7). As the chronic BP-lowering effects of exercise are presumed at least in part to be precipitated by the BP reduction associated with an acute bout of exercise (termed *post*exercise *hypotension*, or PEH) (12,29), exposure to some aerobic exercise almost every day is most beneficial for the hypertensive adult. In addition, smaller bouts of aerobic exercise, performed more frequently to accumulate >30 minutes per day of activity, is also effective. Equally important is the concept of a gradual progression because individuals with hypertension may

FITT

TABLE 15.7 FITT RECOMMENDATIONS FOR INDIVIDUALS WITH METABOLIC AND CARDIOVASCULAR CONDITIONS

ACSM FITT Principle of the ExR_x

Chronic Medical Condition	Frequency (How often?)	Intensity (How hard?)	Time	Type (What kind?) Primary	Resistance	Flexibility	Special Considerations
Healthy Adult	≥5 d · wk^{-1} of moderate exercise, or ≥3 d · wk^{-1} of vigorous exercise, or a combination of moderate and vigorous exercise on ≥3–5 d · wk^{-1} is recommended.	Moderate to vigorous. Light-to-moderate intensity exercise may be beneficial in deconditioned individuals.	If moderate intensity: ≥30 min · d^{-1} to total 150 min · wk^{-1}. If vigorous intensity: ≥20 min · d^{-1} to total 75 min · wk^{-1}.	Regular, purposeful exercise that involves major muscle groups and is continuous and rhythmic in nature is recommended.	Muscle strengthening 2–3 d · wk^{-1} (nonconsecutive) Moderate-to-vigorous intensity; 2–4 sets of 8–12 repetitions	2–3 d · wk^{-1}; static stretch 10–30 s; 2–4 repetitions of each exercise	Sedentary behaviors can have adverse health effects, even among those who regularly exercise. Adding short physical activity breaks throughout the day may be considered as a part of the exercise.
Hypertension	5–7 d · wk^{-1}	Moderate	≥30 min · d^{-1} of continuous or accumulated exercise with a minimum of 10 min bouts	Aerobic	Muscle strengthening 2–3 d · wk^{-1} (nonconsecutive) Moderate-to-vigorous intensity; 2–4 sets of 8–12 repetitions	2–3 d · wk^{-1}; static stretch 10–30 s; 2–4 repetitions of each exercise	Encourage patients to exercise in the morning to benefit from the immediately BP–lowering effects throughout the day. Emphasis should be on aerobic exercise activities.
Dyslipidemia	≥5 d · wk^{-1} to maximize caloric expenditure	Moderate	30–60 min · d^{-1} with greater benefits with weight loss (*i.e.*, 50–60 min · d^{-1})	Aerobic	Muscle strengthening 2–3 d · wk^{-1} (nonconsecutive) Moderate-to-vigorous intensity; 2–4 sets of 8–12 repetitions	2–3 d · wk^{-1}; static stretch 10–30 s; 2–4 repetitions of each exercise	A special focus should be on exercise that uses large muscle groups and maximizes caloric expenditure. Lipid-lowering medication (*i.e.*, statins and fibric acid) may cause muscle weakness and soreness (*i.e.*, myalgia).
Overweight and Obesity	≥5 d · wk^{-1}	Moderate to vigorous	30 min · d^{-1} to total 150 min · wk^{-1} increasing to 60 min · d^{-1} to total 250–300 min · wk^{-1}	Aerobic	Muscle strengthening 2–3 d · wk^{-1} moderate-to-vigorous intensity; 2–4 sets of 8–12 repetitions	2–3 d · wk^{-1}; static stretch 10–30 s; 2–4 repetitions of each exercise	Target a minimal reduction in body weight of at least 3%–10% over 3–6 mo. A reduction of energy intake by 500–1,000 kcal · d^{-1} is adequate to elicit weight loss of 1–2 lb · wk^{-1}. Prior history of orthopedic injuries should be assessed to reduce risk of injury.

ExR_x, exercise prescription

Based on the FITT Recommendations present in *ACSM's Guidelines for Exercise Testing and Prescription.* 10th ed. Philadelphia (PA): Wolters Kluwer; 2018. 480 p.

exhibit both exaggerated increases in BP during exercise as well as sudden drops in BP following exercise (the latter a particular concern among individuals medicated for hypertension using multiple BP-lowering drugs).

Similar to the exercise prescription for dyslipidemia, the exercise prescription for hypertension emphasizes aerobic exercise over resistance exercise. The emphasis placed on aerobic exercise represents the inconsistent evidence regarding the impact of resistance training on lowering resting BP (11). However, it should be noted that resistance training is safe and effective in adults with hypertension, although engaging in a prolonged Valsalva maneuver during resistance training (or any type of exercise) should be avoided because it transiently results in extremely high BP responses. In addition, 80% of individuals with hypertension are obese (19,20), and the caloric expenditure that can be maximized with aerobic exercise is another consideration for exercise prescription in adults with hypertension. Finally, because hypertension is the most important CVD risk factor, accounting for 40% of all CVD deaths (19), adults with hypertension may exhibit signs and symptoms of other cardiovascular pathologies. In addition, antihypertensive medications may impair thermoregulation and/or alter heart rate and fluid balance during exercise. Therefore, higher risk patient populations may warrant extra caution when designing and implementing exercise programs.

Dyslipidemia

The FITT principles for dyslipidemia encourage an emphasis on healthy weight maintenance such that energy expenditure during exercise training should be maximized for weight loss (see Table 15.7). Whereas guidelines for adults who are overweight/obese actually set standards for a reduction in body weight of at least 3%–10% over 3–6 months (by reducing energy intake 500–1,000 kcal $\cdot$ d^{-1}), guidelines for dyslipidemia simply emphasize whole-body, large muscle mass aerobic exercise on a regular basis, which facilitates greater caloric expenditure. It is worthwhile to note that the guidelines for dyslipidemia consider resistance training an adjunct to aerobic training, as data regarding the impact of resistance exercise on changes in blood lipids are equivocal and often confounded by concurrent changes in body weight and diet. However, in a systematic review of resistance training studies, 9 of 23 studies showed significant reductions in LDL-C ranging from 5% to 23% with at least 12 weeks of resistance training in otherwise healthy adults (31). Similarly, other meta-analyses have reported statistically significant reductions in both LDL-C and TG with resistance training (although no change in HDL-C) (17). Of note, emerging evidence suggests that a combination of aerobic and resistance training may evoke the most favorable alterations in lipid lipoproteins by concurrently augmenting HDL-C and lowering LDL-C (17,24). Consequently, resistance exercise training performed 2–3 days a week in addition to large muscle mass aerobic exercise may substantially improve blood lipid levels in individuals with dyslipidemia.

One other consideration for patients with dyslipidemia is the impact that statin therapy may have on skeletal muscle. Although statins are relatively well tolerated with few serious side effects, they are associated with a variety of muscle complaints such as weakness, pain, and cramps in approximately 5%–10% of patients (5,27). In addition, these statin-associated muscle symptoms (SAMS) may be exacerbated by exercise based on several reports indicating that athletes and/or physically active individuals are less likely to tolerate statin therapy (5) and creatine kinase levels (indicative of muscle damage) after exercise may be higher in athletes using statin therapy than those not using statin therapy (26,33). Therefore, adults using statin therapy who are initiating or increasing their exercise routine and experience unusual muscle symptoms repeatedly should be advised to consult with their physician because there are alternative dosing strategies/types of statin drugs that may mitigate SAMS.

Case Study 15-1 Quiz:

Exercise Prescription Considerations

6. Is the frequency of Mr. Case Study-BP's exercise prescription effective for treating his dyslipidemia and hypertension? Why or why not?
7. Should Mr. Case Study-BP have been advised to limit his resistance training to only body weight exercises such as sit-ups and push-ups? Why or why not?

SUMMARY

In general, exercise prescription for individuals with metabolic syndrome, hypertension, and dyslipidemia is safe and effective particularly because physical activity is a cornerstone of lifestyle treatment for all three conditions and prevents further progression into cardiovascular or metabolic disease. Indeed, these individuals stand to benefit the most from large amounts of routine aerobic physical activity to increase caloric expenditure and exposure to postexercise hypotension, and resistance training in conjunction with aerobic training maximizes metabolic benefits from habitual physical activity. Specific points include the following:

- Diet and lifestyle modifications may be as, if not more, important than pharmacological treatments for metabolic syndrome, hypertension, and dyslipidemia.
- Regular aerobic exercise of sufficient dose and frequency such as to encourage weight loss and daily postexercise hypotension form the basis of exercise prescription for these diseases.
- Resistance exercise, although less stringently quantified, may have equally important benefits, particularly for the treatment of dyslipidemia.
- Exercise preparticipation screening guidelines indicate that most asymptomatic individuals with these conditions are able to begin a low- to moderate-intensity exercise routine without additional medical clearance.
- Clinician oversight for the management of additional risk factors and concomitant medications can be helpful because metabolic syndrome, hypertension, and dyslipidemia are often comorbid with other cardiovascular and metabolic risk factors.

REFERENCES

1. Alberti KG, Eckel RH, Grundy SM, et al. Harmonizing the metabolic syndrome: a joint interim statement of the International Diabetes Federation Task Force on Epidemiology and Prevention; National Heart, Lung, and Blood Institute; American Heart Association; World Heart Federation; International Atherosclerosis Society; and International Association for the Study of Obesity. *Circulation*. 2009;120(16):1640–5.
2. American College of Sports Medicine. *Guidelines for Exercise Testing and Prescription*. 10th ed. Philadelphia (PA): Wolters Kluwer; 2018. 480 p.
3. American Diabetes Association. Standards of medical care in diabetes-2016 abridged for primary care providers. *Clin Diabetes*. 2016;34(1):3–21.
4. Arnarson A, Ramel A, Geirsdottir OG, Jonsson PV, Thorsdottir I. Changes in body composition and use of blood cholesterol lowering drugs predict changes in blood lipids during 12 weeks of resistance exercise training in old adults. *Aging Clin Exp Res*. 2014;26(3):287–92.

5. Bruckert E, Hayem G, Dejager S, Yau C, Bégaud B. Mild to moderate muscular symptoms with high-dosage statin therapy in hyperlipidemic patients — the PRIMO study. *Cardiovasc Drugs Ther.* 2005;19(6):403–14.
6. Cheng S, Xanthakis V, Sullivan LM, Vasan RS. Blood pressure tracking over the adult life course: patterns and correlates in the Framingham heart study. *Hypertension.* 2012;60(6):1393–9.
7. Chobanian AV, Bakris GL, Black HR, et al. The Seventh Report of the Joint National Committee on Prevention, Detection, Evaluation, and Treatment of High Blood Pressure: the JNC 7 report. *JAMA.* 2003;289(19):2560–71.
8. Colberg SR, Sigal RJ, Fernhall B, et al. Exercise and type 2 diabetes: the American College of Sports Medicine and the American Diabetes Association: joint position statement. *Diabetes Care.* 2010;33(12):e147–67.
9. Crim MT, Yoon SS, Ortiz E, et al. National surveillance definitions for hypertension prevalence and control among adults. *Circ Cardiovasc Qual Outcomes.* 2012;5(3):343–51.
10. Downs JR, Clearfield M, Weis S, et al. Primary prevention of acute coronary events with lovastatin in men and women with average cholesterol levels: results of AFCAPS/TexCAPS. *JAMA.* 1998;279(20):1615–22.
11. Eckel RH, Jakicic JM, Ard JD, et al. 2013 AHA/ACC guideline on lifestyle management to reduce cardiovascular risk: a report of the American College of Cardiology/American Heart Association Task Force on Practice Guidelines. *Circulation.* 2014;129(25 suppl 2):S76–99.
12. Eicher JD, Maresh CM, Tsongalis GJ, Thompson PD, Pescatello LS. The additive blood pressure lowering effects of exercise intensity on post-exercise hypotension. *Am Heart J.* 2010;160(3):513–20.
13. Expert Panel on Detection, Evaluation, and Treatment of High Blood Cholesterol in Adults. Executive summary of the third report of the National Cholesterol Education Program (NCEP) Expert Panel on Detection, Evaluation, and Treatment of High Blood Cholesterol in Adults (Adult Treatment Panel III). *JAMA.* 2001;285(19):2486–97.
14. Gami AS, Witt BJ, Howard DE, et al. Metabolic syndrome and risk of incident cardiovascular events and death: a systematic review and meta-analysis of longitudinal studies. *J Am Coll Cardiol.* 2007;49(4):403–14.
15. Grundy SM, Cleeman JI, Daniels SR, et al. Diagnosis and management of the metabolic syndrome: an American Heart Association/National Heart, Lung, and Blood Institute scientific statement. *Circulation.* 2005;112(17):2735–52.
16. James PA, Oparil S, Carter BL, et al. 2014 Evidence-based guideline for the management of high blood pressure in adults: report from the panel members appointed to the Eighth Joint National Committee (JNC 8). *JAMA.* 2014;311(5):507–20.
17. Kelley GA, Kelley KS. Impact of progressive resistance training on lipids and lipoproteins in adults: a meta-analysis of randomized controlled trials. *Prev Med.* 2009;48(1):9–19.
18. Kokkinos PF, Faselis C, Myers J, Panagiotakos D, Doumas M. Interactive effects of fitness and statin treatment on mortality risk in veterans with dyslipidaemia: a cohort study. *Lancet.* 2013;381(9864):394–9.
19. Lavie CJ, Milani RV, Ventura HO. Obesity and cardiovascular disease: risk factor, paradox, and impact of weight loss. *J Am Coll Cardiol.* 2009;53(21):1925–32.
20. Leon BM, Maddox TM. Diabetes and cardiovascular disease: epidemiology, biological mechanisms, treatment recommendations and future research. *World J Diabetes.* 2015;6(13):1246–58.
21. Mozaffarian D, Benjamin EJ, Go AS, et al. Heart disease and stroke statistics — 2016 update: a report from the American Heart Association. *Circulation.* 2016;133(4):e38–60.
22. Naci H, Ioannidis JP. Comparative effectiveness of exercise and drug interventions on mortality outcomes: metaepidemiological study. *Br J Sports Med.* 2015;49(21):1414–22.
23. National Center for Health Statistics Web site [Internet]. Atlanta (GA): Centers for Disease Control and Prevention; [cited 2015 Nov 20]. Available from: www.cdc.gov/nhs
24. Paoli A, Pacelli QF, Moro T, et al. Effects of high-intensity circuit training, low-intensity circuit training and endurance training on blood pressure and lipoproteins in middle-aged overweight men. *Lipids Health Dis.* 2013;12:131.
25. Parikh NI, Pencina MJ, Wang TJ, et al. A risk score for predicting near-term incidence of hypertension: the Framingham heart study. *Ann Intern Med.* 2008;148(2):102–10.
26. Parker BA, Augeri AL, Capizzi JA, et al. Effect of statins on creatine kinase levels before and after a marathon run. *Am J Cardiol.* 2012;109(2):282–7.
27. Parker BA, Capizzi JA, Grimaldi AS, et al. Effect of statins on skeletal muscle function. *Circulation.* 2013;127(1):96–103.
28. Pencina MJ, Navar-Boggan AM, D'Agostino RB Sr, et al. Application of new cholesterol guidelines to a population-based sample. *N Engl J Med.* 2014;370(15):1422–31.
29. Pescatello LS, Franklin BA, Fagard R, Farquhar WB, Kelley GA, Ray CA. American College of Sports Medicine position stand. Exercise and hypertension. *Med Sci Sports Exerc.* 2004;36(3):533–53.
30. Riebe D, Franklin BA, Thompson PD, et al. Updating ACSM's recommendations for exercise preparticipation health screening. *Med Sci Sports Exerc.* 2015;47(11):2473–9.
31. Scandinavian Simvastatin Survival Study Group. Randomised trial of cholesterol lowering in 4444 patients with coronary heart disease: the Scandinavian Simvastatin Survival Study (4S). *Lancet.* 1994;344(8934):1383–9.
32. Stone NJ, Robinson JG, Lichtenstein AH, et al. 2013 ACC/AHA guideline on the treatment of blood cholesterol to reduce atherosclerotic cardiovascular risk in adults: a report of the American College of Cardiology/American Heart Association Task Force on Practice Guidelines. *Circulation.* 2014;129(25 suppl 2):S1–45.

33. Thompson PD, Zmuda JM, Domalik LJ, Zimet RJ, Staggers J, Guyton JR. Lovastatin increases exercise-induced skeletal muscle injury. *Metabolism.* 1997;46(10):1206–10.
34. Wald DS, Law M, Morris JK, Bestwick JP, Wald NJ. Combination therapy versus monotherapy in reducing blood pressure: meta-analysis on 11,000 participants from 42 trials. *Am J Med.* 2009;122(3):290–300.
35. Wood D, De Backer G, Faergeman O, Graham I, Mancia G, Pyörälä K. Prevention of coronary heart disease in clinical practice. Summary of recommendations of the second joint task force of European and other societies on coronary prevention. *Blood Press.* 1998;7(5–6):262–9.

CHAPTER 16

Special Considerations for Chronic Obstructive Pulmonary Disease

INTRODUCTION

This chapter presents background, special considerations related to exercise testing, prescription, and progression for individuals with chronic obstructive pulmonary disease (COPD). The case study that follows outlines the results for an **older adult** woman with COPD who participated in a 12-week exercise program as part of a local hospital-based outpatient pulmonary rehabilitation (PR) program that included unsupervised exercise at home. This case study presents guidance for the design of a progressive **aerobic** conditioning and resistance training program with a primary goal of fully optimized exercise capacity, participation in **activities of daily living (ADL)**, adherence to long-term fitness training and **physical activity**, and maximum control and adaptation to disabling symptoms for an individual with stable COPD.

Case Study 16-1

Mrs. Case Study-COPD

Mrs. Case Study-COPD is a 66-year-old woman weighing 72 kg (158.7 lb) with a height of 152 cm (60 in) (**body mass index [BMI]** 31.2 kg · m^{-2}). She has a history of moderate COPD diagnosed 8 months ago following hospitalization for acute exacerbation of COPD. She has a history of hypertension, hyperlipidemia, hypothyroidism, gastroesophageal reflux disease (GERD), mild depression, and moderate obstructive sleep apnea (OSA). All comorbidities currently undergo regular evaluation, management, and follow-up by her primary care practitioner and are treated with medication. OSA is treated with nocturnal bilevel positive airway pressure. She denies any history of acute cardiovascular disease (CVD), diabetes, or cancer. She reports she has gained 10 lb since retiring 1 year ago. She is negative for α_1-antitrypsin deficiency. Risk factors for chronic lung disease include a 60 pack-year cigarette smoking history. She quit smoking 8 months ago during hospitalization and underwent cessation support in the community. She continues to take bupropion and has weaned off nicotine patch and gum without relapse, urge for relapse, or cravings. She denies any family history of heart disease, diabetes, or cancer. Her mother and brother died of COPD in their 70s. She retired 1 year ago as a stockbroker at a local firm to spend time with her aging father. Prior to retirement, she was physically active including walking 30 minutes most days. Her primary goal for an **exercise** program is to improve function and symptom control and reduce risk of disease worsening, physical decline, and/or hospitalization. She is divorced and attributes a high stress level to managing her finances postretirement. She lives alone and has 12 stairs at home. She feels unsteady at times and denies any history of falls. In addition to a history of smoking, her ex-husband and family "were all heavy smokers." She has no pets. She thinks she may be sensitive to pollen but has never undergone allergy testing. She currently reports being very short of breath when around secondhand smoke or perfume. Her respiratory medications at hospital discharge include tiotropium dry powder inhaler (DPI) 18 μg one inhalation daily, indacaterol 75 μg one inhalation daily, and albuterol metered-dose inhaler (MDI) at two inhalations every 4 hours as needed for dyspnea. She tapered off oral prednisone 2 weeks postdischarge. Other medications include hydrochlorothiazide, lisinopril, pravastatin, levothyroxine, pantoprazole, and bupropion. She has performed 12 weeks of exercise as part of outpatient PR combined with self-reported home exercise. She uses a wireless activity monitor to measure steps walked. Results from this training are presented as follows.

She was asymptomatic until 1 year ago, at which point she noticed dyspnea when walking up inclines and stairs. She attributed this to getting older and being out of shape following retirement. She notes an increase in fatigue over the past few months. She denies any history of chest discomfort or dizziness. During hospitalization, electrocardiogram (ECG) showed sinus rhythm with no ectopy. Transthoracic echo was unremarkable. Two weeks following hospital discharge, she underwent pulmonary evaluation with full pulmonary function testing and 6-minute walk test (6MWT) (Table 16.1 and Box 16.1). On her current medication, she denies dyspnea at rest and has 2–3/10 category/ratio (CR) dyspnea with walking, 6–7/10 during bending over, carrying groceries, vacuuming, house work, gardening, bathing, and dressing. Her dyspnea is 7–8/10 with stairs and inclines.

Table 16.1 Pulmonary Function Testing Results: Mrs. Case Study-COPD

	Prebronchodilator		Postbronchodilator		
	Predicted	Measured	% Predicted	Measured	% Change
FVC (L)	4.41	3.32	76	75	−1
$FEV_{1.0}$ (L)	3.17	2.07	65	2.10	2
$FEV_{1.0}$/FVC	72	62		63	1

(continues)

Case Study 16-1 (continued)

Box 16.1 Six-Minute Walk Test Results: Mrs. Case Study-COPD

A series of two 6MWTs were administered. During the initial 6MWT, Mrs. Case Study-COPD had a resting SpO_2 of 94% on room air; however, she experienced desaturation to 85% on room air after 1 minute of walking. The test was stopped and, following 20 minutes of rest, was restarted exclusively to adjust her oxygen levels. Her oxygen flow rate was titrated to a setting of 3 obtained from an intermittent oxygen delivery device; yielding an SpO_2 of 90%–91% during the 6MWT.

Following 20 minutes of rest, a 6MWT was performed to evaluate functional capacity. She walked 287 m (943 ft) using pulse flow oxygen while carrying a portable M6 oxygen tank. Testing followed ATS/ERS field test standards and protocol (1). Average speed was approximately 1.79 mph. Her resting HR was 72 bpm and peak HR was 123 bpm. SpO_2 at an oxygen setting of 3 fell to 90%. Maximum dyspnea was 6/10 Borg CR dyspnea scale.

Muscle **strength** was measured using **one repetition maximum (1-RM)** method according to accepted standards for leg press, shoulder press, leg extension, latissimus dorsi pull-down, and biceps curl exercises.

Mrs. Case Study-COPD performed the following exercise prescription/progression for 12 weeks at PR and was given a home exercise prescription based on her exercise results in the PR program. She plans to exercise at a local gym and agrees to attend PR maintenance exercise monthly.

Her PR exercise training program consisted of supervised aerobic and resistance training 2 days a week for 12 weeks. During the PR training program, oxygen saturation (SpO_2), dyspnea, heart rate (HR), and blood pressure (BP) were monitored preexercise, during, and postexercise. Aerobic exercise was performed with warm-up and cool-down periods in which exercise intensity was gradually increased and decreased over 5 minutes prior to and at the end of the endurance training period. She progressed over 12 weeks to walking 20 minutes on the treadmill at maximum speed of 2.2 mph (59 m · min^{-1}) and stationary bike for 10 minutes at a dyspnea score level of 2/10 on a 10-point Borg CR scale. Exercise intensity and tolerance were evaluated and maintained using a CR dyspnea rating of 4–6/10 during exercise. Increases in aerobic exercise were initially made in duration until a total duration of all aerobic modes of 30 minutes per session was achieved, followed by incremental increase in intensity. Only one variable was increased at each time with increases followed by reassessment of SpO_2, dyspnea, HR, and BP. Resistance exercises included arm and ankle weights, sit-to-stand exercises, and wall push-ups. Wall push-ups were progressed to table push-ups after 3 weeks. Hand and leg weight training included shoulder press, lateral pull-down, biceps curl, sitting row, and leg extension with the following percentages of 1-RM intensity: week 1 at 50%, week 2 at 60%, week 3 at 70%, and weeks 4–12 at 80% (Table 16.2). Given her history of deconditioning, balance training exercises were added.

Table 16.2 describes the exercise program guidelines recommended for Mrs. Case Study-COPD during transition from PR to her fitness center. Her maintenance exercise was augmented by monthly "tune-up" visits at her local PR maintenance program. She continues to track daily steps using a wireless step counter and meets with her former PR classmates weekly for a 30-minute mall walk followed by coffee. At the PR maintenance 2 months following PR, dumbbell lunges were added at five repetitions, each to be used 3 nonconsecutive days per week. Ongoing adherence to exercise prescription is a significant clinical concern and requires behavior change and ongoing re-evaluation to promote long-term benefits. Although this area requires further research, considerations for long-term adherence include group exercise such as PR maintenance programs, community-based exercise programs, and home exercise programs that include clinical ongoing follow-up, support, problem solving, and consideration of activity monitoring.

Case Study 16-1 (continued)

Table 16.2 Progressive Resistance Training Program for Weeks 1–12 for Mrs. Case Study-COPD

Week	Monday (% RM, Sets × Repetitions)	Friday (% RM, Sets × Repetitions)
1	Baseline 1-RM testing	50, 2 × 12 of above upper and lower extremity exercises
2	60, 2 × 10	60, 2 × 10
3	70, 2 × 8	80, 2 × 8
4[a]	80, 2 × 8	80, 2 × 8
5	80, 1 × 8	1-RM testing
6–8	60, 2 × 8	70, 2 × 8
9	80, 1 × 8	80, 2 × 8
10–11	60, 2 × 8	70, 3 × 8
12	80, 1 × 8	1-RM testing

[a]Resistance exercises included arm and ankle weights, sit-to-stand exercises, and wall push-ups. Note that wall push-ups were progressed to table push-ups after 3 weeks. Hand and leg weight training included shoulder press, lateral pull-down, biceps curl, sitting row, and leg extension.

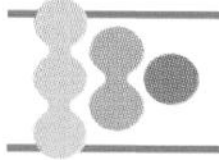

Description, Prevalence, and Etiology

COPD is a common, treatable, preventable, progressive disorder characterized by chronic airway inflammation and progressive airflow limitation (14). Pathological changes have an impact on airways, lung parenchyma, and pulmonary vasculature depending on the COPD subtype (*e.g.*, chronic bronchitis and/or emphysema) (14). The World Health Organization estimates that 65 million people worldwide have moderate-to-severe COPD (39). COPD is a major cause of morbidity and mortality (14); it is now the third leading cause of death in the United States and the only major cause that is on the rise (18). A history of smoking tobacco is the most important risk factor for COPD; other less common risk factors include biomass exposure and occupational exposures. Exacerbations and comorbidities may contribute to disease impact. Common comorbidities include CVD, osteoporosis, anxiety/depression, lung cancer, infections, and diabetes mellitus (14). A clinical diagnosis of COPD should be considered in persons aged ≥40 years with dyspnea, chronic cough or sputum production, and a history of exposure to risk factors (tobacco smoke, occupational smoke, dust, chemicals, indoor air pollution, and/or family history of COPD) (14). Accurate diagnosis and assessment of severity requires spirometry and, often, full pulmonary function testing. The presence of significant expiratory airflow limitation, the hallmark of the disease, is assessed by spirometry. Forced expiratory volume in 1 second ($FEV_{1.0}$)/forced vital capacity (FVC) ratio <0.7 is considered diagnostic of COPD and the severity or degree of airflow impairment as defined by the percentage of the predicted value of $FEV_{1.0}$ (Table 16.3).

Once COPD has been diagnosed, questionnaires may be used to assess symptoms and health status. The Global Initiative for Chronic Obstructive Lung Disease (GOLD) guidelines (14) recommend the modified British Medical Research Council (mMRC) questionnaire (20) to assess dyspnea and the COPD Assessment Test (5) to evaluate the impact of symptoms on patient health status.

Table 16.3 Global Initiative for Chronic Obstructive Pulmonary Disease Spirometric Classification of Severity in COPD Based on the $FEV_{1.0}$

Severity	Postbronchodilator $FEV_{1.0}$/FVC	Postbronchodilator $FEV_{1.0}$ Percentage
Mild	<0.70	$FEV_{1.0}$ ≥80% predicted
Moderate	<0.70	50% ≤$FEV_{1.0}$ <80% predicted
Severe	<0.70	30% ≤$FEV_{1.0}$ <50% predicted
Very severe	<0.70	$FEV_{1.0}$ <30% of predicted or $FEV_{1.0}$ <50% predicted + respiratory failure

From Global Initiative for Chronic Obstructive Lung Disease. Global strategy for the diagnosis, management and prevention of COPD 2015 [Internet]. Fontana (WI): Global Initiative for Chronic Obstructive Lung Disease; [cited 2015 Jul 12]. Available from: http://www.goldcopd.org/

In terms of exercise limitations, COPD is associated with disabling symptoms including dyspnea and fatigue, which are often worse with exertion (14). Clinical abnormalities include skeletal muscle dysfunction, exercise intolerance, and significant morbidity and mortality (19,28,32,33). These impairments may be worsened by and negatively affect physical activity (12). Decline in regular physical activity and exercise over time results in **deconditioning** (disuse atrophy of the muscles of ambulation), increased dyspnea at lower levels of exertion, and greater functional impairment and disability (27,34,38). Exposure to systemic corticosteroids may also contribute to muscle dysfunction. Deconditioning due to **physical inactivity** is a major rationale for exercise training as part of comprehensive PR.

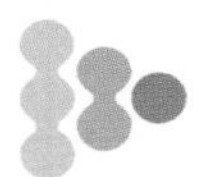

Preparticipation Health Screening, Medical History, and Physical Examination

Accurate diagnosis begins with history and physical examination, including history of irritant (smoking, etc.) and allergen exposure, symptoms including dyspnea (rest and/or with exertion), cough and/or wheeze, fatigue, dizziness, and pain. A recent physical examination by a physician and, at a minimum, a recent 12-lead ECG are required. An echocardiogram or similar testing should be obtained in any patient at risk for heart disease. Current or recent CVD requires diagnostic testing and cardiology evaluation with clearance prior to beginning an exercise program. All identified comorbidities should be optimally managed prior to initiating an exercise program.

Optimizing pulmonary mechanics before implementing an exercise program is essential for patients with COPD. Medication management, adherence, and side effects should be assessed. Inhalation is the route of choice for bronchodilators and maintenance corticosteroids. Standard medical therapy for mild COPD includes, at a minimum, a rescue short-acting bronchodilator (usually albuterol, levalbuterol, and/or combination albuterol/ipratropium). Pharmacological management of moderate COPD includes at least one long-acting bronchodilator (usually a long-acting β-agonist and/or a long-acting anticholinergic inhaler) (14). A growing number of long-acting β-agonists, anticholinergics, and inhaled corticosteroids alone or in combination are available to improve both effectiveness and convenience of care tailored to severity of COPD and related symptoms. Those with severe COPD or who are experiencing frequent exacerbations are generally additionally treated with inhaled corticosteroids. Ongoing patient training and assessment to insure effective inhaler technique and adherence to medication regimen is required. Patients unable to demonstrate proper inhaler technique should be considered for a holding chamber.

Patients with COPD may experience hypoxemia during rest, ADL, exercise, and/or sleep. Hypoxemia can result from ventilation/perfusion mismatch, diffusion defect, right-to-left shunt, or alveolar hypoventilation. In COPD, hypoxemia at rest or during low-level exertion is typically caused by ventilation/perfusion mismatch (37). At high exercise intensities, a diffusion deficit may become a contributing factor (16). Supplemental oxygen is usually capable of restoring normal oxygenation. Patients with a right-to-left shunt have a more limited response to supplemental oxygen (9). Hypoxemia may also be triggered by depressed ventilatory drive and is typically accompanied by hypercapnia and low pH. Chronically low ventilatory drive (chronic respiratory acidosis) is associated with hypercapnia and near-normal pH. Hypoxemia is often aggravated with exposure to high altitude or during disease exacerbation. Evaluation of hypoxemia begins with a comprehensive history and physical examination and includes arterial blood gas (ABG) sampling or, at a minimum, noninvasive measurement of arterial oxygen saturation level with a pulse oximeter. Pulse oximetry, however, does not provide information about acid–base balance, carbon dioxide, or bicarbonate levels. Evaluation of hypoxemia during exercise may be performed using either ABG sampling or, more commonly, pulse oximetry (24).

During exercise, demand for oxygen by working muscle increases in proportion to the level of work performed (2). This results in a higher cardiopulmonary demand to deliver oxygen to muscle fibers. For normal individuals, delivery of oxygen (cardiac output × arterial oxygen content) to tissues is regulated by changing cardiac output to meet the metabolic demand of exercise; pulmonary ventilation is increased to prevent decreases in arterial oxygen content. In chronic lung disease, the ability of the lungs to maintain arterial oxygen content may be impaired, resulting in impaired oxygen delivery and reduced exercise ability.

Supplemental oxygen can increase arterial oxygen content (thereby improving tissue oxygen delivery), decrease carotid body stimulation (thereby reducing pulmonary ventilation, respiratory muscle work, and dyspnea), and relieve pulmonary vasoconstriction (thereby alleviating cardiac output restriction). Oxygen improves the effectiveness of short- and long-term exercise training in hypoxemic patients with COPD by reducing dyspnea, hypoxic ventilatory drive, and hyperinflation and by delaying acidosis. Supplemental oxygen allows rehabilitation participants to exercise at higher work rates during their training program. Ambulatory oxygen equipment has the potential to increase mobility, adherence, exercise tolerance, and autonomy in hypoxemic patients. Patients requiring oxygen should undergo titration as part of PR, preferably using the patient's own ambulatory oxygen system.

Case Study 16-1 Quiz:

Preparticipation Health Screening, Medical History, and Physical Examination

1. Describe criteria for diagnosis and severity of COPD.
2. Identify three factors that affect COPD diagnosis and/or progression.

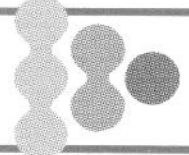

Exercise Testing Considerations

Evaluation of exercise tolerance may be provided by use of a cardiopulmonary exercise test (CPET) or field test such as 6MWT. Although the rationale for CPET is substantial, many programs lack access to this testing and use 6MWT to evaluate functional performance. After medical evaluation and optimization of bronchodilator and oxygen therapy, a CPET may offer important insights into limitations to exercise, potential safety of exercise, and information for developing the exercise prescription. Testing is done on a treadmill or an electronically braked cycle ergometer. Incremental exercise tests may be used to assess cardiopulmonary function with modifications of traditional protocols (*e.g.*, slower work rate increments) depending on functional limitations and the onset of dyspnea. A test duration of 8–12 minutes is optimal in those with mild-to-moderate COPD (7); a somewhat shorter duration may be satisfactory for patients with severe and very severe disease (4). During testing, subjects breathe through a mouthpiece allowing ventilation and gas exchange to be measured breath by breath. Continuous measurements of pulse oximetry and 12-lead ECG are commonly obtained. Diagnostic algorithms have been established to allow detection of cardiovascular, ventilator, and gas exchange limitations to exercise.

If a CPET is not an option, **submaximal** field testing such a 6MWT or shuttle walk test (15) can provide some helpful information for establishing the exercise prescription and for ongoing monitoring of progress. The 6MWT is a simple, inexpensive method to assess functional exercise performance and response to PR in persons with COPD. The test is considered valid, reliable, and responsive to rehabilitative interventions (15). The American Thoracic Society (ATS)/European Respiratory Society (ERS) 2014 protocol should be followed carefully (15). All variables should be consistent during the initial and post-rehabilitation tests, including test location, track layout and length, staffing, time of day, oxygen (flow rate, system, and transport), medications, use of usual walking aides, encouragement, and indications for stopping the test. The protocol includes patient instruction, scripts, and standardized encouragement. According to the ATS/ERS field test statement, the 6MWT has an excellent safety profile when standard protocols are used, including test cessation if the SpO_2 is below 80%. Contraindications and precautions for field walking tests are the same as CPET (1). It deserves mention, however, that 6MWT will not detect cardiac abnormalities (*e.g.*, exercise-induced hypertension, cardiac ischemia, and arrhythmias) that might be important considerations when initiating an exercise program.

The 6MWT is a self-paced test of walking performance; the distance walked is the primary test outcome. The patient is instructed to walk as far as possible in 6 minutes along a flat hallway (14). The SpO_2 and HR are measured continuously during testing, and the SpO_2 nadir and end-test HR are recorded. SpO_2 measurements during 6MWT are reliable provided that an adequate pulse signal is present (1). Dyspnea and subjective fatigue are measured before and after the 6MWT using validated measurement scales, such as the Borg CR scale. The 6MWT report should include the distance walked, number of rests during the test, total time stopped, SpO_2 nadir, and end-test pulse rate. The 6MWT is associated with considerable learning effect; therefore, two tests should be performed during initial testing with the greatest distance of the two tests used. The minimal important difference for the 6MWT in adults with chronic respiratory disease is between 25 m (82 ft) and 33 m (106 ft) with a median value across trials of 30 m (98 ft) (1).

The shuttle walk test also described in the ATS/ERS 2014 field test statement requires only a 10-m (32-ft) course; however, it does involve the addition of a prerecorded audio signal in order to cue the patient to an increasing pace. Assessment of its validity and reliability has been primarily in patients with COPD (1).

Case Study 16-1 Quiz:

Exercise Testing

3. What are the intended actions and their potential impact on clinical management of the three inhaled respiratory medications prescribed for the case study patient for control of her pulmonary disease?
4. Describe the rationale for performing a 6MWT in this patient. Was the protocol followed correctly?
5. What monitoring and interventions are needed for a patient with COPD and history of hypoxemia for exercise to be safe?

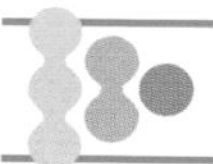

Exercise Prescription and Progression Considerations

General guidelines for **exercise prescription** and progression for individuals with COPD are presented in frequency, intensity, time, and type (FITT) table (Table 16.4). A comprehensive exercise program for persons with COPD should include individualized application of the FITT methodology based on the patient's exercise testing results, functional and cognitive capabilities, disease-specific limitations, and clinical and patient goals. Intensity and duration guidelines should be considered together because they dictate the total energy expenditure of an exercise session.

Appropriate warm-up and cool-down are essential for this population and should include whole-body and low- to moderate-intensity cardiorespiratory and local muscle endurance exercise to provide a gradual transition to higher intensity exercise performed during the conditioning phase. Stretching exercise should be considered as a distinct segment and performed before warm-up and after cool-down exercise. Three to 5 days per week of endurance exercise training is recommended (35,40), and at least two sessions (35) per week should be supervised by clinical exercise professionals (35).

CPET provides symptom scores, symptom-limited maximum HR, and maximum work rate that may be used to develop exercise intensity prescription. The anaerobic or lactate threshold (the oxygen uptake at which lactic acidosis becomes prominent) may also be utilized (8). When CPET is not available, symptom scores (*e.g.*, rating of perceived exertion [RPE], dyspnea scales) may be used to establish training intensities. Dyspnea scores provide self-adjusting anchors for intensity prescriptions. Intensity targets of 12–14 on the traditional 0–20 Borg RPE scale or 4–6 on the Borg 0–10 CR scale (2–4,6,7,9,16,24,26,30,37) have been used (26). Regular monitoring of SpO_2 is needed and should be maintained at ≥88% by the use of supplemental oxygen if needed (40). This enables higher intensity exercise to be sustained for longer periods.

In terms of duration, no specific guidelines for exercise duration have been established for patients with COPD beyond the initial goal of 30 (range 20–60) minutes progressing to 60–90 minutes as tolerated. Individuals with moderate or severe COPD may only tolerate a few minutes initially.

Lower extremity exercise such as walking, including use of treadmills, has practical value in improving performance of the muscles of ambulation. Cycle ergometry can be used to vary the exercise mode and may be preferred in patients with arthritis, joint deformities, impaired balance, or morbid obesity because of its low impact on the musculoskeletal system. Other modes of endurance exercise training include indoor or outdoor walking, rowing, arm ergometry, stepping, swimming, water aerobics, modified aerobic dance, and seated aerobics (40). In COPD, arm exercise may be poorly tolerated because the auxiliary muscles of respiration are involved in performing tasks using the arms. Current guidelines (35) support the use of upper extremity exercise specifically for developing upper limb exercise capacity, upper extremity ADL performance, and reducing ventilation and oxygen cost (22). Although evidence is limited, both free-weight exercises and arm ergometry are recommended for improving ADL. No studies have identified an optimal upper extremity training regimen (22). The exercise prescription for resistance training should follow the FITT principle for healthy adults and/or older adults.

Recent evidence-based and scientific guidelines for PR (40) emphasize the importance of resistance exercise training for increasing muscle strength and mass of both upper and lower extremities. There is no consensus regarding the characteristics of an optimal resistance training program for patients with COPD. The current recommendation for resistance training intensity in older individuals is 60%–70% of 1-RM or a weight that allows the individual to perform 10–15 repetitions. These intensities have been shown to be safe in patients with COPD when provided by experienced personnel (21). The 1-RM is a highly effort-dependent measure requiring **maximal** force production. An alternative strategy calls for guiding resistance training intensity using perceptual ratings in which moderate exercise is rated at 5–6 and high intensity at 7–8 on a 10-point scale (25).

FITT

TABLE 16.4 FITT RECOMMENDATIONS FOR INDIVIDUALS WITH CHRONIC OBSTRUCTIVE PULMONARY DISEASE

ACSM FITT Principle of the ExR_x

Chronic Medical Condition	Frequency (How often?)	Intensity (How hard?)	Time	Type (What kind?) Primary	Resistance	Flexibility	Special Considerations
Healthy Adult	≥5 d · wk^{-1} of moderate exercise, or ≥3 d · wk^{-1} of vigorous exercise, or a combination of moderate and vigorous exercise on ≥3–5 d · wk^{-1} is recommended.	Moderate to vigorous. Light-to-moderate intensity exercise may be beneficial in deconditioned individuals.	If moderate intensity: ≥30 min · d^{-1} to total 150 min · wk^{-1}. If vigorous intensity: ≥20 min · d^{-1} to total 75 min · wk^{-1}.	Regular, purposeful exercise that involves major muscle groups and is continuous and rhythmic in nature is recommended.	2–3 d · wk^{-1} (nonconsecutive)	2–3 d · wk^{-1}; static stretch 10–30 s; 2–4 repetitions of each exercise	Sedentary behaviors can have adverse health effects, even among those who regularly exercise. Adding short physical activity breaks throughout the day may be considered as a part of the exercise.
Chronic Obstructive Pulmonary Disease	3–5 d · wk^{-1}	Moderate-to-vigorous intensity (60%–80% peak work rate or 4–6 on the Borg CR-10 scale)	20–60 min · d^{-1} at moderate-to-high intensities as tolerated. If the 20–60 min durations are not achievable, accumulate ≥20 min of exercise interspersed with intermittent exercise/rest periods of lower intensity work or rest.	Common aerobic modes including walking (free or treadmill), stationary cycling, and upper ergometry	2–3 d · wk^{-1} at 60%–70% 1-RM for beginners Experienced weight trainers: ≥80% Endurance: <50% of 1-RM Strength: 2–4 sets, 8–12 reps Endurance: ≤2 sets 15–20 reps Weight machines, free weights, or body weight exercises	≥2–3 d · wk^{-1} with daily being the most effective Static, dynamic, and/or PNF stretching Stretch to the point of feeling tightness or slight discomfort. 10–30 s hold for static stretching 2–4 repetitions of each exercise	Preexercise assessment of the patient should include dyspnea, SpO_2, HR, and BP in addition to recording body weight, unusual dyspnea, fatigue with usual activity, and pain. The use of oximetry is recommended for the initial exercise training sessions to evaluate possible exercise-induced oxyhemoglobin desaturation and to identify the work rate at which desaturation occurs.

ExR_x, exercise prescription; PNF, proprioceptive neuromuscular facilitation.

Based on the FITT Recommendations present in *ACSM's Guidelines for Exercise Testing and Prescription*. 10th ed. Philadelphia (PA): Wolters Kluwer; 2018. 480 p.

The resistance training portion of a comprehensive PR program can be completed within 20–40 minutes, assuming one set of 8–12 repetitions performed for 8–10 exercises interspersed with 2–3 minutes rest between sets (36). This estimate may be modified based on disease severity and program design. The number and choice of exercises should be based on patient goals and needs assessment (*e.g.*, improving ability to climb stairs) and contraindications such as arthritic joints or osteoporosis. A seated leg press exercise or repetitions of sit to stand while holding progressively heavier weights may be more appropriate than weight squats. The rest interval between sets should typically be 2–3 minutes in duration.

Choice of equipment for resistance training is often dictated by availability, patient tolerance, and safety. Some types of weight machines have excessive resistances or weights that are in increments that are too large for some patients with significant **sarcopenia**, weakness, and/or disabling symptoms.

The functional and clinical benefits of enhanced **flexibility** are not well established, and no specific guidelines for persons with chronic respiratory diseases are available. A summary of exercise training and prescription considerations for individuals with COPD is presented as follows:

- Preexercise assessment of the patient should include dyspnea, SpO_2, HR, and BP in addition to recording body weight, unusual dyspnea, fatigue with usual activity, and pain.
- Pay attention to providing sufficient warm-up and cool-down for patients with COPD.
- Higher intensities yield greater physiological benefits (*e.g.*, reduced minute ventilation and HR at a given work rate) and should be encouraged when appropriate (1,11).
- For patients with mild COPD, intensity guidelines for healthy older adults are appropriate. For those with moderate-to-severe COPD, intensities representing >60% peak work rate in an incremental test have been recommended (35).
- Light-intensity aerobic exercise may be appropriate initially for persons with severe COPD or significant deconditioning. Intensity may be increased as tolerated within the target time window.
- As an alternative to using peak work rate or peak oxygen uptake ($\dot{V}O_{2peak}$) to determine exercise intensity, dyspnea ratings of between 4 and 6 on the Borg CR10 scale may be used (17,35). A dyspnea rating between 3 and 6 on the Borg CR10 scale has been shown to correspond, on average, to 53% and 80% of $\dot{V}O_{2peak}$, respectively (17).
- The use of oximetry is recommended for the initial exercise training sessions to evaluate possible exercise-induced oxyhemoglobin desaturation and to identify the work rate at which desaturation occurs.
- Regardless of the prescribed exercise intensity, the exercise professional should closely monitor initial exercise sessions and adjust intensity and duration according to individual responses and tolerance. In many cases, the presence of symptoms, particularly dyspnea/breathlessness, supersedes objective methods of exercise prescription.
- Peripheral muscle dysfunction contributes to exercise intolerance (23) and is significantly and independently related to increased use of health care resources and poorer prognosis (10,31).
- Maximizing pulmonary function using bronchodilators before exercise training in those with airflow limitation can reduce dyspnea and improve exercise tolerance (35).
- Because individuals with COPD may experience greater dyspnea while performing ADL involving the upper extremities, include resistance exercises for the muscles of the upper body.
- Supplemental oxygen is indicated for patients with a partial pressure of arterial oxygen (P_aO_2) $\leq$55 mm Hg or an SpO_2 $\leq$88% while breathing room air (29), including during exercise. In patients using ambulatory supplemental oxygen, flow rates will likely need to be increased during exercise to maintain SpO_2 >88%. There is evidence to suggest that the administration of supplemental oxygen to those who do not experience exercise-induced hypoxemia may lead to greater gains in exercise endurance, particularly during high-intensity exercise (13,30,35).

Case Study 16-1 Quiz:

Exercise Prescription and Progression Considerations

6. Compare and contrast the application of the FITT principle in the given case study with the recommendations as presented in the *ACSM's Guidelines for Exercise Testing and Prescription, 10th edition* (*GETP10*) (Chapter 9). Identify any significant differences and discuss whether you agree or disagree with these different applications of the FITT recommendations. Justify your answer.
7. Can you suggest other exercises that would be beneficial for this patient given the goal to reduce disability and symptoms?

SUMMARY

This chapter presents relevant information regarding exercise testing, prescription, and progression recommendations for individuals with COPD.

- Exercise in COPD, particularly as part of PR, is the standard of care for COPD and is associated with improvement in function, dyspnea, health-related quality of life, and mood.
- Behavior change assuring long-term adherence to exercise is required.
- Patients require complete preexercise evaluation that includes evaluation and optimization of lung disease and comorbidities.
- The cornerstone of effective medication management of COPD is bronchodilation with long-acting anticholinergics and/or β-agonists.
- Safe exercise in the PR setting requires risk stratification, physician supervision, and staff competency in effective management of clinical abnormalities and facility support for an emergency response scenario.
- A case study is presented as a means to clarify the concepts discussed. It should be noted that COPD often exists with other comorbidities such as CVD (see Chapter 10), diabetes (see Chapter 14), and aging (see Chapter 9), so the clinician working with patients with COPD should be familiar with the exercise testing, prescription, and progressions for these other special populations.

REFERENCES

1. American College of Sports Medicine. *ACSM's Guidelines for Exercise Testing and Prescription*. 10th ed. Philadelphia (PA): Wolters Kluwer; 2018. 480 p.
2. Astrand PO, Rodahl K. *Textbook of Work Physiology: Physiological Bases of Exercise*. New York (NY): McGraw Hill; 1977. 456 p.
3. Beauchamp MK, Nonoyama M, Goldstein RS, et al. Interval versus continuous training in individuals with chronic obstructive pulmonary disease — a systematic review. *Thorax*. 2010;65(2):157–64.
4. Benzo RP, Paramesh S, Patel SA, Slivka WA, Sciurba FC. Optimal protocol selection for cardiopulmonary exercise testing in severe COPD. *Chest*. 2007;132(5):1500–5.
5. Bestall JC, Paul EA, Garrod R, Garnham R, Jones PW, Wedzicha JA. Usefulness of the Medical Research Council (MRC) dyspnoea scale as a measure of disability in patients with chronic obstructive pulmonary disease. *Thorax*. 1999;54(7):581–6.
6. Borg G. *Borg's Perceived Exertion and Pain Scales*. Champaign (IL): Human Kinetics; 1998. 104 p.

7. Buchfuhrer MJ, Hansen JE, Robinson TE, Sue DY, Wasserman K, Whipp BJ. Optimizing the exercise protocol for cardiopulmonary assessment. *J Appl Physiol Respir Environ Exerc Physiol.* 1983;55(5):1558–64.
8. Casaburi R, Patessio A, Ioli F, Zanaboni S, Donner CF, Wasserman K. Reductions in exercise lactic acidosis and ventilation as a result of exercise training in patients with obstructive lung disease. *Am Rev Respir Dis.* 1991;143(1):9–18.
9. Chetty KG, Dick C, McGovern J, Conroy RM, Mahutte CK. Refractory hypoxemia due to intrapulmonary shunting associated with bronchioloalveolar carcinoma. *Chest.* 1997;111(4):1120–1.
10. Decramer M, Gosselink R, Troosters T, Verschueren M, Evers G. Muscle weakness is related to utilization of health care resources in COPD patients. *Eur Respir J.* 1997;10:417–23.
11. Després JP, Lamarche B. Low-intensity endurance exercise training, plasma lipoproteins and the risk of coronary heart disease. *J Intern Med.* 1994;236(1):7–22.
12. Divo M, Cote C, de Torres JP, et al. Comorbidities and risk of mortality in patients with chronic obstructive pulmonary disease. *Am J Respir Crit Care Med.* 2012;186(2):155–61.
13. Emtner M, Porszasz J, Burns M, Somfay A, Casaburi R. Benefits of supplemental oxygen in exercise training in nonhypoxemic chronic obstructive pulmonary disease patients. *Am J Respir Crit Care Med.* 2003;168(9):1034–42.
14. Global Initiative for Chronic Obstructive Lung Disease. Global strategy for the diagnosis, management and prevention of COPD 2015 [Internet]. Fontana (WI): Global Initiative for Chronic Obstructive Lung Disease; [cited 2015 Jul 12]. Available from: http://www.goldcopd.org/
15. Holland AE, Spruit MA, Thierry T, et al. An official European Respiratory Society/American Thoracic Society technical standard: field walking tests in chronic respiratory disease. *Eur Respir J.* 2014;44:1428–46.
16. Hopkins SR. Exercise induced arterial hypoxemia: the role of ventilation-perfusion inequality and pulmonary diffusion limitation. *Adv Exp Med Biol.* 2006;588:17–30.
17. Horowitz MB, Littenberg B, Mahler DA. Dyspnea ratings for prescribing exercise intensity in patients with COPD. *Chest.* 1996;109(5):1169–75.
18. Hoyert DL, Xu JQ. Deaths: preliminary data for 2011. *Natl Vital Stat Rep.* 2012;61(6):1–65.
19. Jones PW, Brusselle G, Dal Negro RW, et al. Health-related quality of life in patients by COPD severity within primary care in Europe. *Respir Med.* 2011;105(1):57–66.
20. Jones PW, Harding G, Berry P, Wiklund I, Chen WH, Kline Leidy N. Development and first validation of the COPD Assessment Test. *Eur Respir J.* 2009;34(3):648–54.
21. Kaelin ME, Swank AM, Adams KJ, Barnard KL, Berning JM, Green A. Cardiopulmonary responses, muscle soreness, and injury during the one repetition maximum assessment in pulmonary rehabilitation patients. *J Cardiopulm Rehabil.* 1999;19(6):366–72.
22. Langer D, Hendriks E, Burtin C, et al. A clinical practice guideline for physiotherapists treating patients with chronic obstructive pulmonary disease based on a systematic review of available evidence. *Clin Rehabil.* 2009;23(5):445–62.
23. Maltais F, Decramer M, Casaburi R, et al. An official American Thoracic Society/European Respiratory Society statement: update on limb muscle dysfunction in chronic obstructive pulmonary disease. *Am J Respir Crit Care Med.* 2014;189(9):e15–62.
24. Mengelkoch LJ, Martin D, Lawler J. A review of the principles of pulse oximetry and accuracy of pulse oximeter estimates during exercise. *Phys Ther.* 1994;74(1):40–9.
25. Nelson ME, Rejeski WJ, Blair SN, et al. Physical activity and public health in older adults: recommendation from the American College of Sports Medicine and the American Heart Association. *Med Sci Sports Exerc.* 2007;39(8):1435–45.
26. Nici L, Donner C, Wouters E, et al. American Thoracic Society/European Respiratory Society statement on pulmonary rehabilitation. *Am J Respir Crit Care Med.* 2006;173(12):1390–413.
27. Polkey MI, Moxham J. Attacking the disease spiral in chronic obstructive pulmonary disease: an update. *Clin Med (Lond).* 2011;11(5):461–4.
28. Porszasz J, Emtner M, Goto S, et al. Exercise training decreases ventilatory requirements and exercise-induced hyperinflation at submaximal intensities in patients with COPD. *Chest.* 2005;128(4):2025–34.
29. Qaseem A, Wilt TJ, Weinberger SE, et al. Diagnosis and management of stable chronic obstructive pulmonary disease: a clinical practice guideline update from the American College of Physicians, American College of Chest Physicians, American Thoracic Society, and European Respiratory Society. *Ann Intern Med.* 2011;155:179–91.
30. Ries AL, Bauldoff GS, Carlin BW, et al. Pulmonary rehabilitation: joint ACCP/AACVPR evidence-based clinical practice guidelines. *Chest.* 2007;131:4S–42S.
31. Schols AM, Soeters PB, Dingemans AM, Mostert R, Frantzen PJ, Wouters EF. Prevalence and characteristics of nutritional depletion in patients with stable COPD eligible for pulmonary rehabilitation. *Am Rev Respir Dis.* 1993;147(5):1151–6.
32. Seymour JM, Spruit MA, Hopkinson NS, et al. The prevalence of quadriceps weakness in COPD and the relationship with disease severity. *Eur Respir J.* 2010;36(1):81–8.
33. Sillen MJ, Franssen FM, Delbressine JM, et al. Heterogeneity in clinical characteristics and co-morbidities in dyspneic individuals with COPD GOLD D: findings of the DICES trial. *Respir Med.* 2013;107(8):1186–94.
34. Spruit MA, Polkey MI, Celli B, et al. Predicting outcomes from 6-minute walk distance in chronic obstructive pulmonary disease. *J Am Med Dir Assoc.* 2012;13(3):291–7.
35. Spruit MA, Singh SJ, Garvey C, et al. An official American Thoracic Society/European Respiratory Society statement: key concepts and advances in pulmonary rehabilitation. *Am J Respir Crit Care Med.* 2013;188(8):e13–64.

36. Storer TW. Exercise in chronic pulmonary disease: resistance exercise prescription. *Med Sci Sports Exerc*. 2001;33(7 suppl):S680–92.
37. Wagner PD, Dantzker DR, Dueck R, Clausen JL, West JB. Ventilation-perfusion inequality in chronic obstructive pulmonary disease. *J Clin Invest*. 1977;59(2):203–16.
38. Waschki B, Spruit MA, Watz H, et al. Physical activity monitoring in COPD: compliance and associations with clinical characteristics in a multicenter study. *Respir Med*. 2012;106(4):522–30.
39. World Health Organization. Chronic respiratory diseases: burden of COPD [Internet]. Geneva (Switzerland): World Health Organization; [cited 2015 Oct 9]. Available from: http://www.who.int/respiratory/copd/burden/en/
40. ZuWallack R, Crouch R. *AACVPR's Guidelines for Pulmonary Rehabilitation Programs*. 4th ed. Champaign (IL): Human Kinetics; 2011. 192 p.

CHAPTER 17

Special Considerations for Asthma and Interstitial Lung Disease

INTRODUCTION

This chapter presents the background and special considerations for assessing and developing exercise prescriptions for individuals with asthma and interstitial lung disease (ILD). The following will provide awareness about the vastly different disease profiles, symptoms, treatments, and nuances for establishing exercise programs in this important population. The case study presents a patient with persistent asthma symptoms and provides an overview of the assessment and pulmonary rehabilitation (PR) experience.

ASTHMA

Case Study 17-1

Ms. Case Study-Asthma

Ms. Case Study-Asthma is a 46-year-old nonsmoking woman with a history of adult-onset asthma and allergic rhinitis 10 years ago. She is 87 kg (191 lb) in body weight and 167 cm (65.7 in) in height for a **body mass index (BMI)** of 31.2 kg $\cdot$ m^{-2} (moderate obesity). Most recently, she experienced an "asthma attack" and called 911. She was admitted via the emergency department and hospitalized for 5 days; no intubation or mechanical ventilation was required. Prior to the hospitalization, she visited the emergency department on two other occasions for exacerbations. Since her hospital discharge 4 months ago, she complains she has not yet recovered and has been unable to return to her normal activities. She reports having gained 10 lb since her hospitalization. She has a notable history of anxiety and long-standing clinical depression. She is treated with medication and sees her psychiatrist monthly. Ms. Case Study-Asthma reports significant anxiety since the hospitalization and fears having another asthma attack. She has been relatively sedentary since the hospitalization.

Ms. Case Study-Asthma estimates her exercise tolerance to be less than a half a block and rates dyspnea as category rating of 3–4 with walking on the level. She frequently stops to catch her breath when walking up one flight of stairs to get to her apartment. She is no longer able to take her dog for daily walks. She is able to openly express being afraid to walk around the block for fear she will not make it back home. She reports to having two to three exacerbations on the average per year, all of which have required oral corticosteroids for prolonged periods. She is currently taking 20 mg of prednisone daily. She is prescribed inhaled corticosteroids (ICS) in combination with a long-acting β_2-agonist (LABA) as well as a short-acting β_2-agonist (SABA) to be used as needed. Her gastroesophageal reflux disease (GERD) is being well managed. There are no orthopedic concerns or use of any assistive devices. She has an individualized asthma action plan (AAP) and several peak expiratory flow (PEF) meters which she received from her physician at hospital discharge. She is not using either at present. She does share that her primary care physician has discussed the importance of monitoring her symptoms to detect changes and to notify him earlier to avoid trips to the emergency department. She says she feels overwhelmed and asks for help to return to walking her dog every day. Additionally, she feels she could benefit by having a review of her medications and use of her PEF.

The patient was instructed and performed two 6-minute walk tests (6MWT) following recommended standards with 20-minute rest between tests. The patient was observed incorrectly administering two actuations during one breath of the SABA, albuterol. Poor coordination between breath and actuation was noted with administration midway into the inspiratory effort. She did not administer her controller or maintenance dose of ICS and β-agonist (as prescribed) on the morning of testing as she perceives use to yield little-to-no benefit. No supplemental oxygen has been prescribed. She walked 315 m (1,033.5 ft) and rested a total of 44 seconds. Oxygen saturation was 96% pre- and 98% post-6MWT. Resting heart rate (HR) was 88 bpm and increased to 110 bpm. She rated dyspnea as (C-R) 4, leg muscle fatigue as (C-R) 3, and very slight low back pain. There was no use of pursed lips breathing, shoulders were slightly elevated, and no accessory muscle use was observed. Balance was adequate, and gait was even. No safety concerns were assessed. Mild-to-moderate audible wheezing was assessed upon test completion and resolved within 5 minutes posttesting. See Table 17.1 for pulmonary function test results.

Case Study 17-1 (continued)

Table 17.1 Pulmonary Function Test Results: Ms. Case Study-Asthma

	Prebronchodilator		Postbronchodilator		
	Predicted	**Measured**	**Predicted**	**Measured**	**% Change**
FVC (L)	3.77	2.94	78	2.89	−2
$FEV_{1.0}$ (L)	3.14	2.02	64	2.25	12%
$FEV_{1.0}$/FVC (%)	83	68			

FVC, forced vital capacity.

The patient was enrolled in an 8-week PR program that included supervised exercise, individualized education, and weekly peer psychosocial support sessions with a psychologist. The PR team provided individualized education on inhaled medication and techniques and peak flow meter and nebulizer use. Teach-back methods were used for medication delivery and PEF devices to assure comprehension and verify skill. The patient was asked to perform home daily PEF testing and bring logs for review and discussion to sessions. In addition, exacerbation prevention was discussed, and an individualized AAP was developed.

After 2 weeks of supervised exercise training, the patient was provided with a home exercise program and instructions to track her activity. Her home exercise program included the use of free weights for strength training twice weekly and taking her dog for daily walks, as this was an important patient goal established at the initial evaluation.

Supervised exercise consisted of both resistance and aerobic exercise twice weekly for 8 weeks. Resistance training consisted of three upper extremity exercises and two lower from a seated position and one standing. An overview of exercise training can be seen in Tables 17.2 and 17.3. The following exercises were used for strength training: shoulder press, bicep curls, side lateral raises, leg extension, hip flexor raises, and hamstring curls. She also trained using an upper body cycle ergometer and walked on the treadmill. Her training target was set to a symptom limit using a category scale (C-R) of 3–6 for dyspnea and muscle fatigue.

Ms. Case Study-Asthma was encouraged to use her albuterol puffer 10–15 minutes before exercise and to gradually warm up for 5 minutes at a lower level of intensity. She was also encouraged to extend her cool-down period to include walking an additional 5 minutes at a lower intensity. Throughout training, her oxygenation remained above 90% breathing room air. Her back pain remained slight and did not impede progress.

Ms. Case Study-Asthma began using her albuterol puffer 10–15 minutes before exercise with symptom improvement. She decided to purchase a treadmill for home use during her 8-week PR training to support walking for longer durations on a level surface and in a climate-controlled environment. Under physician supervision, oral systemic corticosteroid doses were tapered and eventually withdrawn midway into training.

In summary, postprogram assessments showed an improvement of 70 m (229.7 ft) in her 6MWT. Walking durations improved significantly as well as intensity levels of 1.5–2.8 mph for up to 35 minutes. Additionally, resistance levels and durations improved with cycle ergometer use from 5 minutes at baseline to 15. She found the group support sessions to be valuable in helping her to better cope and manage recent health changes. She opted to join the postprogram maintenance exercise group weekly for added support and to maintain contact with rehab team members. Of note, measures of self-efficacy and standardized shortness of breath scores improved significantly postprogram. Depression scores showed some improvement but remained elevated postprogram.

(continues)

Case Study 17-1 (continued)

Table 17.2 Weekly Average Aerobic Endurance Training for Ms. Case Study-Asthma

Week	BP (mm Hg)	Sat/HR	TM (mph)	Time (min)	Sat/HR	Dyspnea	MF	Comments
1	108/67	94/86	1.5 2.0 1.5	5 15 3	95/86	3	1	SABA used 15 min before session 1:1 Coaching on pursed-lip breathing (PLB) and shoulder relaxation Constant encouragement provided PEF trending at 250–300 L · s^{-1}
2	109/66	95/88	1.5 2.2 1.5	5 20 5	94/87	3	5	Patient reports slight quad muscle soreness. SABA 30 min prior, 100% cuing required with PLB No PEF monitoring by patient
3	115/79	95/88	1.5 2.2	5 7	95/90	Unable to obtain	—	Stopped session: patient crying; met 1:1 to discuss feelings of depression, no suicidal thoughts Appointment with psychiatrist later today
4	106/73	94/95	2.3	30	94/100	3	2	SABA used 30 min prior; 50% cuing required with PLB/PEF 430 this AM
5	110/71	94/86	2.2 dropped to 1.8	26	93/88	4	0.5	Complained of increased breathlessness before session SABA used 15 min prior with some relief PEF 400 this AM Patient encouraged to track PEF and follow AAP
6	108/70	96/72	2.3	30	95/123	3	3	PEF 300 with audible wheezing SABA administered with subjective improvement before exercise
7	110/71	93/87	2.4	30	95/115	3	2	Patient administered nebulizer with SABA 1 h prior to session
8	114/73	97/88	2.5	35	95/115	3	2	SABA prior to session; PEF 350
9	110/69	96/88	2.5	30	93/129	4	4	SABA prior to session; PEF 325
10	105/70	98/85	2.7	30	93/125	4	3	SABA prior to session; PEF 400
11	114/79	95/83	2.5–2.7	30	96/114	3	4	Woke up short of breath at 4:00 AM. Administered SABA via nebulizer; improved wheezing SABA taken 15 min prior to walking
12	110/68	96/92	2.7	35	94/117	3	3	Feeling good today; SABA 20 min prior to session

All training was done on room air. No reported pain throughout training. Dyspnea and muscle fatigue were rated using a symptom category scale. BP, blood pressure; Sat, oxygen saturation; TM, treadmill; MF, muscle fatigue, 0–4 scale; AM, morning.

Case Study 17-1 (continued)

Table 17.3 Progressive Resistance Training for Ms. Case Study-Asthma

Week	UBE Min. 60 RPM at 400 kg · m^{-1} · min^{-1}	Dyspnea	Fatigue	U/L Weights	Reps/Sets
1	5	4	4	2/2	8/1
2	7	0	4	2/2	12/1
3	Not done[a]	—	—	2/2	12/2
4	10	4	4	3/2	12/2
5–7	15	3	4	3/2	12/2
6–8	16	3–4	4	3/3	12/2
10–12	20	4	5	3/3	12/2

Min., minutes; RPM, rev/min.
Clinic equipment and space limitations allowed a program of seated exercise using an upper body ergometer (UBE), hand (upper or U) and ankle (lower or L) weights. Training progression was targeted to a symptom limit of symptom category rating (CR) of 4–6.
[a]No reported pain. Exercise deferred; patient visibly upset and crying, expressed feeling of sadness. No thoughts of self-harm. Has appointment with psychiatrist later today.

Case Study 17-1 Quiz:

Ms. Case Study-Asthma

1. How is the diagnosis of asthma made?
2. Why is assessing and observing inhaled medication use important in people with asthma?
3. Is there a disparity between the patient's perceptions of her baseline exercise tolerance in comparison to the C-R rating with the 6MWT?

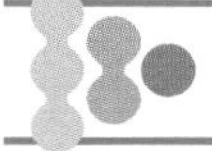

Description, Prevalence, and Etiology

Asthma is a heterogeneous disease usually characterized by chronic airway inflammation (13). The Global Initiative for Asthma (GINA) Guidelines supports confirming a diagnosis by a positive history of respiratory symptoms of wheezing, shortness of breath, chest tightness, and cough that varies over **time** and in **intensity** and presents with variable expiratory airflow limitation (13). Variations in symptoms and airflow obstruction are often triggered by factors such as **exercise**, allergen or irritant exposure, changes in weather, or viral respiratory infections (13). Asthma continues to be a major public health concern (13,35). The World Health Organization (WHO) estimates that 334 million people are affected by asthma with a majority living in low- and middle-income countries worldwide (8,35).

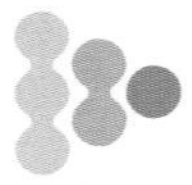

Preparticipation Health Screening, Medical History, and Physical Examination

The diagnosis of asthma is made through a medical history, physical examination, and objective assessment of lung function (7,13). An assessment of symptom patterns and evidence of airflow limitation are essential in confirming asthma (7,13).

Airway hyperresponsiveness and chronic airway inflammation may persist despite the absence of symptoms or when lung function is within normal limits (13). Episodes of wheezing, chest tightness, shortness of breath, and coughing are common and typically resolve spontaneously or with appropriate treatment (7,13,26). According to GINA, some patients with asthma will have normal physical assessments (13). Dougherty and Fahy (7), cites the presence of wheezing with auscultation as being the most common abnormal physical finding. There are several risk factors for poor asthma outcomes, among them are uncontrolled asthma symptoms, high SABA use, inadequate use of ICS, incorrect metered dose inhaler use, comorbid conditions such as obesity and GERD, and major psychological or socioeconomic concerns (13). Some data suggest that even patients with mild disease may limit or avoid activities that may be perceived as triggering asthma symptoms (13). It is not uncommon for exercise and strenuous activity to diminish when symptoms worsen either acutely or in progressive chronic asthma (21).

Asthma diagnosis, treatment, and symptom control are crucial prior to initiating a program of exercise and **physical activity**. Patients should avoid known triggers and adhere to prescribed medications. Asthma treatment goals target controlling symptoms, supporting normal physical activity, and preventing exacerbations (8,13).

Patients with asthma are prescribed controller or maintenance medications for regular use to reduce airway inflammation, control symptoms, and reduce future risks for exacerbations and threats to declining lung function (3,13,27). GINA guidelines recommend the use of ICS and leukotriene receptor antagonists (LTRA) to reduce airway inflammation (13). Inhaled SABA, LABA, and anticholinergic bronchodilators (*i.e.*, anti-muscarinic antagonists, or long-acting muscarinic antagonists [LAMA]) are added to relieve airflow limitation (3,9,13,27). Expert consensus supports the use of reliever or rescue medications (SABA) for all patients for relief when needed and with those experiencing exercise-induced bronchospasm (EIB) (13,19). Add-on therapies are used with severe asthma when symptoms persist or exacerbations occur despite optimized treatment (Box 17.1) (13,19).

Box 17.1 Exercise Benefits for Adult Patients with Asthma

The following are exercise benefits for adult patients with asthma:

- Improved anxiety and depression (23)
- Improved quality of life (23,24)
- Reduced exacerbation events (10)
- Improved maximal volume of oxygen consumed per unit time ($\dot{V}O_{2max}$) (10,24)
- Improved symptom-free days (10)

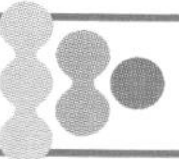

Symptom Monitoring and Asthma Action Plan Use

The use of AAPs has been identified by GINA as a key component to exacerbation prevention and is recommended for all patients with asthma (3,8,13,26). There are currently no studies or recommendations to guide physical activity based on symptom control with the use of AAP staging. AAPs are written sets of instructions developed by patient and provider to recognize worsening asthma symptoms. Action plan instructions help patients to urgently modify treatment and seek appropriate medical attention when warranted (26). Patients and their providers collaborate to develop plans that include recommendations to adjust or add medications when symptoms increase. Involving patients to share in making treatment decisions has been shown to improve adherence and asthma outcomes (13).

AAPs may include color categories to symbolize stages of symptom control (Fig. 17.1). Asthma symptoms are generally well controlled within the green zone. The yellow zone signifies caution as symptoms are less controlled with regard to increased cough, and/or wheezing, with possibly reduced activity tolerance. Changes to medications are advised to provide relief and control symptoms (3,13). The red zone is serious and represents the most severe breathing impairment. When patients are assessed within this zone, it often means symptoms have failed to respond to prior treatment adjustments, management is elusive, and acute care intervention is necessary. Exercise should be deferred during this period until symptom control can be restored.

There are currently no studies or recommendations to guide exercise intensity based on symptom assessment with the use of action plans or PEF monitoring. PEF monitoring has been recommended once asthma has been diagnosed to assess pharmacological treatment response for up to 3 months (13). Monitoring PEF may also be helpful in earlier detection of exacerbations mainly in patients with "poor perception of airflow limitation" (13). Lung function, as defined by forced expiratory volume in one second ($FEV_{1.0}$), has not been shown to correlate well with asthma symptoms in adults and children (13). For this reason, GINA recommends long-term PEF monitoring for some patients with severe asthma and for those with impaired perception of airflow limitation (13).

It can take up to several days or longer to recover from airway inflammation and clearance of excess secretions as a result of an exacerbation of asthma (32). This is an important factor for patients and health care providers to keep in mind. Returning to baseline function and gaining symptom control may be slower in some and quicker in other patients. Coaching patients to return to baseline physical activity levels should include a review of current medications (*i.e.*, oral corticosteroids) and the use of rescue or fast-acting bronchodilators. Patients who are weaning onto lower systemic corticosteroid doses and eventual withdrawal may note increasing symptoms of breathlessness. Patients need to return to regular exercise when they are able for overall general health. It is important to note that Garcia-Aymerich and colleagues (10) demonstrated reductions in exacerbations in patients who participated in regular exercise. Clinicians who support exercise in patients with asthma should be familiar with action plans and engage patients in conversations about their plans. Reviewing symptom status and plans with patients may also help to gain insight into the patient's understanding of asthma control and variability with medication use.

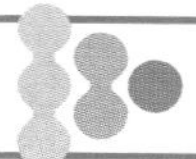

Exercise Testing Considerations

The *ACSM's Guidelines for Exercise Testing and Prescription, 10th edition* (*GETP10*) reviews the most common methods for assessing exercise in asthma and related airflow limitations of EIB (2). "Exercise-induced bronchospasm is a phenomenon of the airways that occurs during or after exercise or physical exertion" (25). The mechanism of EIB is poorly understood. Molis and Molis (25) provide a succinct description of EIB as airway cooling and dryness during periods of hyperventilation

ASTHMA ACTION PLAN

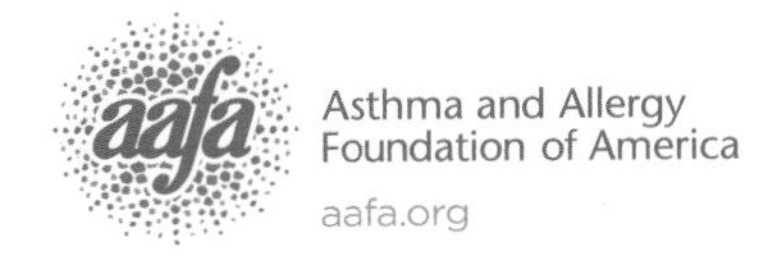

Name:	Date:
Doctor:	Medical Record #:
Doctor's Phone #: Day	Night/Weekend
Emergency Contact:	
Doctor's Signature:	

Personal Best Peak Flow: ____________

The colors of a traffic light will help you use your asthma medicines.

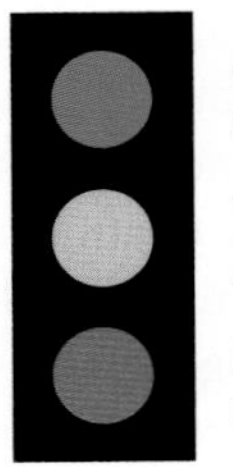

GREEN means Go Zone! Use preventive medicine.

YELLOW means Caution Zone! Add quick-relief medicine.

RED means Danger Zone! Get help from a doctor.

GO

You have *all* of these:
- Breathing is good
- No cough or wheeze
- Sleep through the night
- Can work & play

Peak flow: from ______ to ______

Use these daily preventive anti-inflammatory medicines:

MEDICINE	HOW MUCH	HOW OFTEN/WHEN
For asthma with exercise, take:		

CAUTION

You have *any* of these:
- First signs of a cold
- Exposure to known trigger
- Cough
- Mild wheeze
- Tight chest
- Coughing at night

Peak flow: from ______ to ______

Continue with green zone medicine and add:

MEDICINE	HOW MUCH	HOW OFTEN/ WHEN
CALL YOUR PRIMARY CARE PROVIDER.		

DANGER

Your asthma is getting worse fast:
- Medicine is not helping
- Breathing is hard & fast
- Nose opens wide
- Ribs show
- Can't talk well

Peak flow: reading below ______

Take these medicines and call your doctor now.

MEDICINE	HOW MUCH	HOW OFTEN/WHEN

GET HELP FROM A DOCTOR NOW! Do not be afraid of causing a fuss. Your doctor will want to see you right away. It's important! If you cannot contact your doctor, go directly to the emergency room. DO NOT WAIT. Make an appointment with your primary care provider within two days of an ER visit or hospitalization.

FIGURE 17.1 Asthma action plan. (Reprinted with permission from the Asthma and Allergy Foundation of America.)

(with exercise) leading to airway dehydration and the release of cellular inflammatory mediators (26). EIB in elite athletes is well documented as well as in patients with asthma and can be managed with pharmacotherapy (2,25,29). The use of SABA is the recommended treatment of choice for EIB (2,25,29). Spirometry testing is recommended before and after exercise along with cardiopulmonary capacity and noninvasive monitoring of oxygenation (2). American College of Sports Medicine (ACSM) guidelines recommends some level of vigorous activity for 10–15 minutes while breathing dry air (13,25). An $FEV_{1.0}$ decrease of ≥15% from baseline is often considered as a positive result for EIB (2,25,29). 6MWTs may be used in those with moderate-to-severe persistent asthma when other testing is unavailable. Additional testing methods are reviewed in the *GETP10* (2).

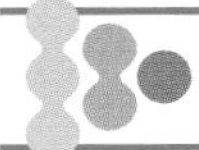

Exercise Prescription and Progression Considerations

Exercise is recommended for patients with asthma for general health benefits (13). Physical training is well tolerated among people with asthma, and those with stable asthma should be encouraged to participate in regular exercise training, without fear of symptom exacerbation (4). Morton and Fitch (26) contend that those with well-controlled asthma should be able to exercise normally and derive physiologic benefits. There is little evidence to recommend one form of exercise over another (2,13).

Patients with asthma who are experiencing acute symptom changes will have reduced exercise abilities. Those patients with unstable symptoms may require more medical oversight and changes in medications or dosages to provide relief and control symptoms (3,13). Symptom stabilization and disease management is crucial for optimizing exercise.

Data availability on exacerbation airway recovery in asthma is limited. Singhal and colleagues (32) found similar patterns of postexacerbation recovery in patients with chronic obstructive pulmonary disease (COPD) and asthma of 10–12 days posthospital admission. Depending on the severity of the exacerbation and baseline airway status, airway hyperresponsiveness may take several days to return to preexacerbation levels (32). Airway recovery should be taken into consideration for those facilitating exercise in patients with moderate-to-severe exacerbations (32).

Specific evidence-based training guidelines for people with asthma are not available at this time (2). The avoidance of irritants and pollutants is always recommended especially when ventilation is high during periods of exercise (2,4,25,26). ACSM guidelines and system reviews support frequency, intensity, time, and type (FITT) recommendations in people with asthma when individualized to patient capabilities (2,4,25) (FITT table, Table 17.4). ACSM guidelines also recognize training to an intensity graded 3–6 on the C-R 10 scale (25).

Recommendations for preexercise may include the administration of SABA 15 minutes prior and a gradual warm-up to minimize EIB (13,33). Additional recommendations include a warm-up period of low-level "rhythmic" activity and a "warm-down" postexercise especially in those with EIB (26). Monitoring for postexercise bronchospasm should occur as well. See Box 17.2 for benefits of exercise for adults with asthma.

Case Study 17-1 Quiz:

Exercise Prescription and Progression Considerations

4. What purpose does it serve to perform a warm-up period prior to achieving target training levels?
5. Can you suggest other exercises that may benefit this patient?
6. Does having depression impact the ability to optimally care and self-manage a chronic breathing condition?

FITT

TABLE 17.4 FITT RECOMMENDATIONS FOR INDIVIDUALS WITH ASTHMA

ACSM FITT Principle of the ExR_x

Chronic Medical Condition	Frequency (How often?)	Intensity (How hard?)	Time	Type (What kind?) Primary	Resistance	Flexibility	Special Considerations
Healthy Adult	≥5 d · wk^{-1} of moderate exercise, or ≥3 d · wk^{-1} of vigorous exercise, or a combination of moderate and vigorous exercise on ≥3–5 d · wk^{-1} is recommended.	Moderate to vigorous. Light-to-moderate intensity exercise may be beneficial in deconditioned individuals.	If moderate intensity: ≥30 min · d^{-1} to total 150 min · wk^{-1}. If vigorous intensity: ≥20 min · d^{-1} to total 75 min · wk^{-1}.	Regular, purposeful exercise that involves major muscle groups and is continuous and rhythmic in nature is recommended.	2–3 d · wk^{-1} (nonconsecutive)	2–3 d · wk^{-1}; static stretch 10–30 s; 2–4 repetitions of each exercise	Sedentary behaviors can have adverse health effects, even among those who regularly exercise. Adding short physical activity breaks throughout the day may be considered as a part of the exercise.
Asthma	3–5 d · wk^{-1}	Moderate (40%–59% HRR or $\dot{V}O_2R$). If tolerated, progress to 60%–70% HRR or $\dot{V}O_2R$ after 1 mo.	Progressively increase to at least 30–40 min.	Aerobic activities using large muscle groups, such as walking, cycling, swimming, or pool exercise	2–3 d · wk^{-1} at 60%–70% 1-RM (lower intensity to start) Experienced weight trainers: ≥80% Endurance: <50% of 1-RM strength: 2–4 sets, 8–12 reps Endurance: ≤2 sets, 15–20 reps Weight machines, free weights, or body weight exercises	≥2–3 d weekly with daily being the most effective Static, dynamic, and/or PNF stretching Stretch to the point of feeling tightness or slight discomfort. 10–30 s hold for static stretching 2–3 repetitions of each exercise	FITT guidelines for patients with ILD are similar to those for patients with COPD. For this population, moderate-intensity exercise is suggested, and vigorous exercise is generally contraindicated, particularly for those with PPH. Resistance exercise may be added after aerobic training parameters have been established. Intensity of exercise should be below levels that provoke oxygen desaturation, dyspnea, or hypertension.

ExR_x, exercise prescription; HRR, heart rate reserve; $\dot{V}O_2R$, oxygen uptake reserve; 1-RM, one repetition maximum; PNF, proprioceptive neuromuscular facilitation; PPH, primary pulmonary hypertension.

Based on the FITT Recommendations present in *ACSM's Guidelines for Exercise Testing and Prescription*. 10th ed. Philadelphia (PA): Wolters Kluwer; 2018. 480 p.

Box 17.2 Exercise Benefits for Adult Patients with Interstitial Lung Disease

The following are exercise benefits for adult patients with asthma:

- Improved functional exercise capacity (16)
- Improved quality of life (16)
- Improvement in dyspnea (16)
- Improvement in psychological distress (9)

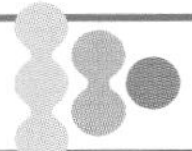

Asthma Exercise Summary

This chapter segment presents pertinent information on how patients with asthma should exercise and be monitored. It is well-known that patients with asthma often limit their activities to avoid uncomfortable symptoms. Exercise programs should be individualized and include assessment of inhaled medication use and levels of symptom control. Helping patients to identify and understand their airway changes may promote better management and increased exercise. Clinicians working with patients with asthma should be familiar with asthma medications, exacerbations, and special conditions in testing and exercise training.

Specific points to consider should include episodes of wheezing, chest tightness, shortness of breath, and coughing are the most common signs and symptoms associated with asthma, most commonly treated with SABA, and the additional use of ICS and LTRA to reduce airway inflammation (13). Inhaled SABA, LABA, and anticholinergic bronchodilators (*i.e.*, LAMAs) are added to relieve airflow limitation.

Physical training is well tolerated among people with asthma, and those with stable asthma should be encouraged to participate in regular exercise training without fear of symptom exacerbation. Highlights for FITT recommendations include administration of SABAs 15 minutes prior, a gradual warm-up to minimize EIB with a warm-up period that includes low-level "rhythmic" activity, and a "warm-down" postexercise, especially in those with EIB. Monitoring for postexercise bronchospasm should occur as well.

INTERSTITIAL LUNG DISEASE

Unlike with COPD, confirming an ILD diagnosis requires a more extensive workup and may take considerable time to conclude from symptom onset. Early and accurate diagnosis is crucial for aligning appropriate treatments, staging disease, and monitoring progression through pulmonary function testing. This section focuses on the exercise limitations of patients while highlighting important clinical considerations for exercise assessment and training.

Case Study 17-2

Mr. Case Study-ILD

Mr. Case Study-ILD is a 64-year-old male who is disabled with a negative smoking history and complaints of significant progressive dyspnea for the past 6 months. He was diagnosed with ILD 14 months ago. He worked in a shipyard and was exposed to several airborne inorganic substances for over 30 years. He also complains of a per-

(continues)

Case Study 17-2 (continued)

sistent dry cough that worsens with exercise and a lack of stamina. He is treated for GERD and is asymptomatic at present. He has been treated with the maximum dose of an oral antifibrotic to slow the progression of lung function loss for the past 3 months. Other than ILD and GERD, he is otherwise healthy. Mr. Case Study-ILD does report an old back (disc) injury from lifting but is not currently limited by pain. He is highly engaged in his care and has good family support. He estimates his exercise tolerance to be one-half to three-fourth block on the level and states to have breathlessness with all **activities of daily living**, including dressing and bathing. Supplemental oxygen is prescribed at 3 L $\cdot$ m^{-1} via an oxygen concentrator (maximum flow setting 5 L $\cdot$ m^{-1}) for use with sleep and when at home. He uses an inspiratory pulse dose oxygen conservation device with a small cylinder (M6), which he carries in a shoulder bag. He reports no oxygen use during showering. He has reduced showering to every other day due to severe dyspnea and fatigue and has recently started using a chair for energy conservation. His BMI is 25 kg $\cdot$ m^{-2}, he has had no weight changes, and his appetite is fair. On physical examination, clubbing is noted and there is no pedal edema. Lung sounds reveal bibasilar inspiratory crackles with a resting respiratory rate of 26. Infrequent nonproductive coughing is observed at rest only. The electrocardiogram shows normal sinus rhythm, and echocardiography results show a pulmonary arterial pressure of 35 mm Hg. As part of the lung transplant work-up, a heart catheterization, ventilation and perfusion scan, and a repeat echocardiogram will be performed.

Pulmonary Function Results

Pulmonary function test results are seen in Table 17.5. A 6MWT was used to assess functional capacity. Percent saturation (SpO_2) is an indirect measure of arterial oxygen saturation. The patient walked a total of 346 m (1,135 ft), averaging 2.1 mph, SpO_2 dropped to 83%, whereas HR increased from 98 to 133 bpm. The patient rated perceived dyspnea as 7 out of 10 (maximum) via modified category scale (C-R) and muscle fatigue as severe (C-R) 5, without pain. An additional assessment was needed to determine the level of supplemental oxygen that would be required to support an SpO_2 of ≥90% approximating the patient's walking speed and activity level.

Oxygen Assessment and Titration

Oxygen assessment and titration results are shown in Table 17.6. Mr. Case Study-ILD's exercise and activity tolerance is limited by severe hypoxemia, dyspnea, and leg muscle fatigue. His goal is lung transplantation. The lung transplant team has recommended Mr. Case Study-ILD attended PR to improve his understanding about his lung disease and begin an exercise program.

Table 17.5 Pulmonary Function Test Results: Mr. Case Study-ILD

	Predicted	Measured	% Predicted
FVC (L)	4.28 L	1.98 L	46
$FEV_{1.0}$ (L)	3.23 L	1.56 L	48
$FEV_{1.0}$/FVC (%)	75	79	
TLC	6.04 L	2.60 L	43
RV	2.22 L	0.56 L	68
DLCO	27.1	7.1	26

FVC, forced vital capacity; TLC, total lung capacity; RV, residual volume; DLCO, diffusion capacity of the lung.

Table 17.6 Oxygen Assessment and Titration Results

	Oxygen Flow (SpO_2)	Resting Heart Rate	Treadmill Speed (C-R)	Duration (min)
5 L • m^{-1} nasal cannula	99% HR 100	1.3 mph	3	SpO_2, 86%, HR 128 bpm Dyspnea (6) Muscle fatigue (6) No pain
Recovered Rested 5–7 min 8 L • m^{-1}	100% HR 104	1.3 mph	10	SpO_2 92%, HR 128 bpm Dyspnea (5) Muscle fatigue (4) No pain

The PR team follows an oxygen titration policy to increase flow rate settings to support and maintain an oxygen saturation of ≥90% during supervised training. When oxygen saturation levels drop to ≤88%, exercise will be terminated and flow rates will be increased. Patients are rested between flow setting changes for equilibration to occur. The **exercise prescription** requires **submaximum** training due to hypoxemia. The category ratio (C-R) of 3–6 similar to ACSM recommendations for COPD were considered as a reference guide. If SpO_2 levels remain at ≥90%, durations may be targeted for up to 30 minutes, three to five times weekly. Limb strength training was initiated using 2-lb hand and ankle weights. Fatigue was a considerable factor and was compounded by side effects from the oral antifibrotic medication.

Mr. Case Study-ILD performed the following exercise prescription/progression for 8 weeks at PR. His exercise program consisted of submaximum endurance training using a treadmill twice weekly for short durations with an eventual goal of 20–30 minutes while maintaining an SpO_2 ≥90%. **Strength** training was done twice weekly, three upper extremity exercises and two lower from a seated position and one standing. Supplemental oxygen at 8 L • m^{-1} was needed with exercise. The sequence in which strength and endurance training was conducted was also assessed. Starting the session with strength training was preferred by Mr. Case Study-ILD; when done in reverse, he was unable to progress in repetitions following the walk as he complained of higher fatigue levels. The following exercises were used for strength training: shoulder press, bicep curls, side lateral raises, leg extension, hip flexor raises, and hamstring curls (standing). Table 17.7 presents a review of strength

Table 17.7 Mr. Case Study-ILD Strength Training Review

Week	Resistance Weight Upper/Lower (no.)	Reps	Sets
1	2/2	12	1
2	2/2	12	1
3	3/2	8	2
4	3/3	12	2
5	4/3	8/12	2
6	4/3	12/2	2
7	5/3	12/2	2
8	5/3	12/2	2

Table 17.8 Mr. Case Study-ILD Exercise Training Overview

Week	BP	Pre-SpO_2 and HR	During SpO_2 and HR	Treadmill Speed (mph)	C-R Dyspnea	C-R Muscle Fatigue
1	138/68	96/88	92/138	1.3 × 3:30 min Rested 5 min 1.3 × 6 min	6 5	6 4
2	136/65	100/90	89/137	1.4 × 7 min Rested 6 min 1.4 × 5 min	6 5	0 3
3	130/83	100/95	93/138	1.5 × 10 min Rested 5 min 1.5 × 7 min	6 5	5 5
4	137/80	99/89	94/133	1.5 × 18 min No rests	7	3
5	138/82	100/90	96/126	1.0 × 25 min	4	2
6	130/78	96/92	94/130	1.0 × 30 min	4	1
7	131/81	100/88	94/116	1.0 × 20 min limited by cough, sinus congestion	4	1
8	130/67	100/78	91/127	1.1 × 25 min	5–6	2

training and progression based on symptom report and patient tolerance. Endurance exercise was progressed by symptom assessment of dyspnea and fatigue as well as oxygenation status. Mr. Case Study-ILD received training for a home exercise program which included strength training and short walk intervals and SpO_2 of ≥90%. He purchased weights and an oximeter monitor for home exercise training (see Tables 17.8 and 17.9).

Table 17.9 Mr. Case-Study-ILD Comparison of the 6-Minute Walk Test Pre- and Postpulmonary Rehabilitation Training

	Pretraining Program	Posttraining Program
BP	130/68	138/88
HR	98–133	87–124
SpO_2	99%–83%	99%–85%
O_2 Setting	No. 3	$8 L \cdot m^{-1}$
Distance	346 m (1135 ft)	344 m (1128 ft)
Rests	0	0
Speed	2.1	2.1
Dyspnea	7	4–5
Muscle fatigue	5	3
Pain	0	0

Preprogram, the patient carried an M6 O_2 cylinder in a shoulder pack and used a pulsed dose oxygen device. Postprogram, the patient used an E-sized cylinder and pulled it in a two-wheeled cart.

Description, Prevalence, and Etiology

ILDs are characterized by involvement of the lung parenchyma, the development of inflammation and fibrosis, loss of alveolar-capillary integrity, and eventual gas exchange impairment (16,18). ILD conditions cause restrictive pulmonary function and circulatory limitations that contribute to a high degree of disability (15,33). ILD encompasses a vast diversity of diseases, the etiology of which — for many — remains unclear. ILD includes idiopathic pulmonary fibrosis (IPF), sarcoidosis, acute and chronic interstitial pneumonias, and connective tissue diseases (CTD) such as rheumatoid arthritis (RA), scleroderma, and many others (16,18). Patients generally present with dyspnea upon exertion, limited exercise tolerance, and fatigue, although some will complain of cough. Increasing dyspnea and decreasing exercise tolerance leads to disability and reduces health-related quality of life (15,16,33). As with other chronic progressive lung diseases, patients often experience muscle **deconditioning** due to avoidance of exercise (15,28). The impact of hypoxemia on exercise with ILD is profound (11,12,14–16). Impairment of respiratory muscle function is further appreciated by the presence of resting and/or exertional hypoxemia resulting in increased work of breathing, thus "rendering the respiratory muscles prone to hypoxia" (28). The multiplicity of ILD makes for challenging study of exercise training limitations.

As lung function worsens, some patients may encounter dyspnea at relatively low levels of exercise, whereas others may exhibit moderate exercise tolerance. Ventilatory limitation and skeletal muscle dysfunction are present in both COPD and ILD, whereas hypoxemia and pulmonary hypertension (PH) may be more important in some patients with ILD (12,15,16,18,28,33). Assessing oxygenation during exertion and treating hypoxemia is crucial in patients with ILD (15,28,33,34). Harris-Eze and colleagues (14) concluded that arterial hypoxemia, not respiratory mechanics, led to limits in **maximal** incremental exercise. Exercise limitation is varied within this diverse population of people with chronic respiratory impairment. There is consensus that some level of exercise is important (Box 17.3).

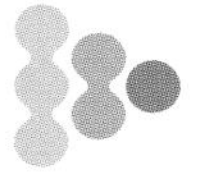

Preparticipation Health Screening, Medical History, and Physical Examination

Before initiating a program of exercise and rehabilitation, medical histories should be reviewed for validation of an accurate diagnosis and to detect the presence of comorbid conditions. Given the diverse scope of ILD, comorbid conditions should be scrutinized with respect to the specific ILD diagnosis whenever possible. For example, patients with RA have greater risks for developing increased rates of cardiovascular disease (CVD), infection, and hyperglycemia events (6). In the

Box 17.3 Respiratory Physiology Considerations in Interstitial Lung Disease

The following are respiratory physiology considerations related to interstitial lung disease:

- Alveolar injury — inflammation
- Destruction of alveolar-capillary integrity — loss of gas exchange units
- Reduced diffusion capacity
- Hypoxemia (at rest and/or with exertion)
- Poor lung compliance — increased elastic recoil
- Lower lung tidal volumes
- Increased respiratory rates
- Ventilatory and circulatory limitation with exercise

Box 17.4 Activity Limitations Considerations for Patients with Interstitial Lung Disease

The following are exercise limitations considerations for patients with interstitial lung disease:

- Dry cough worsening with exercise
- Severe exercise-induced hypoxemia
- Fatigue
- Muscle aches and joint pain with some autoimmune and connective tissue disorders, that is, sarcoidosis, rheumatoid arthritis, and scleroderma
- Lack of activity and confidence
- Activity avoidance due to progressive dyspnea
- Poor exercise tolerance
- Limited oxygen storage capability
- Fear of running out of oxygen

same international study of over 4,500 patients with RA, risk factors for developing comorbidities were unassessed or suboptimally managed in 30%–50% of the population (6). IPF international guidelines underscore the presence of multiple comorbidities of PH, pulmonary embolus (PE), lung cancer, and coronary artery disease (CAD) (20,30). More than half of patients with sarcoidosis had comorbid conditions, which increased with multiorgan involvement and in older age (22).

Medication use varies widely in ILD, thus providing opportunities for clinicians to gain knowledge and become aware of potential side effects that may interfere with regular exercise.

Obtaining an appraisal of exercise and gaining insight into the patients' perception about their physical capabilities is necessary as pulmonary function values and dyspnea do not correlate well. Patients with high levels of anxiety, fatigue, muscles aches, and joint pain will have added limitations to consider. Physical examination often reveals higher resting respiratory rates, accessory muscle recruitment (at rest or with exertion), clubbing, and pedal edema in some patients. Patients should be closely assessed for severe exercise-induced hypoxemia (Boxes 17.4 and 17.5).

Box 17.5 Preexercise Assessment of the Patient with Interstitial Lung Disease

Preexercise assessment of a patient with interstitial lung disease include the following:

- *Cough*

  Changes in severity or frequency
  Nonproductive versus productive
  Identify factors that worsen and relieve coughing.

- *Oxygen use*

  At rest
  With sleep
  With exertion/activity

  Engage patients who do self-oximetry monitoring to ask about any changes in flow settings between supervised training sessions, that is, increases in flow to support an SpO_2 of ≥90% with activity.

- *Pain*

  Changes and severity of muscle or joint pain

- *Acute changes in dyspnea*

Some patients with mixed obstructive and restrictive lung disease may be prescribed fast-acting β-agonists. Use before exercise may or may not be helpful. A subjective assessment of use obtaining the patient's perception of benefits may be important preexercise.

Case Study 17-2 Quiz:

Preparticipation Health Screening, Medical History, and Physical Examination

1. Describe the value of knowing the diffusing capacity of the lungs for carbon monoxide (DLCO) prior to exercise testing.
2. What monitoring and interventions are needed to support exercise goals?

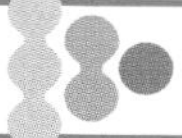

Exercise Testing Considerations

There are limited data and no consensus on how to evaluate and prescribe exercise in patients with ILD. This may be in part related to the fact that ILD encompasses over 300 diseases (28). The use of cardiopulmonary exercise testing (CPET) and **field tests** such as the 6-minute and shuttle walk tests have been deemed valuable for assessing impairment (2,11). *There is agreement that monitoring oxygen saturation is imperative. GETP10* (2) (Chapters 4 and 5) provides a comprehensive overview of exercise testing options as does the special populations chapter on COPD (Chapter 9).

Case Study 17-2 Quiz:

Exercise Testing Considerations

3. Why did not the 6-minute walk distance (6MWD) improve significantly?
4. Was the treadmill oxygen titration assessment helpful in determining O_2 flow setting?

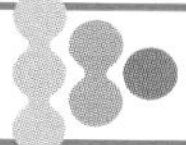

Exercise Prescription and Progression Considerations

The optimum exercise prescription for persons with ILD is not yet known (17). Rochester et al. (31) support a disease-relevant approach-setting training based on individual patient needs. There is consensus across all studies that supports monitoring by oximetry and treating hypoxemia with supplemental oxygen. Most all studies stress the need for exercise programs to be individually tailored to the patient's needs. Patients with severe hypoxemia, coughing, and fatigue may require interval training and closer supervision (17).

In a Cochrane Review, Holland and Hill (16) concluded that physical training is safe in patients with ILD. Their results showed improvements in functional exercise capacity, dyspnea, and quality of life immediately following training with benefits in patients with IPF as well. Huppmann and colleagues (18) assessed **aerobic** and resistance training five times weekly in over 400 patients with ILD. After a month of training, a 46-m (151-ft) improvement in 6MWD was observed, with no changes in dyspnea. About 14% of patients showed a decline in 6MWD due to acute exacerbations and cardiac decompensation. Patients with PH started with lower 6MWD and showed benefits similar to patients with ILD with no PH. Roughly 80% of the cohort received supplemental oxygen. The study showed improvements in functional capacity (as noted by an increase in their distance walked) and quality of life supporting the addition of PR (and supervised exercise training) as an adjunct therapy to the treatment of patients with ILD (18).

Ferreira and colleagues (9) studied a cohort of 113 patients with ILD and showed improvements in 6MWD, dyspnea, and psychological distress post-PR. In addition, Spruit and colleagues (33), in an international statement on the advances in PR, summarized the importance of PR for patients with ILD despite limited research.

Exercise and Idiopathic Pulmonary Fibrosis

A group of international experts defines IPF as a specific form of chronic, progressive fibrosing interstitial pneumonia of unknown cause, occurring primarily in **older adults**, limited to the lungs, and associated with a radiographic pattern of usual interstitial pneumonia (UIP) (30). Evidence-based guidelines support a multidisciplinary approach to diagnosis, which includes pulmonologists, radiologists, and pathologists (30). Large-scale studies are lacking on the incidence or prevalence of IPF; however, Raghu and colleagues (30) note increased incidence presenting in the sixth or seventh decade of life. Risk factors include a history of cigarette smoking, environmental exposure to a variety of inorganic dusts, microbial agents such as chronic viral infections, GERD, and genetic factors (30).

Experts describe IPF as a fatal disease that can progress unpredictably (30). The decline of lung function varies with most patients experiencing a gradual worsening over a number years, whereas others may experience more acute episodes of decline (30). Recommendations are strong for the use of long-term oxygen therapy in IPF (30). Assessment of oxygenation is recommended for all patients with IPF at rest and with exertion at baseline and at 3- to 6-month intervals (30). Although current guidelines rated PR as weak in terms of support, treatment was still recommended in a majority of patients but not in an important minority of patients with IPF (30). These include patients with PH, GERD, and worsening symptoms of shortness of breath (30).

Swigris and colleagues (34) studied PR in a small cohort of patients with IPF. Supervised exercise consisted of aerobic and resistance training over 6–8 weeks. The aerobic training started at 60% of predicted maximum HR based on age. Intensity and duration were gradually increased to build tolerance and confidence with a goal of reaching a maximum for 30 minutes. Breathing training, oxygen use, psychosocial support, and energy-saving instruction were included. Oxygen saturation levels of 89% or less were treated with supplemental oxygen. Functional capacity and fatigue improved post-PR (34).

Vainshelboim et al. (36) conducted a randomized controlled trial of physical activity in a group of patients with IPF following 12 weeks of supervised training. Patients were trained twice weekly for 30–60 minutes most days of the week. Significant improvements in physical activity was seen at 12 weeks; however, activity levels diminished by the 11-month follow-up. Researchers suggested that a program of exercise maintenance could benefit patients with IPF (36).

There are a limited number of studies researching the benefits of nonpharmacological treatments in patients with ILD, and research to date does demonstrate improvements similar to those found in COPD. Patients with ILD who are limited by dyspnea and poor exercise tolerance should be considered for exercise training and PR intervention (2,9,11,16,17,30,31).

Case Study 17-2 Quiz:

Exercise and Idiopathic Pulmonary Fibrosis

5. What are some compounding exercise limitations for patients with IPF and ILD?

Oxygen Assessment and Prescription in Interstitial Lung Disease

There is no single standardized method for assessing oxygenation in patients with chronic lung disease. This poses a problem for both clinicians and patients. All patients with pulmonary disease get regular assessment of resting oxygen saturation levels when vital signs are obtained with physician visits. There are missed opportunities to assess oxygenation using standardized methods during exertion as oxygen desaturation is common in patients diagnosed with ILD. Exercise tolerance is further limited by hypoxemia, and if patients with ILD are to experience improved functional abilities, hypoxemia must be detected and treated (2,11,22).

The Centers for Medicare & Medicaid Services (CMS) have established criteria for coverage of long-term oxygen therapy for Medicare beneficiaries (5). These coverage rules are often followed by other health care payers. CMS criteria describe an assessment by oximetry or arterial blood gas at rest and with exercise. Initially, patients are assessed at rest breathing room air. When the partial pressure of arterial oxygen (P_aO_2) is $\leq$55 mm Hg or the SpO_2 is $\leq$88% at rest by noninvasive oximetry, the patient is provided supplemental oxygen and tested during exercise. When the resting SpO_2 is above 88%, the patient is generally walked, and if the SpO_2 falls below 88% while walking, another assessment is required with supplemental oxygen to demonstrate SpO_2 levels of $\geq$90% with exertion. In addition, CMS Group I coverage extends supplemental oxygen to patients with SpO_2 levels below 88% for longer than 5 minutes while sleeping (5). Group II coverage has a provision for qualifying patients with an SpO_2 of 89% or a P_aO_2 between 56 and 59 mm Hg with dependent pedal edema, PH, or cor pulmonale (5). When patients require supplemental oxygen to treat exercise-induced hypoxemia, oxygen is prescribed and provided by durable medical equipment companies. Oxygen at flow rates of 1–6 $L \cdot min^{-1}$ is most commonly delivered via disposable nasal cannula at a concentration of 24%–40% (1). It is important to take into consideration that varied respiratory rates can influence the fractional concentration of oxygen (1). Patients will likely need home supply systems and portable sources. Oxygen concentrators are commonly used for home, whereas small oxygen cylinders (size M6) are carried in portable shoulder or backpacks when active outside the home. Patients with more severe hypoxemia may require high-flow concentrators for home use that deliver up to 10 $L \cdot min^{-1}$ and larger oxygen cylinders (size E) with carts for trips beyond the home. These systems can be heavy and cumbersome. Clinicians should be aware that more patients are purchasing oximeters to self-monitor and titrate oxygen. Patients are often lacking instruction and provider support for self-monitoring and oxygen titration. Many providers are reluctant to support patient-initiated oxygen titration changes. In the absence of guidance and training, many patients will lack the information needed to use oximetry in ways that promote adequate oxygenation. Self-monitoring may help some patients to understand when to use oxygen despite not feeling breathless and help others to slow their walking pace or when to stop an activity.

Case Study 17-2 Quiz:

Oxygen Assessment and Prescription in Interstitial Lung Disease

6. Is it important to assess patients on their own portable oxygen products during exercise?
7. In your opinion, would this patient benefit from ongoing emotional and exercise support beyond completion of his PR treatment?
8. Can you suggest other exercises that would be beneficial for this patient to keep him engaged in activity until he receives a transplant?

SUMMARY

This chapter presents relevant information regarding the assessment and training of the patients with asthma and ILD. Many patients with asthma may experience wheezing with exercise, whereas patients with ILD are more likely to exhibit hypoxemia, many despite having supplemental oxygen prescriptions. Patients with ILD who are candidates for lung transplantation can benefit from monitoring and ongoing exercise support not only to bridge them to transplant but also to help modify training levels and oxygen settings as disease worsens. Specific points to consider include:

ILDs are characterized by involvement of the lung parenchyma, the development of inflammation and fibrosis, loss of alveolar-capillary integrity, and eventual gas exchange impairment (16). ILD conditions cause restrictive pulmonary function and circulatory limitations that contributes to a high degree of disability. ILD encompasses a vast diversity of diseases, the etiology for which several remains unclear. For patients with ILD, although no consensus regarding exercise prescription exists, maintaining saturation and treating hypoxemia are key, with saturation levels of ≥90% with exertion maintained.

A summary of exercise prescription and progression considerations for patients with asthma and ILD is listed as follows:

- General considerations for exercise in the patient with asthma include the use of SABA 10–15 minutes before exercise (29).
- Gradually warm up at lower intensity for 5–15 minutes (7,26).
- Use breathing techniques (13).
- Gradually cool down postexercise (7,26).
- Monitor for the presence of postsymptoms such as wheezing, chest tightness, or cough.
- Avoid exercising in areas of pollution, cold air, or strong odors (3,13).
- Patients who regularly monitor PEF may trend results and use measurements to help determine when to modify intensity or defer exercise entirely.
- ILD encompasses a vast variety of diseases with no clear consensus regarding exercise prescription and progression. What is critical for this group of patients is the use of supplemental oxygen and the monitoring of saturation levels through the use of pulse oximetry.

REFERENCES

1. American Association for Respiratory Care. AARC clinical practice guideline. Oxygen therapy in the home or alternate site health care facility — 2007 revision & update. *Respir Care*. 2007;52:1063–8.
2. American College of Sports Medicine. *ACSM's Guidelines for Exercise Testing and Prescription*. 10th ed. Philadelphia (PA): Wolters Kluwer; 2018. 480 p.
3. British Thoracic Society, Scottish Intercollegiate Guidelines Network. British guideline on the management of asthma. *Thorax*. 2014;69(suppl 1):1–192.
4. Carson K, Chandratilleke M, Picot J, Brinn M, Esterman A, Smith B. Physical training for asthma. *Cochrane Database Syst Rev*. 2013;(9):CD001116.
5. Centers for Medicare & Medicaid Services. *National Coverage Determination (NCD) for Home Use of Oxygen* (NCD 240.2, Pub. No. 100-3, Version No. 1) [Internet]. Baltimore (MD): Centers for Medicare & Medicaid Services; [cited 2016]. Available from: https://www.cms.gov
6. Dougados M, Soubrier M, Antunez A, et al. Prevalence of comorbidities in rheumatoid arthritis and evaluation of their monitoring: results of an international, cross-sectional study (COMORA). *Ann Rheum Dis* [Internet]. 2013 [cited 2013 Oct 4];73(1):62–8. Available from: http://ard.bmj.com/content/early/2013/10/04/annrheumdis-2013-204223.full
7. Dougherty RH, Fahy JV. Acute exacerbations of asthma: epidemiology, biology and the exacerbation-prone phenotype. *Clin Exp Allergy*. 2009;39(2):193–202.
8. Evans D, Rushton A, Halcovitch N, Whitley G, Gatheral T, Spenser S. Personalised asthma action plans for adults with asthma. *Cochrane Database Syst Rev* [Internet]. 2015 [cited 2015 Sept 8];(9):CD011859. Available from: http://onlinelibrary.wiley.com

9. Ferreira A, Garvey C, Connors GL, et al. Pulmonary rehabilitation in interstitial lung diseases: benefits and predictors of response. *Chest.* 2009;135(2):442–7.
10. Garcia-Aymerich J, Varraso R, Antó J, Camargo CA Jr. Prospective study of physical activity and risk of asthma exacerbations in older women. *Am J Respir Crit Care Med.* 2009;179:999–1003.
11. Garvey C. Interstitial lung disease and pulmonary rehabilitation. *J Cardiopulm Rehab Prev.* 2010;30:141–6.
12. Gläser S, Noga O, Koch B, et al. Impact of pulmonary hypertension on gas exchange and exercise capacity in patients with pulmonary fibrosis. *Respir Med.* 2009;103(2):317–24.
13. Global Initiative for Asthma. *Global Strategy for Asthma Management and Prevention* [Internet]. Edgewater (NJ): MCR Vision; [cited 2015 Jul 30]. Available from: http://ginasthma.org
14. Harris-Eze AO, Sridhar G, Clemens RE, Zintel TA, Gallagher CG, Marciniuk DD. Role of hypoxemia and pulmonary mechanics in exercise limitation in interstitial lung disease. *Am J Respir Crit Care Med.* 1996;154:994–1001.
15. Holland AE. Exercise limitation in interstitial lung disease — mechanisms, significance and therapeutic options. *Chron Respir Dis.* 2010;7(2):101–11.
16. Holland AE, Hill CJ. Physical training for interstitial lung disease. *Cochrane Database Syst Rev.* 2008;(4):CD006322. doi:10.1022/14651858.CD006322.pub2.
17. Holland AE, Wadell K, Spruit M. How to adapt the pulmonary rehabilitation programme to patients with chronic respiratory disease other than COPD. *Eur Respir Rev.* 2013;22:577–86.
18. Huppmann P, Sczepanski B, Boensch M, et al. Effects of inpatient pulmonary rehabilitation in patients with interstitial lung disease. *Eur Respir J.* 2013;42(2):444–53.
19. Kim H, Mazza J. Asthma. *Allergy Asthma Clin Immunol.* 2011;7(suppl 1):S2.
20. King C, Nathan SD. Identification and treatment if comorbidities in idiopathic pulmonary fibrosis and other fibrotic lung diseases. *Curr Opin Pulm Med.* 2013;19(5):466–73.
21. Mancuso CA, Sayles W, Robbins L, et al. Barriers and facilitators to healthy physical activity in asthma patients. *J Asthma.* 2006;43(2):137–43.
22. Martusewicz-Boros MM, Boros PW, Wiatr E, Roszkowski-Śliż K. What comorbidities accompany sarcoidosis? A large cohort (n = 1779) patients analysis. *Sarcoidosis Vasc Diffuse Lung Dis.* 2015;32(2):115–20.
23. Mendes FA, Gonçalves R, Nunes MP, et al. Effects of aerobic training on psychosocial morbidity and symptoms in patients with asthma: a randomized clinical trial. *Chest.* 2010;138(2):331–7.
24. Meyer A, Günther S, Volmer T, Taube K, Baumann HJ. A 12-month, moderate-intensity exercise training program improves fitness and quality of life in adults with asthma: a controlled trial. *BMC Pulm Med* [Internet]. 2015 [cited 2015 May 7];15:56. Available from: http://www.ncbi.nlm.nih.gov/pubmed/25947010
25. Molis MA, Molis WE. Exercise-induced bronchospasm. *Sports Health.* 2010;2(4):311–7.
26. Morton AR, Fitch KD. Australian Association for Exercise and Sports Science position statement on exercise and asthma. *J Sci Med Sport.* 2011;14(4):312–6.
27. National Clinical Guideline Centre. *Asthma: Diagnosis and Monitoring in Adults, Children and Young People* [Internet]. London (United Kingdom); National Institute for Health and Care Excellence [cited 2016 Jan 18]. Available from: https://www.nice.org.uk/guidance/gid-cgwave0640/resources/asthma-diagnosis-and-monitoring-draft-guideline2
28. Panagiotou M, Polychronopoulos V, Strange C. Respiratory and lower limb muscle function in interstitial lung disease. *Chron Respir Dis.* 2016;13(2):162–72. doi:10.1177/1479972315626014.
29. Parsons JP, Hallstrand TS, Mastronarde JG, et al. An official American Thoracic Society clinical practice guideline: exercise-induced bronchoconstriction. *Am J Respir Crit Care Med.* 2013;187(9):1016–27.
30. Raghu G, Collard H, Egan JJ, et al. An official ATS/ERS/JRS/ALAT statement: idiopathic pulmonary fibrosis: evidence-based guidelines for diagnosis and management. *Am J Respir Crit Care Med.* 2011;183(6):788–824.
31. Rochester CL, Fairburn C, Crouch RH. Pulmonary rehabilitation for respiratory disorders other than chronic obstructive pulmonary disease. *Clin Chest Med.* 2014;35(2):369–89.
32. Singhal P, Kumar R, Gaur S. Assessment of time course for recovery of patient with acute exacerbations in chronic obstructive pulmonary disease and bronchial asthma. *Indian J Allergy Asthma Immunol.* 2006;20(1):29–36.
33. Spruit MA, Singh SJ, Garvey C, et al. An official American Thoracic Society/European Respiratory Society statement: key concepts and advances in pulmonary rehabilitation. *Am J Respir Crit Care Med.* 2013;188(8):e13–64.
34. Swigris J, Fairclough D, Morrison M, et al. Benefits of pulmonary rehabilitation in idiopathic pulmonary fibrosis. *Respir Care.* 2011;56(6):783–9.
35. To T, Stanojevic S, Moores G, et al. Global asthma prevalence in adults: findings from the cross-sectional world health survey. *BMC Public Health* [Internet]. 2012 [cited 2012 Mar 19];12:204. Available from: http://onlinelibrary.wiley.com
36. Vainshelboim B, Fox BD, Kramer MR, Izhakian S, Gershman E, Oliveira J. Short-term improvement in physical activity and body composition after supervised exercise training program in idiopathic pulmonary fibrosis. *Arch Phys Med Rehabil.* 2016;97(5):788–97.

CHAPTER 18

Special Considerations for Weight Management

INTRODUCTION

This chapter discusses special considerations relevant to **exercise** testing, prescription, and progression for individuals who are overweight or obese. The case study focuses on a middle-aged woman with obesity who was screened prior to participation in a 4-month exercise training program. She completed baseline testing, including anthropometric measurements, a submaximal exercise test, and assessments of muscular fitness and flexibility. This case study presents direction for the formulation of an appropriate exercise prescription to result in weight loss and a reduction in chronic disease risk factors for a patient with obesity.

Case Study 18-1

Ms. Case Study-WM

Ms. Case Study-WM is a 48-year-old woman who works 5 days per week as a bank executive. She previously walked up the stairs to her third floor office but has started to use the elevator because in the past month, she has experienced shortness of breath when walking up the stairs. The patient was physically active throughout college as a club lacrosse player but has not exercised regularly since she gave birth to her children who are now 16 and 14 years old. Ms. Case Study-WM is 167.6 cm (66 in), weighs 102.7 kg (226 lb), and drinks one to two glasses of wine per day due to the stress of her job and divorce 1 year ago. Lab results from her physical examination 1 month ago revealed total blood cholesterol: 230 mg · dL^{-1}, low-density lipoprotein (LDL): 150 mg · dL^{-1}, high-density lipoprotein (HDL): 48 mg · dL^{-1}, and blood glucose: 110 mg · dL^{-1}. Her blood pressure (BP) was recorded as 132/84 mm Hg at this doctor's visit. Ms. Case Study-WM has a family history of heart disease with her father dying at 53 years of age of a myocardial infarction and her brother's coronary revascularization at 48 years of age. She is a nonsmoker. Current medications for Ms. Case Study-WM include Atorvastatin (Lipitor) for hypercholesterolemia and Lisinopril for high BP.

Ms. Case Study-WM's body fat percentage was obtained using bioelectrical impedance analysis (BIA). Waist circumference (WC) was measured at the narrowest circumference above the umbilicus and below the xiphoid process. Height was measured using a wall-mounted stadiometer, and weight was measured on a calibrated balance beam scale (Box 18.1). **Submaximal** exercise test results obtained from a modified Balke protocol are presented in Table 18.1. Muscle **strength**, seen in Box 18.2, was assessed by a five repetition maximum (5-RM) protocol using plate-loading resistance training machines. **Flexibility** testing results are shown in Box 18.3.

Box 18.1 Anthropometric Measurements for Ms. Case Study-WM with Obesity

Following are anthropometric measurements for Ms. Case Study-WM with obesity:

- Height: 167.6 cm
- Weight: 102.7 kg
- BMI: 36.5 kg · m^{-2}
- Body fat: 32.4%
- Waist circumference: 98 cm

Table 18.1 Submaximal Exercise Test Results from a Modified Balke Protocol

Stage	Minute	Grade (%)	Speed (mph)	HR (bpm)	BP (mm Hg)	Rating of Perceived Exertion (6–20 Borg Scale)
1	1	0	3.0	98		
	2	0	3.0	102	152/86	11
2	3	2.5	3.0	126		
	4	2.5	3.0	127	164/86	14
3	5	5	3.0	140	180/88	16

Preexercise HR: 78 bpm; preexercise BP: 134/86 mm Hg; recovery BP: 152/82 mm Hg.

(continues)

Case Study 18-1 (continued)

Box 18.2 Five Repetition Maximum, Muscular Fitness Testing Results for Ms. Case Study-WM with Obesity

Following are 5-RM, muscular fitness testing results for Ms. Case Study-WM with obesity:

- Chest press: 35 lb
- Leg press: 165 lb
- Biceps curl: 12.5 lb
- Leg extension: 50 lb
- Latissimus dorsi pull-down: 35 lb
- Leg curl: 30 lb
- Triceps extension: 15 lb

Box 18.3 Flexibility Testing Results for Ms. Case Study-WM with Obesity

Following are flexibility testing results for Ms. Case Study-WM with obesity:

- Trunk forward flexion using a sit-and-reach box: 21 cm
- Shoulder and upper arm flexibility: fail for both right (−7 cm) and left (−10 cm) sides

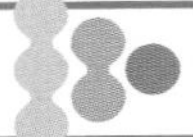

Description, Prevalence, and Etiology

Data suggest that obesity continues to be a significant public health concern in the United States, with 68.5% of adults in the United States classified as overweight or obese (**body mass index** [BMI] $\geq$25.0 kg · m^{-2}) and 34.9% categorized as obese (BMI $\geq$30.0 kg · m^{-2}) (9). Overweight and obesity are associated with an increased risk of Type 2 diabetes, hypertension, dyslipidemia, coronary heart disease (CHD), stroke, some forms of cancer, musculoskeletal problems, respiratory problems, and elevated risk of all-cause and cardiovascular disease (CVD) mortality (7). Additionally, there are negative psychosocial, biomedical, and economic implications of overweight and obesity for the U.S. population (7). Maintenance of body weight is primarily determined by the energy balance equation (Energy Intake = Energy Expenditure) (1). Although this concept of weight management appears to be straightforward, there is a constellation of causes contributing to overweight and obesity. Contributing factors include, but are not limited to, genetic, epigenetic, social and physical environment, biological, and psychological variables that can lead to positive energy balance (9). Evidence suggests that even a minimal weight loss of 2%–3% can reduce cardiovascular risk factors (3,7,9). Furthermore, maintaining a weight loss of 3%–5% may result in the lowering of risk factors associated with overweight and obesity comorbidities (*e.g.*, blood glucose and glycolated hemoglobin [HbA1C] test levels) (7). **Physical activity** is a target focus of interventions that are linked to an improvement in health outcomes and increased success with weight loss when combined with caloric restriction (5,7). Additionally, physical activity is found to be one of the best predictors of long-term weight maintenance after weight loss (1,2,5,7). Through increasing physical activity levels, individuals who are overweight or obese can expend more calories, thus aiding in a negative

Table 18.2 American College of Sports Medicine Recommendations on Physical Activity and Weight Loss

Physical Activity Amount	Potential Magnitude of Weight Loss
<150 min · wk^{-1}	Minimal weight loss
>150 min · wk^{-1}	~2–3 kg
>225–420 min · wk^{-1}	5–7.5 kg

energy balance. Table 18.2 contains American College of Sports Medicine (ACSM) recommendations on physical activity and weight loss (4).

Preparticipation Health Screening, Medical History, and Physical Examination

Minimally, in order to be consistent with ACSM's updated exercise preparticipation health screening recommendations, individuals with overweight and obesity should be assessed first for current exercise participation; known cardiovascular, metabolic, or renal disease or signs or symptoms of these diseases; and planned exercise intensity level (1,11).

In order to individualize treatment appropriately, other pertinent information to collect prior to initiating an exercise program for an individual who is overweight or obese may include a thorough medical history due to an increased risk of associated comorbidities (*e.g.*, hypertension, dyslipidemia, diabetes, CHD, stroke, gallbladder disease, osteoarthritis, sleep apnea, respiratory problems, and certain cancers) (7).

Additional information to collect as part of the preparticipation exercise screening would be height, weight, BP, heart rate (HR), waist circumference, medications, musculoskeletal/orthopedic problems, psychological conditions, and amount of sedentary time (7,11). Supplementary factors for the clinician to assess prior to program participation for individuals with overweight or obesity are history of weight gain and loss over time, dietary habits, physical activity history, family history of obesity, barriers to weight loss (*e.g.*, low social support, readiness for change, low self-efficacy, time constraints, financial concerns), and individual weight and physical activity goals (7). Because of the complex etiology of overweight and obesity, considering a multitude of factors in prescreening will provide the health care provider with useful information to create a safe and effective **exercise prescription**. Based on the *ACSM's Guidelines for Exercise Testing and Prescription, 10th edition* (*GETP10*) (1), perhaps some of the most important information to obtain from this group of individuals is a clear understanding of the person's current level of physical activity and the presence of signs; symptoms; and/or known cardiovascular, metabolic, or renal disease.

Case Study 18-1 Quiz:

Preparticipation Health Screening, Medical History, and Physical Examination

1. Is medical clearance recommended for this individual prior to exercise testing and prescription? Why or why not?
2. What additional information is important to consider from the review of this patient's case study for the exercise preparticipation health screening?
3. What further questions would be helpful prior to initiating an exercise program?

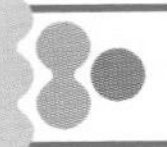

Exercise Testing Considerations

A primary consideration for exercise testing for individuals with overweight and obesity is the presence of other comorbidities (*e.g.*, hypertension, diabetes, dyslipidemia) which can be associated with increased cardiovascular risk and decreased exercise performance (1,7,10). Due to the presence and degree of severity of these comorbidities, there is a potential for a low exercise capacity in individuals with overweight and obesity (1). Therefore, a low initial workload and a conservative progression may be warranted in these individuals (1). Moreover, non–weight-bearing modes of testing, such as cycle ergometer tests, should also be considered for this population (1). Traditional physiological test termination criteria may not be valid due to the possibility of individuals with overweight and obesity ending the test early based on symptoms associated with comorbidities (1). Examples of appropriate exercise tests for individuals with overweight or obesity include, but are not limited to, the modified Balke, 6-minute walk, modified Naughton, and YMCA cycle ergometry (1). For these protocol details, as well as additional test examples, please refer to Chapters 4 and 5 of *GETP10* (1). A summary of considerations for individuals with overweight or obesity prior to exercise testing are as follows (1):

- Assess the presence of comorbidities (*e.g.*, hypertension, diabetes, dyslipidemia) which are associated with cardiovascular risk and exercise performance.
- If no known cardiovascular, metabolic, or renal disease is present, an exercise test may not be required for a low- to moderate-intensity exercise program.
- Reduced exercise capacity may require submaximal exercise testing protocols considering the initial workload (*e.g.*, 2–3 **metabolic equivalents** [**METs**]) and progression of **maximal** intensity protocols (0.5–0.1 MET increase/testing stage).
- Various musculoskeletal (*e.g.*, osteoarthritis) or orthopedic conditions may require alternate testing modalities to the treadmill such as leg or arm ergometry.
- Medications that may alter HR or BP response at rest or during exercise (*e.g.*, β-blockers).
- Additional medications to treat comorbidities (*e.g.*, antidiabetic medications) or obesity itself (*e.g.*, appetite suppressant such as Qsymia [phentermine and topiramate])
- Exercise equipment should be assessed for maximal weight capacity and patient fit to ensure the safety and comfort of the participant.
- Assessment equipment should be appropriate to accurately determine weight (*e.g.*, maximal weight limit), BP (*e.g.*, appropriate cuff size), HR (monitor vs. palpation), and body fat percentage (*e.g.*, BIA vs. skinfolds).
- Environmental factors should be considered to ensure a temperature regulated climate as heat intolerance is often common in this population.

Case Study 18-1 Quiz:

Exercise Testing Considerations

4. Why was the modified Balke protocol chosen for Ms. Case Study-WM? What protocol would you have chosen for this patient? Justify your response.
5. What are the potential side effects of her medications that could potentially have an impact on exercise testing?
6. Why was the 5-RM used to assess muscular strength in Ms. Case Study-WM? Do you agree or disagree? Justify your answer.

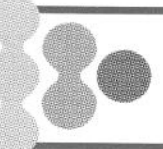

Exercise Prescription and Progression Considerations

Frequency, intensity, time, and type (FITT) recommendations for individuals with overweight and obesity are listed in FITT table (Table 18.3) (1). The main goal for these individuals is to progress to 250–300 minutes per week of moderate- to vigorous-intensity **aerobic** exercise in order to achieve clinically significant weight loss. However, low fitness levels are commonly observed in this population (1,5). Therefore, this often translates into an initial exercise prescription that is a low volume of aerobic exercise with a goal to progress time, intensity, and

TABLE 18.3 FITT RECOMMENDATIONS FOR INDIVIDUALS WITH OVERWEIGHT AND OBESITY

FITT

ACSM FITT Principle of the ExR_x

Chronic Medical Condition	Frequency (How often?)	Intensity (How hard?)	Time	Type (What kind?) Primary	Resistance	Flexibility	Special Considerations
Healthy Adult	$\geq$5 d · wk^{-1} of moderate exercise, or $\geq$3 d · wk^{-1} of vigorous exercise, or a combination of moderate and vigorous exercise on $\geq$3–5 d · wk^{-1} is recommended.	Moderate to vigorous. Light-to-moderate intensity exercise may be beneficial in deconditioned individuals.	If moderate intensity: $\geq$30 min · d^{-1} to total 150 min · wk^{-1}. If vigorous intensity: $\geq$20 min · d^{-1} to total 75 min · wk^{-1}.	Regular, purposeful exercise that involves major muscle groups and is continuous and rhythmic in nature is recommended.	2–3 d · wk^{-1} (nonconsecutive)	2–3 d · wk^{-1}; static stretch 10–30 s; 2–4 repetitions of each exercise	Sedentary behaviors can have adverse health effects, even among those who regularly exercise. Adding short physical activity breaks throughout the day may be considered as a part of the exercise.
Obesity and Overweight	$\geq$5 d · wk^{-1}	Initial intensity should be moderate (40%–59% HRR or $\dot{V}O_2R$). If tolerated, progress to 60%–70% HRR or $\dot{V}O_2R$ for greater health benefits.	30 min · d^{-1} (150 min · wk^{-1}); increase to 60 min · d^{-1} or more (250–300 min · wk^{-1}).	Prolonged, rhythmic activities using large muscle groups (*e.g.*, walking, cycling, swimming)	2–3 d · wk^{-1} at 60%–70% 1-RM; gradually increase to enhance strength and muscle mass 2–4 sets, 8–12 reps of each major muscle groups Resistance machines and/or free weights	$\geq$2–3 d · wk^{-1} Static, dynamic, and/or PNF stretching Stretch to the point of feeling tightness or slight discomfort. Stretch for 10–30 s; hold for static stretching. 2–3 repetitions of each exercise	The main goal of the exercise program should be to maximize caloric expenditure. For example, progressing to 250–300 min · wk^{-1} of moderate- to vigorous-intensity exercise will equate to approximately >2,000 kcal · wk^{-1}. Consider lifestyle and behavioral factors that may alter the exercise prescription and progression (*e.g.*, lack of time; multiple short bouts of physical activity each day may be an appropriate strategy).

ExR_x, exercise prescription; HRR, heart rate reserve; $\dot{V}O_2R$, oxygen uptake reserve; 1-RM, one repetition maximum; PNF, proprioceptive neuromuscular facilitation.

Based on the FITT Recommendations present in *ACSM's Guidelines for Exercise Testing and Prescription.* 10th ed. Philadelphia (PA): Wolters Kluwer; 2018. 480 p.

frequency appropriate for the individual. One useful strategy to progress the volume of physical activity for individuals with overweight and obesity is to prescribe multiple daily bouts of at least 10 minutes in duration (6,8). Another reason this strategy can be useful is that it can assist individuals with making physical activity a regular lifestyle behavior. Overweight and obesity treatment often requires a comprehensive lifestyle intervention program (7). Thus, establishing a diverse team of health care providers (*e.g.*, registered dietitians, psychologists, physicians), in addition to the exercise professional, is useful for improving weight loss and maintenance and overall health outcomes for these individuals (1,7). Exercise professionals should pay special consideration to the information obtained from the preparticipation health screening and lifestyle behavior information when formulating an exercise prescription. Refer to Table 18.4 for an example aerobic exercise prescription and progression for Ms. Case Study-WM that was appropriate based on her preparticipation health screening, lifestyle information, and exercise testing results.

Resistance training for individuals with overweight and obesity does not result in a clinically significant weight loss (4). However, the benefits of resistance training for these individuals include a potential increase in **muscular strength** and physical functioning as well as a reduction in risk factors associated with CVD, diabetes, and other chronic diseases (3). It may be worth mentioning that resistance training assists in the preservation of lean body mass, which has metabolic consequences (2).

Based on these considerations, resistance training was prescribed 2 days per week during the 4-month personal training program. Each session includes six to eight multijoint exercises that target major muscle groups of the upper and lower body. The first 2 weeks include one set of 10–12 repetitions for each exercise, using a weight to elicit fatigue within the prescribed repetition range. One set for initial resistance training may be appropriate due to Ms. Case Study-WM's low level of muscular fitness and lack of familiarity with resistance training. After week 2, the prescription progresses with an additional set for each exercise and the weight increases appropriately due to her neuromuscular adaptations from completing the prescribed resistance training exercises. Table 18.5 presents the resistance training prescription for Ms. Case Study-WM.

Flexibility exercises are prescribed following a 5-minute aerobic exercise cool-down. Each static stretch is to be performed two times for 20 seconds and held to a mild discomfort level. The targeted major muscle groups for Ms. Case Study-WM include pectoralis, rotator cuff, hamstrings, quadriceps, and gastrocnemius.

Table 18.4 Example Aerobic Exercise Prescription/Progression for Ms. Case Study-WM

Week	Frequency	Intensity	Time	Type
1–3	Two times per week	40%–50% HRR	20 min	Walking
4	Two times per week	40%–50% HRR	25 min	Walking
5	Three times per week	40%–50% HRR	30 min	Walking, stationary cycling
6–7	Three times per week	45%–55% HRR	32 min	Walking
8–9	Four times per week	50%–60% HRR	32 min	Walking, elliptical
10–11	Four times per week	55%–65% HRR	35 min	Walking, elliptical
12–14	Five times per week	55%–65% HRR	35 min	Walking
15–16	Five times per week	60%–70% HRR	40 min	Walking

Table 18.5 Example Resistance Training Exercise Prescription for Ms. Case Study-WM

Exercise	Muscle Groups Utilized	Intensity
Chest press	Pectoralis, deltoids, triceps	Two sets per exercise utilizing a weight that elicits fatigue within 10–12 repetitions; 1 min rest between sets
Row	Latissimus dorsi, biceps	
Overhead press	Deltoids, triceps	
Latissimus dorsi pull-down	Latissimus dorsi, biceps	
Trunk flexion	Rectus abdominis	
Back extension	Erector spinae	
Leg press	Quadriceps, hamstrings, glutes	

A summary of exercise prescription and progression for individuals with overweight and obesity include the following (1):

- The main goal of the exercise program should be to maximize caloric expenditure. For example, progressing to 250–300 minutes per week of moderate- to vigorous-intensity exercise will equate to approximately ≥2,000 kcal per week. In order to specifically calculate the energy expenditure of a bout of exercise, refer to Chapter 6 of *GETP10* (1).
- An initial low volume of physical activity (*e.g.*, multiple daily 10-min bouts of moderate-intensity activity) may be required to enhance adherence to and engagement with the exercise prescription.
- Exercise intensity may be gauged by using simplified methods such as the rating of perceived exertion or the talk test. Please refer to Chapter 6 of *GETP10* (1).
- Inclusion of a 5- to 10-minute warm-up and cool-down is recommended when prescribing aerobic exercise.
- Assess the presence of comorbidities (*e.g.*, hypertension, diabetes, dyslipidemia) and orthopedic or musculoskeletal problems that will have an impact on the exercise prescription and progression.
- Consider lifestyle and behavioral factors that may alter the exercise prescription and progression (*e.g.*, lack of time; multiple short bouts of physical activity each day may be an appropriate strategy).

Case Study 18-1 Quiz:

Exercise Prescription and Progression Considerations

7. Compare the FITT principle for Ms. Case Study-WM with the recommendations presented in the *GETP10* (1) (see FITT table, Table 18.3). Discuss components of her exercise prescription and progression that are not congruent with *GETP10* and provide the rationale for why you agree or disagree with these differences.
8. Estimate approximately how many calories Ms. Case Study-WM is expending through her aerobic exercise prescription in week 2 (assume 2.8 mph, 0% grade) versus week 15 (assume 3.5 mph, 3% grade) for her walking.
9. Identify some potential barriers to Ms. Case Study-WM completing the exercise prescription. What are some behavioral strategies you could potentially utilize to help her overcome these barriers?

SUMMARY

This chapter contains considerations for exercise testing, prescription, and progression recommendations for individuals with overweight or obesity:

- The main goals of the exercise prescription and progression for these individuals are to maximize caloric expenditure for weight loss; reduce cardiovascular, diabetes, and other chronic disease risk factors; and promote long-term maintenance of weight loss (1,2,7).
- Physical activity by itself has a modest impact on the magnitude of weight loss observed in an intervention (4).
- The combination of reducing energy intake, coupled with increased energy expenditure through physical activity, can result in clinically significant weight loss and maintenance of the weight lost (1,7).

REFERENCES

1. American College of Sports Medicine. *ACSM's Guidelines for Exercise Testing and Prescription*. 10th ed. Philadelphia (PA): Wolters Kluwer; 2018. 480 p.
2. Clark JE, Goon DT. The role of resistance training for treatment of obesity related health issues and for changing health status of the individual who is overfat or obese: a review. *J Sports Med Phys Fitness*. 2015;55(3):205–22.
3. Donnelly JE, Blair SN, Jakicic JM, Manore MM, Rankin JW, Smith BK. American College of Sports Medicine position stand. Appropriate physical activity intervention strategies for weight loss and prevention of weight regain for adults. *Med Sci Sports Exerc*. 2009;41(2):459–71.
4. Donnelly JE, Jakicic JM, Pronk NP, et al. Is resistance exercise effective for weight management? *Evid Based Prev Med*. 2004;1(1):21–9.
5. Jakicic JM, Marcus BH, Lang W, Janney C. Effect of exercise on 24-month weight loss in overweight women. *Arch Intern Med*. 2008;168(14):1550–9.
6. Jakicic JM, Wing RR, Butler BA, Robertson RJ. Prescribing exercise in multiple short bouts versus one continuous bout: effects on adherence, cardiorespiratory fitness, and weight loss in overweight women. *Int J Obes Relat Metab Disord*. 1995;19(12):893–901.
7. Jensen MD, Ryan DH, Apovian CM, et al. 2013 AHA/ACC/TOS guideline for the management of overweight and obesity in adults: a report of the American College of Cardiology/American Heart Association Task Force on Practice Guidelines, and The Obesity Society. *J Am Coll Cardio*. 2014;63(25 Pt B):2985–3023.
8. Macfarlane DJ, Taylor LH, Cuddihy TF. Very short intermittent vs. continuous bouts of activity in sedentary adults. *Prev Med*. 2006;43(4):332–6.
9. Mitchell NS, Catenacci VA, Wyatt HR, Hill JO. Obesity: overview of an epidemic. *Psychiatr Clin North Am*. 2011;34(4):717–32.
10. Ogden CL, Carroll MD, Kit BK, Flegal KM. Prevalence of childhood and adult obesity in the United States, 2011–2012. *JAMA*. 2014;311(8):806–14.
11. Riebe D, Franklin BA, Thompson PD, et al. Updating ACSM's recommendations for exercise preparticipation health screening. *Med Sci Sports Exerc*. 2015;47(11):2473–9.

CHAPTER 19

Special Considerations for Chronic Pain

INTRODUCTION

The most recent U.S. statistics, from 2012, showed that the total cost for treating chronic pain disorders ranged between $560 and $635 billion annually (47). This number was estimated to increase to $873.8 billion per year by 2014 (119). The emerging prevalence of chronic pain disorders among individuals requires the health and fitness professional to have a basic understanding regarding the recognition, management, and safe exercise prescription for common chronic pain conditions. This chapter presents three common conditions: chronic nonspecific low back pain, fibromyalgia, and rheumatoid arthritis. The information presented is intended to provide the reader with an empirical perspective on management of these conditions.

CHRONIC NONSPECIFIC LOW BACK PAIN

Case Study 19-1:

Mr. Case Study-LBP

Mr. Case Study-LBP is a 54-year-old man weighing 100 kg (220 lb) with a height of 175 cm (69 in) and with a history of chronic nonspecific low back pain (CNSLBP) treated with naproxen sodium, a nonsteroidal anti-inflammatory drug (NSAID), as needed per his physician. His risk factors for cardiovascular disease (CVD) included obesity (waist circumference of 40.5 in/103 cm) and dyslipidemia (total cholesterol of 204 mg · dL^{-1}). In addition, his triglycerides, low-density lipoprotein (LDL), and high-density lipoprotein (HDL) were 165 mg · dL^{-1}, 126 mg · dL^{-1}, and 45 mg · dL^{-1}, respectively. He is a nonsmoker, and his blood pressure (BP) and fasting glucose are 136/84 mm Hg and 90 mg · dL^{-1}, respectively. His father and mother are both 74 years old and are apparently healthy. He is an assistant chief of police in a large mid-Atlantic suburb and reports working primarily at his desk and computer most of the day. He has been taking his dog on a 1.5-mile walk each day (23 min), approximately a 4–**metabolic equivalent (MET)** activity. He used to be an avid rock climber and also competed in weekly softball tournaments. He has had occasional episodes of low back pain throughout his adulthood. His physician told him that he has slight degeneration of a disc in his low back and is overweight. He wants him to "get in shape" and "lose weight" before he considers placing him on medications (Crestor [rosuvastatin], Lopressor SR [metoprolol], and Zestril [lisinopril]) and has cleared him medically to do so. Mr. Case Study-LBP stated that his dog is very energetic, is growing rapidly, and requires a lot of **strength** to control and "I'm often tired and I hurt all over after walking him." He has no contraindications to **exercise** and does not currently have back pain. He was successfully discharged from 6 weeks of physical therapy for an episode of pain across his low back and buttocks 2 months ago. Shortly after discharge from physical therapy, his physician stopped his treadmill exercise test (Bruce protocol) after 6 minutes at approximately a 7-MET level without any signs or symptoms of hemodynamic intolerance. He did have back and leg pain and described the severity as being 8 out of 10 on a visual pain scale. He was able to dissipate the pain immediately by supporting his low back with his hands and leaning backward gently. One week later, he completed another treadmill test with a ramp protocol at an estimated level of 10 METs while reporting a pain severity of 4 out of 10.

His fitness assessment and respective results included the Young Men's Christian Association (YMCA) cycle ergometer test (estimated 10 METs), **one repetition maximum (1-RM)** and 10 repetition maximum (10-RM) bench press (150 lb and 120 lb) and horizontal (supine) leg press (300 lb and 240 lb) tests, push-ups (9 repetitions), American College of Sports Medicine (ACSM) abdominal crunch test (23 repetitions), sit and reach (14 in) and a 10-RM latissimus pull-down (110 lb), and seated scapular row (80 lb) on selectorized resistance machines. He reported a 10 out of 10 (Extremely Hard) effort on the OMNI Perceived Exertion Scale for Resistance Exercise (OMNI-RES) during each strength test and reported that he would not be able to complete another repetition without using improper form. He experienced some pain across his low back after the bike, abdominal crunch, and sit-and-reach tests, which was alleviated very shortly after each of these tests by gentle standing back extension stretches.

He then performed 16 weeks of supervised exercise with a personal trainer at a medical fitness center where his physician sent him. Details from this program follow. Table 19.1 presents the exercise program recommended for Mr. Case Study-LBP by his personal trainer. During the first 4 weeks, his exercise training program consisted of cardiovascular endurance training 3 days a week and full-body resistance training 2 days a week on selected machines. He trained 10 minutes on the recumbent bike, Nu-Step (recumbent arm and leg ergometer) and elliptical trainer (foot pedal-only model), and treadmill (no elevation), respectively, at between 50% and 70% of heart rate (HR) reserve, which in his case coincided with an **intensity** of 6–7 METs. He also performed two sets of trunk stability exercises, which included opposite arm/leg raises in the quadruped position (bird dogs) and two isometric half-side (knees flexed approximately 90°) and half-prone (knees, shins and feet on the ground) bridges/planks for 10 seconds each. **Flexibility** exercises for the hamstrings and pectorals in an upright position were emphasized. Although the percentage of 1-RM is frequently used to assign load intensities during resistance exercise sessions, the 10-RM, an

Case Study 19-1 (continued)

acceptable alternative, was used instead to help him increase his strength and endurance while avoiding the need for frequent interruptions for testing.

Mr. Case Study-LBP increased his **aerobic** endurance training time to 45 minutes, **frequency** to five times per week, added the elliptical trainer with arm rails to his routine, and began selecting exercises he enjoyed and could tolerate from the Compendium of Physical Activities. The complexity of the workout for Mr. Case Study-LBP was increased over time by substituting standing exercises with free weights, stability ball exercises, advanced trunk/core stability exercises, sled pushing and pulling activities, and assisted pull-ups. He added curl-up exercises to the trunk stability part of his workout and stated that his back felt good after doing them. Table 19.1 provides a description of his exercise program.

Table 19.1 16-Week Progressive Resistance Training Program for Mr. Case Study-LBP

Week	Monday (Sets × Repetitions and OMNI-RES)	Friday (Sets × Repetitions and OMNI-RES)
1 2	Baseline 1-RM and multiple-RM testing 1 × 10 with actual 10-RM at an OMNI-RES of 9	1 × 10 with actual 10-RM and OMNI-RES of 10 1 × 10 with actual 10-RM at an OMNI-RES of 8 1 × 5 for trunk stability exercises
3 4	2 × 10-RM and at an OMNI-RES of 8 2 × 10-RM and at an OMNI-RES of 7	2 × 12 with 10-RM and OMNI-RES of 7 at the end of week 3 2 × 14 with 10-RM at an OMNI-RES of 6
5 6	2 × 10-RM with newly established 10-RM and at an OMNI-RES of 10 2 × 10-RM and at an OMNI-RES of 8 Increased trunk stability exercises to 2 sets of 10	2 × 10-RM and at an OMNI-RES of 9 2 × 10-RM and OMNI-RES of 7
7 8	3 × 10-RM and at an OMNI-RES of 8 at the end of third set on Monday of week 7 3 × 10-RM and at an OMNI-RES of 7	3 × 10-RM and at an OMNI-RES of 8 Increased trunk stability exercises to 3 × 10 Repetitions increased to 12 and OMNI-RES dropped to 6
9 10	3 sets with newly established 10-RM for machines and new free weight and standing exercises and with an OMNI-RES of 10 3 × 10-RM and with an OMNI-RES of 9	3 × 10-RM with an OMNI-RES of 9 3 × 10-RM and with an OMNI-RES of 8
11 12	3 × 12 with 10-RM and an OMNI-RES of 7 Adjusted exercise and load intensities during week 12 3 × 10 with newly established 10-RM and at an OMNI-RES of 10	3 × 14 with 10-RM and an OMNI-RES of 7 3 × 10-RM established on the previous Monday at an OMNI-RES of 9
13 14	3 × 10 at an OMNI-RES of 8 added sled push/pull and assisted pull-ups 3 × 8 with a newly established 8-RM and at an OMNI-RES of 10	3 × 10 at an OMNI-RES of 7 3 × 8 at an OMNI-RES of 10
15 16	3 × 9 with the 8-RM loads established the previous week and with an OMNI-RES of 9 3 × 10 with the same loads as previous week and at an OMNI-RES of 8	3 × 9 with the same loads as Monday and at an OMNI-RES of 8 3 × 10 with the same 8-RM at an OMNI-RES of 7

(continues)

Case Study 19-1 (continued)

Table 19. 2 provides a functional rationale for Mr. Case Study-LBP's specific resistance exercises. He was able to meet and exceed his weekly exercise duration and MET-min goals of >300 minutes per week and ≥1,000 MET-min per week for improving his health and for helping him manage his weight.

Table 19.2 Resistance Exercises and Functional Rationale

Exercise	Muscle Groups Involved	ADL Impacted by Exercise
Leg press	Glutes, quadriceps, hamstrings	Walking uphill; walking a big dog
Squats	Glutes, quadriceps, hamstrings	Proper floor-to-waist lifting
Lunges	Glutes, quadriceps, hamstrings	Resisting a large dog pulling Walking up/down elevations
Sled pushes/pulls	Glutes, quadriceps, hamstrings	Maintain a stable trunk when a large dog pulls its leash; walking up/down elevations
Knee extensions	Quadriceps	Walking up/down elevations/stairs
Knee flexion	Hamstrings	Walking up/down elevations/stairs
Shoulder press	Deltoids, triceps	Putting heavy loads on overhead surfaces
Row with machines or cables	Latissimus dorsi, rhomboids, Trapezius, biceps	Pulling a leash to control a large dog, rock climbing
Lat pull-down	Latissimus dorsi, teres major	Rock climbing
Assisted pull-up	Rhomboids, brachialis, biceps	
Chest press	Pectorals, deltoids, triceps	Pulling a big dog inward or in front of the body on a leash or pushing a lawn mower up a hill
Biceps curl	Brachialis, biceps	Rock climbing
Seated triceps dip	Triceps	Pushing a lawnmower up a hill

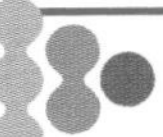

Description, Prevalence, and Etiology

Low back pain (LBP) is a common musculoskeletal condition affecting between 49% and 70% of persons living in Westernized nations and 70% and 85% of persons living in the United States during their lifetimes. It is often attributed to either nociceptive (sensitization of pain receptors within spinal/mechanical structures and myofascial tissues), neuropathic (radicular or nerve-related pain), or central (sensitization within the brain) sources (98). Persons aged 45–64 years have the highest reporting rate for LBP (22). One in four adults experiences chronic LBP lasting more than 12 months, and approximately 14% of them (58.8 million) also report having difficulty performing **activities of daily living (ADL)** (32,120). The annual U.S. cost for treatment and lost wages due to back pain increased by 91% from $132.4 during the periods of 1996–1998 to $253 billion during the period of 2009–2011 (1). Generally, back pain is categorized by its etiology, location, and duration of symptoms and classified as being either of the following:

- *Specific*: pain caused by unique or unusual pathophysiologic mechanisms (disc herniation, tumor, osteoporosis, arthritis, diseases, trauma, mechanical disorders or spinal pathology)
- *Nonspecific*: pain not caused by a specific disease or spine pathology

- *Acute*: pain lasting less than 6 weeks
- *Subacute*: pain lasting 6–12 weeks
- *Chronic*: pain lasting longer than 12 weeks

CNSLBP is generally defined as pain, muscle tension, or stiffness localized below the costal margins (ribs) and above the inferior gluteal folds with or without leg pain (sciatica) lasting ≥12 months (33,73). CNSLBP is the second leading cause of physician's visits, the leading cause of lost work time, the second leading cause of disability, and most common cause of **physical activity** limitations in persons younger than the age of 45 years.

Evidence indicates that persons with LBP experience intolerance and avoidance of physical activity, and lower levels of **physical fitness** and function, and thus engage in a more sedentary lifestyle than age- and gender-matched persons without CNSLBP (35,36,51,77,114,123,128,129).

LBP can also contribute to lost work time, reduced health-related quality of life, decreased neuromuscular function and strength, and fear/avoidance of physical activity secondary to anticipation of pain (34,36,51,55,61,66,67,88,113,114).

The reader is directed to two resources providing examples that list a number of "red flags" (identified by qualified health care providers) as conditions often accompanying specific LBP that can indicate possible underlying spinal pathology, nerve root problems, and a need to consult the patient's physician or health care provider (42,125–127). LBP is generally diagnosed or "ruled in" when red flags, magnetic resonance imaging, and radiograph results are found to be negative for spine or nerve pathology, respectively (129).

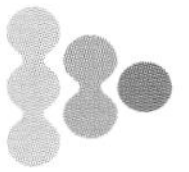

Preparticipation Health Screening, Medical History, and Physical Examination

Case Study 19-1 Quiz:

Preparticipation Health Screening, Medical History, and Physical Examination

1. What other conditions beside LBP need to be addressed in the exercise program? How can this be accomplished?
2. What motion(s) and position(s) seem to cause and reduce Mr. Case Study-LBP's back pain?

Many persons with LBP are sedentary and experience physical activity intolerance. Other health issues (*e.g.*, overweight, obesity, metabolic syndrome, hypertension, and Type 2 diabetes) may be present in this population. Exercise professionals should conduct a thorough preactivity screening and determine patients' exercise and history of physical activity, presence of or signs suggestive of cardiovascular, metabolic, or renal disease as well as the risks for adverse events during exercise according to the guidelines set by the ACSM (6). Depending on the level of risk, the patient may require a medical examination and/or potentially a physician-supervised **graded exercise test** prior to exercise program initiation. Persons with LBP are typically treated with NSAIDs and acetaminophen (nonopioid analgesic) and are advised to stay active and avoid bed rest (129). Occasionally, muscle relaxants and narcotic analgesics, which can cause drowsiness, increased reaction time, and impaired judgment, are prescribed for severe pain (129).

NSAIDs are used to relieve pain and inflammation, but long-term use of them has been associated with gastrointestinal irritation, ulcers, heartburn, diarrhea, fluid retention, and, in rare cases, kidney dysfunction and CVD. Nonopioid analgesics are used to reduce pain, but long-term use in some cases has been associated with liver damage.

Although many persons with LBP are less physically active and physically fit than apparently healthy age-matched cohorts, it is believed that LBP does not by itself exert specific effects on the exercise response (113). Exercise responses and activity limitations are typically affected by individual pain severity and location, physical fitness and strength, and body positions required during exercise testing and training. Some individuals with LBP are intolerant of specific motions such as trunk flexion or extension, and some positions such as prolonged standing and sitting can cause discomfort, which can prevent them from producing their best exercise and/or testing efforts and results.

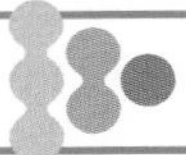

Exercise Testing Considerations

Case Study 19-1 Quiz:

Exercise Testing Considerations

3. How is maximal effort during multiple-repetition maximum testing ensured?
4. Why did the patient not achieve as high an aerobic capacity during the graded exercise test with the Bruce protocol? Why was a second protocol attempted later?

Cardiorespiratory fitness testing using either a treadmill, a bicycle, or a step ergometer with a ramp or incremental protocol, as well as **field tests** such as the 6-minute walk test (6MWT), have been well-tolerated, effective assessments for persons with LBP (36,100). Multiple repetition maximum testing is an effective alternative to 1-RM testing for determining **muscular strength**, exercise training loads, and postprogram strength increases in persons with LBP (61,67,68). The standard rating of perceived exertion (RPE) and the OMNI-RES can approximate intensity of patients' effort during cardiorespiratory fitness and musculoskeletal testing and training (7,17,107).

An OMNI-RES rating of 9 and 10 approximate near-maximal and **maximal** effort during multiple repetition testing (107). The "timed up and go" (TUG) and multiple repetition sit-to-stand (STS) tests are appropriate tools for measuring neuromotor performance in older individuals (60 yr and older) with LBP (6). The inability to tolerate prolonged sitting, standing, frequent bending (trunk flexed postures), and pain exacerbations can negatively affect patient test tolerance and performance efforts (36,77,100,113).

Exercise Prescription and Progression Considerations

Case Study 19-1 Quiz:

Exercise Prescription and Progression Considerations

5. What precaution(s) need to be taken to enhance safety during workouts for persons with LBP?
6. How can strength be increased while ensuring patient safety?
7. Can you suggest other exercises that would be beneficial for this patient given the strong desire to return to rock climbing, walking a big dog, and competing in court sports?

General guidelines for **exercise prescription** and progression for individuals with LBP resemble those of apparently healthy persons without it, which are presented in Tables 6.5, 6.6, and 6.7 in *ACSM's Guidelines for Exercise Testing and Prescription, 10th edition* (*GETP10*) (6,100). Exercise program goals should be individualized and address overall health and fitness requirements. Exercise selections should be determined by patients' comfort and activity tolerance (2,34,46,67,100). The Compendium of Physical Activities can help patients with CNSLBP select exercises they can perform comfortably while meeting their exercise goals (2,6,46).

Persons with LBP should follow resistance training guidelines for apparently healthy sedentary individuals (6,46,100). In terms of resistance training, the "two for two" rule of intensity load progression (increase intensity after two or more repetitions per exercise set are performed beyond the goal repetitions for two consecutive sessions) is appropriate (7). Proper technique and posture should be maintained during each exercise (106). Equipment type (machines, body weight, tubing, free weights) and exercise position (sitting, standing, prone, supine) should be dictated by patients' tolerance or directional preference (52,58,76).

Case Study 19-1 Quiz:

Exercise Prescription and Progression Considerations

8. What are appropriate core/trunk conditioning exercises? How can they be progressed?

Trunk/core conditioning exercise, like most resistance training exercises, can be modified and performed in standing sitting, prone, or supine (hook lying) positions. Some patients are more intolerant of trunk/spine movements like flexion or extension and often find trunk conditioning exercises with extension and flexion bias, respectively, more comfortable (52,58,76). **Isometric** activities such as side and prone bridges, pelvic tilts, supine bridges, and derotation exercises can precede more dynamic activities (52,58,76,88,113,136).

Extension exercises can be progressed from easier (lying prone on floor with arms at sides) to more challenging (the swimmer and superman on the floor or a stability ball), to "bird-dogs" on the floor in quadruped position (87–89,100,135).

Stretches should be preceded by light aerobic activity (11–13 RPE or 4–5 OMNI-RES) for 8–10 minutes. Static, dynamic, and proprioceptive neuromuscular facilitation stretching are all acceptable as tolerated (6,40). Hamstring, hip flexors, and anterior shoulder girdle muscle flexibility exercises should be emphasized (6,100).

A summary of exercise training and prescription considerations for individuals with LBP are found in frequency, intensity, time, and type (FITT) table (Table 19.3) and is presented as follows:

- Exercise program should be individualized, and goals should address all health and fitness needs of persons with LBP.
- Comorbid health conditions might be present and should also dictate exercise program development decisions.
- If present, movement directional preferences/biases can dictate the positions in which continuous resistance training, resistance training, and flexibility exercises are performed.
- Exercises causing pain during or after workout sessions should be eliminated and substituted with alternative activities.
- New or worsening symptoms warrant exercise termination and communication with a physician and/or health care provider.
- Exercises/activities that are high-impact (*e.g.*, running) should be avoided or introduced gradually with caution.
- Persons with LBP should learn fundamental movement patterns like squatting, hip hinging, and lifting from the floor and should avoid sitting for long periods (89,113).

FITT

TABLE 19.3 FITT RECOMMENDATIONS FOR EXERCISE PRESCRIPTION MODIFICATIONS AND SPECIAL CONSIDERATIONS FOR INDIVIDUALS WITH LOW BACK PAIN, FIBROMYALGIA, AND RHEUMATOID ARTHRITIS

ACSM FITT Principle of the ExR_x

Chronic Medical Condition	Frequency (How often?)	Intensity (How hard?)	Time	Type (What kind?) Primary	Resistance	Flexibility	Special Considerations
Healthy Adult	$\geq$5 d · wk^{-1} of moderate exercise, or $\geq$3 d · wk^{-1} of vigorous exercise, or a combination of moderate and vigorous exercise on $\geq$3–5 d · wk^{-1} is recommended.	Moderate to vigorous. Light-to-moderate intensity exercise may be beneficial in deconditioned individuals.	If moderate intensity: $\geq$30 min · d^{-1} to total 150 min · wk^{-1}. If vigorous intensity: $\geq$20 min · d^{-1} to total 75 min · wk^{-1}.	Regular, purposeful exercise that involves major muscle groups and is continuous and rhythmic in nature is recommended.	Muscle strengthening 2–3 d · wk^{-1} (nonconsecutive) Moderate-to-vigorous intensity; 2–4 sets of 8–12 repetitions	2–3 d · wk^{-1}; static stretch 10–30 s; 2–4 repetitions of each exercise	Sedentary behaviors can have adverse health effects, even among those who regularly exercise. Adding short physical activity breaks throughout the day may be considered as a part of the exercise.
Low Back Pain	$\geq$5 d · wk^{-1} of moderate exercise or $\geq$3 d · wk^{-1} of vigorous exercise or a combination of moderate and vigorous exercise $\geq$3–5 d · wk^{-1}	Moderate or vigorous	$\geq$30 min · d^{-1} of continuous or accumulated exercise with a minimum of 10-min bouts	Aerobic exercises in body positions best tolerated	2–3 d · wk^{-1} (nonconsecutive); 2–4 sets of 8–12 repetitions with 60%–70% 1-RM intensity for most adults; 10–15 repetitions with 40%–50% 1-RM for novice or elderly; for strength and power	2–3 d · wk^{-1}; stretch to point of slight discomfort 10–30 s in most adults and 30–60 s in older individuals; 2–4 repetitions of each exercise according to patient tolerance	An individualized approach to exercise program development that addresses all health-related fitness variables, comorbidities (if present), and movement directional preferences can enhance program compliance, effectiveness, and health-related quality of life and contribute to the adoption of a more physically active lifestyle.
Fibromyalgia	3 d · wk^{-1}	Light to moderate	20–30 min; improvements are observed after 4 wk	Aerobic Low-impact weight-bearing exercise (*e.g.*, water exercise, cycling, walking, swimming) initially to minimize pain	2–3 d · wk^{-1} 40%–80% of 1-RM exercises for all major muscle groups using a variety of equipment and body weight; 1–3 sets, 5–20 repetitions; an individualized approach to rest between sets and workouts based on patient tolerance is warranted.	2–3 d · wk^{-1} mild-to-moderate intensity within pain-free range 10–30 s in most adults and 30–60 s in older individuals; flexibility exercise for each major muscle–tendon unit 2–4 repetitions, preceded by light-to-moderate aerobic activity warm-up	Patients with FM should use their subjective pain ratings to adjust the intensity and volume of each exercise session, be encouraged to stay as active as possible during exacerbations, and be instructed regularly to use proper exercise technique and avoid exercising when they are excessively fatigued.
Rheumatoid Arthritis	3–5 d · wk^{-1} increasing to >5 · wk^{-1}	Moderate to vigorous	150 min · wk^{-1} if moderate or 75 min · wk^{-1} if vigorous or a combination of moderate and vigorous activity	Activities with low joint stress, such as walking, cycling, swimming, or aquatic exercise	2–3 d · wk^{-1} initial intensity of 50%–60% 1-RM to 60%–80% 1-RM; all major muscle groups using elastic bands, dumbbells, machines, free weights, and body weight exercises 8–12 repetitions per set 2–4 repetitions per major muscle group	2 d · wk^{-1}; static stretch 10–30 s; 2–4 repetitions of each exercise	Exercise testing and program development should be individualized, and goals should address all physical health, fitness, and functional needs of persons with RA. Recognizing barriers such as fatigue, lower baseline activity levels, and a fear of detrimental effects from exercise (inflammation and accelerated joint erosion) is necessary to affect a lifestyle change that incorporates exercise.

ExR_x, exercise prescription.

Based on the FITT Recommendations present in *ACSM's Guidelines for Exercise Testing and Prescription.* 10th ed. Philadelphia (PA): Wolters Kluwer; 2018. 480 p.

FIBROMYALGIA

This section discusses the management and special considerations for fibromyalgia (FM). The discussion begins with a case study outlining an exercise program for a 45-year-old woman diagnosed with FM 6 months ago. The case study illustrates a common program for these individuals, which often may be influenced by their current level of symptoms (*e.g.*, pain) and disability (19).

Case Study 19-2:

Mrs. Case Study-FM

Mrs. Case Study-FM is a sedentary, 48-year-old woman, 5 ft 2 in (157.5 cm) and 165 lb (75 kg) with a **body mass index (BMI)** of 30 kg · m^{-2}. She is a kindergarten teacher and was recently diagnosed by her rheumatologist with FM. She is a nonsmoker and was an avid early morning mall walker, tennis player, and ballroom dancer but has become sedentary since developing the symptoms of FM about a year ago. Her parents are both 73 years of age and are obese with Type 2 diabetes, hypertension, and dyslipidemia controlled by medications. Her school has a pool and a student and faculty fitness center which has fully equipped cardiovascular and resistance training areas. She reports awakening after 3–4 hours of interrupted sleep every morning feeling groggy, exhausted, stiff, and depressed. She has had chronic, diffuse bilateral pain in her trunk and extremities for the last year. Laboratory tests for rheumatoid arthritis (RA) and x-rays for osteoarthritis were negative. Her pain has limited her at school from kneeling and squatting down at her students' desks and tables, getting up and down from the floor, and participating in active games on the playground with her class. In addition, lifting heavy grocery bags and carrying laundry baskets up and down her stairs have become difficult. She gave up walking, tennis, and ballroom dancing as well. Her pain, insomnia, and depression are being managed by Lyrica (pregabalin), Flexeril (cyclobenzaprine), Lunesta (eszopiclone), and Zoloft (sertraline), respectively. She gained 10 lb in a year due to relative inactivity and overeating. Her resting HR was 80 bpm, and latest BP, cholesterol, and triglycerides were 140/84 mm Hg, 260 mg · dL^{-1}, and 170 mg · dL^{-1}, respectively. Fasting glucose was within normal limits. Since being diagnosed with FM, her physician had her complete a Bruce protocol treadmill test with a 12-lead electrocardiogram (ECG), which she stopped at just more than 7 minutes and at an estimated peak volume of oxygen consumed per unit time ($\dot{V}O_2$) of 28 mL · kg^{-1} · min^{-1} (8 METs) due to general fatigue and diffuse leg pain. Her perceived exertion and pain were each rated 8 out of 10 on category-ratio (CR) intensity and pain scales, respectively. She also had a dual-energy x-ray absorptiometry (DEXA) test that indicated the presence of reduced bone mineral density (BMD), however, not to a level constituting a diagnosis of osteopenia or osteoporosis. She achieved a peak HR of 155 bpm (90% of age-predicted maximal HR) and BP of 180/80 mm Hg. Her physician considered the test to be "normal" and unremarkable yet at a relatively low MET level. Her grip strength and 1-RM bench press and leg press scores were all below average and within the 40th, 35th, and 30th percentiles, respectively. Her physician has cleared her to participate in a comprehensive exercise program to improve her strength, stamina, cardiovascular fitness, and BMD while helping manage her risk factors for CVD. She has also been referred to a registered dietitian to address weight loss, CVD risk reduction, and bone health.

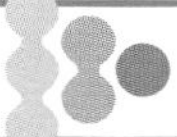

Description, Prevalence, and Etiology

FM is a chronic pain disorder that affects the joints, muscles, tendons, and soft tissue of the body. It is estimated that more than 5 million Americans have FM with a higher presence among women ages 35–60 years (25,81). FM is often underdiagnosed with 1 in 5 receiving an accurate diagnosis within an average of 5 years (132,133).

Traditionally, FM has been categorized as a rheumatic-like disorder with accompanying psychological factors such as anxiety and depression (107). More current hypotheses suggest that FM is caused by neurochemical imbalances in the central nervous system that are associated with a heightened pain perception (24,31). FM can be considered a central processing disorder where the ascending and descending neurological pathways operate abnormally which create amplified pain sensations. This creates a heightened sensitivity to stimuli called *allodynia* and a heightened response to painful stimuli called *hyperalgesia* (24,50). Individuals with FM may also suffer from myofascial pain syndrome. Research has suggested a connection between the two conditions in which 50% of individuals with FM may also suffer from myofascial pain syndrome or vice versa (83).

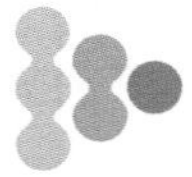

Preparticipation Screening, Medical History, and Physical Examination

Case Study 19-2 Quiz:

Preparticipation Screening, Medical History, and Physical Examination

1. What are the primary symptoms of FM that could significantly affect a patient's exercise program?

According to the American College of Rheumatology guidelines, individuals often present with the primary triad of symptoms: (a) bilateral widespread musculoskeletal pain above and below the waist with pain in the axial skeleton that lasted longer than 3 months, (b) fatigue, and (c) sleep disturbances (8,112,134). The musculoskeletal pain is the hallmark symptom that is often described as a "diffuse ache" with specific "tender points" along the body. Eighteen specific points have been identified along the upper and lower body. Individuals must have palpable pain in 11 of 18 tender points to be diagnosed (134). Individuals may also report other related conditions such as depression, anxiety, cognitive difficulties (*e.g.*, poor concentration), balance problems, irritable bowel syndrome, headaches, tenderness, stiffness, tingling and numbness, and restless leg syndrome (12,116). Thus, the diagnosis of FM is dependent on the patient history and clinical examination because medical tests and imaging are inconclusive (48,101). Associated risk factors include a familial predisposition with first relatives having the highest risk, physical trauma or injury, stress, and infections such as hepatitis C (8,121).

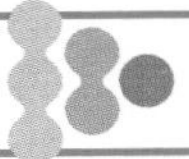

Exercise Testing Considerations

Case Study 19-2 Quiz:

Exercise Testing Considerations

2. Is the 1-RM test necessary for assessing strength in persons with FM?
3. What effect can symptoms have on exercise testing?
4. What tools can enhance exercise testing sessions for individuals with FM?
5. Why were the Åstrand cycle and walking tests recommended?

The fitness professional must recognize that the individual's symptoms of FM may fluctuate each day. The patient may report multiple areas of pain that affect overall function. The patient's symptoms (*e.g.*, pain and fatigue) should be reviewed prior to fitness testing in order to develop an individualized testing protocol. The types of tests and order of testing should reflect the individual's wiliness and current physical abilities.

For **submaximal** aerobic capacity, the Åstrand cycle ergometer test and walking test (5, 6, and 10 min) have shown good validity and reliability for individuals with FM (103). For resistance training, the 1-RM test has been shown to be valid and reliable measure of strength (64,108). Pain and fatigue levels should be monitored throughout the testing process using the numeric pain rating scale (0 = no pain and 10 = worst pain ever experienced) or visual analog scale (95). The Borg CR-10 scale can also be used to track a patient's perceived exertion level during exercise (17,64). The Fibromyalgia Impact Questionnaire is often used to assess symptoms, physical function, and overall well-being (64).

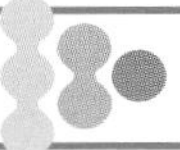

Exercise Prescription and Progression Considerations

Case Study 19-2 Quiz:

Exercise Prescription and Progression Considerations

6. Why would overtraining be common in individuals with FM?
7. How does fear affect ability to exercise in individuals with FM?
8. How can overtraining be avoided for individuals with FM?
9. Why should exercise prescriptions for individuals with FM be individualized?

The initial management of FM may include referral to physical therapy, pharmacological therapy, acupuncture, lifestyle changes (*e.g.*, eliminate stressors, improve sleep routines), dietary changes such as avoiding caffeine, and pain management such as cognitive-behavioral therapy or support groups (8,28,117). A successful exercise prescription requires effective communication between the patient and the fitness professional. Poor exercise adherence is common among individuals with FM due to their pain and functional level (19). Understanding potential predictors of high physical function in these patients may provide some insight for the fitness professional. Also, understanding the patient's overall perception toward physical activity is important. More specifically, determining how the patient learns and stays motivated and the person's level of self-efficacy (*e.g.*, ability to complete a task and reach goals) is important to a successful program.

Exercise has also been shown to an effective intervention in the maintenance of this chronic condition. The best evidence supports a multimodal exercise program (aerobic training, strength training, and flexibility) with the following parameters: (a) an exercise frequency of three times a week, (b) exercise session duration of 30–60 minutes, (c) aerobic exercise intensity of 57%–75% of maximum HR, (d) resistance training load of 40%–80% of 1-RM, and (e) an overall program duration of more than 7 weeks (13,64).

The following sections discuss each component of the multimodal program as a single mode of exercise. Some patients may not be able to participate in a multimodal program due to their pain or functional limitations. FITT guidelines for patients with FM can be found in FITT table (see Table 19.3).

For aerobic exercise, a light-to-moderate (57%–76% of maximum HR) intensity is recommended for these individuals. Aerobic exercise has been shown to reduce pain, fatigue, and depression and improve physical fitness in individuals with FM (13,19,53,70). Further recommendations for aerobic activity includes the following: (a) Activity should consist of land-based or aquatic exercises, (b) exercise should last for 20–30 minutes, (c) intensity should be light to moderate, and (d) the frequency of exercise should be two to three times per week for at least 4 weeks (53).

For strength training, a resistance training load of 40%–80% of 1-RM, one to three sets of 5–20 repetitions is recommend for individuals with FM (16,18,20,21,72). Strength gains have been found with programs that have lasted 12–21 weeks in duration (64,72,121). The patient's ability to participate may fluctuate due to the variability in muscle discomfort that can occur with FM.

For flexibility, there is no consensus on the ideal flexibility program for FM. Patients often require an individualized flexibility prescription because they will have their own unique myofascial issues.

A summary of exercise training and prescription considerations for individuals with FM is presented as follows:

- Symptoms of pain and fatigue may fluctuate daily in individuals with FM and can directly affect the rate of progression as well as the intensity, type, and volume of exercise/physical activity tolerated at any given time.
- Exercise testing and training of patients with FM should be individualized in order to maximize their comfort, minimize or prevent pain and fatigue, and enhance their physical performance.
- A complement of exercise modes including endurance, resistance, and flexibility training are appropriate components of exercise programs for persons with FM; can contribute to improvements in their symptoms, physical fitness, and functional performance; and should each be part of their exercise program.
- Patients with FM should learn how to use their subjective pain ratings to adjust the intensity and volume of each exercise session.
- Patients with FM should be encouraged to stay as active as possible during exacerbations (flare-ups of symptoms) and select alternate activities as tolerated to maintain their baseline physical fitness and function
- In order to prevent injuries and exacerbations of symptoms in persons with FM, they should be instructed regularly to use proper exercise technique and also to avoid exercising when they are excessively fatigued.
- Best evidence supports a multimodal exercise program consisting of aerobic training, strength training, and flexibility exercise.

Other forms of exercise such as aquatic therapy, Pilates, tai chi, and yoga have low- to moderate-quality evidence supporting their efficacy for patients with FM (5,14,43,80).

RHEUMATOID ARTHRITIS

This section presents special considerations related to the exercise assessment and programming for adults with RA who have been medically cleared to exercise. The case study is followed throughout this section to provide insight into condition-specific strategies for increasing fitness levels, reducing disease-based risk factors and comorbidities, enhancing physical activity tolerance, and improving function for an individual with RA.

Case Study 19-3:

Mrs. Case Study-RA

Mrs. Case Study-RA is a 60-year-old woman diagnosed with RA 5 years ago based on the 2010 American College of Rheumatology/European League Against Rheumatism classification criteria (3). At the time of diagnosis, she had tenderness and swelling at >10 joints, and laboratory testing confirming that she is seropositive for the rheumatoid factor and had an abnormally high erythrocyte sedimentation rate.

Mrs. Case Study-RA has been employed as an accountant for the past 30 years and lives in a two-storey residence with her spouse. Her community has a heated pool and fitness center. Her current pharmacological therapies include methotrexate, a disease-modifying antirheumatic drug (DMARD), as well as an oral glucocorticoid for short-term use when she experiences an RA flare (aggravation of her condition). Medical history is unremarkable with the exception of early osteopenia diagnosed on a DEXA test.

Her rheumatologist placed her on 1,000 mg of calcium and 800 IU per day of vitamin D as a result of the DEXA test and known risk for osteopenia among individuals with RA (91). Although a risk of cardiovascular events and subclinical atherosclerosis is present among individuals with RA (131), her laboratory profile indicates an absence of hypercholesterolemia and hyperlipidemia. She is a nonsmoker, and her BP and fasting glucose are 125/74 mm Hg and 90 mg · dL^{-1}, respectively. Although generally sedentary, her physical activity includes taking her 15-kg (about 33 lb) dog on an estimated walk daily (about 150 ft) and walking up and down stairs in her residence. She is reluctant to exercise as she fears worsening of her condition. The patient's rheumatologist recommended that she complete a treadmill test (Bruce protocol) with a ramp protocol; however, her test was discontinued shortly after initiation due to bilateral knee pain.

Mrs. Case Study-RA presents for an exercise assessment and prescription following **medical clearance** from her rheumatologist who has been managing her RA. Currently, her RA is in remission, and symptoms are controlled with pharmacological therapy. She has not participated in formal exercise for approximately 10 years. She verbalizes concern that exercise may have detrimental effects on her condition as she read a document that stated exercise accelerates joint degradation and increases inflammation. Currently, her average pain is a 2 out of 10 with normal ADL in her wrists, hands, knees, and elbows. She reports that pain has the potential to increase substantially during flares and with strenuous activities such as opening a new jar or bottle. Mrs. Case Study-RA reports general fatigue and reduced sleep, difficulty with stairs in her residence, limited ability to carry grocery bags, difficulty opening jars, and an inability to perform and sustain a deep squat as needed for gardening activities. She reports a fear of walking her dog as she has had difficulty controlling her dog's tendency to pull on the leash. She works in a metropolitan area and has been challenged with crossing the street given the time allotment of the crossing light. Her goals are to improve her physical conditioning to a level that alleviates her functional limitations, improves BMD or attenuates further loss, and reduces fatigue. She would like to begin a walking program using the heated pool in her community and cautiously begin strength training.

An evidence-informed exercise program was designed for Mrs. Case Study-RA based on findings from the exercise assessment and established guidelines for exercise and physical activity for **older adults** (23,38).The routine consisted of aerobic exercise, muscle performance training, and flexibility. Aerobic training was initiated in a heated pool at waist-high level to minimize impact on the knee, foot, and ankle joints. A progression to land-based walking or cycling was tolerated at the 3-week point. Sessions lasted approximately 30 minutes with a rating of 5–6 on the CR-10 scale. At week 9, stair-based training was added for specificity given stair demands of the patient. Irrespective of the patient's activity choice, land-based walking or stairs was performed at least three times per week as this would be beneficial for BMD. At week 9, intensity was increase additionally to include more vigorous performance. The exception to the dosing plan was gripping and adduction activities as this was performed with putty and was completed at conclusion of each session for 3–5 minutes. Gripping and adduction was advanced by changing the putty resistance level. At week 6, it was recommended that one to two sets of each exercise be performed 3 times a week on nonconsecutive days. At week 9, three sets of each exercise were performed every other day. The "two for two" rule of intensity load progression (increase intensity after two or more repetitions per exercise set) is performed beyond the goal repetitions for two consecutive sessions. Modifications to restrict shoulder positioning were made for the chest press and military press to avoid shoulder injury (74,75).

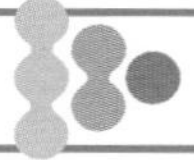

Description, Prevalence, and Etiology

Case Study 19-3 Quiz:

Description, Prevalence, and Etiology

1. What factors, in addition to age and gender, may explain the finding of reduced BMD?

RA is a chronic inflammatory disease that primarily affects the synovial joints and is a leading cause of disability. Although the prevalence of RA is low compared with osteoarthritis, it is considered the most common systemic inflammatory arthritis among adults (54). The onset of RA is most prevalent in the fourth decade, with women being affected 2.5–5 times more than men (54,82).

Although the etiology of RA is largely unknown, the disease process is triggered by an autoimmune response, which results in the body attacking its own healthy tissues (27). The autoimmune process triggers inflammation of the synovial joints, with evidence that a 3- to 100-fold increase in proinflammatory cytokines is present (27,90). This inflammatory response is known to spread to tissues that surround the joint, which results in erosion and destruction of the articular cartilage and leads to pain and associated morbidities (104). The course of RA is typically one of exacerbations (flares) and remission. Exacerbations are episodes whereby an increase in disease activity is present, which often coincides with increased pain, swelling, and tenderness. It has been estimated that persisting synovial inflammation results in erosion and destruction of the articular cartilage at a rate of 2% per year (110). Predominant features of RA include joint pain, swelling, tenderness, and eventual destruction of the synovial joints; however, extra-articular manifestations and comorbidities may develop over time (26). Although formal diagnosis is made based on established criteria (3), the manifestations of the condition itself vary between individuals as does its impact and progression. Box 19.1 presents the more common signs and symptoms associated with RA.

Although more common characteristics are used for diagnosis and evaluation of disease activity, comorbidities such as CVD, rheumatoid cachexia, osteopenia, and functional impairments occur in well over one-half of individuals diagnosed with RA (26,94,110,118). The increased risk for CVD is thought to be the result of systemic inflammation (87). Evidence suggests that individuals with RA underestimate their CVD risk and have aerobic capacities 20%–30% lower than age-matched controls (93,122).

Box 19.1 Functional Limitations Reported by the Patient

Functional limitations reported by the patient included the following:

- Carrying grocery bags
- Opening jars
- Walking her dog (controlling leash)
- Walking speed for crossing street
- Ascending stairs
- Descending stairs
- Squatting to floor for gardening

Rheumatoid cachexia is defined by a loss of skeletal mass with concomitant increases in adiposity (84,85). It affects approximately two-thirds of individuals with RA, often a result of catabolic factors (*e.g.*, proinflammatory cytokines, corticosteroid use), reduced anabolic profiles, poor nutrition, as well as the sequela of reduced physical activity levels (26,84,130). Rheumatoid cachexia may affect changes beyond **body composition** as a loss of muscle mass contributes to impaired strength and fatigue and increased adiposity may augment the risk of diabetes and CVD.

Reduced BMD may initially present as osteopenia and over time lead to osteoporosis. The etiology of reduced BMD is multifactorial and includes reduced weight-bearing exercise, corticosteroid use, as well as systemic inflammation (91).

As a consequence of the aforementioned signs and symptoms, disease state, and comorbidities, these individuals will often present with reduced physical activity and associated functional limitations (97). As such, reduced physical activity perpetuates the risk of CVD, rheumatoid cachexia, and osteopenia (94). From a prognostic perspective, many of the more common comorbidities are seemingly amenable to risk mitigation. Thus, recognizing common comorbidities lends insight into appropriate test selection, exercise programming, and preventative efforts.

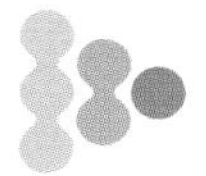

Preparticipation Health Screening, Medical History, and Physical Examination

Case Study 19-3 Quiz:

Preparticipation Health Screening, Medical History, and Physical Examination

2. Is the assessment of BMI an accurate depiction of an individual's body composition? In the case of Mrs. Case Study-RA, what changes may occur in body composition and how will these changes affect for BMI?

The exercise assessment should commence with collection of demographic data, patient limitations and goals, completion of questionnaires, and a familiarization trial for the physical tests and outcome measures. A familiarization trial is included as many of the selected tests have a learning effect. Prior to engaging in any testing, the exercise professional should have patients complete the Physical Activity Readiness Questionnaire for Everyone (PAR-Q+) assessment which, in this case study, indicate appropriateness for exercise. The Swedish Exercise Self-Efficacy Scale (ESES-S) was used as well. The ESES-S is a self-reported 6-item instrument that measures an individual's self-efficacy to perform exercise when barriers are present and has been partially validated in a population with RA (96). The ESES-S asks the patient about exercise confidence in the presence of six different scenarios. A total score for the six items is calculated with scores ranging from 6 (low efficacy) to 60 (high efficacy). The ESES-S has a low administrative burden (*e.g.*, six questions) and may offer the exercise specialist an understanding of an individual's perceived barriers to exercise.

In this case, the scale was administered as a result of evidence suggesting that individuals with RA fear detrimental effects from exercise as well as the patient's verbalization of exercise reluctance. Performance testing was selected based on the patient's subjective reports,

Table 19.4 Baseline Patient Assessment and Goals with Functional Relevance

Test	Baseline Assessment	Goals	Functional Activity Relevance
ESES-S self-report	18	60	N/A
Waist circumference (in)	40	35 ↓ CVD risk	N/A
Waist-to-hip ratio	0.99	Reduce to 0.90 ↓ CVD risk	N/A
TUG	14 s	9 s	Safely crossing street
6MWT	460 m	600 m	Walking endurance
Right handgrip strength (dominant hand)	21 kg	26 kg	Carrying groceries Control of dog leash Opening jars
Left handgrip strength	20 kg	25 kg	Carrying groceries Control of dog leash Opening jars
30-s STS	9 reps	17 reps	Stair activities Control of dog leash Squat ability
30-s Bicep curl (2 kg right)	15 reps	25 reps	Carrying groceries Control of dog leash
Chair sit and reach	−4 cm	0 cm	Functional bending
Weight-bearing lunge measure of ankle dorsiflexion ROM	5 cm bilaterally	13 cm	Normal ankle dorsiflexion is required for stair descent (87), normal walking, and performing a deep squat (68).

ROM, range of motion.

impairments and comorbidities related to RA, and persistent limitations from her physical therapy discharge note. See Table 19.4 for testing results, established goals, and functional relevance. Specifically, nine tests were performed in the following order: (a) observation, (b) anthropometrics and body composition, (c) TUG, (d) 6MWT, (e) grip strength, (f) 30-second STS, (g) 30-second bicep curl, (h) chair sit and reach for lower extremity flexibility, and (i) weight-bearing lunge for ankle dorsiflexion mobility.

Prior to physical testing, the exercise professional observed the patient's posture and physical appearance (see Box 19.2). Mrs. Case Study-RA had no apparent structural deformities and ambulated independently without an assistive device. The exercise specialist measured the patient's body mass and height, and from these measurements, a BMI was documented. The waist-to-hip ratio (WHR) was conducted to determine visceral obesity which is a risk factor for CVD. Based on available equipment, skinfold analysis was conducted to determine body fat percentage. This technique was undertaken with awareness that it is only an estimate of body fat, and the cluster of tests (skinfold, WHR, BMI) would provide a more accurate depiction of the patient's body composition and risk for CVD.

Box 19.2 Rheumatoid Arthritis: Characteristic Signs and Symptoms

- Characteristic signs and symptoms of rheumatoid arthritis (RA) include the following: pain, swelling, inflammation, and tenderness affecting multiple joints (polyarticular)
- Joint involvement is primarily bilateral.
- Small joints of wrist and hands affected first (60, 105,106)
- Joint deformities (*e.g.*, subluxation, ulnar drift, swan-neck) (15)
- Firm, painless growths under the skin near the joints (RA nodules)
- Stiffness in joints after rest and in morning hours
- General feeling of fatigue (11,37)
- Sleep disturbances (37)
- Fear of physical activity and depression (49,69, 106,111)
- Radiographic evidence of joint erosion and destruction
- Laboratory values positive for rheumatoid factor
- Laboratory values positive for anti-citrullinated protein antibody
- Abnormal C-reactive protein during acute phase
- Abnormal elevation of erythrocyte sedimentation rate

From Aletaha D, Neogi T, Silman AJ, et al. 2010 Rheumatoid arthritis classification criteria: an American College of Rheumatology/European League Against Rheumatism collaborative initiative. *Arthritis Rheum.* 2010;62(9):2569–81. doi:10.1002/art.27584; Belza BL. Comparison of self-reported fatigue in rheumatoid arthritis and controls. *J Rheumatol.* 1995;22(4):639–43; Bielefeld T, Neumann DA. The unstable metacarpophalangeal joint in rheumatoid arthritis: anatomy, pathomechanics, and physical rehabilitation considerations. *J Orthop Sports Phys Ther.* 2005;35(8):502–20. doi:10.2519/jospt.2005.35.8.502; Durcan L, Wilson F, Cunnane G. The effect of exercise on sleep and fatigue in rheumatoid arthritis: a randomized controlled study. *J Rheumatol.* 2014;41(10):1966–73. doi:10.3899/jrheum.131282; Grover HS, Gaba N, Gupta A, Marya CM. Rheumatoid arthritis: a review and dental care considerations. *Nepal Med Coll J.* 2011;13(2):74–6; Iversen MD, Brandenstein JS. Do dynamic strengthening and aerobic capacity exercises reduce pain and improve functional outcomes and strength in people with established rheumatoid arthritis? *Phys Ther.* 2012;92(10):1251–7. doi:10.2522/ptj.20110440; Iversen MD, Brawerman M, Iversen CN. Recommendations and the state of the evidence for physical activity interventions for adults with rheumatoid arthritis: 2007 to present. *Int J Clin Rheumtol.* 2012;7(5):489–503. doi:10.2217/ijr.12.53; Kelley GA, Kelley KS. Effects of exercise on depressive symptoms in adults with arthritis and other rheumatic disease: a systematic review of meta-analyses. *BMC Musculoskelet Disord.* 2014;15:121. doi:10.1186/1471-2474-15-121; Rindfleisch JA, Muller D. Diagnosis and management of rheumatoid arthritis. *Am Fam Physician.* 2005;72(6):1037–47; and Scott DL, Wolfe F, Huizinga TW. Rheumatoid arthritis. *Lancet.* 2010;376(9746):1094–108. doi:10.1016/S0140-6736(10)60826-4.

Case Study 19-3 Quiz:

Preparticipation Health Screening, Medical History, and Physical Examination

3. What tests may be conducted in lieu of the treadmill test?
4. Why would the 6MWT be more desirable than a treadmill test for a patient with RA?

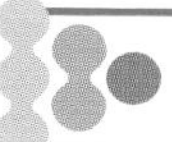

Exercise Testing Considerations

The TUG test was selected as it mirrors the distance of crossing a metropolitan street and possessed a component of walking speed. The test was performed according to previously established guidelines (86). The TUG test is performed by having the patient sit in a stationary chair (approximately 44 cm [17 in]). The patient then stands and walks a distance of 3 m at a brisk speed and then turns around and returns to chair. The activity is timed using a standard stopwatch from the time the patient initiates rising from chair to the point of returning to the chair. Moderate-to-high correlations of the TUG have been observed when comparing this test with other functional tests of balance, walking speed, and stair climbing (45,56,102). Previous research on individuals with RA has shown improvements in TUG scores from quadriceps and hamstring strengthening, indicating test responsiveness (109). Cardiorespiratory fitness testing using either a treadmill, a bicycle, or a step ergometer with a ramp or incremental protocol can be considered, but the 6MWT is a viable alternative to the standardized treadmill test and reflects ADL and self-reported function.

Individuals with RA may risk a flare of their condition from a treadmill test. One may equate 6MWT performance with **muscular endurance** and secondary measures may be obtained to include exertion using the Borg CR-10 scale and cardiovascular response such as O_2 saturation, BP, and HR. The Borg CR-10 RPE has a point range from 0 to 10 where 0 means "nothing at all" and 10 means "very very hard" (99). Relative contraindications for the test include HR $>$120 bpm or uncontrolled hypertension. The distance walked during the 6MWT may be entered into the Enright and Sherrill formula (40,41) to determine expected distance given age, gender, height, and body mass.

Muscle performance can be tested with assessments such as static handgrip strength, the 30-second STS, and 30-second bicep curl tests in individuals unable to tolerate either 1-RM or multiple-RM testing (71,104). Handgrip strength is important to assess in patients with RA secondary to a known predilection for hand and wrist weakness and instability (15,79). Results may be reliably documented based on one trial for individuals with RA (71). The 30-second STS test assesses quadriceps, gluteal, and hamstring functioning, each being important for ascending and descending stairs and has moderately high correlation with the 1-RM leg press (62).

The chair sit-and-reach test and weight-bearing lunge are valid and reliable measures of ankle dorsiflexion and lower extremity flexibility of the hamstring muscles and plantar flexor musculotendinous structures, respectively (63,78). Testing was carried out according to previously established procedures (63,78). The weight-bearing lunge test provides a functional measure of ankle dorsiflexion and is obtained by determining the patient's ability to lunge toward and contact the wall with the knee of ankle being tested. With the knee in contact with the wall and heel flat on floor, the distance from the great toe to the wall is measured. The farther the great toe from the wall, the greater the patient's dorsiflexion.

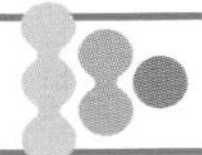

Exercise Prescription and Progression Considerations

Case Study 19-3 Quiz:

Exercise Prescription and Progression Considerations

5. What options exist for improving cardiorespiratory fitness that will also improve BMD?
6. What physical activity changes may help increase BMD?
7. The program provided to Mrs. Case Study-RA was based on both evidence and safety. What advancements should be made to the weight-training resistance program to incorporate muscle groups omitted in the initial program design?

Given the long-term outcomes and ensuing functional impairments associated with RA, appropriately dosed exercise is the cornerstone of conservative care. Appropriate exercise recommendations for individuals with RA are contingent on the results from an individualized fitness assessment as well as recognition of disease-specific precautions. Results, where possible, should be compared with age- and gender-matched normative values as well as authoritative guidelines. The exercise program for the patient with RA will differ from programming for healthy individuals given the risk for flares as well as physical limitations such as grip weakness, joint instability, and mobility restrictions. See Table 19.5 for specific modifications for Mrs. Case Study-RA as well as relevance

Table 19.5 Specific Exercise Modifications and Relevance to Functional Activity

Exercise	Modification	Muscles Involved	Functional implication
Total gym	Begin 45° incline and progress incline. Elastic band around knees to promote hip abduction	Gluteal medius, minimus and maximus, quadriceps, hamstrings	Sit-to-stand, stairs, walking dog, walking speed
Chair squat	May add backpack with weights for resistance	Gluteal maximus, quadriceps, hamstrings	Sit-to-stand, stairs, walking dog, walking speed
Knee extension machine	May work within pain-free range	Quadriceps	Sit-to-stand, stairs, walking dog, walking speed
Hamstring curl	May work within pain-free range	Hamstrings	Stairs, walking dog, walking speed
Shoulder press machine	Use front grip option to avoid shoulder pain.	Deltoids, triceps	Pushing and reaching overhead, carrying groceries
Chest press machine	Limit descent range to minimize depth of elbows past torso.	Deltoids, pectorals, triceps	Pushing activity
Bicep curls	Consider resistance training gloves with elastic wrist strap option for stability.	Biceps, brachialis, brachioradialis	Carrying groceries and controlling dog leash
Triceps extension	Should perform standing as well as overhead to target all heads of triceps	Triceps	Pushing activity
Seated rows	Maintain scapular retraction and lumbar lordosis.	Latissimus dorsi, rhomboids, middle trapezius	Control dog leash, lifting groceries
Time based Gripping putty	Selection of putty colors of progressive intensity	Finger flexors	Opening jars and carrying groceries and joint protection
Time based Finger adduction with putty	Selection of putty colors of progressive intensity	Finger adductors	Opening jars and carrying groceries and joint protection
Brisk land-based or water walking	Flat terrain Water walking waist level	Gluteals, hamstrings, quadriceps	Walking endurance and lower extremity muscle performance
Chair sit and reach Standing lunch calf stretch	Avoid ballistic movement. Calf stretch with knees straight as well as slightly flexed	Hamstring, gastrocnemius, soleus	Functional mobility for stair descent, walking, and deep squat

to functional activities. Moreover, ongoing discomfort or swelling from affected joints may preclude participation in certain exercises. From a safety perspective, these individuals may have joint hyperlaxity from joint erosions and be susceptible to fracture as a result of osteoporosis or osteopenia. Consistently measuring exercise intensity and pain will serve useful to prevent any untoward effects from exercise. A numerical scale, such as the Borg CR-10 RPE, may be used to measure exertion level (137). An 11-point numerical pain rating scale with 0 (no pain) to 10 (worst pain imaginable) can also be used to monitor the effects of exercise (136). The numerical pain rating scale is commonly used to measure pain and fatigue in individuals with RA, which may be beneficial in guiding their exercise programs (39,92).

With respect to the type of exercise, evidence suggests that land-based aerobic training has shown a moderate effect on aerobic capacity, pain, and quality of life, whereas combined aerobic and resistance training has shown a positive effect for aerobic capacity and CVD risk factors (lipids, BP, body composition, systemic inflammation, insulin resistance) among individuals with RA (10,29,115). Moreover, evidence suggests that combined strength and aerobic training has a beneficial effect on 10-year CVD event probability (115). In the aforementioned studies, exercise frequency was approximately two to five times a week at generally greater than 55% maximum HR for up to 12 weeks (60). Water-based exercise may lend improvements in pain, strength, quality of life, and function among individuals with RA (4,57,59,60,65). Aquatic programs generally range from 30 to 60 minutes (moderate aerobic activity) for two to three times per week in a water temperature of 30°–35°C.

With respect to resistance training, systematic reviews have consistently reported increased muscle performance in the upper and lower extremity musculature, including grip strength (9,57). Baillet et al. (9) conducted a systematic review and found that resistance training programs improved isokinetic, isometric, and grip strength in individuals with RA. The resistance training programs ranged from 15 to 60 minutes, 2–7 days per week, for 3–104 weeks. The exercises were performed at a load ranging from 30% to 100% or 1-RM for one to four sets of 5–30 repetitions. Flint-Wagner et al. (44) reported that a 16-week (three times per week) high-intensity resistance training program improved strength, pain, and function among individuals with RA when compared with a matched control group. Lastly, a multimodal program consisting of moderate-intensity cardiovascular activity 5 days per week, resistance training at 40%–50% 1-RM 3 days per week, and daily stretching significantly reduced pain and stiffness, increased function, reduced fatigue, and improved sleep quality when compared with usual care among a group of individuals with RA (37).

With respect to comorbidities, evidence suggests a favorable effect of exercise for attenuating a loss of BMD, improving joint health, and favorably altering body composition. The Rheumatoid Arthritis Patients in Training (RAPIT) program study observed a reduced rate of BMD loss in the hip during 2 years of high-intensity weight-bearing exercise training (30,31). Although it has been postulated that resistance training or high-intensity exercise may accelerate disease activity, evidence has shown otherwise (124).

SUMMARY

A summary of exercise training and prescription considerations for individuals with RA is presented as follows:

- Exercise testing and program development should be individualized, and goals should address all physical health, fitness, and functional needs of persons with RA.
- Comorbid health conditions might be present and should also dictate exercise program development decisions (*e.g.*, osteoporosis, atherosclerosis).
- In many cases, a more gradual rate of progression in exercise intensity and volume is warranted with specific modification.

- Pain levels and, if present, limitations from comorbid conditions and patient tolerance should determine the positions which aerobic, resistance, and flexibility exercises are performed.
- Exercises causing pain during or after workout sessions should be either modified, eliminated, or substituted with alternative activities.
- Pain that is worse 2 hours after exercise termination warrants reductions in intensity and volume during subsequent exercise sessions.
- New or worsening symptoms warrant exercise termination and communication with a physician and/or health care provider.
- A growing body of evidence supports the safety and efficacy of exercise-based interventions for improving function and attenuating comorbidities
- Exercise programs for patients with RA must be efficacious and void of detrimental effects including joint pain, inflammation, and instability.
- Recognizing barriers such as fatigue, lower baseline activity levels, and a fear of detrimental effects from exercise (inflammation and accelerated joint erosion) is necessary to effect a lifestyle change that incorporates exercise.

RECOMMENDED RESOURCES

ACSM/AMA Exercise is Medicine®: http://www.exerciseismedicine.org

American College of Sports Medicine position stand. Progression models in resistance training for healthy adults (Ratamess, Alvar, Evetovich, et al., 2009): http://www.acsm.org

American College of Sports Medicine position stand. Quantity and quality of exercise for developing and maintaining cardiorespiratory, musculoskeletal, and neuromotor fitness in apparently healthy adults: guidance for prescribing exercise (Garber, Blissmer, Deschenes, et al., 2011): http://www.acsm.org

Compendium of Physical Activities: https://sites.google.com/site/compendiumofphysicalactivities/

MedlinePlus, U.S. Library of Medicine, National Institutes of Health: https://www.nlm.nih.gov/medlineplus/backpain.html

National Institute of Neurological Disorders and Stroke: http://www.ninds.nih.gov/disorders/backpain/backpain.htm

National Strength and Conditioning Association: http://www.nsca-lift.org

Rehabilitation Measures Database: http://www.rehabmeasures.org/default.aspx

Physical Activity Guidelines for Americans (U.S. Department of Health and Human Services. 2008 Physical Activity Guidelines for Americans [Internet], 2008): http://www.health.gov/PAguidelines/

REFERENCES

1. Agency for Healthcare Research and Quality. *Medical Expenditure Panel Survey* [Internet]. Rockville (MD): U.S. Department of Health and Human Services; [cited 2016 Feb 25]. Available from: https://meps.ahrq.gov/mepsweb/
2. Ainsworth BE, Haskell WL, Herrmann SD, et al. 2011 Compendium of Physical Activities: a second update of codes and MET values. *Med Sci Sports Exerc*. 2011;43(8):1575–81. doi:10.1249/MSS.0b013e31821ece12.
3. Aletaha D, Neogi T, Silman AJ, et al. 2010 Rheumatoid arthritis classification criteria: an American College of Rheumatology/European League Against Rheumatism collaborative initiative. *Arthritis Rheum*. 2010;62(9):2569–81. doi:10.1002/art.27584.
4. Al-Qubaeissy KY, Fatoye FA, Goodwin PC, Yohannes AM. The effectiveness of hydrotherapy in the management of rheumatoid arthritis: a systematic review. *Musculoskeletal Care*. 2013;11(1):3–18. doi:10.1002/msc.1028.
5. Altan L, Korkmaz N, Bingol U, Gunay B. Effect of Pilates training on people with fibromyalgia syndrome: a pilot study. *Arch Phys Med Rehabil*. 2009;90(12):1983–8. doi:10.1016/j.apmr.2009.06.021.
6. American College of Sports Medicine. *ACSM's Guidelines for Exercise Testing and Prescription*. 10th ed. Philadelphia (PA): Wolters Kluwer; 2018. 480 p.
7. American College of Sports Medicine. American College of Sports Medicine position stand. Progression models in resistance training for healthy adults. *Med Sci Sports Exerc*. 2009;41(3):687–708.
8. Arnold LM, Clauw DJ, McCarberg BH. Improving the recognition and diagnosis of fibromyalgia. *Mayo Clin Proc*. 2011;86(5):457–64. doi:10.4065/mcp.2010.0738.
9. Baillet A, Vaillant M, Guinot M, Juvin R, Gaudin P. Efficacy of resistance exercises in rheumatoid arthritis: meta-analysis of randomized controlled trials. *Rheumatology (Oxford)*. 2012;51(3):519–27. doi:10.1093/rheumatology/ker330.

10. Baillet A, Zeboulon N, Gossec L, et al. Efficacy of cardiorespiratory aerobic exercise in rheumatoid arthritis: meta-analysis of randomized controlled trials. *Arthritis Care Res (Hoboken)*. 2010;62(7):984–92. doi:10.1002/acr.20146.
11. Belza BL. Comparison of self-reported fatigue in rheumatoid arthritis and controls. *J Rheumatol*. 1995;22(4):639–43.
12. Bennett RM. Clinical manifestations and diagnosis of fibromyalgia. *Rheum Dis Clin North Am*. 2009;35(2):215–32. doi:10.1016/j.rdc.2009.05.009.
13. Bidonde J, Busch AJ, Bath B, Milosavljevic S. Exercise for adults with fibromyalgia: an umbrella systematic review with synthesis of best evidence. *Curr Rheumatol Rev*. 2014;10(1):45–79.
14. Bidonde J, Busch AJ, Webber SC, et al. Aquatic exercise training for fibromyalgia. *Cochrane Database Syst Rev*. 2014;(10):CD011336. doi:10.1002/14651858.CD011336.
15. Bielefeld T, Neumann DA. The unstable metacarpophalangeal joint in rheumatoid arthritis: anatomy, pathomechanics, and physical rehabilitation considerations. *J Orthop Sports Phys Ther*. 2005;35(8):502–20. doi:10.2519/jospt.2005.35.8.502.
16. Bircan C, Karasel SA, Akgün B, El O, Alper S. Effects of muscle strengthening versus aerobic exercise program in fibromyalgia. *Rheumatol Int*. 2008;28(6):527–32. doi:10.1007/s00296-007-0484-5.
17. Borg G, Hassmén P, Lagerström M. Perceived exertion related to heart rate and blood lactate during arm and leg exercise. *Eur J Appl Physiol Occup Physiol*. 1987;56(6):679–85.
18. Busch AJ, Schachter CL, Overend TJ, Peloso PM, Barber KA. Exercise for fibromyalgia: a systematic review. *J Rheumatol*. 2008;35(6):1130–44.
19. Busch AJ, Webber SC, Brachaniec M, et al. Exercise therapy for fibromyalgia. *Curr Pain Headache Rep*. 2011;15(5):358–67. doi:10.1007/s11916-011-0214-2.
20. Busch AJ, Webber SC, Richards RS, et al. Resistance exercise training for fibromyalgia. *Cochrane Database Syst Rev*. 2013;(12):CD010884. doi:10.1002/14651858.CD010884.
21. Cazzola M, Atzeni F, Salaffi F, Stisi S, Cassisi G, Sarzi-Puttini P. Which kind of exercise is best in fibromyalgia therapeutic programmes? A practical review. *Clin Exp Rheumatol*. 2010;28(6 suppl 63):S117–24.
22. Centers for Disease Control and Prevention. *2012 Data Release* [Internet]. Atlanta (GA): National Center for Health Statistics; [cited 2016 Feb 25]. Available from: http://www.cdc.gov/nchs//nhis/nhis_2012_data_release.htm
23. Chodzko-Zajko WJ, Proctor DN, Fiatarone Singh MA, et al. American College of Sports Medicine position stand. Exercise and physical activity for older adults. *Med Sci Sports Exerc*. 2009;41(7):1510–30. doi:10.1249/MSS.0b013e3181a0c95c.
24. Clauw DJ, Arnold LM, McCarberg BH. The science of fibromyalgia. *Mayo Clin Proc*. 2011;86(9):907–11. doi:10.4065/mcp.2011.0206.
25. Clauw DJ, Crofford LJ. Chronic widespread pain and fibromyalgia: what we know, and what we need to know. *Best Pract Res Clin Rheumatol*. 2003;17(4):685–701.
26. Cooney JK, Law RJ, Matschke V, et al. Benefits of exercise in rheumatoid arthritis. *J Aging Res*. 2011;2011:681640. doi:10.4061/2011/681640.
27. Cubick EE, Quezada VY, Schumer AD, Davis CM. Sustained release myofascial release as treatment for a patient with complications of rheumatoid arthritis and collagenous colitis: a case report. *Int J Ther Massage Bodywork*. 2011;4(3):1–9.
28. Deare JC, Zheng Z, Xue CC, et al. Acupuncture for treating fibromyalgia. *Cochrane Database Syst Rev*. 2013;(5):CD007070. doi:10.1002/14651858.CD007070.pub2.
29. de Jong Z, Munneke M, Kroon HM, et al. Long-term follow-up of a high-intensity exercise program in patients with rheumatoid arthritis. *Clin Rheumatol*. 2009;28(6):663–71. doi:10.1007/s10067-009-1125-z.
30. de Jong Z, Munneke M, Lems WF, et al. Slowing of bone loss in patients with rheumatoid arthritis by long-term high-intensity exercise: results of a randomized, controlled trial. *Arthritis Rheum*. 2004;50(4):1066–76. doi:10.1002/art.20117.
31. de Jong Z, Munneke M, Zwinderman AH, et al. Is a long-term high-intensity exercise program effective and safe in patients with rheumatoid arthritis? Results of a randomized controlled trial. *Arthritis Rheum*. 2003;48(9):2415–24. doi:10.1002/art.11216.
32. de Jong Z, Munneke M, Zwinderman AH, et al. Long term high intensity exercise and damage of small joints in rheumatoid arthritis. *Ann Rheum Dis*. 2004;63(11):1399–405. doi:10.1136/ard.2003.015826.
33. Delitto A, George SZ, Van Dillen LR, et al. Low back pain. *J Orthop Sports Phys Ther*. 2012;42(4):A1–57. doi:10.2519/jospt.2012.0301.
34. Descarreaux M, Normand MC, Laurencelle L, Dugas C. Evaluation of a specific home exercise program for low back pain. *J Manipulative Physiol Ther*. 2002;25(8):497–503.
35. Di Iorio A, Abate M, Guralnik JM, et al. From chronic low back pain to disability, a multifactorial mediated pathway: the InCHIANTI study. *Spine (Phila Pa 1976)*. 2007;32(26):E809–15. doi:10.1097/BRS.0b013e31815cd422.
36. Duque I, Parra JH, Duvallet A. Maximal aerobic power in patients with chronic low back pain: a comparison with healthy subjects. *Eur Spine J*. 2011;20(1):87–93. doi:10.1007/s00586-010-1561-0.
37. Durcan L, Wilson F, Cunnane G. The effect of exercise on sleep and fatigue in rheumatoid arthritis: a randomized controlled study. *J Rheumatol*. 2014;41(10):1966–73. doi:10.3899/jrheum.131282.
38. Elsawy B, Higgins KE. Physical activity guidelines for older adults. *Am Fam Physician*. 2010;81(1):55–9.
39. Englbrecht M, Tarner IH, van der Heijde DM, Manger B, Bombardier C, Müller-Ladner U. Measuring pain and efficacy of pain treatment in inflammatory arthritis: a systematic literature review. *J Rheumatol Suppl*. 2012;90:3–10. doi:10.3899/jrheum.120335.

40. Enright PL. The six-minute walk test. *Respir Care.* 2003;48(8):783–5.
41. Enright PL, Sherrill DL. Reference equations for the six-minute walk in healthy adults. *Am J Respir Crit Care Med.* 1998;158 (5 pt 1):1384–7. doi:10.1164/ajrccm.158.5.9710086.
42. Ferguson FC, Morison SM, Ryan CG. Physiotherapists' understanding of red flags for back pain. *Musculoskeletal Care.* 2015;13:42–50.
43. Fischer-White TG, Anderson JG, Taylor AG. An integrated methodology to assess compliance with Delphi survey key components of yoga interventions for musculoskeletal conditions as applied in a systematic review of fibromyalgia studies. *Explore (NY).* 2016;12(2):100–12. doi:10.1016/j.explore.2015.12.003.
44. Flint-Wagner HG, Lisse J, Lohman TG, et al. Assessment of a sixteen-week training program on strength, pain, and function in rheumatoid arthritis patients. *J Clin Rheumatol.* 2009;15(4):165–71. doi:10.1097/RHU.0b013e318190f95f.
45. Freter SH, Fruchter N. Relationship between timed 'up and go' and gait time in an elderly orthopaedic rehabilitation population. *Clin Rehabil.* 2000;14(1):96–101.
46. Garber CE, Blissmer B, Deschenes MR, et al. American College of Sports Medicine position stand. Quantity and quality of exercise for developing and maintaining cardiorespiratory, musculoskeletal, and neuromotor fitness in apparently healthy adults: guidance for prescribing exercise. *Med Sci Sports Exerc.* 2011;43(7):1334–59. doi:10.1249/MSS.0b013e318213fefb.
47. Gaskin DJ, Richard P. The economic costs of pain in the United States. *J Pain.* 2012;13(8):715–24.
48. Ge HY, Wang Y, Danneskiold-Samsøe B, Graven-Nielsen T, Arendt-Nielsen L. The predetermined sites of examination for tender points in fibromyalgia syndrome are frequently associated with myofascial trigger points. *J Pain.* 2010;11(7):644–51. doi:10.1016/j.jpain.2009.10.006.
49. Grover HS, Gaba N, Gupta A, Marya CM. Rheumatoid arthritis: a review and dental care considerations. *Nepal Med Coll J.* 2011;13(2):74–6.
50. Gur A, Oktayoglu P. Central nervous system abnormalities in fibromyalgia and chronic fatigue syndrome: new concepts in treatment. *Curr Pharm Des.* 2008;14(13):1274–94.
51. Hammill RR, Beazell JR, Hart JM. Neuromuscular consequences of low back pain and core dysfunction. *Clin Sports Med.* 2008;27(3):449–62, ix. doi:10.1016/j.csm.2008.02.005.
52. Hanney WJ, Pabian PS, Smith MT, Patel CK. Low back pain: movement considerations for exercise and training. Strength *Cond J.* 2008;35(4):99–106. doi:10.1519/SSC.0b013e31829d125a.
53. Häuser W, Klose P, Langhorst J, et al. Efficacy of different types of aerobic exercise in fibromyalgia syndrome: a systematic review and meta-analysis of randomised controlled trials. *Arthritis Res Ther.* 2010;12(3):R79. doi:10.1186/ar3002.
54. Helmick CG, Felson DT, Lawrence RC, et al. Estimates of the prevalence of arthritis and other rheumatic conditions in the United States. Part I. *Arthritis Rheum.* 2008;58(1):15–25. doi:10.1002/art.23177.
55. Hendrick P, Milosavljevic S, Hale L, et al. The relationship between physical activity and low back pain outcomes: a systematic review of observational studies. *Eur Spine J.* 2011;20(3):464–74. doi:10.1007/s00586-010-1616-2.
56. Hughes C, Osman C, Woods AK. Functional reach, and timed up and go tests in older adults. *Issues Aging.* 1998;21:18–22.
57. Hurkmans E, van der Giesen FJ, Vliet Vlieland TP, Schoones J, Van den Ende EC. Dynamic exercise programs (aerobic capacity and/or muscle strength training) in patients with rheumatoid arthritis. *Cochrane Database Syst Rev.* 2009;(4):CD006853. doi:10.1002/14651858.CD006853.pub2.
58. Huynh L, Chimes GP. Get the lowdown on low back pain in athletes. *ACSMs Health Fit J.* 2014;18:15–22.
59. Iversen MD, Brandenstein JS. Do dynamic strengthening and aerobic capacity exercises reduce pain and improve functional outcomes and strength in people with established rheumatoid arthritis? *Phys Ther.* 2012;92(10):1251–7. doi:10.2522/ptj.20110440.
60. Iversen MD, Brawerman M, Iversen CN. Recommendations and the state of the evidence for physical activity interventions for adults with rheumatoid arthritis: 2007 to present. *Int J Clin Rheumtol.* 2012;7(5):489–503. doi:10.2217/ijr.12.53.
61. Jackson JK, Shepherd TR, Kell RT. The influence of periodized resistance training on recreationally active males with chronic nonspecific low back pain. *J Strength Cond Res.* 2011;25(1):242–51. doi:10.1519/JSC.0b013e3181b2c83d.
62. Jones CJ, Rikli RE, Beam WC. A 30-s chair-stand test as a measure of lower body strength in community-residing older adults. *Res Q Exerc Sport.* 1999;70(2):113–9. doi:10.1080/02701367.1999.10608028.
63. Jones CJ, Rikli RE, Max J, Noffal G. The reliability and validity of a chair sit-and-reach test as a measure of hamstring flexibility in older adults. *Res Q Exerc Sport.* 1998;69(4):338–43. doi:10.1080/02701367.1998.10607708.
64. Jones KD, Adams D, Winters-Stone K, Burckhardt CS. A comprehensive review of 46 exercise treatment studies in fibromyalgia (1988-2005). *Health Qual Life Outcomes.* 2006;4:67. doi:10.1186/1477-7525-4-67.
65. Kamioka H, Tsutani K, Okuizumi H, et al. Effectiveness of aquatic exercise and balneotherapy: a summary of systematic reviews based on randomized controlled trials of water immersion therapies. *J Epidemiol.* 2010;20(1):2–12.
66. Kasuyama T, Sakamoto M, Nakazawa R. Ankle joint dorsiflexion measurement using the deep squatting posture. *J Phys Ther Sci.* 2009;21:195–9.
67. Kell RT, Asmundson GJ. A comparison of two forms of periodized exercise rehabilitation programs in the management of chronic nonspecific low-back pain. *J Strength Cond Res.* 2009;23(2):513–23. doi:10.1519/JSC.0b013e3181918a6e.
68. Kell RT, Risi AD, Barden JM. The response of persons with chronic nonspecific low back pain to three different volumes of periodized musculoskeletal rehabilitation. *J Strength Cond Res.* 2011;25(4):1052–64. doi:10.1519/JSC.0b013e3181d09df7.

69. Kelley GA, Kelley KS. Effects of exercise on depressive symptoms in adults with arthritis and other rheumatic disease: a systematic review of meta-analyses. *BMC Musculoskelet Disord.* 2014;15:121. doi:10.1186/1471-2474-15-121.
70. Kelley GA, Kelley KS, Hootman JM, Jones DL. Exercise and global well-being in community-dwelling adults with fibromyalgia: a systematic review with meta-analysis. *BMC Public Health.* 2010;10:198. doi:10.1186/1471-2458-10-198.
71. Kennedy D, Jerosch-Herold C, Hickson M. The reliability of one vs. three trials of pain-free grip strength in subjects with rheumatoid arthritis. *J Hand Ther.* 2010;23(4):384–90. doi:10.1016/j.jht.2010.05.002.
72. Kingsley JD, McMillan V, Figueroa A. The effects of 12 weeks of resistance exercise training on disease severity and autonomic modulation at rest and after acute leg resistance exercise in women with fibromyalgia. *Arch Phys Med Rehabil.* 2010;91(10):1551–7. doi:10.1016/j.apmr.2010.07.003.
73. Koes BW, van Tulder MW, Thomas S. Diagnosis and treatment of low back pain. *BMJ.* 2006;332(7555):1430–4. doi:10.1136/bmj.332.7555.1430.
74. Kolber MJ, Beekhuizen KS, Cheng MS, Hellman MA. Shoulder injuries attributed to resistance training: a brief review. *J Strength Cond Res.* 2010;24(6):1696–704. doi:10.1519/JSC.0b013e3181dc4330.
75. Kolber MJ, Corrao M, Hanney WJ. Characteristics of anterior shoulder instability and hyperlaxity in the weight-training population. *J Strength Cond Res.* 2013;27(5):1333–9. doi:10.1519/JSC.0b013e318269f776.
76. Kolber MJ, Hanney WJ. The dynamic disc model: a systematic review of the literature. *Phys Ther Rev.* 2009;14(3):181–9. doi:10.1179/174328809X452827.
77. Kongsted A, Kent P, Jensen TS, Albert H, Manniche C. Prognostic implications of the Quebec Task Force classification of back-related leg pain: an analysis of longitudinal routine clinical data. *BMC Musculoskelet Disord.* 2013;14:171. doi:10.1186/1471-2474-14-171.
78. Konor MM, Morton S, Eckerson JM, Grindstaff TL. Reliability of three measures of ankle dorsiflexion range of motion. *Int J Sports Phys Ther.* 2012;7(3):279–87.
79. Lamb SE, Williamson EM, Heine PJ, et al. Exercises to improve function of the rheumatoid hand (SARAH): a randomised controlled trial. *Lancet.* 2015;385(9966):421–9. doi:10.1016/S0140-6736(14)60998-3.
80. Lauche R, Cramer H, Häuser W, Dobos G, Langhorst J. A systematic overview of reviews for complementary and alternative therapies in the treatment of the fibromyalgia syndrome. *Evid Based Complement Alternat Med.* 2015;2015:610615. doi:10.1155/2015/610615.
81. Lawrence RC, Felson DT, Helmick CG, et al. Estimates of the prevalence of arthritis and other rheumatic conditions in the United States. Part II. *Arthritis Rheum.* 2008;58(1):26–35. doi:10.1002/art.23176.
82. Lawrence RC, Helmick CG, Arnett FC, et al. Estimates of the prevalence of arthritis and selected musculoskeletal disorders in the United States. *Arthritis Rheum.* 1998;41(5):778–99. doi:10.1002/1529-0131(199805)41:5<778::aid-art4>3.0.co;2-v.
83. Leblebici B, Pektaş ZO, Ortancil O, Hürcan EC, Bagis S, Akman M. Coexistence of fibromyalgia, temporomandibular disorder, and masticatory myofascial pain syndromes. *Rheumatol Int.* 2007;27(6):541–4. doi:10.1007/s00296-006-0251-z.
84. Lemmey AB, Jones J, Maddison PJ. Rheumatoid cachexia: what is it and why is it important? *J Rheumatol.* 2011;38(9):2074; author reply 2075. doi:10.3899/jrheum.110308.
85. Lemmey AB, Marcora SM, Chester K, Wilson S, Casanova F, Maddison PJ. Effects of high-intensity resistance training in patients with rheumatoid arthritis: a randomized controlled trial. *Arthritis Rheum.* 2009;61(12):1726–34. doi:10.1002/art.24891.
86. Livingston LA, Stevenson JM, Olney SJ. Stairclimbing kinematics on stairs of differing dimensions. *Arch Phys Med Rehabil.* 1991;72(6):398–402.
87. Maradit-Kremers H, Nicola PJ, Crowson CS, Ballman KV, Gabriel SE. Cardiovascular death in rheumatoid arthritis: a population-based study. *Arthritis Rheum.* 2005;52(3):722–32. doi:10.1002/art.20878.
88. Maul I, Läubli T, Oliveri M, Krueger H. Long-term effects of supervised physical training in secondary prevention of low back pain. *Eur Spine J.* 2005;14(6):599–611. doi:10.1007/s00586-004-0873-3.
89. McGill SM. *Low Back Disorders: Evidence-Based Prevention and Rehabilitation.* 3rd ed. Human Kinetics; 2016. 424 p.
90. McInnes IB. Rheumatoid arthritis. From bench to bedside. *Rheum Dis Clin North Am.* 2001;27(2):373–87.
91. Mikuls TR. Co-morbidity in rheumatoid arthritis. *Best Pract Res Clin Rheumatol.* 2003;17(5):729–52.
92. Minnock P, Kirwan J, Bresnihan B. Fatigue is a reliable, sensitive and unique outcome measure in rheumatoid arthritis. *Rheumatology (Oxford).* 2009;48(12):1533–6. doi:10.1093/rheumatology/kep287.
93. Minor MA, Hewett JE. Physical fitness and work capacity in women with rheumatoid arthritis. *Arthritis Care Res.* 1995;8(3):146–54.
94. Munsterman T, Takken T, Wittink H. Are persons with rheumatoid arthritis deconditioned? A review of physical activity and aerobic capacity. *BMC Musculoskelet Disord.* 2012;13:202. doi:10.1186/1471-2474-13-202.
95. Najm WI, Seffinger MA, Mishra SI, et al. Content validity of manual spinal palpatory exams — a systematic review. *BMC Complement Altern Med.* 2003;3:1. doi:10.1186/1472-6882-3-1.
96. Nessen T, Demmelmaier I, Nordgren B, Opava CH. The Swedish Exercise Self-Efficacy Scale (ESES-S): reliability and validity in a rheumatoid arthritis population. *Disabil Rehabil.* 2015;37(22):2130–4. doi:10.3109/09638288.2014.998780.
97. Ngian GS. Rheumatoid arthritis. *Aust Fam Physician.* 2010;39(9):626–8.
98. Nijs J, Apeldoorn A, Hallegraeff H, et al. Low back pain: guidelines for the clinical classification of predominant neuropathic, nociceptive, or central sensitization pain. *Pain Physician.* 2015;18(3):E333–46.

99. Noble BJ, Borg GA, Jacobs I, Ceci R, Kaiser P. A category-ratio perceived exertion scale: relationship to blood and muscle lactates and heart rate. *Med Sci Sports Exerc*. 1983;15(6):523–8.
100. Perkins J, Zipple JT. Nonspecific low back pain. In: Ehrman JK, Gordon PM, Visich PS, Keteyian SJ, editors. *Clinical Exercise Physiology*. 2nd ed. Champaign (IL): Human Kinetics; 2009. p. 497–520.
101. Perrot S, Dickenson AH, Bennett RM. Fibromyalgia: harmonizing science with clinical practice considerations. *Pain Pract*. 2008;8(3):177–89. doi:10.1111/j.1533-2500.2008.00190.x.
102. Podsiadlo D, Richardson S. The timed "up & go": a test of basic functional mobility for frail elderly persons. *J Am Geriatr Soc*. 1991;39(2):142–8.
103. Ratter J, Radlinger L, Lucas C. Several submaximal exercise tests are reliable, valid and acceptable in people with chronic pain, fibromyalgia or chronic fatigue: a systematic review. *J Physiother*. 2014;60(3):144–50. doi:10.1016/j.jphys.2014.06.011.
104. Rikli RE, Jones CJ. Development and validation of a functional fitness test for community-residing older adults. *J Aging Phys Act*. 1999;7:129–61.
105. Rikli RE, Jones CJ. The reliability and validity of a 6-minute walk test as a measure of physical endurance in older adults. *J Aging Phys Act*. 1998;6:363–75.
106. Rindfleisch JA, Muller D. Diagnosis and management of rheumatoid arthritis. *Am Fam Physician*. 2005;72(6):1037–47.
107. Robertson RJ, Goss FL, Rutkowski J, et al. Concurrent validation of the OMNI Perceived Exertion Scale for Resistance Exercise. *Med Sci Sports Exerc*. 2003;35(2):333–41. doi:10.1249/01.MSS.0000048831.15016.2A.
108. Rooks DS, Silverman CB, Kantrowitz FG. The effects of progressive strength training and aerobic exercise on muscle strength and cardiovascular fitness in women with fibromyalgia: a pilot study. *Arthritis Rheum*. 2002;47(1):22–8.
109. Schwartz AV, Villa ML, Prill M, et al. Falls in older Mexican-American women. *J Am Geriatr Soc*. 1999;47:1371–8.
110. Scott DL, Steer S. The course of established rheumatoid arthritis. *Best Pract Res Clin Rheumatol*. 2007;21(5):943–67. doi:10.1016/j.berh.2007.05.006.
111. Scott DL, Wolfe F, Huizinga TW. Rheumatoid arthritis. *Lancet*. 2010;376(9746):1094–108. doi:10.1016/S0140-6736(10)60826-4.
112. Silverman S, Sadosky A, Evans C, Yeh Y, Alvir JM, Zlateva G. Toward characterization and definition of fibromyalgia severity. *BMC Musculoskelet Disord*. 2010;11:66. doi:10.1186/1471-2474-11-66.
113. Simmonds MJ, Derghazarian T. Lower back pain syndrome. In: Durstine JL, Moore GE, Painter PL, Roberts SO, editors. *ACSM's Exercise Management for Persons With Chronic Diseases and Disabilities*. 3rd ed. Champaign (IL): Human Kinetics; 2009. p. 266–9.
114. Smeets RJ, Wittink H, Hidding A, Knottnerus JA. Do patients with chronic low back pain have a lower level of aerobic fitness than healthy controls? Are pain, disability, fear of injury, working status, or level of leisure time activity associated with the difference in aerobic fitness level? *Spine (Phila Pa 1976)*. 2006;31(1):90–7.
115. Stavropoulos-Kalinoglou A, Metsios GS, Veldhuijzen van Zanten JJ, Nightingale P, Kitas GD, Koutedakis Y. Individualised aerobic and resistance exercise training improves cardiorespiratory fitness and reduces cardiovascular risk in patients with rheumatoid arthritis. *Ann Rheum Dis*. 2013;72(11):1819–25. doi:10.1136/annrheumdis-2012-202075.
116. Sumpton JE, Moulin DE. Fibromyalgia: presentation and management with a focus on pharmacological treatment. *Pain Res Manag*. 2008;13(6):477–83.
117. Theadom A, Cropley M, Smith HE, Feigin VL, McPherson K. Mind and body therapy for fibromyalgia. *Cochrane Database Syst Rev*. 2015;(4):CD001980. doi:10.1002/14651858.CD001980.pub3.
118. Turesson C, O'Fallon WM, Crowson CS, Gabriel SE, Matteson EL. Extra-articular disease manifestations in rheumatoid arthritis: incidence trends and risk factors over 46 years. *Ann Rheum Dis*. 2003;62(8):722–7.
119. United States Bone and Joint Initiative. *The Burden of Musculoskeletal Diseases in the United States*. 3rd ed. Rosemont (IL): United States Bone and Joint Initiative; [cited 2014 Apr 19]. Available from: http://www.boneandjointburden.org
120. United States Bone and Joint Initiative Web site [Internet]. Rosemont (IL): United States Bone and Joint Initiative; [cited Feb 25]. Available from: http://www.boneandjointburden.org
121. Valkeinen H, Alen M, Hannonen P, Häkkinen A, Airaksinen O, Häkkinen K. Changes in knee extension and flexion force, EMG and functional capacity during strength training in older females with fibromyalgia and healthy controls. *Rheumatology (Oxford)*. 2004;43(2):225–8. doi:10.1093/rheumatology/keh027.
122. van Breukelen-van der Stoep DF, Zijlmans J, van Zeben D, et al. Adherence to cardiovascular prevention strategies in patients with rheumatoid arthritis. *Scand J Rheumatol*. 2015;44(6):443–8. doi:10.3109/03009742.2015.1028997.
123. van den Berg-Emons RJ, Schasfoort FC, de Vos LA, Bussmann JB, Stam HJ. Impact of chronic pain on everyday physical activity. *Eur J Pain*. 2007;11(5):587–93. doi:10.1016/j.ejpain.2006.09.003.
124. van den Ende CH, Breedveld FC, le Cessie S, Dijkmans BA, de Mug AW, Hazes JM. Effect of intensive exercise on patients with active rheumatoid arthritis: a randomised clinical trial. *Ann Rheum Dis*. 2000;59(8):615–21.
125. van den Ende CH, Vliet Vlieland TP, Munneke M, Hazes JM. Dynamic exercise therapy for rheumatoid arthritis. *Cochrane Database Syst Rev*. 2000;(2):CD000322. doi:10.1002/14651858.CD000322.
126. van den Ende CH, Vliet Vlieland TP, Munneke M, Hazes JM. Dynamic exercise therapy in rheumatoid arthritis: a systematic review. *Br J Rheumatol*. 1998;37(6):677–87.
127. van den Hoogen HJ, Koes BW, Devillé W, van Eijk JT, Bouter LM. The prognosis of low back pain in general practice. *Spine*. 1997;22:1515–21.

128. van Weering M, Vollenbroek-Hutten MM, Kotte EM, Hermens HJ. Daily physical activities of patients with chronic pain or fatigue versus asymptomatic controls. A systematic review. *Clin Rehabil.* 2007;21(11):1007–23. doi:10.1177/0269215507078331.
129. Vlaeyen JW, Linton SJ. Fear-avoidance and its consequences in chronic musculoskeletal pain: a state of the art. *Pain.* 2000;85(3):317–32.
130. Walsmith J, Abad L, Kehayias J, Roubenoff R. Tumor necrosis factor-alpha production is associated with less body cell mass in women with rheumatoid arthritis. *J Rheumatol.* 2004;31(1):23–9.
131. Wasko MC. Rheumatoid arthritis and cardiovascular disease. *Curr Rheumatol Rep.* 2008;10(5):390–7.
132. Weir PT, Harlan GA, Nkoy FL, et al. The incidence of fibromyalgia and its associated comorbidities: a population-based retrospective cohort study based on International Classification of Diseases, 9th Revision codes. *J Clin Rheumatol.* 2006;12(3):124–8. doi:10.1097/01.rhu.0000221817.46231.18.
133. Wolfe F. What use are fibromyalgia control points? *J Rheumatol.* 1998;25(3):546–50.
134. Wolfe F, Clauw DJ, Fitzcharles MA, et al. The American College of Rheumatology preliminary diagnostic criteria for fibromyalgia and measurement of symptom severity. *Arthritis Care Res (Hoboken).* 2010;62(5):600–10. doi:10.1002/acr.20140.
135. Youdas JW, Boor MM, Darfler AL, Koenig MK, Mills KM, Hollman JH. Surface electromyographic analysis of core trunk and hip muscles during selected rehabilitation exercises in the side-bridge to neutral spine position. *Sports Health.* 2014;6(5):416–21. doi:10.1177/1941738114539266.
136. Young IA, Cleland JA, Michener LA, Brown C. Reliability, construct validity, and responsiveness of the neck disability index, patient-specific functional scale, and numeric pain rating scale in patients with cervical radiculopathy. *Am J Phys Med Rehabil.* 2010;89(10):831–9. doi:10.1097/PHM.0b013e3181ec98e6.
137. Zamunér AR, Moreno MA, Camargo TM, et al. Assessment of Subjective Perceived Exertion at the anaerobic threshold with the Borg CR-10 Scale. *J Sports Sci Med.* 2011;10(1):130–6.

CHAPTER 20

Special Considerations for Cancer

INTRODUCTION

This chapter presents background information and special considerations for exercise testing, prescription, and progression for individuals with cancer. The case study that follows outlines the personal and health history of a middle-aged woman diagnosed with and treated for breast cancer. This background information will be used as a guide for exercise testing and development of a progressive aerobic and resistance training program with the primary goal of return to work and recreational activities for this patient.

Case Study 20-1

Mrs. Case Study-CA

Mrs. Case Study-CA is a 58-year-old woman weighing 89.5 kg (197 lb) with a height of 165 cm (5 ft 5 in). She has a history of stage IIA hormone receptor–positive breast cancer, diagnosed 7 months ago. She also has a family history of breast cancer in her maternal grandmother and in an older sister. Mrs. Case Study-CA has a history of prediabetes and is taking a stable dose of metformin. She does not smoke and drank alcohol moderately (four to six drinks per week) up to the time of her breast cancer diagnosis. As her course of treatment, Mrs. Case Study-CA received neoadjuvant chemotherapy for the first 3 months to shrink the breast tumor followed by breast-conserving surgery (BCS; sometimes called *lumpectomy* or *partial mastectomy*) in the left breast. She then received local radiation therapy during months 5 and 6. Adjuvant hormone therapy (tamoxifen, an estrogen receptor antagonist) was initiated at the time of surgery and will continue, once daily, for at least 5 years.

Prior to her cancer diagnosis, Mrs. Case Study-CA was working full-time as an accountant at a large corporation. Although she regularly worked 10 hours per day, 5 days per week, Mrs. Case Study-CA made an effort to go for daily 15-minute walks on her lunch break and tended to her garden 1 hour per night, 3 days per week. Since her diagnosis, she has not had the energy for her daily walks, and her husband has taken over gardening duties in addition to cooking and cleaning, adding stress to the marriage. Mrs. Case Study-CA's primary goals for an exercise program are to facilitate her return to work and to mitigate the side effects of treatments, allowing her to return to gardening and cooking.

At a recent visit with her primary care physician, Mrs. Case Study-CA expressed interest in returning to work, adding in her daily walks, and starting to garden again. Her physician conducted a physical exam and noted mild swelling in her left axillary lymph nodes (lymphedema; localized fluid retention and tissue swelling), reduced **range of motion (ROM)** in the left shoulder, and muscular weakness in the left arm compared with the right arm. Mrs. Case Study-CA did not report any dizziness or shortness of breath when walking but did report being easily fatigued when climbing stairs and doing housework.

While in the clinic, Mrs. Case Study-CA's physician sent her to the heart center for exercise testing. Before testing, she was fitted with a compression sleeve to help control the lymphedema in her left arm. After a warm-up, she completed a **submaximal** exercise test on the treadmill using the modified Bruce protocol. The results of the exercise test are presented in Table 20.1. The test was stopped after 2 minutes of stage 3 due to patient-reported fatigue.

Mrs. Case Study-CA's physician told her that it was safe for her to begin light- to moderate-intensity exercise, such as walking. She sought guidance from an exercise professional to help her safely add exercise back into her routine. During the initial consultation, Mrs. Case Study-CA performed simple ROM exercises to determine her ability to perform different exercises. Then, she completed **one repetition maximum** (1-RM) testing on the bench press, leg press, and lateral raise. Her estimated 1-RM was determined to be 85.0 kg (187 lb) for the leg press, 31.5 kg (69 lb) for the bench press, 8.0 kg (17 lb) for the right lateral raise, and 5.5 kg (12 lb) for the left lateral raise based on workload from 8-RM.

Table 20.1 Results of Graded Exercise Treadmill Test (Modified Bruce Protocol)

Stage	Time (min)	Speed (mph)	Incline (%)	Heart Rate (bpm)	Blood Pressure (mm Hg)	Rating of Perceived Exertion
Rest	3	0	0	74	118/82	6
0	3	1.5	0	98	130/82	8
0.5	3	1.5	0	106	138/82	9
1	3	1.7	0	112	150/82	12
2	3	1.7	5	146	168/82	13
3	2	1.7	10	162	176/82	15
Recovery	2	0	0	116	136/82	6
Recovery	3	0	0	80	122/82	6

Description, Prevalence, and Etiology

Cancer is a general term encompassing over 200 unique disease states. Cancer is broadly defined as uncontrolled cell growth, usually as a result of genetic or single-nucleotide mutations, which can occur in epithelial tissue (carcinoma), connective tissue (sarcomas), bone (blastoma), blood (leukemia), or lymph nodes (lymphoma) (21). Each cancer is further classified by the size and spread of the tumor(s), indicated by a staging system. There are several staging systems, but a five-stage system is often used (1). Stage 0 indicates presence of abnormal cells that are localized. Stages 1–4 indicate the presence of tumors, with increasing size and spread represented by a higher stage number. Stage 4 indicates that tumors have spread to other tissues or organ systems in the body from the primary tumor site called *metastasis*. Each tumor may also be evaluated for appearance and assigned a grade based on cellular differentiation within the tumor. In general, tumor grading systems range from 1 to 4, with "1" indicating well-differentiated tumor cells that are likely to grow and spread slowly and "4" indicating undifferentiated cells that are likely to grow and spread rapidly. The grade of the tumor, along with the organ or tissue site and stage, will determine the timing and aggressiveness of cancer treatment. Thus, these tumor characteristics should be considered when developing an **exercise prescription**.

The current U.S. prevalence for all types of cancer is 13.7 million (20). The most common cancer sites are female breast, lung, male prostate, and colon and rectum (20). These cancers result from a combination of exposures, including environmental agents (*e.g.*, cigarette smoke), lifestyle factors (*e.g.*, diet, **physical activity**), and host factors (*e.g.*, genetics, body weight). Understanding how these risk factors have an impact on disease progression and recurrence is important for developing exercise prescriptions for individuals with cancer. The National Coalition for Cancer Survivorship's definition of cancer survivor, identified from time of diagnosis to the rest of life, including cancer treatment, will be used in this text (13).

Engaging in a regular physical activity program has been shown to reduce risk for recurrence, cancer-specific mortality, and all-cause mortality among adults with a history of cancer (2,8,12,23). A regular **exercise** program can also help delay or control other chronic conditions which are common among cancer survivors (4,6,7,10,11,14,25), such as diabetes or cardiovascular disease (CVD), discussed in more detail in other chapters of this textbook. There is ample evidence that exercise training can help mitigate cancer-related fatigue and can improve physical function and quality of life for cancer survivors (5,15–17). Recently, the short- and long-term cardiovascular health benefits of exercise among cancer survivors have been investigated (18).

Overview of Preparticipation Health Screening, Medical History, and Physical Examination

The American College of Sports Medicine (ACSM) recommendations for exercise preparticipation health screening (1) can be followed for patients with a personal history of cancer. Each patient's current physical activity levels, time since diagnosis, course of treatment, symptoms and side effects, and other personal health factors will determine what steps should be taken prior to beginning an exercise program.

The patient's health history should be considered when determining if additional evaluation is necessary. Cancer-related side effects will vary by treatment modality (*e.g.*, chemotherapy, radiation, surgery, immune therapy, hormone therapy) and host factors, such as age and presence of comorbidities. The number of treatment options and agents, and their potential side effects, is as varied as the cancers themselves. Common immediate side effects of treatment include pain, fatigue, nausea and vomiting, change in appetite, and localized swelling or lymphedema (19). Long-term effects, or side effects that occur during or shortly after treatment is completed, can include changes in cognition, body weight and composition, cardiovascular health, immune function, and nerve function. Cognitive side effects are often referred to as *chemo brain* by patients and can include changes in memory and comprehension. Patients may experience unintentional increases or decreases in body weight depending on their phase of treatment, type of therapy, or experience with other symptoms or side effects. Loss of muscle mass, or cachexia (wasting), or increases in fat mass may occur with or without changes in body weight. Cardiovascular health can be affected by changes in metabolic profile (*e.g.*, dyslipidemia), in **body composition**, or in vascular structure and function resulting from treatment. Treatment agents that target the immune response, such as inflammation, or specific immune receptor cells can have an impact on a patient's ability to respond to antigens or recover from infection. Peripheral neuropathies may result from damage to nerves during surgery and can manifest as pain, numbness, or ataxia in the affected tissues or joints. Patients may experience muscle weakness and/or balance issues related to treatment incurred neuropathies. Reduced ROM around affected joints during and after treatment (*e.g.*, shoulder joint following breast surgery) is also common. Patients undergoing hormone therapy can experience loss in bone mass and bone mineral density, thus increasing risk for bone break and fractures. Hormone therapy for cancer is aimed at reducing circulating hormones (*e.g.*, androgen deprivation therapy for prostate cancer, estrogen reduction for breast cancer) in order to deprive the tumor cells. This has an opposite effect on bone health than hormone replacement therapy used to relieve symptoms of menopause in women. Additionally, surgical removal of hormone-producing glands or organs as part of cancer treatment can result in reduction in bone mass and density.

Advances in treatment, screening, and diagnosis have led to increased 5- and 10-year survival rates for a number of cancer sites (2). Due to these improvements, new late effects, or side effects appearing months to years after the end of treatment, are appearing in patients with a history of cancer. The cardiotoxic effects of chemotherapies are being increasingly recognized and can lead to complications such as cardiomyopathy, left ventricular dysfunction, and heart failure (HF) (3,17). Factors increasing the risk of chemotherapy cardiotoxic effects include the presence of other CVD risk factors (*e.g.*, age, family history, hypertension, smoking) and the number and dose of concomitant chemotherapy agents administered (3). Patients who display or report signs or symptoms of cardiac arrhythmias or HF such as shortness of breath, rapid onset of fatigue, or light-headedness/dizziness with moderate-intensity activity should undergo additional medical evaluation before beginning an exercise program in order to determine exercise safety. If the patient has confirmed HF, the guidelines for exercise testing and prescription for HF should be followed (see Chapter 12).

The immediate and long-term side effects of treatment should be assessed prior to or during medical examination in order to guide exercise testing, prescription, and progression. A medical examination may need to be repeated after completion of cancer treatments, after any major changes in medication (type or dose), or if the patient reports changes in symptoms or side effects. Furthermore, exercise should be discontinued temporarily after major changes in symptoms or side effects and until a medical evaluation is performed and the patient is cleared to safely resume exercise.

Case Study 20-1 Quiz:

Preparticipation Health Screening, Medical History, and Physical Examination

1. What type of preparticipation health screening is necessary for this patient prior to engaging in moderate-intensity exercise?
2. What specific host factors should be considered for their impact on cancer treatment and exercise tolerance?

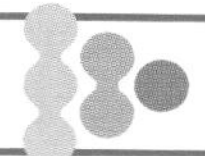

Exercise Testing Considerations

The exercise testing guidelines for cancer survivors follow those recommended for healthy adults wishing to begin a program of moderate- or vigorous-intensity aerobic activity (1,24). No exercise testing is required prior to beginning a light walking program or before **flexibility** or progressive resistance training (24). Requiring an exercise test can create an unnecessary barrier for cancer survivors to begin activity after diagnosis and treatment. However, the individual patient's current health status, symptoms, treatment side effects, and other host factors should be considered carefully when determining if exercise testing is needed. For instance, if a patient reports becoming fatigued after light-to-moderate exercise, an exercise test may provide beneficial information on how cancer treatments may be affecting aerobic capacity and heart rate (HR) response and to determine if and how exercise is exacerbating side effects.

If aerobic exercise testing is performed, the same guidelines should be followed for healthy adults (see Chapter 8). Patients should be monitored for abnormal changes in HR and blood pressure (BP) and presence of signs or symptoms of cardiovascular events. Additionally, the patient should be monitored for abnormal changes in treatment side effects such as sudden or worsening pain, swelling, bruising, or fatigue. If selecting a stage-based exercise test, consider the length of each stage and workload increment between stages when determining which test is appropriate. For some patients, using a modified protocol or fitness battery designed for **older adults** (see Aging, Chapter 9) may be more suitable. Changes in balance and cognition (chemo brain) should be considered when selecting the mode of aerobic exercise testing. For those with neuropathies, ataxia, or balance issues, a cycle ergometer provides a safer option over a treadmill. If a patient is receiving hormone therapy or has metastatic disease to the bone, aerobic exercise testing may be performed on a cycle ergometer to reduce the risk for breaks and fractures.

Maximal strength testing (1-RM) has been demonstrated to be safe in breast cancer survivors with and at risk for lymphedema (22). Patients with or who are at risk for lymphedema should be fit with an appropriate pressure garment before exercise testing to prevent swelling from worsening. Patients should be guided through each exercise without resistance to determine if they have appropriate ROM to safely perform 1-RM testing. If 1-RM evaluation is not appropriate by direct testing, the 1-RM workload can be estimated using workloads that correspond to 6–10-RM. If a patient reports or presents with balance issues, 1-RM testing may be performed on resistance machines to allow for full control throughout the ROM. Similarly, if a patient has received hormone therapy or has metastatic disease to the bone, alternative or reduced-load testing methods should be considered to minimize the risk of breaks or fractures. Exercise and exercise testing should not be performed if patients are experiencing extreme fatigue, anemia, ataxia, or any other signs and symptoms of serious illness.

Patients who are at risk for cardiotoxicity may be taking medications to prevent ventricular dysfunction or HF (9). These medications include β-blockers (*e.g.*, carvedilol), renin-angiotensin inhibitors (*e.g.*, enalapril), and aldosterone antagonists (*e.g.*, spironolactone). These medications can lower the resting HR and alter the HR response to exercise and exercise testing. An exercise test can help determine a new target HR using heart rate reserve (%HRR) and maximal heart rate (%HR_{max}) methods; however, rating of perceived exertion (RPE) methods are encouraged to monitor intensity in these patients. Patients who complete an exercise test and display decreased functional capacity (*e.g.*, low maximal volume of oxygen consumed per unit time [$\dot{V}O_{2max}$] for age and sex); abnormal electrocardiogram (ECG)/arrhythmias; or previously unreported shortness of breath, dizziness, etc., may have undetected cardiotoxic side effects of chemotherapy treatment. These patients should be referred back to their health care provider for follow-up medical evaluation.

Additional exercise testing can be performed at the discretion of the exercise professional based on symptoms or issues the patient raises during the initial evaluation. If the patient is experiencing difficulties with balance, assessments such as the semitandem stand, full-tandem stand, or single-leg stand may be used. If the patient is presenting with ROM or flexibility issues, testing such as the sit-and-reach or back-scratch tests may be implemented. Coordination drills may be useful in assessing the extent of cognition changes (chemo brain) or neuropathy.

Case Study 20-1 Quiz:

Exercise Testing Considerations

3. What is the potential impact on exercise testing of the medications and treatments prescribed for Mrs. Case Study-CA?
4. Was exercise testing necessary for the patient? Why or why not?
5. Regardless of your answer in the previous question, was the choice of a submaximal treadmill test using the modified Bruce protocol appropriate? Why or why not?

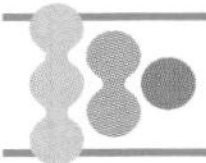

Exercise Prescription and Progression Considerations

In general, patients being treated for cancer can begin progression with light- and moderate-intensity physical activity as recommended for healthy adults (see Chapter 8). Each patient will be unique in exercise and health history, where they are in the treatment, and what symptoms or side effects are being experienced that may limit exercise or exercise progression. There is no one established frequency, intensity, time, and type (FITT) guideline for exercise prescription for cancer survivors; however, general exercise prescription guidelines for cancer survivors are presented in FITT table (Table 20.2) (1). Each patient's unique health history, treatments, and symptom and side effect presentation should be considered when determining the best method to monitor and progress aerobic exercise intensity. Although %HRR and %HR_{max} methods are provided in FITT table (see Table 20.2), monitoring exercise intensity may be best achieved using RPE, especially for patients taking medications to prevent or mitigate cardiotoxic side effects. A target RPE of 12–13 for **moderate intensity** and 14–17 for **vigorous intensity** on the Borg scale is recommended.

As with healthy adults, resistance and weight training is encouraged on 2–3 days per week. Patients should begin at a very low resistance (<30% 1-RM) and progress in small increments (24). **Strength** and weight training has been determined to be safe for breast cancer survivors, even in the presence of lymphedema (24). Patients with or who are at risk for lymphedema should wear an appropriate pressure garment during exercise to prevent swelling from worsening and be monitored closely for changes in swelling. Patients taking hormone therapy, which can decrease bone density and increase risk for breaks and fractures, should incorporate low-intensity weight bearing and functional tasks into their exercise routine to help mitigate the negative effects of treatment. Survivors with metastatic disease to the bone may need to begin at an intensity lower than 30% 1-RM, at a lower volume, and avoid high-impact movements (*e.g.*, jumping) to reduce risk of breaks and fractures. For those with very frail bone structure, body weight exercises or light elastic bands can be used.

FITT

TABLE 20.2 RECOMMENDATIONS FOR INDIVIDUALS WITH CANCER

ACSM FITT Principle of the ExR_x

Chronic Medical Condition	Frequency (How often?)	Intensity (How hard?)	Time	Type (What kind?) Primary	Resistance	Flexibility	Special Considerations
Healthy Adult	≥5 d · wk^{-1} of moderate exercise, or ≥3 d · wk^{-1} of vigorous exercise, or a combination of moderate and vigorous exercise on ≥3–5 d · wk^{-1} is recommended.	Moderate to vigorous. Light-to-moderate intensity exercise may be beneficial in deconditioned individuals.	If moderate intensity: ≥30 min · d^{-1} to total 150 min · wk^{-1}. If vigorous intensity: ≥20 min · d^{-1} to total 75 min · wk^{-1}.	Regular, purposeful exercise that involves major muscle groups and is continuous and rhythmic in nature is recommended.	2–3 d · wk^{-1} (nonconsecutive)	2–3 d · wk^{-1}; static stretch 10–30 s; 2–4 repetitions of each exercise	Sedentary behaviors can have adverse health effects, even among those who regularly exercise. Adding short physical activity breaks throughout the day may be considered as a part of the exercise.
Cancer	3–5 d · wk^{-1}	Moderate (40%–59% HRR or VO_2R; 64%–75% HR_{max}; RPE of 12–13) to vigorous (60%–89% VO_2R; 76%–95% HR_{max}; RPE of 14–17	75 min · wk^{-1} of vigorous intensity or 150 min · wk^{-1} of moderate-intensity activity or an equivalent combination of the two.	Prolonged, rhythmic activities using large muscle groups (*e.g.*, walking, cycling, swimming)	2–3 d · wk^{-1} At least 1 set of 8–12 repetitions Free weights, resistance machines, or weight-bearing functional tasks (*e.g.*, sit-to-stand) targeting all major muscle groups	>2–3 · wk^{-1} with daily being the most effective Move through ROM as tolerated. 10–30 hold for static stretching Stretching or ROM exercises for all major muscle groups. Address specific areas of joint or muscle restriction that may have resulted from treatment with steroids, radiation, or surgery.	Patients with cancer often deal with the debilitating effects of treatment (chemotherapy and radiation) with side effects such as extreme fatigue, anemia, and ataxia. Adjustments to exercise should be made based on signs and symptoms on days following treatment. For some patients, swimming may be contraindicated.

ExR_x, exercise prescription; HR_{max}, maximal heart rate; $\dot{V}O_2R$, oxygen uptake reserve.

Based on the FITT Recommendations present in *ACSM's Guidelines for Exercise Testing and Prescription*. 10th ed. Philadelphia (PA): Wolters Kluwer; 2018. 480 p.

Cancer survivors may progress in duration, frequency, and intensity at a slower rate than healthy adults and should progress as tolerated. For some patients, maintenance of physical function or fitness may be a goal of exercise therapy due to changes in body composition (cachexia) or decreased aerobic capacity resulting from cancer treatments. Patients should be monitored closely for changes in symptoms and side effects, such as fatigue, muscle weakness, and swelling. Exercises should be stopped according to symptom response, such as unusual swelling/lymphedema or pain. If exercise is discontinued for a period, the intensity level or resistance should be decreased and progressed slowly back to where it was when the patient stopped.

For patients who display issues with balance or who may have reduced bone mineral density, extra safety precautions should be taken during aerobic, resistance, and flexibility exercises. **Aerobic** training can be performed on a stationary cycle or recumbent stepper or by swimming or doing water aerobics instead of on a treadmill to reduce the risk of falling and ease pain symptoms. If opting for water-based aerobic activity, ensure that the patient is completing load-bearing activities and adhering to recommended resistance and weight training FITT principles in order to maintain bone health. Resistance exercises can be performed on machines to help the patient maintain control of the movement through the entire ROM. Flexibility exercises can be modified to be completed in the sitting position to reduce risk of falling. Balance exercises, such as tandem and single-leg stands, and coordination drills can be added 2–3 days per week alongside resistance and flexibility exercises in order to improve patient balance and confidence to perform daily tasks. The patient can progress to treadmill walking, free weights, and standing stretches as balance and bone health improves.

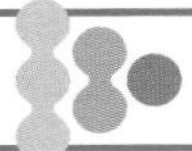

Special Considerations and Contraindications to Exercise

The following are special considerations for and contraindications to exercise for cancer survivors:

- Exercise or exercise testing should not be performed if the patient is displaying severe side effects (*e.g.*, extreme fatigue, anemia, ataxia) or signs or symptoms of serious illness.
- Some patients should not exercise on the day of chemotherapy, and adjustments in duration and intensity of exercise are implicated during active treatment in accordance with reported or observed symptoms and side effects. The body's response to chemotherapy (*e.g.*, irregular HR) can vary over time, so allowing adequate time for the patient to adjust and respond to treatment is necessary in order to safely engage in exercise training.
- Patients taking an immunosuppressant or who are immunocompromised may be advised to exercise in a private or medical facility rather than a public fitness facility to avoid harmful exposures or triggers. Regardless of immune function, cleaning equipment with sanitary wipes or sprays and clean towels before and after use is recommended to limit risk of infection.
- Swimming should be avoided for patients with catheters, ostomies, or other external devices; recent surgery; skin eruptions from radiation therapy; or an immunosuppressed state.
- Core strengthening and flexibility exercises should be adapted for patients with recent gastrointestinal or genitourinary cancer treatment or any patient with recent abdominal surgery. As with any population, avoid the Valsalva maneuver and emphasize proper breathing during exercise.

Case Study 20-1 Quiz:

Exercise Prescription and Progression Considerations

6. What weight/resistance should Mrs. Case Study-CA begin at for upper body exercises?
7. What additional exercises would you recommend to facilitate Mrs. Case Study-CA's return to work and recreational activities?
8. How would you recommend progressing the case study patient's aerobic routine?

SUMMARY

This chapter presents relevant information regarding exercise testing, prescription, and progression recommendations for individuals with cancer. A case study is presented as a means to clarify the concepts discussed. It should be noted that each cancer diagnosis is unique, and often, the patient will present with other comorbidities such as diabetes (see Chapter 14), CVD (see Chapter 10), obesity (Chapter 18), and aging (see Chapter 9). The clinician and exercise professional working with this population should be familiar with exercise testing, prescription, and progression for these special populations in addition to the considerations for each patient with cancer.

A summary of exercise training and prescription considerations for individuals with cancer is as follows:

- Each diagnosis, treatment, and patient need will be unique; therefore, a thorough evaluation of past medical history, treatments, and medications should be conducted prior to exercise testing, training, and progression.
- Common side effects of cancer treatment include fatigue, changes in cognition, balance issues possibly due to neuropathies (pain or numbness from peripheral nerve damage) and/or muscle weakness, reduced ROM, and bone fractures. These should be adapted for and monitored during exercise training.
- Cancer treatment will impact the patient/survivor's ability to perform aerobic, resistance, and flexibility exercises. The patient's capabilities can vary widely from day to day, especially during active treatment. The exercise prescription and progression should be modified accordingly, avoiding inactivity.
- Removal of lymph nodes exposes a cancer survivor to the risk of lymphedema (a condition of localized fluid retention and tissue swelling). If the survivor has any changes in their shoulder, breast, arm, hand, trunk, leg, or foot, including swelling, stop the exercises and have the survivor see a lymphedema specialist. If the cancer survivor has been diagnosed with lymphedema, it is recommended that a well-fitted compression garment is worn to exercise.
- If a patient experiences a change in treatment, disease status, symptoms, or side effects or experiences another medical event, it is prudent to reevaluate the patient using the ACSM guidelines for exercise preparticipation health screening and determine whether a physician exam or **medical clearance** is required prior to continuing an exercise program.

REFERENCES

1. American College of Sports Medicine. *ACSM's Guidelines for Exercise Testing and Prescription*. 10th ed. Philadelphia (PA): Wolters Kluwer; 2018. 480 p.
2. Arem H, Moore SC, Park Y, et al. Physical activity and cancer-specific mortality in the NIH-AARP Diet and Health Study cohort. *Int J Cancer*. 2014;135(2):423–31.
3. Bloom MW, Hamo CE, Cardinale D, et al. Cancer therapy-related cardiac dysfunction and heart failure: part 1: definitions, pathophysiology, risk factors, and imaging. *Circ Heart Fail*. 2016;9(1):e002661.
4. Brown BW, Brauner C, Minnotte MC. Noncancer deaths in white adult cancer patients. *J Natl Cancer Inst*. 1993;85(12):979–87.
5. Brown JC, Huedo-Medina TB, Pescatello LS, Pescatello SM, Ferrer RA, Johnson BT. Efficacy of exercise interventions in modulating cancer-related fatigue among adult cancer survivors: a meta-analysis. *Cancer Epidemiol Biomarkers Prev*. 2011;20(1):123–33.
6. Calip GS, Malone KE, Gralow JR, Stergachis A, Hubbard RA, Boudreau DM. Metabolic syndrome and outcomes following early-stage breast cancer. *Breast Cancer Res Treatment*. 2014;148(2):363–77.
7. De Bruijn KM, Arends LR, Hansen BE, Leeflang S, Ruiter R, van Eijck CH. Systematic review and meta-analysis of the association between diabetes mellitus and incidence and mortality in breast and colorectal cancer. *Br J Surg*. 2013;100(11):1421–9.

8. Garcia DO, Thomson CA. Physical activity and cancer survivorship. *Nutr Clin Pract.* 2014;29(6):768–79.
9. Hamo CE, Bloom MW, Cardinale D, et al. Cancer therapy-related cardiac dysfunction and heart failure: part 2: prevention, treatment, guidelines, and future directions. *Circ Heart Fail.* 2016;9(2):e002843.
10. Haque R, Prout M, Geiger AM, et al. Comorbidities and cardiovascular disease risk in older breast cancer survivors. *Am J Manag Care.* 2014;20(1):86–92.
11. Hawkes AL, Lynch BM, Owen N, Aitken JF. Lifestyle factors associated concurrently and prospectively with co-morbid cardiovascular disease in a population-based cohort of colorectal cancer survivors. *Eur J Cancer.* 2011;47(2):267–76.
12. Lemanne D, Cassileth B, Gubili J. The role of physical activity in cancer prevention, treatment, recovery, and survivorship. *Oncology (Williston Park).* 2013;27(6):580–5.
13. Ligibel JA, Denlinger CS. New NCCN guidelines for survivorship care. *J Natl Compr Canc Netw.* 2013;11(5 suppl):640–4.
14. Lipscombe LL, Chan WW, Yun L, Austin PC, Anderson GM, Rochon PA. Incidence of diabetes among postmenopausal breast cancer survivors. *Diabetologia.* 2013;56(3):476–83.
15. McNeely ML, Courneya KS. Exercise programs for cancer-related fatigue: evidence and clinical guidelines. *J Natl Compr Canc Netw.* 2010;8(8):945–53.
16. Mishra SI, Scherer RW, Geigle PM, et al. Exercise interventions on health-related quality of life for cancer survivors. *Cochrane Database Syst Rev.* 2012;(8):CD007566.
17. Mishra SI, Scherer RW, Snyder C, Geigle PM, Berlanstein DR, Topaloglu O. Exercise interventions on health-related quality of life for people with cancer during active treatment. *Cochrane Database Syst Rev.* 2012;(8):CD008465.
18. Muppidi R, Spranklin L, Scialla W, Islam N, Freudenberger R, Malacoff R. Cardiotoxicity of anticancer therapies. *Rev Cardiovasc Med.* 2015;16(4):225–34.
19. National Cancer Institute. Side effects [Internet]. Bethesda (MD): National Cancer Institute; [cited 2015]. Available from: https://www.cancer.gov/about-cancer/treatment/side-effects
20. National Cancer Institute. Surveillance, Epidemiology, and End Results Program [Internet]. Bethesda (MD): National Cancer Institute; [cited 2016]. Available from: https://www.seer.cancer.gov/
21. National Cancer Institute. What is cancer? [Internet]. Bethesda (MD): National Cancer Institute; [cited 2015]. Available from: https://www.cancer.gov/about-cancer/understanding/what-is-cancer
22. Rock CL, Doyle C, Demark-Wahnefried W, et al. Nutrition and physical activity guidelines for cancer survivors. *CA Cancer J Clin.* 2012;62(4):243–74.
23. Schmid D, Leitzmann MF. Association between physical activity and mortality among breast cancer and colorectal cancer survivors: a systematic review and meta-analysis. *Ann Oncol.* 2014;25(7):1293–311.
24. Schmitz KH, Courneya KS, Matthews C, et al. American College of Sports Medicine roundtable on exercise guidelines for cancer survivors. *Med Sci Sports Exerc.* 2010;42(7):1409–26.
25. Singh S, Earle CC, Bae SJ, et al. Incidence of diabetes in colorectal cancer survivors. *J Natl Cancer Inst.* 2016;108(6):djv402.

CHAPTER 21

Special Considerations for Bone Health and Osteoporosis

INTRODUCTION

This chapter presents an overview of osteoporosis and discuss special considerations related to exercise testing, prescription, and progression for individuals diagnosed with osteoporosis. The case study presented focuses on a woman diagnosed with osteoporosis who would like to begin an exercise program at her local fitness facility. This case study provides guidance for the design of a program that includes progressive resistance training, **aerobic** conditioning, and balance training, with the primary goal of preventing falls and fracture in an individual with diagnosed osteoporosis, or low bone mineral density (BMD).

Case Study 21-1

Mrs. Case Study-BH

Mrs. Case Study-BH is a 65-year-old woman weighing 61.2 kg (134.6 lb) and with a height of 167.6 cm (66 in); her **body mass index (BMI)** is 21.8 kg · m^{-2}. She was diagnosed with osteoporosis, or low BMD, at her most recent physical examination. Her vertebral T-score was −2.7, and her hip T-score was −2.0. (The World Health Organization defines osteoporosis as a T-score less than 2.5.) After ruling out secondary causes of osteoporosis (*e.g.*, malabsorptive disorders, hyperparathyroidism), her physician prescribed a bisphosphonate (anti-bone resorption drug) to improve her bone density, and she has been taking this medication for the past 2 months. She reports no previous falls or nontraumatic fractures, but her mother suffered an osteoporotic thoracic spine vertebral fracture in her mid-70s that left her with a kyphotic posture (rounding or curvature of the thoracic and cervical spine). Mrs. Case Study-BH is a semiretired elementary school counselor who currently works part-time where she spends the majority of her time sitting at her desk. When she is not working, she enjoys walking and gardening. She reports walking in her neighborhood and on the school's outdoor track on average 3 days per week for approximately 30 minutes. She has no history of resistance training.

Mrs. Case Study-BH began menopause at age 48 years and is not taking a hormone replacement therapy. She reports having periodically taken a multivitamin supplement in the past but does not take any other dietary supplements. She has been a nonsmoker for approximately 20 years after beginning smoking at 17 years of age and consumes alcohol 2–3 days per week and wears corrective lenses. She is an otherwise healthy individual. In addition to the bisphosphonate prescription, Mrs. Case Study-BH's physician recommended that she visit her local fitness facility and begin participating in an exercise program.

Mrs. Case Study-BH's goal in pursuing an exercise program is to prevent a future fracture and maintain her current mobility and quality of life. She expressed concern over her osteoporosis diagnosis and fears that she will suffer a vertebral fracture and acquire a hunched posture like her mother or will fall and fracture a hip.

Based on Mrs. Case Study-BH's **Physical Activity Readiness Questionnaire for Everyone (PAR-Q+)** responses, she currently engages in light-to-moderate levels of regular physical activity (walking 30 min on 3 d · wk^{-1} for the past 5 yr) and does not have cardiovascular, metabolic, or renal disease and has no signs or symptoms suggestive of these diseases (*ACSM's Guidelines for Exercise Testing and Prescription, 10th edition* [*GETP10*]). As part of her goal to prevent further bone loss and osteoporotic fracture, Mrs. Case Study-BH would like to continue her current activity level and also aims to incorporate physical activities that promote bone health. Mrs. Case Study-BH's PAR-Q+ outcomes indicated that she is not required to seek medical clearance before initiating her exercise program. However, the exercise professional still may choose to request medical clearance from the physician of an individual with osteoporosis. Mrs. Case Study-BH's exercise professional requested medical clearance, and her physician recommended avoiding any exercise that includes spinal flexion (*e.g.*, toe touches). Her physician also recommended resistance training activities that load the spine and hip regions but to begin with light resistance at first and to progress only when Mrs. Case Study-BH can perform the exercises correctly with good form.

Given Mrs. Case Study-BH's concern for osteoporotic fracture and kyphosis, her exercise program should aim to minimize bone loss, reduce fall risk, and improve her current **physical fitness**. Her exercise professional devised a 24-week program including progressive aerobic, resistance, and balance training progressions across three 8-week cycles.

Mrs. Case Study-BH has engaged in a regular, 3-day-per-week walking program of approximately 30 minutes per day for the past several years. Therefore, the initial goal of her 24-week aerobic training program was to progressively increase activity from light-to-moderate intensity over the first 8 weeks of her exercise program through moderate-intensity walking intervals of increasing duration.

During the second 8-week cycle, Mrs. Case Study-BH progressively increased her exercise frequency by 1 day per week with a dance class that met osteogenic (bone forming) requirements of generating unaccustomed loading patterns by performing multiaxial dance steps. Over the final 8-week cycle, Mrs. Case Study-BH gradually increased her time spent in each exercise bout from 30 to 45 minutes per day. The additional osteogenic component was

Case Study 21-1 (continued)

met with short bouts of stair climbing in her home three times per day. Over the 24-week aerobic exercise program, Mrs. Case Study-BH progressively increased both frequency and time spent in aerobic endurance activities to achieve American College of Sports Medicine (2) guidelines for **older adults** by engaging in 30–45 minutes per day of moderate-intensity aerobic activity (accumulating 120–180 min · wk^{-1}).

Because Mrs. Case Study-BH reported no previous experience with resistance training, her resistance and balance program began with body weight exercises with a primary focus on proper form and spinal alignment. Across three 8-week cycles, Mrs. Case Study-BH's exercises were aimed at improving strength and balance and progressed from body weight exercises toward incorporating resistance with bands, free weights, and resistance machines. The exercises addressed all the major muscle groups, and emphasis was placed on progressive overload through increasing numbers of sets, resistance, and exercise difficulty. Exercise difficulty included progressions from partial to full **range of motion** (avoid full spinal flexion), supported to unsupported movements, and body weight to loaded resistance. Endurance training for postural muscles began with **isometric** exercises performed in the supine position and progressed to daily spinal extensor training with progressions to prone and seated positions with resistance bands. Mrs. Case Study-BH began each 8-week cycle with one set of each exercise and gradually increased one set every 2–3 weeks. During the first 8-week cycle, Mrs. Case Study-BH's balance training began with static positions (*e.g.*, supported semitandem stance) with challenging progressions that reduced contact with support and shifted weight as she was able to demonstrate stance holding for each position (*e.g.*, 30 s). During the subsequent cycles, she performed progressively challenging dynamic activities (*e.g.*, semitandem walk and obstacle courses with cones). Once she demonstrated stability during the movement, increasingly challenging dual tasks were introduced (*e.g.*, turning head toward a visual target during walking). Following Mrs. Case Study-BH's 24-week exercise program, she reported feeling stronger; having increased endurance; and feeling less worried about falling, suffering, and fracture, which might leave her kyphotic like her mother.

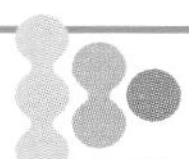

Description, Prevalence, and Etiology

Osteoporosis is a skeletal disorder characterized by compromised bone **strength** that results in an increased susceptibility to fracture (11,28). It is estimated that approximately 200 million women worldwide currently have osteoporosis (34), and the prevalence among all adults is expected to rise with the increase in life expectancy and aging population (16). Osteoporosis and related fractures are more common in women than men, with 1 in 2 women suffering a fracture over the age of 50 years (11,35,45). The greater prevalence of fractures in women is the basis for the false belief that osteoporosis is a health concern only for women. Men are also at risk for fracture, with approximately 25% of all men over the age of 50 years suffering an osteoporotic fracture in their lifetime (33).

This increase in risk of fracture with low bone mass is the clinical relevance of osteoporosis. More than 1.5 million fractures are associated with osteoporosis each year. Osteoporotic fractures are low-trauma fractures that occur with forces generated by a fall from a standing height or lower and are most common at the spine, hip, and wrist. Regardless of the initial fracture site, adults who fracture have a much greater risk of fracturing again at any location (19). After the age of 50 years, it is estimated that approximately 1 in 2 women and 1 in 5 men will suffer from an osteoporosis-related fracture in their lifetime (11,35,45).

Etiology of Osteoporosis

Hip fractures are considered to be the most devastating consequences of osteoporosis because they are associated with severe disability and increased mortality (6). Osteoporosis is a silent disease (*i.e.*, often not accompanied by symptoms) and is commonly first detected by clinical screening or by experiencing an osteoporotic fracture. As a result, much of the attention in osteoporosis is focused on early prevention, detection, and treatment.

Fractures occur when the magnitude of a load on a bone is greater than the strength of a bone (14). Therefore, although osteoporosis denotes skeletal fragility, osteoporotic fractures are the result of both skeletal fragility and the load that occurs from a fall. Because most hip and wrist fractures occur as a consequence of falling, factors influencing both bone fragility and risk of falling should be considered when discussing the pathophysiology of osteoporotic fractures.

The characteristics of bone that determine its strength include the quantity of bone material present, the quality of the material, and the distribution of the material in space (*i.e.*, the structure of the bone). These factors are determined by the dynamic cellular activities known as *bone modeling* and *remodeling*, which are regulated by bone's hormonal and mechanical environments. Modeling is the *independent* action of osteoclasts (bone-resorbing cells) and osteoblasts (bone-forming cells) on the surfaces of bone, whereby new bone is added along some surfaces and removed from others. Modeling affects the size and shape of bones and is especially important for reshaping long bones as they grow in length during adolescence. Remodeling is a localized process that involves the *coupled* action of osteoclasts and osteoblasts, in which osteoclasts first resorb a pit of older bone, and osteoblasts are subsequently recruited to the site to form and mineralize new bone. This process happens throughout the lifespan and occurs diffusely throughout the skeleton. An important role of remodeling is to replace damaged bone with new, healthy bone. Like any material subjected to repetitive loading, bone experiences fatigue damage in the form of very small cracks. However, unlike inert materials, bones are able to replace damaged bone with new bone tissue through the process of targeted bone remodeling (52).

Characteristics of Bone Strength

As mentioned earlier, many skeletal characteristics contribute to bone strength and, consequently, bone fragility, including the quantity of bone material present, the quality of the material, and the structure of the material. It is important to understand how each of these features of bone strength change with age in order to understand why our bones become weaker and are more susceptible to fracture in later life.

Bone Quantity

Bone quantity refers to the amount of bone material present. The average pattern of change in bone mass across the lifespan is displayed graphically in Figure 21.1, although the actual pattern of bone mass change is more dynamic than shown both during growth and in later life. For example, approximately 26% of total adult bone mass is accrued in a 2-year period during adolescence (5). This is approximately equivalent to the entire amount of bone lost in later life (21). Overall, global bone formation continues at a faster pace than bone resorption until peak bone mineral accretion is attained sometime in the second or third decade of life (depending on site, region, and sex). In later life, the amount of bone formation within each remodeling site no longer equals the amount of bone that was resorbed, and thus, a small amount of bone is lost with each new remodeling cycle. This is referred to as a negative bone balance.

In later life, gonadal hormones (*e.g.*, testosterone and estrogen) decrease in both men and women. Estrogen, in particular, suppresses activation of new remodeling cycles, and thus, low estrogen levels partially contribute to an increased rate of remodeling (67). As resorption precedes formation in the process of remodeling, and formation and subsequent mineralization are time-intensive processes, an increase in the rate of remodeling results in temporary decreases in

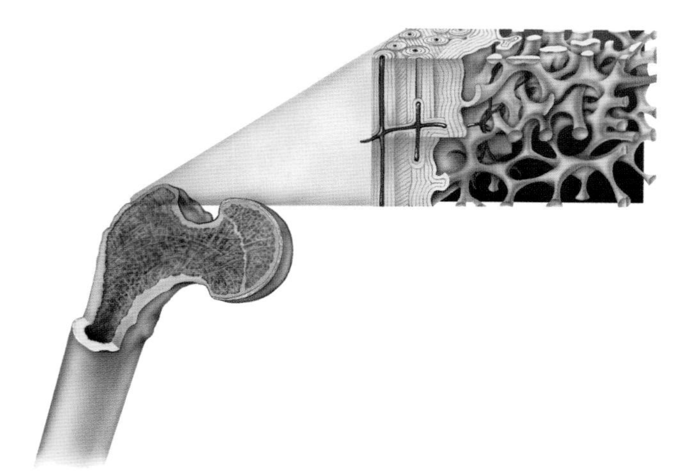

FIGURE 21.1. Bone is a dynamic tissue that is vascularized and innervated. *Cortical* bone is dense and stiff and makes up the shaft of long bones. Cortical bone also provides a shell of protection around *trabecular* bone, which is more porous and flexible and is found at the ends of long bones and in vertebrae. (Reprinted from American College of Sports Medicine. *ACSM's Resource Manual for Exercise Testing and Prescription.* 7th ed. Philadelphia [PA]: Lippincott Williams & Wilkins; 2014. 896 p. Figure 42.1.)

bone mass. Although temporary losses in bone mass lead to a transient increase in bone fragility, increased rates of remodeling with a negative bone balance lead to sustained bone loss of approximately 9%–13% during the first 5 years after menopause (53). Bone turnover eventually slows to a rate similar to premenopausal years. Men also experience age-related bone loss but usually not until later in life than women (17).

Bone Quality

Although the amount of bone in the human skeleton decreases with menopause and advancing age, there is evidence that properties of the remaining bone material may change with age in a way that increases susceptibility to fracture. Bone material from older individuals is less able to absorb energy before failure likely because of an increase in the proportion of mineral within bone tissue compared to collagen as well as changes in collagen properties that are associated with advancing age (18). Also, with advancing age comes susceptibility to fatigue damage. Microcracks have been shown to increase in number and length with age (69). This microdamage accumulation is associated with reduced bone strength (48).

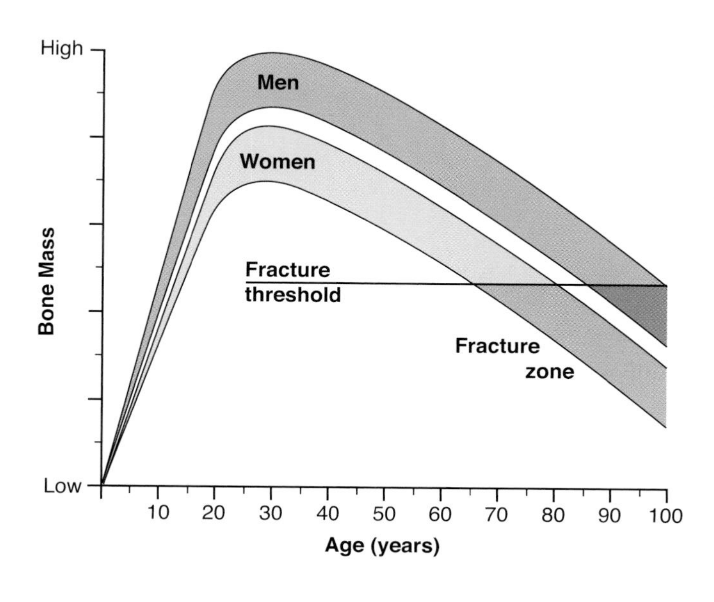

FIGURE 21.2. Normal pattern of bone mineral accretion and loss throughout the lifespan in men and women. (Reprinted from American College of Sports Medicine. *ACSM's Resource Manual for Exercise Testing and Prescription.* 7th ed. Philadelphia [PA]: Lippincott Williams & Wilkins; 2014. 896 p. Figure 42.3).

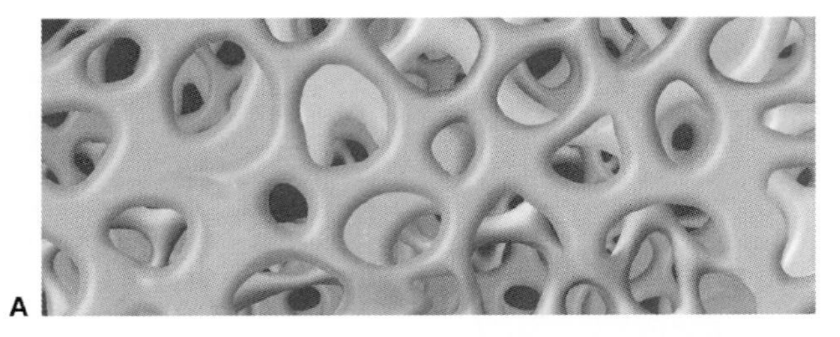

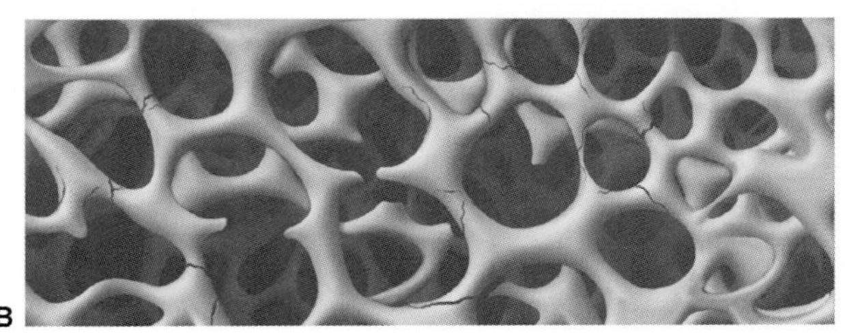

FIGURE 21.3. Slice of trabecular bone in a normal **(A)** and an individual with osteoporosis **(B)** showing loss of trabecular connectivity and increased microdamage with aging. (Reprinted from American College of Sports Medicine. *ACSM's Resource Manual for Exercise Testing and Prescription.* 7th ed. Philadelphia [PA]: Lippincott Williams & Wilkins; 2014. 896 p. Figure 42.4)

Bone Structure

Another important component of bone strength is the structure of bone, that is, how the material is distributed in space. Subtle changes in cross-sectional geometry can markedly increase or decrease bone strength with little or no changes in bone mass or density. Structural differences in cortical bone geometry may partially explain some of the differences in fracture rates between men and women. During growth, the long bones of boys have greater gains in periosteal (outer) diameter of the diaphyses, resulting in a greater overall bone size in boys that remains throughout life, whereas girls have a narrowing of the endocortical (inner) surface of the bone (62). In later life, bone is lost primarily from the endosteal surfaces (inner surface of long bones and intracortical surfaces within the cortex). Thus, the cortex becomes more porous, and the cortices become thinner and more fragile. To offset these losses, bone may be added to the periosteum (outside surface of bone), thereby increasing the diameter of bone and maintaining the strength of the structure in bending (9,62,63). However, as more bone is resorbed from the endocortical surface than is formed on the periosteal surface, the cortices continue to thin, becoming fragile, and are more likely to fracture.

Microarchitecture of trabecular bone is also an important contributor to skeletal fragility (15). For example, if the resorption phase of remodeling is aggressive, as is seen at menopause and thereafter, trabeculae may be penetrated, and the trabecular element may be lost (Fig. 21.3). In these cases, the loss in structural strength disproportionately exceeds the amount of bone lost (54). Furthermore, trabeculae that remain intact may be thinned by excessive remodeling, creating a declining ability to bear loads.

Risks for and Prevention of Fracture

Although skeletal fragility increases susceptibility to fracture, it would be of little concern if damaging loads, such as those generated in a fall, were prevented. Most hip fractures occur after a sideways fall and landing upon the hip (49,68). The incidence of falls increases with age because several sensory systems that control posture (vestibular, visual, and somatosensory) become compromised with advancing age. Furthermore, muscle mass and strength, which prevent instability, decline 30%–50% between the ages of 30 and 80 years (39).

Although bones become more susceptible to fracture, and people become more susceptible to falls with advancing age, fortunately, there are several management tools for prevention and treatment of the condition. Management strategies involve both pharmacological therapy and lifestyle modifications. In this chapter, the focus on lifestyle management, with a particular emphasis on exercise.

Many lifestyle behaviors can be modified to offset risk of osteoporosis and related fractures. For example, all postmenopausal women and older men, regardless of fracture risk, should be encouraged to engage in behaviors that may reduce their risk for skeletal fragility and falls, including adequate calcium (1,000–1,500 mg $\cdot$ d^{-1}) and vitamin D (600–800 IU $\cdot$ d^{-1}) intake, regular exercise, smoking cessation, avoidance of excessive alcohol intake, and visual correction to decrease risk of falling. Of these lifestyle behaviors, exercise is the only one that can simultaneously ameliorate low BMD, augment muscle mass, promote strength gain, and improve dynamic balance — all of which are independent risk factors for fracture (36). Although there is currently no direct evidence that exercise reduces the risk of osteoporotic fracture, clinicians and exercise professionals are encouraged to embrace the theoretical basis behind **exercise prescription** for osteoporosis prevention and treatment (39).

Bone is a dynamic tissue that is capable of continually adapting to its changing mechanical environment. When a bone is loaded in compression, tension, or torsion, bone tissue is deformed. Deformation of bone tissue, or the relative change in bone length, is referred to as *strain*. Bone tissue strain can result in movement of fluid within the bone which may perturbs bone's resident cells — osteocytes. These bone cells are embedded throughout bone tissue and are connected with one another, to other bone cells, and with the bone marrow through slender dendritic processes. The current prevailing theory is that this fluid flow along the osteocyte and its cell processes causes a release of molecular signals that lead to osteoclast and osteoblast recruitment (13,61). This process of turning a mechanical signal into a biochemical signal is called *mechanotransduction*. Mechanotransduction stimulates the physiological processes of modeling and remodeling that creates anatomical changes in bone, resulting in a bone that is better suited to its new mechanical environment.

It has been suggested that the response of bone to its mechanical environment is controlled by a "mechanostat" that aims to keep bone tissue strain at an optimal level by homeostatically altering bone structure (26). Indeed, when bone is subjected to lower than customary loads (as in space flight and immobilization), bone can adapt by ridding itself of excess mass. Alternately, when bone is subjected to greater loads such as uncustomary exercise, bone can become stronger by altering its structure and forming new bone on existing surfaces. Although mechanotransduction is an acute response to exercise, the adaptation of bone structure through modeling and remodeling takes several months to complete. In the case of bone modeling, bone does not respond to exercise by solely adding mass randomly to the skeleton. Rather, animal studies suggest that bone is added where strains are the highest — typically on the periosteal surface in long bones (56). This has the effect of increasing the diameter of long bones, making them more resistant to deformation with loading.

The prevalence of remodeling in bone is also increased with exercise. With the increase in bone tissue strain that occurs with exercise, there is an increase in the number of microcracks in bone. This damage is thought to be targeted for removal by osteoclasts, and new bone is formed in its place (10,53). Thus, one of the proposed chronic effects of exercise on the skeleton involves the maintenance of bone tissue quality through targeted remodeling.

Although osteoporosis is a disease associated with advancing age, there is almost universal consensus that healthy behaviors in youth are important for reducing the risk of osteoporosis in later life (21). The observation that more than 25% of adult bone mineral is laid down during the 2 years surrounding the age of peak linear growth emphasizes the importance of the **adolescent** years in optimizing bone mineral accrual (5). It is estimated that as much bone mineral is laid down during this period as an adult will lose from 50 to 80 years of age (3). Thus, optimizing bone mineral accrual during the growing years is an essential ingredient for the prevention of osteoporosis later in life.

Several reviews have concluded that appropriate physical activity augments bone development (4,7,41). Retrospective human studies clearly indicate that bone responds more favorably to physical activity that were undertaken during childhood and adolescence than during adulthood (23,50). Numerous randomized controlled intervention studies have also been conducted to investigate the change in bone mass and bone strength in children secondary to an exercise intervention.

In general, the magnitude of the augmented response over 7–10 months of exercise intervention varied from 1% at the trochanteric region of the proximal femur (44) to ~3% at the femoral neck for a high-impact jumping intervention (27,47). When moderate activity was increased through daily physical education, a positive effect on bone accretion in prepubertal girls was noted (66). In a school-based intervention with a 10-minute, moderate-impact circuit training three times per week, the benefit doubled if the intervention continued for a second school year (41,42). In these studies, bone mass benefits increased from 2% to approximately 4% at the femoral neck and lumbar spine in both boys and girls. These and other studies suggest that the bone response to loading is optimized in prepuberty and early puberty (12,32,37).

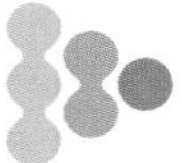

Preparticipation Health Screening, Medical History, and Physical Examination

Prior to beginning an exercise program, anyone with osteoporosis should fill out a physical activity readiness questionnaire. **Medical clearance** may be obtained from the individual's physician, who should assess factors including past and current medical health, fall or fracture risk (*e.g.*, FRAX or CAROC assessments; see recommended resources list at the end of this chapter), physical function (*i.e.*, coordination, balance, and mobility), and any barriers to physical activity participation (*e.g.*, physical and psychological).

Case Study 21-1 Quiz:

Preparticipation Health Screening, Medical History, and Physical Examination

1. Determine Mrs. Case Study-BH's preparticipation health assessment as well as medical clearance guidelines prior to exercise testing and prescription.
2. How would her medical clearance guidelines change if she had reported suffering a vertebral fracture 5 years ago?
3. What signs (physical or from her health history) for osteoporosis and risk for an osteoporosis-related fracture does Mrs. Case Study-BH display?

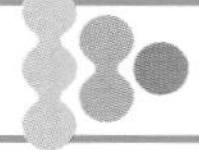

Exercise Testing Considerations

By itself, a diagnosis of osteoporosis is not a contraindication for a symptom-limited exercise test. When exercise tests to assess cardiorespiratory or muscular fitness are performed in individuals with osteoporosis, the following should be considered:

- Use of cycle ergometry as an alternative to treadmill exercise testing to assess cardiovascular function may be indicated in patients with severe vertebral osteoporosis for whom walking is painful.
- Vertebral compression fractures leading to a loss of height and spinal deformation can compromise ventilatory capacity and result in a forward shift in the center of gravity. The latter may affect balance during treadmill walking.
- **Maximal** muscle strength testing is contraindicated in patients with severe osteoporosis given concerns of fracture during testing.

Osteoporosis can preclude detection of abnormal responses associated with heart diseases during an exercise test because performance may be limited by the symptoms of osteoporosis, thus preventing the individual from achieving an adequate heart rate (HR) and blood pressure (BP) response necessary for an accurate diagnosis. Severe kyphosis (rounding of the upper spine) is one such example unique to osteoporosis that may limit an exercise test because of an imposed mechanical limitation on respiratory muscle function. Ideally, data from a symptom-limited exercise test will be available for the calculation of an exercise target HR range using the HR reserve method. If a maximal exercise test is contraindicated or cannot be performed, ratings of perceived exertion can be used to guide exercise intensity in this population. However, if the participant is at moderate or high risk for cardiovascular disease (CVD), it would be prudent to closely assess the patient for indications of ischemia (*e.g.*, angina) or excessive exercise intensity (*e.g.*, excessive HR or BP responses).

Exercise Prescription and Progression Considerations

The goal of exercise in adulthood should be to gain bone strength and to offset bone loss that is observed during this time in life. Trials of exercise lasting 8–12 months in premenopausal women generally show increases in BMD of 1%–3% at loaded sites (usually the spine and hip) compared with controls (25,31,40,64). Differences between exercisers and controls in the premenopausal cohorts are attributed to gains in bone mineral in exercisers (8,31), attenuation of bone loss in exercisers, or a combination of bone gain in exercisers and bone loss in controls (25). Trials of exercise in premenopausal women (ages 22–49 yr) have shown favorable outcomes as a result of jogging, strength training, aerobics, and jumping exercises (39).

Marques et al. (43) published a meta-analysis suggesting that exercise is effective at improving BMD in older adults at the lumbar spine and femoral neck, particularly if exercise was more intense and included loading activities that were multidirectional. Characteristics of exercise are highlighted that will make exercise as osteogenic as possible in the skeletons of older adults, along with considerations for fall prevention.

Several studies have shown that loads applied dynamically and that generate greater magnitude strains result in proportionally greater gains in bone formation (1,20,57,58). What this means is that higher intensity, weight-bearing exercise may be more beneficial for stimulating greater gains in bone mass or, alternatively, greater reductions in bone mass loss with age.

Of the few studies performed in men, most found positive effects of resistance training on BMD at loaded sites. Sixteen weeks of resistance training in men (mean age = 59 yr) resulted in a 3.8% increase in femoral neck BMD compared with controls (46). Similarly, Ryan et al. (59) found that 16 weeks of resistance training in men (mean age = 61 yr) resulted in a 2.8% increase in femoral neck BMD compared with controls. Overall, studies in adults indicate that exercise, if done with adequate loading such as resistance and impact training, is effective at attenuating bone loss observed with advancing age (39).

Several meta-analyses and reviews have determined that exercise is generally less effective in older age than in youth and early adulthood (23,43,50). Skeletal benefits with exercise in older populations are very modest, with reports of an increase in BMD at the lumbar spine of $0.011 \text{ g} \cdot \text{cm}^{-2}$ and at the femoral neck of $0.016 \text{ g} \cdot \text{cm}^{-2}$ on average following an exercise intervention (43). Nevertheless, although exercise may not be as potent at building stronger bones in older age, exercise has been shown to offset the *loss* of bone in older adults (38). Another important benefit of exercise in older age is improvement in balance, coordination, and muscle mass and strength — all of which are critical for reducing the likelihood of falling (22,24,30). Therefore, an overview of general health concepts regarding principles of exercise to improve bone health is provided. Exercise professionals must be also cautious to balance safety concerns with principles of osteogenic exercise.

The exercise professional must balance safety concerns with the desire to improve bone health. Therefore, other loading characteristics that are outlined next may help improve the osteogenic nature of exercise while bypassing the need for exercise to be of high intensity.

Loading Characteristics

One such characteristic is unaccustomed loading. When physical activities are different from everyday activities in the sense that forces on the bone are abnormally distributed, the response of bone to exercise can be greatly improved. For example, in a study of loads applied to turkey bones, when the loads were applied to the wing bones in directions that were different from customary activities, the dynamic exercise resulted in bone mineral content increases of between 133% and 143% of the original value (57). These observations may help explain why the "unaccustomed" actions seen in soccer may be more osteogenic than repetitive, uniaxial activities such as cycling (51).

Another characteristic of loading that may increase osteogenesis is rest-inserted loading. Several animal studies have demonstrated that seconds (65), hours (55), and even weeks (60) of rest inserted between loading cycles and bouts make bone much more sensitive to exercise. For instance, loading the forelimbs of turkeys with 100 cycles per day with low-magnitude loading and 10 seconds of rest inserted between each load cycle resulted in 21.9% of the periosteum (outside surface of long bones) being "activated" with bone formation compared with the forelimb loaded with the same number of cycles at the same low magnitude for the same number of days but without rest inserted between each loading cycle (only 3.8% of the periosteum was activated). These results suggest that partitioning the same number of loading cycles into different bouts throughout the day may make exercise more effective for bone health.

Guidelines for Exercise Prescription

The following guidelines for exercise prescription align with recommendations for older adults, with special considerations for physical activity and bone health. In designing the exercise prescription, the exercise professional should aim to achieve frequency, intensity, time, and type (FITT) recommendations using principles of specificity and progressive overload for prescribing exercises for individuals with osteoporosis, without a vertebral fracture (FITT table [Table 21.1]). The goal of exercise prescription for people with osteoporosis is to select osteogenic and balance activities that are specific to the individual's goals and capabilities. Within these parameters, the following program guidelines should be considered to optimize safety and minimize fall and fracture risk:

- Individuals with limited tolerance for weight-bearing exercise may benefit from aquatic and stationary cycling exercises to improve **muscular strength** and **endurance**. Weight-bearing activities may be gradually introduced as tolerated.
- Instruction to maintain neutral spinal alignment and proper form should be provided throughout the progressive exercise prescription and during **activities of daily living**. Modifications may be necessary to improve body mechanics for safe movement and fall and fracture prevention, particularly for the following:
  - Exercises and activities involving end-range trunk flexion or rotation (*e.g.*, some yoga poses), in combination (*e.g.*, golf swing), or dynamic abdominal exercises (*e.g.*, sit-ups) because they may generate relatively large forces on weak bone (29)
  - Activities involving abrupt or explosive loading, or high-impact loading, or quick, repetitive movements, or those with a high fall risk should be avoided or modified to a slower, more controlled pace or lower impact activities.
  - Lifting and lowering heavy objects from the floor and above the head and holding heavy objects with outstretched hands in front of the body (*e.g.*, reaching to place a heavy box onto a shelf), particularly if exerting maximal strength which increases loads on the spine

FITT

TABLE 21.1 FITT RECOMMENDATIONS FOR INDIVIDUALS WITH OSTEOPOROSIS

ACSM FITT Principle of the ExR_x

Chronic Medical Condition	Frequency (How often?)	Intensity (How hard?)	Time	Type (What kind?) Primary	Resistance	Flexibility	Special Considerations
Healthy Adult	≥5 d · wk^{-1} of moderate exercise, or ≥3 d · wk^{-1} of vigorous exercise, or a combination of moderate and vigorous exercise on ≥3–5 d · wk^{-1} is recommended.	Moderate to vigorous. Light-to-moderate intensity exercise may be beneficial in deconditioned individuals.	If moderate intensity: ≥30 min · d^{-1} to total 150 min · wk^{-1}. If vigorous intensity: ≥20 min · d^{-1} to total 75 min · wk^{-1}.	Regular, purposeful exercise that involves major muscle groups and is continuous and rhythmic in nature is recommended.	2–3 d · wk^{-1} (nonconsecutive)	2–3 d · wk^{-1}; static stretch 10–30 s; 2–4 repetitions of each exercise	Sedentary behaviors can have adverse health effects, even among those who regularly exercise. Adding short physical activity breaks throughout the day may be considered as a part of the exercise.
Osteoporosis	4–5 d · wk^{-1}	Moderate (40%–59% HRR or $\dot{V}O_2R$). Use of the CR-10 scale (0–10) with ratings of 3–4 might be a more appropriate method of establishing intensity.	Begin with 20 min; gradually progress to a minimum of 30 min (with a maximum of 45–60 min).	Walking, cycling, or other individually appropriate aerobic activity(weight bearing preferred)	Start with 1–2 nonconsecutive d · wk^{-1}; may progress to 2–3 d · wk^{-1}. Adjust resistance so that last 2 repetitions are challenging to perform. High-intensity training is beneficial in those who can tolerate it. Begin with 1 set of 8–12 repetitions; increase to 2 sets after about 2 wk; no more than 8–10 exercises/sessions. Standard equipment can be used with adequate instruction and safety considerations.	5–7 d · wk^{-1}. Stretch to the point of feeling tightness or slight discomfort. Hold static stretch for 10–30 s. Hold for static stretching 2–3 repetitions of each exercise. Static stretching of all major joints.	Exercise prescription should align with recommendations for older adults. One important goal is to select osteogenic and balance activities while optimizing safety and minimizing fall and fracture risk. Resistance, flexibility, and neuromotor training should be included in this population.

ExR_x, exercise prescription; HRR, heart rate reserve; $\dot{V}O_2R$, oxygen uptake reserve; CR-10 scale, category ratio scale.

Based on the FITT Recommendations present in *ACSM's Guidelines for Exercise Testing and Prescription*. 10th ed. Philadelphia (PA): Wolters Kluwer; 2018. 480 p.

Programming should be consistent with the FITT recommendations for older individuals with osteoporosis without a fracture (see FITT table [Table 21.1]). This can be accomplished through a 24-week program (separated into three 8-week cycles) of progressive aerobic, balance, and strength training, which is describe as follows.

The primary reasons for prescribing aerobic exercise are to improve aerobic fitness and work capacity and to decrease CVD risk. For individuals with osteoporosis, aerobic exercise should primarily involve weight-bearing modes of exercise such as walking. Other activities could include hill walking, stair climbing, dancing, or other exercises that generate unaccustomed forces and loading patterns. For those with more significant osteoporosis-related pain who cannot tolerate weight-bearing activities, cycling, swimming, or water aerobics are possible alternatives. If the individual is severely limited by pain, his or her physician should be consulted prior to exercise participation.

For individuals who were previously sedentary, an initial goal of 20–30 minutes per session at a very light or light intensity is reasonable but may be shorter (*e.g.*, bouts of 10 min each) at the beginning of a program in cases of extreme **deconditioning**. Improving muscle strength may help to conserve bone and muscle mass and enhance dynamic balance. A progressive resistance training prescription for those with osteoporosis should generally aim to meet recommended guidelines for older adults of more than 2 days per week of training, using 8–12 repetitions at an intensity that causes fatigue but not complete exhaustion for two to four sets per exercise using a sufficient number of exercises to involve the major muscle groups, with the exception of the spinal musculature. The Too Fit To Fracture consensus suggests training postural muscles (*e.g.*, spinal extensors) for endurance through isometric exercises (29). Previously sedentary individuals or those unaccustomed to resistance training should begin training at a lower intensity with slow and controlled movements, with one set per exercise of each of the major muscle groups. Initially, exercises should focus on correct form and postural alignment.

For resistance training and balance exercises that use body weight, elastic bands, free weights, machines, or calisthenics, emphasis should be placed on achieving correct form and spinal alignment. Sit-to-stand, squatting, reaching, and abdominal bracing exercises should be promoted to maintain overall functional performance. For individuals with a history of vertebral fracture (particularly with kyphosis), it is advisable for the exercise professional to consult or refer these individuals to an occupational or physical therapist with training in osteoporosis. History of vertebral fracture may preclude resistance exercises beyond those that utilize body weight.

Balance training for fall prevention may be performed daily for up to 20 minutes and combined with both resistance and aerobic training activities (*e.g.*, dancing). Exercises should begin in supported static standing positions (*e.g.*, hand on a chair or wall) with challenge progressions that might include increased stance holding, reducing contact with support, minimizing the base of support, reducing vision, and introducing dual tasks. Once stability is demonstrated, dynamic exercises with challenge progressions can be introduced (see "Recommended Resources" for evidence-based fall prevention programs).

A program to increase **flexibility** may benefit patients with osteoporosis because decreased flexibility may contribute to poor posture; however, scientific evidence is limited. Furthermore, many of the commonly prescribed exercises for increasing flexibility, especially of the hamstring muscles, involve spinal flexion and should be avoided. There is little consensus on the optimal training program for increasing flexibility in individuals with osteoporosis.

Case Study 21-1 Quiz:

Exercise Prescription and Progression Considerations

4. What are the primary goals of the exercise program for Mrs. Case Study-BH?
5. Identify the contraindications for exercise prescription with this individual.
6. If Mrs. Case Study-BH had reported poor vision and problems with her balance, how would you restructure her exercise prescription?

SUMMARY

Many of the risk factors for both osteoporosis and falls can be prevented or at least attenuated by lifestyle modifications. In particular, exercise builds bone strength in youth, helps maintain bone strength in adulthood, and prevents the loss of bone strength in old age. Exercise also increases muscle strength, improves posture and balance, and improves overall coordination, which all help to prevent falls. Therefore, there is a critical role for the exercise professional in preventing osteoporotic fractures and, therefore, helping people maintain a high quality of life. A summary of special considerations for exercise prescription and programming for individuals with osteoporosis are presented as follows:

- The clinical relevance of osteoporosis is the dramatic increase in risk of fracture, with increases functional limitations and mortality.
- Exercise is very important in this population to reduce fracture risk as a result of its potential to improve low BMD, augment muscle mass, promote strength gain, and improve dynamic balance.
- Exercise prescription guidelines for a person with osteoporosis align with recommendations for older adults, with special considerations for physical activity and bone health.
- In designing the exercise prescription, the exercise professional should aim to achieve FITT recommendations using principles of specificity and progressive overload for prescribing exercises for individuals with osteoporosis, without a vertebral fracture.
- The goal of exercise prescription for people with osteoporosis is to select osteogenic and balance activities that are specific to the individual's goals and capabilities while optimizing safety and minimizing fall and fracture risk.
- Resistance, flexibility, and neuromotor training should be added to weight-bearing aerobic conditioning.

RECOMMENDED RESOURCES

Action Schools! BC: http://www.actionschoolsbc.ca/Content/Home.asp
American Academy of Physical Medicine and Rehabilitation: How PM&R Physicians Use Exercise to Prevent and Treat Osteoporosis: http://www.aapmr.org/patients/conditions/rheumatology/Pages/osteotreat.aspx
American Society of Bone and Mineral Research Webcasts: "Bone Quality: What Is It and Can We Measure It?": http://app2.capitalreach.com/esp1204/servlet/tc?cn=asbmr&c=10169&s=20292&e=4521&&
"Forum on Aging and Skeletal Health": http://www.asbmr.org/TopicalMeetings/Webcasts.aspx
American Society of Bone and Mineral Research: Bone Curriculum: http://www.asbmr.org/Education/BoneCurriculum.aspx
Canadian Association of Radiologist and Osteoporosis (CAROC): http://www.osteoporosis.ca/multimedia/pdf/CAROC.pdf
International Osteoporosis Foundation: http://www.iofbonehealth.org/
Mayo Clinic: Exercising with Osteoporosis: http://www.mayoclinic.com/health/osteoporosis/HQ00643
National Council on Aging: Evidence-Based Fall Prevention Programs: https://www.ncoa.org/healthy-aging/falls-prevention/falls-prevention-programs-for-older-adults/
National Institutes of Health: Osteoporosis and Related Bone Diseases National Resource Center: http://www.niams.nih.gov/bone/
National Osteoporosis Foundation: http://www.nof.org/
Osteofit: http://www.osteofit.org/
Prevention of Falls Network Earth (ProFaNE): http://www.profane.co/
Strongwomen: http://www.strongwomen.com/
U.S. Bone and Joint Initiative: http://www.usbji.org/

REFERENCES

1. Ackerman KE, Nazem T, Chapko D, et al. Bone microarchitecture is impaired in adolescent amenorrheic athletes compared with eumenorrheic athletes and nonathletic controls. *J Clin Endocrinol Metab*. 2011;96(10):3123–33.
2. American College of Sports Medicine. *ACSM's Guidelines for Exercise Testing and Prescription*. 10th ed. Philadelphia (PA): Wolters Kluwer; 2018. 480 p.

3. Arlot ME, Sornay-Rendu E, Garnero P, Vey-Marty B, Delmas PD. Apparent pre- and postmenopausal bone loss evaluated by DXA at different skeletal sites in women: the OFELY cohort. *J Bone Miner Res*. 1997;12(4):683–90.
4. Bailey DA, Faulkner RA, McKay HA. Growth, physical activity, and bone mineral acquisition. *Exerc Sport Sci Rev*. 1996;24: 233–66.
5. Bailey DA, McKay HA, Mirwald RL, Crocker PR, Faulkner RA. A six-year longitudinal study of the relationship of physical activity to bone mineral accrual in growing children: the University of Saskatchewan Bone Mineral Accrual Study. *J Bone Miner Res*. 1999;14(10):1672–9.
6. Barbour KE, Lui LY, McCulloch CE, et al. Trajectories of lower extremity physical performance: effects on fractures and mortality in older women. *J Gerontol A Biol Sci Med Sci*. 2016;71(12):1609–15.
7. Barr SI, McKay HA. Nutrition, exercise, and bone status in youth. *Int J Sport Nutr*. 1998;8(2):124–42.
8. Bassey EJ, Ramsdale SJ. Increase in femoral bone density in young women following high-impact exercise. *Osteoporos Int*. 1994;4(2):72–5.
9. Beck TJ, Oreskovic TL, Stone KL, et al. Structural adaptation to changing skeletal load in the progression toward hip fragility: the study of osteoporotic fractures. *J Bone Miner Res*. 2001;16(6):1108–19.
10. Bentolila V, Boyce TM, Fyhrie DP, Drumb R, Skerry TM, Schaffler MB. Intracortical remodeling in adult rat long bones after fatigue loading. *Bone*. 1998;23(3):275–81.
11. Black DM, Rosen CJ. Clinical practice. Postmenopausal osteoporosis. *N Engl J Med*. 2016;374(3):254–62.
12. Blimkie CJ, Rice S, Webber CE, Martin J, Levy D, Gordon CL. Effects of resistance training on bone mineral content and density in adolescent females. *Can J Physiol Pharmacol*. 1996;74(9):1025–33.
13. Bonewald LF, Johnson ML. Osteocytes, mechanosensing and Wnt signaling. *Bone*. 2008;42(4):606–15.
14. Bouxsein ML. Determinants of skeletal fragility. *Best Pract Res Clin Rheumatol*. 2005;19(6):897–911.
15. Bouxsein ML. Technology insight: noninvasive assessment of bone strength in osteoporosis. *Nat Clin Pract Rheumatol*. 2008;4(6):310–8.
16. Burge R, Dawson-Hughes B, Solomon DH, Wong JB, King A, Tosteson A. Incidence and economic burden of osteoporosis-related fractures in the United States, 2005–2025. *J Bone Miner Res*. 2007;22(3):465–75.
17. Burger H, de Laet CE, van Daele PL, et al. Risk factors for increased bone loss in an elderly population: the Rotterdam Study. *Am J Epidemiol*. 1998;147(9):871–9.
18. Currey JD. *Bones: Structure and Mechanics*. Princeton (NJ): Princeton University Press; 2002. 436 p.
19. Delmas PD, Genant HK, Crans GG, et al. Severity of prevalent vertebral fractures and the risk of subsequent vertebral and nonvertebral fractures: results from the MORE trial. *Bone*. 2003;33(4):522–32.
20. Ellman R, Spatz J, Cloutier A, Palme R, Christiansen BA, Bouxsein ML. Partial reductions in mechanical loading yield proportional changes in bone density, bone architecture, and muscle mass. *J Bone Miner Res*. 2013;28(4):875–85.
21. Faulkner RA, Bailey DA. Osteoporosis: a pediatric concern? *Med Sport Sci*. 2007;51:1–12.
22. Fisher J, Steele J, McKinnon P, McKinnon S. Strength gains as a result of brief, infrequent resistance exercise in older adults. *J Sports Med (Hindawi Publ Corp)*. 2014;2014:731890.
23. Forwood MR, Burr DB. Physical activity and bone mass: exercises in futility? *Bone Miner*. 1993;21(2):89–112.
24. Fragala MS, Dam TT, Barber V, et al. Strength and function response to clinical interventions of older women categorized by weakness and low lean mass using classifications from the Foundation for the National Institute of Health Sarcopenia Project. *J Gerontol A Biol Sci Med Sci*. 2015;70(2):202–9.
25. Friedlander AL, Genant HK, Sadowsky S, Byl NN, Glüer CC. A two-year program of aerobics and weight training enhances bone mineral density of young women. *J Bone Miner Res*. 1995;10(4):574–85.
26. Frost HM. Bone's mechanostat: a 2003 update. *Anat Rec A Discov Mol Cell Evol Biol*. 2003;275(2):1081–101.
27. Fuchs RK, Bauer JJ, Snow CM. Jumping improves hip and lumbar spine bone mass in prepubescent children: a randomized controlled trial. *J Bone Miner Res*. 2001;16(1):148–56.
28. Genant HK, Cooper C, Poor G, et al. Interim report and recommendations of the World Health Organization Task-Force for Osteoporosis. *Osteoporos Int*. 1999;10(4):259–64.
29. Giangregorio LM, McGill S, Wark JD, et al. Too Fit To Fracture: outcomes of a Delphi consensus process on physical activity and exercise recommendations for adults with osteoporosis with or without vertebral fractures. *Osteoporos Int*. 2015;26(3):891–910.
30. Gianoudis J, Bailey CA, Ebeling PR, et al. Effects of a targeted multimodal exercise program incorporating high-speed power training on falls and fracture risk factors in older adults: a community-based randomized controlled trial. *J Bone Miner Res*. 2014;29(1):182–91.
31. Heinonen A, Kannus P, Sievänen H, et al. Randomised controlled trial of effect of high-impact exercise on selected risk factors for osteoporotic fractures. *Lancet*. 1996;348(9038):1343–7.
32. Heinonen A, Sievänen H, Kannus P, Oja P, Pasanen M, Vuori I. High-impact exercise and bones of growing girls: a 9-month controlled trial. *Osteoporos Int*. 2000;11(12):1010–7.
33. Johnell O, Kanis JA. An estimate of the worldwide prevalence and disability associated with osteoporotic fractures. *Osteoporos Int*. 2006;17(12):1726–33.

34. Kanis J. *Assessment of Osteoporosis at the Primary Health Care Level*. Technical Report. Sheffield (United Kingdom): University of Sheffield; 2007. 339 p.
35. Kanis JA, Johnell O, Oden A, et al. Long-term risk of osteoporotic fracture in Malmö. *Osteoporos Int*. 2000;11(8):669–74.
36. Kannus P. Preventing osteoporosis, falls, and fractures among elderly people. Promotion of lifelong physical activity is essential. *BMJ*. 1999;318(7178):205–6.
37. Kannus P, Haapasalo H, Sankelo M, et al. Effect of starting age of physical activity on bone mass in the dominant arm of tennis and squash players. *Ann Intern Med*. 1995;123(1):27–31.
38. Karinkanta S, Heinonen A, Sievänen H, et al. A multi-component exercise regimen to prevent functional decline and bone fragility in home-dwelling elderly women: randomized, controlled trial. *Osteoporos Int*. 2007;18(4):453–62.
39. Khan K, McKay H, Kannus P, Bailey D, Wark J, Bennell K. *Physical Activity and Bone Health*. Champaign (IL): Human Kinetics; 2001. 288 p.
40. Lohman T, Going S, Pamenter R, et al. Effects of resistance training on regional and total bone mineral density in premenopausal women: a randomized prospective study. *J Bone Miner Res*. 1995;10(7):1015–24.
41. MacKelvie KJ, Khan KM, McKay HA. Is there a critical period for bone response to weight-bearing exercise in children and adolescents? A systematic review. *Br J Sports Med*. 2002;36(4):250–7.
42. MacKelvie KJ, McKay HA, Khan KM, Crocker PR. A school-based exercise intervention augments bone mineral accrual in early pubertal girls. *J Pediatr*. 2001;139(4):501–8.
43. Marques EA, Mota J, Carvalho J. Exercise effects on bone mineral density in older adults: a meta-analysis of randomized controlled trials. *Age (Dordr)*. 2012;34(6):1493–515.
44. McKay HA, Petit MA, Schutz RW, Prior JC, Barr SI, Khan KM. Augmented trochanteric bone mineral density after modified physical education classes: a randomized school-based exercise intervention study in prepubescent and early pubescent children. *J Pediatr*. 2000;136(2):156–62.
45. Melton LJ III, Chrischilles EA, Cooper C, Lane AW, Riggs BL. Perspective. How many women have osteoporosis? *J Bone Miner Res*. 1992;7(9):1005–10.
46. Menkes A, Mazel S, Redmond RA, et al. Strength training increases regional bone mineral density and bone remodeling in middle-aged and older men. *J Appl Physiol (1985)*. 1993;74(5):2478–84.
47. Morris FL, Naughton GA, Gibbs JL, Carlson JS, Wark JD. Prospective ten-month exercise intervention in premenarcheal girls: positive effects on bone and lean mass. *J Bone Miner Res*. 1997;12(9):1453–62.
48. Nagaraja S, Couse TL, Guldberg R. E. Trabecular bone microdamage and microstructural stresses under uniaxial compression. *J Biomech*. 2005;38(4):707–16.
49. Nawathe S, Akhlaghpour H, Bouxsein ML, Keaveny TM. Microstructural failure mechanisms in the human proximal femur for sideways fall loading. *J Bone Miner Res*. 2014;29(2):507–15.
50. Nikander R, Sievänen H, Heinonen A, Daly RM, Uusi-Rasi K, Kannus P. Targeted exercise against osteoporosis: a systematic review and meta-analysis for optimising bone strength throughout life. *BMC Med*. 2010;8:47.
51. Nikander R, Sievänen H, Heinonen A, Kannus P. Femoral neck structure in adult female athletes subjected to different loading modalities. *J Bone Miner Res*. 2005;20(3):520–8.
52. Parfitt AM. Targeted and nontargeted bone remodeling: relationship to basic multicellular unit origination and progression. *Bone*. 2002;30(1):5–7.
53. Ravn P, Hetland ML, Overgaard K, Christiansen C. Premenopausal and postmenopausal changes in bone mineral density of the proximal femur measured by dual-energy X-ray absorptiometry. *J Bone Miner Res*. 1994;9(12):1975–80.
54. Recker RR. Skeletal fragility and bone quality. *J Musculoskelet Neuronal Interact*. 2007;7(1):54–5.
55. Robling AG, Burr BD, Turner CH. Recovery periods restore mechanosensitivity to dynamically loaded bone. *J Exp Biol*. 2001;204(pt 19):3389–99.
56. Robling AG, Castillo AB, Turner CH. Biomechanical and molecular regulation of bone remodeling. *Annu Rev Biomed Eng*. 2006;8:455–98.
57. Rubin CT, Lanyon LE. Regulation of bone formation by applied dynamic loads. *J Bone Joint Surg Am*. 1984;66(3):397–402.
58. Rubin CT, Lanyon LE. Regulation of bone mass by mechanical strain magnitude. *Calcif Tissue Int*. 1985;37(4):411–7.
59. Ryan AS, Treuth MS, Rubin MA, et al. Effects of strength training on bone mineral density: hormonal and bone turnover relationships. *J Appl Physiol* (1985). 1994;77(4):1678–84.
60. Saxon LK, Robling AG, Alam I, Turner CH. Mechanosensitivity of the rat skeleton decreases after a long period of loading, but is improved with time off. *Bone*. 2005;36(3):454–64.
61. Scott A, Khan KM, Duronio V, Hart DA. Mechanotransduction in human bone: in vitro cellular physiology that underpins bone changes with exercise. *Sports Med*. 2008;38(2):139–60.
62. Seeman E. From density to structure: growing up and growing old on the surfaces of bone. *J Bone Miner Res*. 1997;12(4):509–21.
63. Seeman E. Pathogenesis of bone fragility in women and men. *Lancet*. 2002;359(9320):1841–50.
64. Snowharter C, Bouxsein ML, Lewis BT, Carter DR, Marcus R. Effects of resistance and endurance exercise on bone mineral status of young women: a randomized exercise intervention trial. *J Bone Miner Res*. 1992;7(7):761–9.

65. Srinivasan S, Weimer DA, Agans SC, Bain SD, Gross TS. Low-magnitude mechanical loading becomes osteogenic when rest is inserted between each loading cycle. *J Bone Miner Res*. 2002;17(9):1613–20.
66. Valdimarsson O, Linden C, Johnell O, Gardsell P, Karlsson MK. Daily physical education in the school curriculum in prepubertal girls during 1 year is followed by an increase in bone mineral accrual and bone width — data from the prospective controlled Malmö pediatric osteoporosis prevention study. *Calcif Tissue Int*. 2006;78(2):65–71.
67. Vanderschueren D, Venken K, Ophoff J, Bouillon R, Boonen S. Clinical review: sex steroids and the periosteum — reconsidering the roles of androgens and estrogens in periosteal expansion. *J Clin Endocrinol Metab*. 2006;91(2):378–82.
68. Wei TS, Hu CH, Wang SH, Hwang KL. Fall characteristics, functional mobility and bone mineral density as risk factors of hip fracture in the community-dwelling ambulatory elderly. *Osteoporos Int*. 2001;12(12):1050–5.
69. Zioupos P. Accumulation of in-vivo fatigue microdamage and its relation to biomechanical properties in ageing human cortical bone. *J Microsc*. 2001;201(pt 2):270–8.

CHAPTER 22

Special Considerations for Psychological Health

INTRODUCTION

Depression and anxiety are forms of psychological distress, which are often comorbid with each other and with chronic disease. They are commonly encountered by exercise professionals working with healthy and special populations and can affect the capacity for exercise training and testing among healthy and special populations. Exercise professionals should be able to recognize symptoms of depression and anxiety and provide recommendations based on evidence relevant to each patient's specific needs. This chapter provides a summary of special considerations for exercise testing and training among those with depression and/or anxiety briefly discussed.

Case Study 22-1

Mr. Case Study-PH

Mr. Case Study-PH is a 43-year-old male with a history of hypertension and obesity. After receiving a recommendation from his physician to begin an exercise program, Mr. Case Study-PH visits your exercise facility for a consultation. Mr. Case Study-PH indicates that he is nervous about being more active because he has tried to increase his exercise level in the past but has had difficulty maintaining a routine. He says that he is very motivated to lose weight but that **exercise** is uncomfortable and sometimes painful and that he worries about being judged by others in the gym. Mr. Case Study-PH indicates that he is sedentary and is very concerned about his current and future health if he is unable to follow the physician's recommendations but struggles some days just to find the motivation to get out of bed. Mr. Case Study-PH is not currently taking any psychoactive medications but has considered seeking mental health counseling in the past.

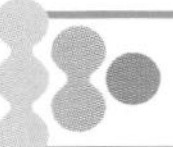

Description, Prevalence, and Etiology

The concept of depression is closely related to loss and involves states of grief or bereavement that would naturally occur after, for example, the death of a loved one or after enduring a catastrophic natural disaster. Sustained clinical depression, however, exists in the absence of such loss. Depression presents cognitively (*e.g.*, negative self-appraisals, a pessimistic view of the world, feelings of helplessness, and hopelessness about the future) and somatically (*e.g.*, extreme fatigue, altered sleep, fluctuations in weight) and significantly affects the ability to function. Distinguishing factors between specific depressive disorders include issues of age of onset/timing, duration, and presumed etiology (2).

Anxiety is a negative affective state characterized by worry, apprehension, or tension in the presence of novel or aversive stimuli. Anxiety is closely related to fear and is a normal protective psychological and physiological response in anticipation of the need for fight-or-flight response. Individuals with disproportionate acute anxiety responses for the level of real or perceived threat as well as individuals who frequently experience anxious symptoms in the absence of any real or perceived threat may be suffering from an anxiety disorder (2). The underlying feature common to anxiety disorders is unwarranted sympathetic nervous system (SNS) activation in response to a perceived future threat. Either chronic or episodic SNS activation under circumstances that pose no immediate danger can be highly debilitating and lead to additional health problems (2).

Depressive and anxiety disorders identified in the *Diagnostic and Statistical Manual of Mental Disorders, 5th edition* (*DSM-5*) are listed in Table 22.1. The *DSM-5* marks a reclassification such that (a) depressive disorders are distinct from bipolar disorders, whereas in the fourth edition, these classes of disorders formed one heterogeneous group of mood disorders, and (b) obsessive/compulsive disorder (OCD) and posttraumatic stress disorder (PTSD) are also reclassified as unique from each other and anxiety disorders, unlike in earlier editions (1,2). Interested readers are encouraged to refer to the *DSM-5* for detailed descriptions of each disorder. Symptoms of depression and anxiety are listed in Table 22.2, although it should be noted that not everyone experiences the same symptoms, and it is unlikely that any one person would present with all symptoms listed. Depressive and anxiety disorders can only be diagnosed by a mental health care professional according to clinical criteria such as those described in the *DSM-5* and are typically treated with pharmacotherapy, psychotherapy, or both.

Anxiety disorders are the most prevalent of mental disorders among adults (2) and are highly comorbid with depression (44). Anxiety disorders and depression are also frequently comorbid

Table 22.1 Depressive and Anxiety Disorders Identified in the *DSM-5*

Depressive Disorders	Anxiety Disorders
Major depressive disorder (MDD)	Generalized anxiety disorder (GAD)
Disruptive mood dysregulation disorder	Separation anxiety
Persistent depressive disorder (a.k.a. dysthymia)	Selective mutism
Premenstrual dysphoric disorder	Specific phobias
Substance/medication-induced depressive disorder	Social anxiety disorder
Depressive disorder due to another medical condition	Panic disorder
	Agoraphobia

with other mental health problems, with about 85% and 76% of cases of generalized anxiety disorder (GAD) and major depressive disorder (MDD), respectively, being comorbid with at least one other mental disorder (44). The United States is ranked highest for 12-month prevalence of anxiety (18.2%) and depression (10%) (67,79), and U.S. citizens have an estimated lifetime risk/lifetime prevalence of 36% and 31.4%, respectively (43). Women are twice as likely to experience anxiety (2) or depression (67) than men. Anxiety and depression are often comorbid with chronic illness, including cardiovascular disease (CVD), hypertension, arthritis, obesity, diabetes, asthma, and chronic obstructive pulmonary disease (COPD). Anxiety and depression increase the risk of morbidity and mortality in clinical samples (15,81), and a recent meta-analysis estimates a 52% increase in the risk of incident CVD in samples reporting clinical or subclinical anxiety at baseline (7). Depression and anxiety represent major public health concerns that are drastically underdiagnosed, as those who do suffer from mental distress often wait many years before seeking treatment (84).

Table 22.2 Common Symptoms of Depression and Anxiety

Depressive Disorders	Anxiety Disorders
▪ Depressed mood	▪ Intense worry, fear, or dread about future outcomes
▪ Decreased interest in all activities	▪ Rumination
▪ Significant weight loss	▪ Avoidant behavior
▪ Persistent psychomotor agitation or retardation (observable by others)	▪ Unwarranted or excessive SNS activation reflected by
▪ Persistent insomnia or hypersomnia	• Elevated heart rate
▪ Persistent indecisiveness or problems concentrating	• Peripheral vasodilation
▪ Persistent fatigue or loss of energy	• Altered breathing
▪ Persistent feelings of guilt or worthlessness	• Diaphoresis (*i.e.*, excessive sweating)
▪ Persistent changes in appetite	▪ Dry mouth
▪ Recurrent suicidal thoughts	▪ Agitation
	▪ Gastrointestinal distress
	▪ Trembling

Although the causes of depression and anxiety are not fully understood, the prevalence of comorbidity between depression and anxiety suggests some common underlying etiology. Generally, neurobiological theories of anxiety and depression specify a role for autonomic dysfunction and often overlap. Central and peripheral evidence of autonomic dysfunction in animals and humans has provided a myriad of candidate mechanisms for anxiety and depression. Most early clinical work in depression and anxiety focused on the norepinephrine (NE) and the serotonin (5-hydroxytryptamine [5-HT]) systems, which modulate brain activity in areas involved in regulating mood and the response to stress. Pharmacological interventions continue to target an increase in the activity level of NE and 5-HT for the treatment of depressive and anxiety disorders. More recently, γ-aminobutyric acid (GABA) and glutamate, which both play a major role in neuroplasticity, have been implicated in the etiology of anxiety (8,62) and depression (40). Investigations focused on GABA were prompted by the observed actions of benzodiazepines, which bind to the $GABA_A$ receptor, and have been successful in treating anxiety disorders. Glutamate mediates fear-conditioning and inhibitory-avoidance memory and has been supported in the etiology of anxiety (8). Neurotropic factors in the brain, specifically brain-derived neurotropic factor (BDNF), are important in proliferation, differentiation, and survival of neurons, as well as neurogenesis, synaptic plasticity, and cognitive function, and have been linked to anxiety and depression (56). A downregulation of BDNF expression in the brain could result in neuronal atrophy and cell loss in brain regions associated with depression and anxiety, such as the hippocampus and prefrontal cortex (21). This hypothesis is supported in animal (54) and human studies (14). A growing body of evidence emphasizes a role for inflammatory dysregulation in the etiology depression (57,59). However, the presence of inflammatory biomarkers is neither necessary nor sufficient for a diagnosis of depression (66), especially among those with CVD in whom this relationship is no longer significant (37). An exhaustive review of the evidence for mechanisms underlying depression and anxiety is beyond the scope of this chapter. Overall, several forms of treatment have been successful in relieving symptoms, but our understanding of underlying mechanisms remains incomplete. It is likely that depression and anxiety result from an interaction of genetic, social, environmental, psychological, cognitive, and physiological factors.

Case Study 22-1 Quiz:

Description, Prevalence, Etiology

1. What are some cognitive symptoms of depression and/or anxiety reported by Mr. Case Study-PH? Somatic symptoms?
2. Are you, as an exercise professional, capable of diagnosing your patients with depression and/or anxiety?

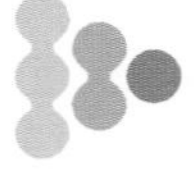

Preparticipation Health Screening, Medical History, and Physical Examination

Exercise professionals should assess risk for depression and anxiety among patients reporting symptoms. Brief screening tools for depression and anxiety used in primary care (*e.g.*, the Brief Patient Health Questionnaire or the Patient Health Questionnaire Depression Scale, the Hospital Anxiety and Depression Scale) can be useful to the exercise professional in assessing patient symptoms (52). Those who indicate more than minimal symptoms of depression and/or anxiety as indicated by scores calculated using the validated scoring criteria for the chosen measure/screening tool or those whose symptoms persist for more than few weeks should be referred for a clinical evaluation by a mental health care professional (52) to rule out other causes for symptoms, check for comorbidities, and develop an appropriate treatment plan. Individuals with any level of symptoms can also be referred to several community resources that are able to provide diagnostic, treatment, or support services, such as family practice or internal medicine physicians, community mental health centers, outpatient clinics, social agencies, family service, self-help groups, or religious organizations. Exercise professionals should make themselves familiar with the resources in their area. As with all personal or sensitive issues, exercise professionals should be tactful, empathetic, and knowledgeable when discussing symptoms of depression and/or anxiety and referring patients to diagnostic screening, counseling, or other forms of assistance.

In the case that someone expresses such hopelessness or depression that suicide risk is suspected, immediate action is necessary. You may call their mental health professional, refer them to a local suicide or crisis center, call the National Hopeline Network (1-800-SUICIDE, available 24 h a day), or have them taken directly to a hospital emergency room. It is important that the person be accompanied to the treatment center and not left alone until professional help is available. Exercise professionals are encouraged to visit https://hopeline.com to learn more about the National Hopeline Network.

Case Study 22-1 Quiz:

Preparticipation Health Screening, Medical History, and Physical Examination

3. How would you determine whether Mr. Case Study-PH is at risk for depression and/or anxiety?
4. Your risk assessment indicates that Mr. Case Study-PH has symptoms of moderate depression and/or anxiety. What should you recommend to him? What else could you provide for him?

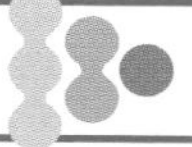

Exercise Testing Considerations

Individuals with depression and/or anxiety are less active than others (13), contributing to a lower level of physical conditioning. A recent meta-analysis reported a modest relationship between MDD and **cardiorespiratory fitness** (CRF) (effect size [ES] = −0.16, 95% confidence interval [CI] = [−0.21, −0.10]), such that greater symptom severity was associated with reduced CRF (64). Anxiety is also inversely related to CRF, and there is some evidence that this relationship is mediated by individual perceptions of anxiety symptoms in response to stress (82). Exercise professionals might expect an individual with symptoms of depression and/or anxiety to perform below average for their age, gender, and health status during **aerobic** exercise testing. Fortunately, the cumulative evidence supports the efficacy of exercise programs for improving CRF in clinically depressed samples (78), and there appear to be no contraindications to participation in regular exercise programs to improve CRF for those suffering from depression and/or anxiety in the absence of other contraindicated conditions.

Of particular relevance to CRF testing among samples with depression and anxiety is the autonomic modulation of the cardiovascular response to exercise. Autonomic balance modulates the cardiovascular response to stress. Measures of heart rate variability (HRV) are accepted as indexes for autonomic balance and regulated emotional responding (4) and provide indices of autonomic tone that have prognostic value (23). Higher levels of variability are related to cardiovascular fitness and reflect a higher level of physical conditioning and autonomic balance. Reduced HRV indicates an autonomic imbalance resulting from reduced parasympathetic drive, increased sympathetic drive to the heart, or both. HRV is related to a number of modifiable and nonmodifiable risk factors for CVD (80) and is thought to be an important factor in assessing cardiovascular risk (23). It could be expected that cardiovascular responses to exercise might be altered among individuals with depressive and/or anxiety disorders, as autonomic dysregulation is implicated in their etiology. Reduced HRVs are reported repeatedly in these clinical populations (25,42,50,51).

An imbalance in autonomic signaling to the heart, indicated by reduced HRV, may result in an elevated resting heart rate (HR), abnormal sinus tachycardia with postural changes (*i.e.*, standing from a recumbent position), and abnormal or inadequate HR responses to exercise (*e.g.*, chronotropic incompetence) (23). Reduced HRV is strongly supported as a robust predictor for the development of abnormal arrhythmias and cardiac mortality in patients with postmyocardial infarction (45). The relationship between reduced HRV among depressed and anxious samples and autonomic regulation of cardiovascular responses during exercise testing is understudied or underreported. Most investigations report on the effect of cardiovascular fitness on the autonomic response to psychological stress (39). Work is needed to test for significant differences in autonomic modulation of cardiovascular responses to graded **maximal** and **submaximal** exercise tests in samples with clinical depression and/or anxiety.

Exercise professionals should use caution when testing and training individuals taking psychoactive medication. Although limited, evidence suggests that there may be interactive effects of exercise and drugs commonly used to treat anxiety and depression. Exercise may have an additive or antagonistic effect on psychological symptoms when combined with pharmacotherapy (9). For example, one report suggests that selective serotonin reuptake inhibitors (SSRIs) may increase the risk of rhabdomyolysis after **eccentric** exercise (47). Of specific relevance to cardiorespiratory exercise testing is the occasional use of β-blockers, which inhibit the HR response to exercise, to minimize physical symptoms when an anxiety-provoking event is anticipated. Exercise professionals should ask their patients if they are currently taking any prescription medications that fall under the classifications listed in Box 22.1, as additional precautions may be necessary to ensure safety during training. Psychoactive medication does not act uniformly between individuals, and the dosage must often be adjusted for optimal therapeutic effect (11). Interactive effects between exercise and antidepressants and anxiolytics are not well understood. More work is necessary to provide clear guidelines for **exercise prescription** among populations taking psychoactive medications (9).

Box 22.1 Classes of Drugs Commonly Used to Treat Depression and Anxiety

Classes of drugs that are commonly used for treatment of depression and anxiety include the following:

- Tricyclic antidepressants
- Monoamine oxidase inhibitors
- Selective serotonin reuptake inhibitors
- Benzodiazepines
- Serotonin antagonists
- Selective noradrenaline reuptake inhibitors
- Barbiturates
- Dopamine agonists
- β-Blockers

Physiological responses to exercise may be misinterpreted by those with high anxiety sensitivity (*i.e.*, the belief that anxiety-related sensations will have negative consequences) who do not regularly exercise. To these individuals, the sensations of physiological arousal (*e.g.*, increased HR, perspiration, respiration) during an exercise test may resemble the unwarranted or excessive SNS activity associated with anxiety and can act as a psychological barrier to exercise. Perceptions of cognitive and somatic symptoms of anxiety have been observed to mediate the relationship between cardiovascular fitness and the **intensity** of those symptoms (85). If a patient reports little or no physical activity, it may be beneficial for the exercise professional to discuss the physiological response to exercise with the patient prior to the exercise test, as this may help the patient reframe their perceptions of the sensations accompanying exercise. Although some patients feel anxious or reluctant to participate in **vigorous** exercise for fear of inducing a panic attack or other negative consequence, there is little evidence to suggest that exercise can induce a panic attack. Moreover, evidence indicates that as little as one session of moderate aerobic exercise can reduce anxiety sensitivity (12).

Case Study 22-1 Quiz:

Exercise Testing Considerations for Depression and Anxiety

5. Mr. Case Study-PH has expressed concern about the exercise test. He says he feels anxious when he thinks about performing a maximal test. What are some things that the exercise professional can do in an attempt to alleviate his anxiety?

Exercise Prescription and Progression Considerations for Depression and Anxiety

In most cases, exercise is a useful adjunctive therapy in the treatment of mental distress and results in both physical and mental health benefits for patients; therefore, exercise prescription and programming should follow guidelines for apparently healthy individuals (frequency, intensity, time, and type [FITT] table, Table 22.3). The beneficial effect of exercise on depression and anxiety has been supported among diverse samples, including otherwise healthy adults (16,17), children and **adolescents** (48), and **older adults** (38), as well as patients with chronic illness (35) and those suffering from clinical depression (69), depression related to pregnancy (18), nonclinical anxiety symptoms (87), and anxiety disorders (6). Exercise can be equally as effective as pharmacotherapy in treating clinical depression (19) and in treating depressive symptoms in patients with coronary heart disease (10,69). Furthermore, exercise is equally as effective as psychotherapy (19,27,69) and better than no treatment, placebo control, and treatment as usual or usual care in treating depression (27). With regard to anxiety, exercise has been observed to perform equally as well as or better than group therapy, yoga or stretching, relaxation or meditation, stress management education, and music therapy (87) and as well as pharmacotherapy (6). Evidence for the comparative effect of exercise compared with cognitive behavioral therapy on anxiety is inconsistent (6,87). Although the cumulative evidence supports a moderate effect of exercise on depression (ES ~.6) and a small effect of exercise on anxiety (ES ~.3), there is still a lack of consensus regarding the optimal dose of exercise for treatment of depression and anxiety (83). More evidence has been generated for the effect of exercise on depression than on anxiety.

TABLE 22.3 FITT RECOMMENDATIONS FOR INDIVIDUALS WITH DEPRESSION AND/OR ANXIETY

FITT

ACSM FITT Principle of the ExR_x

Chronic Medical Condition	Frequency (How often?)	Intensity (How hard?)	Time	Type (What kind?) Primary	Resistance	Flexibility	Special Considerations
Patients Who Have Anxiety and Depression Should Follow Guidelines for Apparently Healthy Adults	$\geq$5 d · wk^{-1} of moderate exercise, or $\geq$3 d · wk^{-1} of vigorous exercise, or a combination of moderate and vigorous exercise on $\geq$3–5 d · wk^{-1} is recommended.	Moderate to vigorous. Light-to-moderate intensity exercise may be beneficial in deconditioned individuals.	If moderate intensity: $\geq$30 min · d^{-1} to total 150 min · wk^{-1}. If vigorous intensity: $\geq$20 min · d^{-1} to total 75 min · wk^{-1}.	Regular, purposeful exercise that involves major muscle groups and is continuous and rhythmic in nature is recommended.	2–3 d · wk^{-1} (nonconsecutive)	2–3 d · wk^{-1}; static stretch 10–30 s; 2–4 repetitions of each exercise	Exercise professionals working with this population should be familiar with symptoms of mental distress and have referral sources available. Tailor the exercise program to the individual needs of the patient and encourage personal responsibility by including the patient in the program planning. Always consider medications effect and any comorbid conditions.

ExR_x, exercise prescription.

Based on the FITT Recommendations present in *ACSM's Guidelines for Exercise Testing and Prescription.* 10th ed. Philadelphia (PA): Wolters Kluwer; 2018. 480 p.

Evidence for the Effects of Exercise on Depression

The evidence for the beneficial effect of exercise on depression in adults is strong (65), although there is some inconsistency reported for effects among some clinical populations (81). The American Psychiatric Association (APA) recently acknowledged the usefulness of exercise as a treatment option for mild depression (3). They elaborate, however, that if symptoms do not improve after a few weeks of exercise alone, then psychotherapy or pharmacotherapy should be prescribed. In cases that warrant psychotherapy or pharmacotherapy, as determined by a mental health care professional, exercise can be an effective add-on strategy (19).

A number of reviews have described what is known regarding properties of exercise prescription that elicit a therapeutic response among those suffering from depressive symptoms or depressive disorders (19,68,69). Exercise interventions for treating clinical depression have primarily used aerobic exercise (*e.g.*, walking, running, cycling), although some reports indicate that programs of resistance training are just as effective (68,69). Most programs have used exercise programs involving three 30- to 45-minute bouts of aerobic exercise per week at 60%–80% of maximum HR for 8 weeks (19). However, effects have been reported from a wide variety of exercise programs lasting 1–52 weeks with as few as two to as many as seven bouts per week of sessions lasting

20–90 minutes at intensities of 50%–88% of maximum HR (69). Evidence-based recommendations for exercise prescription for individuals with MDD indicate that a program of aerobic exercise at 50%–85% of maximum HR three to five times per week for 45–60 minutes per session over a minimum of 10 weeks is most beneficial (68). Conversely, an analysis of effects in samples without depressive disorders indicates the greatest reductions in depressive symptoms from exercise programs lasting 4–16 weeks that combine aerobic and resistance training, rather than one or the other, with sessions that last only 20–29 minutes rather than those lasting 45 minutes or more (69). Emerging evidence suggests that biological factors may predispose some, but not others, to experience symptom reduction with exercise (72). More work is needed to confirm and elaborate these findings.

Evidence for the Effects of Exercise on Anxiety

Although sparse, there is some evidence for samples with clinical anxiety. A meta-analysis including only studies that tested exercise as a treatment for anxiety disorders as defined by the *Diagnostic and Statistical Manual of Mental Disorders, 4th edition* (*DSM-IV*) (except for PTSD) found no significant difference between exercise and other treatments (6). Some evidence suggests that resistance training may yield additional benefit of symptom reduction for anxiety disorders. A randomized controlled trial reported the effects of two exercise conditions on a number of characteristic symptoms of GAD (31) and rate of symptomatic remission (30) in a sample of 30 sedentary women (18–39 yr) diagnosed with GAD. Participants engaged in moderate-intensity resistance exercise or aerobic exercise and were matched in terms of their exercise durations and progression. The exercise duration was twice a week for a total of 6 weeks. Both exercise condition improved symptoms, although the magnitude of effect was larger for resistance exercise than for aerobic exercise for most symptoms (31). Additional evidence suggests that remission rates are greater for resistance exercise (60%) than for wait-list control (30%) and aerobic exercise (40%), although remission rates between exercise conditions did not differ significantly (30).

Most of the support of the anxiolytic effect of exercise comes from samples without clinical anxiety. A recent meta-analysis of the effect of acute exercise on state anxiety (22) reported a small effect (ES = .16), corroborating earlier reviews. Another meta-analysis examined anxiety outcomes after physical activity interventions in healthy samples also indicated a small effect (ES = .22) (16). Moderator analyses indicated that programs that were supervised (rather than unsupervised), delivered individually (rather than in groups), and focused solely on physical activity (rather than on physical activity plus another component, such as diet), resulted in greater reductions in anxiety symptoms. Furthermore, programs that encouraged fitness center–based physical activity after program cessation had greater effects than those encouraging home-based physical activity postintervention. Similar effects have been reported for sample individuals who are chronically ill, who may benefit most from shorter training programs that last 12 weeks or less, with exercise sessions that last at least 30 minutes (34).

Exercise professionals face several challenges in prescribing exercise for patients suffering from depression and anxiety. Despite a wide body of evidence supporting the use of exercise as a treatment for depression and a growing literature regarding anxiety, general practitioners may still be unaware of the effectiveness of using exercise as a treatment strategy for mental distress (73). Those with high anxiety sensitivity, particularly those with panic disorder, may be more likely to experience the physiological arousal of exercise as unpleasant, embarrassing, or even dangerous. Chronic SNS activation may make even modest exercise-induced stimulation feel excessive and unpleasant rather than invigorating. Anxious individuals may also worry about the possibility of injury or other negative outcomes. Nonadherence to therapy is a primary issue for those with depression (41). Patients with depression typically focus on barriers to activity, leaving them overwhelmed and resulting in low self-efficacy for exercise. They also tend to exhibit "all-or-none" thinking and respond quickly to challenges with frustration and self-criticism, making them more likely to give up or drop out (74). Dealing with the cognitively based motivational factors specific to depression and anxiety requires interpersonal skill, sensitivity, and patience. Anticipating and making allowances for cognitively based motivational barriers to progress when initiating exercise programs is especially important for adherence to therapy in populations of those who are mentally ill. Strategies used in behavioral therapy, such as goal setting, action planning, and identification and modification of negative thoughts, can be applied by exercise professionals to prevent nonadherence to therapy or to reengage patients after relapse to inactivity.

Exercise professionals can use motivational interviewing to help them tailor exercise program development to the individual needs and preferences of the patient and maximize program adherence (49). Motivational interviewing is a brief, patient-centered method to enhance readiness through the exploration and resolution of ambivalence about a targeted behavior change. Motivational interviewing is an evidence-based approach for enhancing adherence to treatment recommendations, as it outperforms traditional advice giving in scientific trials targeting physiological, psychological, and behavioral outcomes (36,70). Exercise professionals interested in applying motivational interviewing to their own practice can seek continuing education opportunities (49). Additional training is recommended as proficiency takes time and practice (60).

Exercise professionals have much to gain from discussing exercise with their patients to determine which of the many benefits of exercise is the most salient and what type of activities each patient prefers. Questions to consider include the following:

- What are your current exercise habits?
- Were you ever more active than you currently are?
- What do/did you like about being physically active?
- What is preventing you from being more active currently? How could you incorporate more exercise into your life?
- What is a realistic first step for you in becoming more active? (74)

Preference and tolerance for exercise intensities should also be addressed, as there is evidence that adherence to exercise depends on how one feels during and after exercise (46). Exercise professionals should be cautious not to prescribe exercise at too great a load, or too fast a progression, as this may exacerbate symptoms leading to nonadherence or dropout. It has been suggested that subjective reports of affective responses to exercise hold promise as a means to regulate and monitor exercise intensity (24) and may be especially useful for highly anxious individuals to promote exercise adherence.

Specific recommendations for supervising exercise training of persons with depression have been published and elaborated elsewhere (63) and are summarized in Box 22.2. Exercise professionals should familiarize themselves with these recommendations and apply them when training patients with depressive symptoms. Corresponding recommendations for exercise supervision in anxious populations have not yet been published; however, recommendations listed for depression can also be applied to work with patients with anxiety. Although there remains a lack of consensus regarding an optimal exercise dose for those suffering from depression and anxiety, the cumulative evidence does indicate that some exercise is better than none. Exercise professionals should aim to help patients achieve recommended levels of exercise (28), although it is important that they prescribe a program of exercise to which the patient with depression or anxiety will most likely adhere. In some cases, that may mean reducing total exercise volume in the initial prescription, and/or delaying training progression.

Box 22.2 Recommendations for Supervising Exercise with Patients with Depression

The following are recommendations for exercise professionals who supervise exercise with patients with depression:

- Be familiar with symptoms of mental distress and have referral sources handy.
- Avoid minimizing the person's feelings or concerns.
- Establish rapport with your patients but have clear boundaries.
- Assess current fitness level and physical activity habits.
- Determine the patient's most salient motivators for exercise.
- Make exercise enjoyable and nonthreatening.
- Make exercise accessible.
- Tailor the exercise program to the individual needs of the patient and encourage personal responsibility by including the patient in the program planning.
- Be prepared for nonadherence to treatment and excuses.
- Encourage increased physical activity beyond the exercise program.
- Watch for sabotage and resistance to change.
- Be aware of what behavior is being reinforced.

Case Study 22-1 Quiz:

Exercise Prescription and Progression Considerations

6. In developing a training program for Mr. Case Study-PH, how many times per week might you recommend he train, and how long each session? What types of exercises or activities might you prescribe? Why?

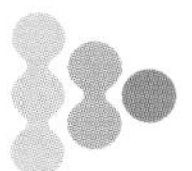

Mechanisms of the Antidepressant and Anxiolytic Effects of Exercise

Several cognitive hypotheses have been presented for the antidepressive and anxiolytic effects of exercise, although there is a dearth of evidence from which to judge their viability. One cognitive hypothesis that has generated some support is that physiological sensations from exercise can help reframe the subjective perception of anxiety-related sensations (12). Another popular explanation with some support is that exercise provides a diversion from stressful stimuli or from depression- or anxiety-provoking thoughts and acts as a "time-out" (5,20). Psychological variables such as self-efficacy (5), self-esteem (33), and personality (86) may mediate or moderate the effects of exercise and exercise on depression and anxiety, although few studies have specifically tested these relationships. More recently, support has been generated for the hypothesis that subjective expectations of the effects of exercise on mood result in a placebo effect (*i.e.*, people expect that exercise will make them feel better and that expectation is partially responsible for their improved mood following exercise). Although studies testing for placebo effects are sparse, the evidence suggests that about half of the psychological effect of exercise is attributable to a placebo effect (53).

It has been suggested that an overall increase in stress resilience may explain the benefits of exercise and exercise for anxiety and depression (71). Several investigations have focused on the cross-stressor adaptation hypothesis, which states that physiological adaptations to the repeated stress of exercise will result in adaptations to the physiological response to mental stress (39). Also, neuroscientific studies using animal models conducted in recent years highlight the central mechanism underlying the hypothalamic–pituitary–adrenal axis adaptations to regular exercise and provide a conceptual backdrop for future directions in human studies (75). Building on evidence of pharmacological effects of antidepressants and benzodiazepines, investigations for the effects of exercise on depression and anxiety focused on functioning of neurotransmitters. Specifically, enhanced 5-HT and neuroendocrine activity in brain areas indicated for animal models of anxiety and depression is supported by a wide body of evidence from animal studies (26,29). Furthermore, human trials support an effect of aerobic exercise training on 5-HT activity similar to the effect of SSRIs (87). Less evidence has been generated for exercise effects on GABA-ergic (transmitting or secreting GABA) and glutaminergic transmission (58). Some evidence points to the benefit of yoga in anxiety reduction corresponding to increased brain GABA levels compared with a metabolically equivalent walking program. Speculation as to the reason for this specific benefit of yoga has been elaborated elsewhere (76,77). There is growing support for a beneficial effect of acute and chronic exercise on BDNF levels, which are associated with improvements in brain function among healthy individuals (79). Furthermore, participation in regular exercise increases resting BDNF levels (ES = .27). This effect is greater for samples with psychiatric disorders (MDD and panic disorder) compared with healthy samples (ES = .40 vs. .19, respectively) (79). **Physical activity** also operates as an anti-inflammatory and antioxidative and nitrogen stress (anti-O&NS) agent, highlighting a possible mechanism through which exercise could exert a positive effect on neuroplasticity, the expression of neurotrophins, and normal neuronal functions, therefore influencing the expression and evolution of anxiety or depressive disorders (29,61). Reductions in depression and anxiety with increased physical activity or after exercise may also be partially explained by mechanisms underlying the effect of exercise on individual symptoms, such as sleep quality (5,32) or energy and fatigue (55). As with the mechanisms proposed in the etiology of depression and anxiety, an exhaustive review of the mechanisms for exercise effects is beyond the scope of this chapter. These and other potential biological mechanisms that have received attention (*e.g.*, dopamine, adenosine, endorphins) have been reviewed elsewhere (5,20,58,63).

SUMMARY

Anxiety and depression are pervasive mental health issues which often go unreported in healthy and special populations. Strong support for a protective effect of regular physical activity against incident depression, and evidence for protection against incident anxiety continues to accumulate. The APA recognizes exercise as an effective first-line treatment for mild depression, and evidence supports the efficacy of exercise as an add-on treatment for moderate-to-severe depression and anxiety symptoms in clinical and nonclinical populations. More work is needed to identify the optimal dose of exercise for symptom reduction, although the existing evidence indicates that some activity is better than none, and participation in physical activity and exercise at levels commensurate with national recommendations is sufficient for alleviating symptoms of depression and anxiety. Mechanisms for these effects remain unclear. The paucity of literature describing the effect of autonomic imbalance on the cardiovascular responses to exercise in depressed and anxious samples reflects a gap in our understanding of the cardiovascular risk associated with depression and anxiety and warrants investigation. The following points are significant:

- Exercise professionals should be familiar with signs and symptoms of depression and anxiety as well as the location and contact information for mental health resources in their area. Community resources as well as emergency resources may both be important to identify. Referral to a mental health care professional should be made for any patient reporting at least moderate symptoms or for whom symptoms persist for more than 2 weeks.
- Special care should be taken by exercise professionals working with patients reporting depression or anxiety to reduce the risk of dropout or nonadherence and to minimize the risk of injury resulting from interactions between exercise and psychoactive medications.
- Exercise professionals working with patients with anxiety or depression should review and apply published recommendations for supervision of exercise for patients with depression (summarized in Box 22.2) to minimize nonadherence to prescribed exercise programs.
- Patients with depression or anxiety should be involved in the development of their exercise prescription. Important information to consider includes which of the many benefits of exercise is most motivationally salient and what properties of physical activity the patients prefer (e.g., preferred intensities or modes).
- Some exercise is better than none for improving symptoms of depression and anxiety. Although exercise professionals should aim to elevate patient exercise levels to the nationally recommended level, reductions in initial work volume and/or delayed progression of an exercise program may be necessary to encourage adherence among patients who report mental distress.

REFERENCES

1. American Psychiatric Association. *Diagnostic and Statistical Manual of Mental Disorders (DSM-IV-TR®)*. 4th ed, text rev. Washington (DC): American Psychiatric Association; 2000. 943 p.
2. American Psychiatric Association. *Diagnostic and Statistical Manual of Mental Disorders (DSM-5®)*. 5th ed. Washington (DC): American Psychiatric Association; 2013. 991 p.
3. American Psychiatric Association. *Practice Guideline for the Treatment of Patients With Major Depressive Disorder* [Internet]. 3rd ed. Washington (DC): American Psychiatric Association; [cited 2016 Mar 4]. Available from: http://www.psychiatry.org/psychiatrists/practice/clinical-practice-guidelines
4. Appelhans BM, Luecken LJ. Heart rate variability as an index of regulated emotional responding. *Rev Gen Psychol*. 2006;10(3):229–40.
5. Asmundson GJ, Fetzner MG, DeBoer LB, Powers MB, Otto MW, Smits JA. Let's get physical: a contemporary review of the anxiolytic effects of exercise for anxiety and its disorders. *Depress Anxiety*. 2013;30(4):362–73.
6. Bartley CA, Hay M, Bloch MH. Meta-analysis: aerobic exercise for the treatment of anxiety disorders. *Prog Neuropsychopharmacol Biol Psychiatry*. 2013;45:34–9.
7. Batelaan NM, Seldenrijk A, Bot M, van Balkom AJ, Penninx BW. Anxiety and new onset of cardiovascular disease: critical review and meta-analysis. *Br J Psychiatry*. 2016;208(3):223–31.
8. Bermudo-Soriano CR, Perez-Rodriguez MM, Vaquero-Lorenzo C, Baca-Garcia E. New perspectives in glutamate and anxiety. *Pharmacol Biochem Behav*. 2012;100(4):752–74.
9. Bernard P, Carayol M. A commentary on the importance of controlling for medication use within trials on the effects of exercise on depression and anxiety. *Ment Health Phys Act*. 2015;9:10–5.
10. Blumenthal JA, Sherwood A, Babyak MA, et al. Exercise and pharmacological treatment of depressive symptoms in patients with coronary heart disease: results from the UPBEAT (Understanding the Prognostic Benefits of Exercise and Antidepressant Therapy) study. *J Am Coll Cardiol*. 2012;60(12):1053–63.
11. Bostwick JM. A generalist's guide to treating patients with depression with an emphasis on using side effects to tailor antidepressant therapy. *Mayo Clin Proc*. 2010;85(6):538–50.
12. Broman-Fulks JJ, Storey KM. Evaluation of a brief aerobic exercise intervention for high anxiety sensitivity. *Anxiety Stress Coping*. 2008;21(2):117–28.

13. Brunes A, Augestad LB, Gudmundsdottir SL. Personality, physical activity, and symptoms of anxiety and depression: the HUNT study. *Soc Psychiatry Psychiatr Epidemiol.* 2013;48(5):745–56.
14. Brunoni AR, Lopes M, Fregni F. A systematic review and meta-analysis of clinical studies on major depression and BDNF levels: implications for the role of neuroplasticity in depression. *Int J Neuropsychopharmacol.* 2008;11(8):1169–80.
15. Chan CMH, Ahmad W, Yusof M, Ho GF, Krupat E. Effects of depression and anxiety on mortality in a mixed cancer group: a longitudinal approach using standardised diagnostic interviews. *Psychooncology.* 2015;24(6):718–25.
16. Conn VS. Anxiety outcomes after physical activity interventions: meta-analysis findings. *Nurs Res.* 2010;59(3):224–31.
17. Conn VS. Depressive symptom outcomes of physical activity interventions: meta-analysis findings. *Ann Behav Med.* 2010; 39(2):128–38.
18. Daley A, Foster L, Long G, et al. The effectiveness of exercise for the prevention and treatment of antenatal depression: systematic review with meta-analysis. *BJOG.* 2015;122(1):57–62.
19. Danielsson L, Noras AM, Waern M, Carlsson J. Exercise in the treatment of major depression: a systematic review grading the quality of evidence. *Physiother Theory Pract.* 2013;29(8):573–85.
20. DeBoer LB, Powers MB, Utschig AC, Otto MW, Smits JA. Exploring exercise as an avenue for the treatment of anxiety disorders. *Expert Rev Neurother.* 2012;12(8):1011–22.
21. Duman RS, Monteggia LM. A neurotrophic model for stress-related mood disorders. *Biol Psychiatry.* 2006;59(12):1116–27.
22. Ensari I, Greenlee TA, Motl RW, Petruzzello SJ. Meta-analysis of acute exercise effects on state anxiety: an update of randomized controlled trials over the past 25 years. *Depress Anxiety.* 2015;32(8):624–34.
23. Freeman JV, Dewey FE, Hadley DM, Myers J, Froelicher VF. Autonomic nervous system interaction with the cardiovascular system during exercise. *Prog Cardiovasc Dis.* 2006;48(5):342–62.
24. Garber CE, Blissmer B, Deschenes MR, et al. Quantity and quality of exercise for developing and maintaining cardiorespiratory, musculoskeletal, and neuromotor fitness in apparently healthy adults: guidance for prescribing exercise. *Med Sci Sports Exerc.* 2011;43(7):1334–59.
25. Gorman JM, Sloan RP. Heart rate variability in depressive and anxiety disorders. *Am Heart J.* 2000;140(4 suppl):77–83.
26. Greenwood BN, Strong PV, Loughridge AB, et al. 5-HT2C receptors in the basolateral amygdala and dorsal striatum are a novel target for the anxiolytic and antidepressant effects of exercise. *PloS One.* 2012;7(9):e46118.
27. Hallgren M, Kraepelien M, Öjehagen A, et al. Physical exercise and Internet-based cognitive-behavioural therapy in the treatment of depression: randomised controlled trial. *Br J Psychiatry.* 2015;207(3):227–34.
28. Haskell WL, Lee I-M, Pate RR, et al. Physical activity and public health: updated recommendation for adults from the American College of Sports Medicine and the American Heart Association. *Circulation.* 2007;116(9):1081–93.
29. Helmich I, Latini A, Sigwalt A, et al. Neurobiological alterations induced by exercise and their impact on depressive disorders. *Clin Pract Epidemiol Ment Health.* 2010;6:115–25.
30. Herring MP, Jacob M, Suveg C, Dishman R, O'Connor P. Feasibility of exercise training for the short-term treatment of generalized anxiety disorder: a randomized controlled trial. *Psychother Psychosom.* 2012;81(1):21–8.
31. Herring MP, Jacob M, Suveg C, O'Connor P. Effects of short-term exercise training on signs and symptoms of generalized anxiety disorder. *Ment Health Phys Act.* 2011;4(2):71–7.
32. Herring MP, Kline C, O'Connor P. Effects of exercise training on self-reported sleep among young women with generalized anxiety disorder (GAD). *Eur Psychiatry.* 2015;30:465.
33. Herring MP, O'Connor P, Dishman R. Self-esteem mediates associations of physical activity with anxiety in college women. *Med Sci Sports Exerc.* 2014;46(10):1990–8.
34. Herring MP, O'Connor PJ, Dishman RK. The effect of exercise training on anxiety symptoms among patients: a systematic review. *Arch Intern Med.* 2010;170(4):321–31.
35. Herring M, Puetz T, O'Connor P, Dishman R. Effect of exercise training on depressive symptoms among patients with a chronic illness: a systematic review and meta-analysis of randomized controlled trials. *Arch Intern Med.* 2012;172(2):101–11.
36. Hettema J, Steele J, Miller WR. Motivational interviewing. *Annu Rev Clin Psychol.* 2005;1:91–111.
37. Hiles SA, Baker AL, de Malmanche T, Attia J. A meta-analysis of differences in IL-6 and IL-10 between people with and without depression: exploring the causes of heterogeneity. *Brain Behav Immun.* 2012;26(7):1180–8.
38. Huang T-T, Liu C-B, Tsai Y-H, Chin Y-F, Wong C-H. Physical fitness exercise versus cognitive behavior therapy on reducing the depressive symptoms among community-dwelling elderly adults: a randomized controlled trial. *Int J Nurs Stud.* 2015;52(10):1542–52.
39. Jackson EM, Dishman RK. Cardiorespiratory fitness and laboratory stress: A meta-regression analysis. *Psychophysiology.* 2006;43(1):57–72.
40. Kalueff AV, Nutt DJ. Role of GABA in anxiety and depression. *Depress Anxiety.* 2007;24(7):495–517.
41. Kangas JL, Baldwin AS, Rosenfield D, Smits JA, Rethorst CD. Examining the moderating effect of depressive symptoms on the relation between exercise and self-efficacy during the initiation of regular exercise. *Health Psychol.* 2015;34(5):556–65.
42. Kemp AH, Quintana DS, Felmingham KL, Matthews S, Jelinek HF. Depression, comorbid anxiety disorders, and heart rate variability in physically healthy, unmedicated patients: implications for cardiovascular risk. *PloS One.* 2012;7(2):e30777.
43. Kessler RC, Angermeyer M, Anthony JC, et al. Lifetime prevalence and age-of-onset distributions of mental disorders in the World Health Organization's World Mental Health Survey Initiative. *World Psychiatry.* 2007;6(3):168–76.

44. Kessler RC, Chiu WT, Demler O, Walters EE. Prevalence, severity, and comorbidity of 12-month DSM-IV disorders in the National Comorbidity Survey Replication. *Arch Gen Psychiatry*. 2005;62(6):617–27.
45. Kleiger RE, Stein PK, Bigger JT Jr. Heart rate variability: measurement and clinical utility. *Ann Noninvasive Electrocardiol*. 2005;10(1):88–101.
46. Kwan BM, Bryan A. In-task and post-task affective response to exercise: translating exercise intentions into behaviour. *Br J Health Psychol*. 2010;15(pt 1):115–31.
47. Labotz M, Wolff TK, Nakasone KT, Kimura IF, Hetzler RK, Nichols AW. Selective serotonin reuptake inhibitors and rhabdomyolysis after eccentric exercise. *Med Sci Sports Exerc*. 2006;38(9):1539–42.
48. Larun L, Nordheim L, Ekeland E, Hagen K, Heian F. Exercise in prevention and treatment of anxiety and depression among children and young people. *Cochrane Database Syst Rev*. 2006;(3):CD004691.
49. Levensky ER, Forcehimes A, O'Donohue WT, Beitz K. Motivational interviewing: an evidence-based approach to counseling helps patients follow treatment recommendations. *Am J Nurs*. 2007;107(10):50–8.
50. Licht CM, de Geus EJ, van Dyck R, Penninx BW. Association between anxiety disorders and heart rate variability in The Netherlands Study of Depression and Anxiety (NESDA). *Psychosom Med*. 2009;71(5):508–18.
51. Licht CM, de Geus EJ, Zitman FG, Hoogendijk WJ, van Dyck R, Penninx BW. Association between major depressive disorder and heart rate variability in The Netherlands Study of Depression and Anxiety (NESDA). *Arch Gen Psychiatry*. 2008;65(12):1358–67.
52. Lichtman JH, Bigger JT Jr, Blumenthal JA, et al. Depression and coronary heart disease recommendations for screening, referral, and treatment: a science advisory from the American Heart Association Prevention Committee of the Council on Cardiovascular Nursing, Council on Clinical Cardiology, Council on Epidemiology and Prevention, and Interdisciplinary Council on Quality of Care and Outcomes Research: endorsed by the American Psychiatric Association. *Circulation*. 2008;118(17):1768–75.
53. Lindheimer JB, O'Connor PJ, Dishman RK. Quantifying the placebo effect in psychological outcomes of exercise training: a meta-analysis of randomized trials. *Sports Med*. 2015;45(5):693–711.
54. Lindholm JSO, Castrén E. Mice with altered BDNF signaling as models for mood disorders and antidepressant effects. *Front Behav Neurosci*. 2014;8:143.
55. Loy BD, O'Connor PJ, Dishman RK. The effect of a single bout of exercise on energy and fatigue states: a systematic review and meta-analysis. *Fatigue Biomed Health Behav*. 2013;1(4):223–42.
56. Martinowich K, Manji H, Lu B. New insights into BDNF function in depression and anxiety. *Nat Neurosci*. 2007;10(9):1089–93.
57. Medina JL, Jacquart J, Smits JAJ. Optimizing the exercise prescription for depression: the search for biomarkers of response. *Curr Opin Psychol*. 2015;4:43–7.
58. Meeusen R, Piacentini MF, Meirleir KD. Brain microdialysis in exercise research. *Sports Med*. 2001;31(14):965–83.
59. Miller AH, Maletic V, Raison CL. Inflammation and its discontents: the role of cytokines in the pathophysiology of major depression. *Biol Psychiatry*. 2009;65(9):732–41.
60. Miller WR, Yahne CE, Moyers TB, Martinez J, Pirritano M. A randomized trial of methods to help clinicians learn motivational interviewing. *J Consult Clin Psychol*. 2004;72(6):1050–62.
61. Moylan S, Eyre H, Maes M, Baune B, Jacka F, Berk M. Exercising the worry away: how inflammation, oxidative and nitrogen stress mediates the beneficial effect of physical activity on anxiety disorder symptoms and behaviours. *Neurosci Biobehav Rev*. 2013;37(4):573–84.
62. Nikolaus S, Antke C, Beu M, Müller H-W. Cortical GABA, striatal dopamine and midbrain serotonin as the key players in compulsive and anxiety disorders — results from in vivo imaging studies. *Rev Neurosci*. 2010;21(2):119–39.
63. O'Neal HA, Dunn AL, Martinsen EW. Depression and exercise. *Int J Sport Psychol*. 2000;31:110–35.
64. Papasavvas T, Bonow RO, Alhashemi M, Micklewright D. Depression symptom severity and cardiorespiratory fitness in healthy and depressed adults: a systematic review and meta-analysis. *Sports Med*. 2016;46(2):219–30.
65. Physical Activity Guidelines Advisory Committee. *Physical Activity Guidelines Advisory Committee Report, 2008*. Washington (DC): U.S. Department of Health and Human Services; 2008. 683 p.
66. Raison CL, Miller AH. Do cytokines really sing the blues? *Cerebrum*. 2013;2013:10.
67. Reeves WC, Strine TW, Pratt LA, et al. Mental illness surveillance among adults in the United States. *MMWR Surveill Summ*. 2011;60(suppl 3):1–29.
68. Rethorst C, Trivedi MH. Evidence-based recommendations for the prescription of exercise for major depressive disorder. *J Psychiatr Pract*. 2013;19(3):204–12.
69. Rethorst C, Wipfli B, Landers D. The antidepressive effects of exercise: a meta-analysis of randomized trials. *Sports Med*. 2009;39(6):491–511.
70. Rubak S, Sandbaek A, Lauritzen T, Christensen B. Motivational interviewing: a systematic review and meta-analysis. *Br J Gen Pract*. 2005;55(513):305–12.
71. Salmon P. Effects of physical exercise on anxiety, depression, and sensitivity to stress: a unifying theory. *Clin Psychol Rev*. 2001;21(1):33–61.
72. Schuch FB, Dunn AL, Kanitz AC, Delevatti RS, Fleck MP. Moderators of response in exercise treatment for depression: a systematic review. *J Affect Disord*. 2016;195:40–9.

73. Searle A, Calnan M, Turner KM, et al. General practitioners' beliefs about physical activity for managing depression in primary care. *Ment Health Phys Act.* 2012;5(1):13–9.
74. Seime RJ, Vickers KS. The challenges of treating depression with exercise: from evidence to practice. *Clin Psychol.* 2006; 13(2):194–7.
75. Stranahan AM, Lee K, Mattson MP. Central mechanisms of HPA axis regulation by voluntary exercise. *Neuromolecular Med.* 2008;10(2):118–27.
76. Streeter CC, Gerbarg PL, Saper RB, Ciraulo DA, Brown RP. Effects of yoga on the autonomic nervous system, gamma-aminobutyric-acid, and allostasis in epilepsy, depression, and post-traumatic stress disorder. *Med Hypotheses.* 2012;78(5):571–9.
77. Streeter CC, Whitfield TH, Owen L, et al. Effects of yoga versus walking on mood, anxiety, and brain GABA levels: a randomized controlled MRS study. *J Altern Complement Med.* 2010;16(11):1145–52.
78. Stubbs B, Rosenbaum S, Vancampfort D, Ward PB, Schuch FB. Exercise improves cardiorespiratory fitness in people with depression: a meta-analysis of randomized control trials. *J Affect Disord.* 2016;190:249–53.
79. Szuhany KL, Bugatti M, Otto MW. A meta-analytic review of the effects of exercise on brain-derived neurotrophic factor. *J Psychiatr Res.* 2015;60:56–64.
80. Thayer JF, Yamamoto SS, Brosschot JF. The relationship of autonomic imbalance, heart rate variability and cardiovascular disease risk factors. *Int J Cardiol.* 2010;141(2):122–31.
81. van der Heijden M, van Dooren F, Pop V, Pouwer F. Effects of exercise training on quality of life, symptoms of depression, symptoms of anxiety and emotional well-being in Type 2 diabetes mellitus: a systematic review. *Diabetologia.* 2013;56(6):1210–25.
82. Watkins LL, Koch GG, Sherwood A, et al. Association of anxiety and depression with all-cause mortality in individuals with coronary heart disease. *J Am Heart Assoc.* 2013;2(2):e000068.
83. Wegner M, Helmich I, Machado S, Nardi A, Arias-Carrión O, Budde H. Effects of exercise on anxiety and depression disorders: review of meta-analyses and neurobiological mechanisms. *CNS Neurol Disord Drug Targets.* 2014;13(6):1002–14.
84. World Health Organization. Prevalence, severity, and unmet need for treatment of mental disorders in the World Health Organization World Mental Health Surveys. *JAMA.* 2004;291(21):2581–90.
85. Williams SE, Carroll D, van Zanten JJV, Ginty AT. Anxiety symptom interpretation: a potential mechanism explaining the cardiorespiratory fitness–anxiety relationship. *J Affect Disord.* 2016;193:151–6.
86. Wilson KE, Das BM, Evans EM, Dishman RK. Structural equation modeling supports a moderating role of personality in the relationship between physical activity and mental health in college women. *J Phys Act Health.* 2016;13:67–78.
87. Wipfli B, Rethorst C, Landers D. The anxiolytic effects of exercise: a meta-analysis of randomized trials and dose-response analysis. *J Sport Exerc Psychol.* 2008;30(4):392–410.

CHAPTER 23

Special Considerations for Physical and Intellectual Disabilities

INTRODUCTION

This chapter presents background information and special considerations related to **exercise** testing, prescription, and progression for individuals with physical and intellectual disabilities (IDs), including spinal cord injuries (SCIs) and autism.

SPINAL CORD INJURY

The case study that follows describes an adult female who, following a traumatic SCI, received 21 weeks of combined acute and postacute rehabilitation before being discharged and returning to her home. This case study presents guidance for the design of a progressive **aerobic** conditioning, resistance training, **flexibility**, and neuromotor training program with the primary goals of returning to work and improving functional capacity and independence. See Box 23.1 for common terminology related to SCI.

Box 23.1 Terminology for Spinal Cord Injury

- **Tetraplegia**: Impairment or loss of motor and/or sensory function in the cervical segments of the spinal cord resulting in impaired function in the arms, trunk, legs, and pelvic organs (7).
- **Paraplegia**: Impairment or loss of motor and/or sensory function in the thoracic, lumbar, or sacral segments of the spinal cord. Arm function is preserved, but trunk, legs, and pelvic organs may be impaired depending on the neurological level of injury (7).
- **Neurological level of injury**: The most caudal segment of the spinal cord with normal sensory and motor function on both sides of the body as determined by clinical neurological examination (7).
- **Complete injury**: No motor or sensory function is preserved in the sacral segments S4–S5 (124).
- **Incomplete injury**: Some preservation of sensory and/or motor function below the neurological level of injury (7).
- **Spasticity**: Disordered sensorimotor control, resulting from an upper motor neuron lesion, presenting as intermittent or sustained involuntary activation of muscles including clinical presentations of hypertonia, hyperreflexia, flexor and extensor spasms, and clonus (98).
- **Hypertonia**: Abnormality in reflex mechanisms resulting from upper motor neuron injuries leading to altered balance of excitation and inhibition of spinal motor neurons and presenting clinically as persistent, involuntary muscle activity and "stiffness" in the trunk and/or extremities (89,91).
- **Clonus**: Involuntary rhythmic muscle contraction resulting in distal joint oscillations, which may be elicited by a sudden rapid muscle stretch (17,65).
- **Autonomic dysreflexia**: Acute severe paroxysmal hypertension caused by uncontrolled sympathetic activity leading to symptoms such as throbbing headaches, profuse sweating, flushing of the skin, and bradycardia (78). Autonomic dysreflexia is most often associated with spinal cord injuries at or above the level of T5 and if left unattended can become a life-threatening medical emergency.
- **Tenodesis grip**: A normal anatomical action whereby, as the wrist extends, the fingers flex and naturally fall against the thumb in a position of lateral pinch.
- **Heterotopic ossification**: The abnormal formation of calcified tissue within the hip, knee, elbow, or shoulder resulting in limited **range of motion** of the involved extremity (18).

Case Study 23-1

Mrs. Case Study-SCI

Mrs. Case Study-SCI is a 32-year-old female weighing 153 lb (69.5 kg) with a height of 67 in (170 cm). Her **body mass index (BMI)** = 24 kg · m^{-2}. She was injured 4 years ago in a diving accident, which resulted in a C5 burst fracture with retropulsion of bone fragments into the spinal canal. Surgical management of the injury included anterior decompression and stabilization at C4–C6. Following surgery, she was transferred to an out-of-state specialty SCI rehabilitation hospital where she completed 5 weeks of inpatient, 8 weeks of outpatient, and 8 weeks of transitional rehabilitation. No cognitive deficits were indicated following her accident, and she reported being able to follow all directions and commands throughout postacute rehabilitation. Upon discharge, a final neurological examination using the American Spinal Injury Association (ASIA) International Standards for Neurological Classification of Spinal Cord Injury (ISNCSCI) was performed. Results from the examination indicated a C5 neurological level of injury with ASIA Impairment Scale (AIS) classification C indicating motor-incomplete tetraplegia. Mrs. Case Study-SCI demonstrates some partial but very weak motor function in the lower extremities as well as present but impaired sensation below her neurological level of injury. Figure 23.1 provides the detailed motor and sensory scores from her neurological examination.

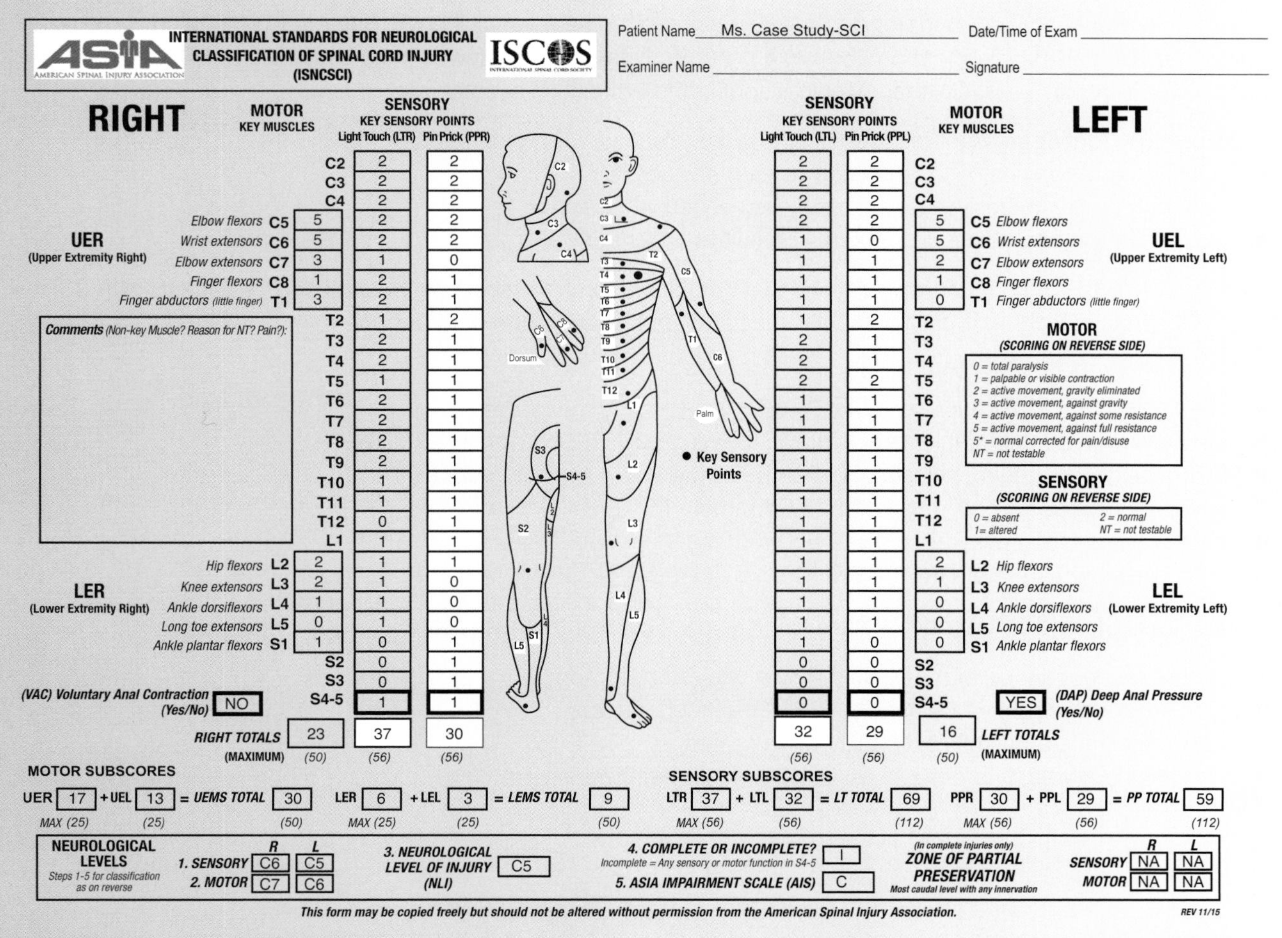

ASIA — AMERICAN SPINAL INJURY ASSOCIATION — INTERNATIONAL STANDARDS FOR NEUROLOGICAL CLASSIFICATION OF SPINAL CORD INJURY (ISNCSCI) — ISCoS

Patient Name: Ms. Case Study-SCI — Date/Time of Exam: ____ — Examiner Name: ____ — Signature: ____

RIGHT Motor Key Muscles	Right Motor	Right Light Touch (LTR)	Right Pin Prick (PPR)	Level	Left Light Touch (LTL)	Left Pin Prick (PPL)	Left Motor	LEFT Motor Key Muscles
		2	2	C2	2	2		
		2	2	C3	2	2		
		2	2	C4	2	2		
Elbow flexors	5	2	2	C5	2	2	5	Elbow flexors
Wrist extensors	5	2	2	C6	1	0	5	Wrist extensors
Elbow extensors	3	1	0	C7	1	1	2	Elbow extensors
Finger flexors	1	2	1	C8	1	1	1	Finger flexors
Finger abductors (little finger)	3	2	1	T1	1	1	0	Finger abductors (little finger)
		1	2	T2	1	2		
		2	1	T3	2	1		
		2	1	T4	2	1		
		1	1	T5	2	2		
		2	1	T6	1	1		
		2	1	T7	1	1		
		2	1	T8	1	1		
		2	1	T9	1	1		
		1	1	T10	1	1		
		1	1	T11	1	1		
		0	1	T12	1	1		
		1	1	L1	1	1		
Hip flexors	2	1	1	L2	1	1	2	Hip flexors
Knee extensors	2	1	0	L3	1	1	1	Knee extensors
Ankle dorsiflexors	1	1	0	L4	1	1	0	Ankle dorsiflexors
Long toe extensors	0	1	0	L5	1	1	0	Long toe extensors
Ankle plantar flexors	1	0	1	S1	1	0	0	Ankle plantar flexors
		0	1	S2	0	0		
		0	1	S3	0	0		
(VAC) Voluntary Anal Contraction (Yes/No): NO		1	1	S4-5	0	0		(DAP) Deep Anal Pressure (Yes/No): YES
RIGHT TOTALS (MAXIMUM)	23 (50)	37 (56)	30 (56)		32 (56)	29 (56)	16 (50)	LEFT TOTALS (MAXIMUM)

UER (Upper Extremity Right); LER (Lower Extremity Right); UEL (Upper Extremity Left); LEL (Lower Extremity Left)

Comments (Non-key Muscle? Reason for NT? Pain?):

MOTOR (SCORING ON REVERSE SIDE)
0 = total paralysis
1 = palpable or visible contraction
2 = active movement, gravity eliminated
3 = active movement, against gravity
4 = active movement, against some resistance
5 = active movement, against full resistance
5* = normal corrected for pain/disuse
NT = not testable

SENSORY (SCORING ON REVERSE SIDE)
0 = absent; 1 = altered; 2 = normal; NT = not testable

• Key Sensory Points

MOTOR SUBSCORES
UER 17 + UEL 13 = UEMS TOTAL 30 — MAX (25) (25) (50)
LER 6 + LEL 3 = LEMS TOTAL 9 — MAX (25) (25) (50)

SENSORY SUBSCORES
LTR 37 + LTL 32 = LT TOTAL 69 — MAX (56) (56) (112)
PPR 30 + PPL 29 = PP TOTAL 59 — MAX (56) (56) (112)

NEUROLOGICAL LEVELS (Steps 1-5 for classification as on reverse)

	R	L
1. SENSORY	C6	C5
2. MOTOR	C7	C6

3. NEUROLOGICAL LEVEL OF INJURY (NLI): C5
4. COMPLETE OR INCOMPLETE? I (Incomplete = Any sensory or motor function in S4-5)
5. ASIA IMPAIRMENT SCALE (AIS): C

ZONE OF PARTIAL PRESERVATION (In complete injuries only) — Most caudal level with any innervation

	R	L
SENSORY	NA	NA
MOTOR	NA	NA

This form may be copied freely but should not be altered without permission from the American Spinal Injury Association. REV 11/15

FIGURE 23.1. ASIA ISNCSCI examination results for Mrs. Case Study-SCI at discharge from rehabilitation. (From American Spinal Injury Association. *International Standards for Neurological Classification of Spinal Cord Injury (ISNCSCI)*. Atlanta [GA]: American Spinal Injury Association; 2015.)

(continues)

Case Study 23-1 (continued)

Mrs. Case Study-SCI reports that she uses a manual wheelchair with power-assisted wheels as her primary means of mobility and lives with her husband in a small, rural community in the Midwest United States. Her home has been modified and made accessible to accommodate her needs. When pushing her wheelchair over long distances or uphill, she complains of arm muscle fatigue, shoulder pain, dizziness, and shortness of breath. She reports feeling "out of shape," and her posture appears kyphotic with rounded shoulders, forward head, and protruding abdomen. In addition, she reports experiencing "stiffness" in the hip and knee extensors as well as the ankle plantar flexors when transferring to and from her wheelchair. Both parents are living and in good health and occasionally assist her with **activities of daily living (ADL)** when her husband is unavailable. Mrs. Case Study-SCI indicated that she smokes infrequently during social occasions, and although she was given a home exercise program and desires to be more physically active, she has not participated in a structured exercise program since discharge from transitional rehabilitation. Upon inquiry, she states lack of energy, lack of accessible facilities in her area, and limited knowledge of appropriate exercises as barriers to exercise participation. She owns an assistive standing device (*i.e.*, an EasyStride standing frame), which she uses to stand approximately 45–60 minutes per day, as well as resistance bands and wrist weights in 2-, 4-, and 6-lb (.90-, 1.81-, and 2.72-kg) increments. On occasion, she notes feeling light-headed and dizzy when moving from a prone to seated or standing position but only when she does not take her orally prescribed 10-mg dose of midodrine.

Three years ago, she completed a course of bisphosphonate (Didronel [etidronate disodium]) and nonsteroidal anti-inflammatory drug (*i.e.*, NSAID [indomethacin]) to treat bilateral hip heterotopic ossification (HO). Her most recent x-ray identified mild, nonprogressive HO inferior to the right femoral neck. She reports being on a consistent bowel and bladder management program and is currently taking the following medications to manage neuropathic pain, lower extremity spasticity, neurogenic bladder, and orthostatic hypotension:

- Imipramine (antidepressant/bladder incontinence): 50 mg orally once per day
- Baclofen (antispasmodic): 20 mg orally three times per day
- Midodrine (antihypotensive): 10 mg orally as needed when active
- Gabapentin (neuropathic pain): 300 mg orally two times per day

See Table 23.1 for common medications that are used to manage secondary conditions for patients with SCI.

Baseline blood work and cardiovascular measures from her most recent annual physical examination revealed the following:

- Total cholesterol: 187 mg · dL^{-1} (4.84 mmol · L^{-1})
- Low-density lipoprotein cholesterol (LDL-C): 103 mg · dL^{-1} (2.67 mmol · L^{-1})
- High-density lipoprotein cholesterol (HDL-C): 35 mg · dL^{-1} (1.35 mmol · L^{-1})
- Fasting blood glucose: 107 mg · dL^{-1} (5.94 mmol · L^{-1})
- Seated resting blood pressure (BP): 94/60 mm Hg
- Seated resting heart rate (HR): 68 bpm

Mrs. Case Study-SCI described the following as her health and fitness goals:

- Improve independence with ADL so that she can return to work.
- Learn an exercise routine that she can perform independently.
- Improve balance and limits of stability while seated.
- Decrease body weight in order to assist with mobility and transfers.

Case Study 23-1 (continued)

Table 23.1 Common Medications Used to Manage Secondary Conditions in Spinal Cord Injury

Generic Drug Name/Brand Name	Use or Condition	Common Side Effects
Amitriptyline/Elavil	Antidepressant	Drowsiness, dizziness, blurred vision, weight gain, dry mouth
Imipramine/Tofranil	Antidepressant and neurogenic bladder	Blurred vision, headache, drowsiness, nausea, weight gain/loss
Nortriptyline/Pamelor	Antidepressant and neuropathic pain	Drowsiness, dizziness, blurred vision, weight gain, dry mouth
Carbamazepine/Tegretol	Anticonvulsant and neuropathic pain	Nausea, dizziness, drowsiness, dry mouth
Pregabalin/Lyrica	Anticonvulsant and neuropathic pain	Drowsiness, dizziness, dry mouth, weight gain, swelling in arms/legs
Gabapentin/Neurontin	Anticonvulsant and neuropathic pain	Drowsiness, dizziness, fatigue, ataxia, sedation, loss of coordination
Baclofen/Lioresal	Antispasmodic	Drowsiness, dizziness, muscle weakness, headache, fatigue
Diazepam/Valium	Antispasmodic	Drowsiness, dizziness, fatigue, blurred vision, headache
Dantrolene sodium/Dantrium	Antispasmodic	Drowsiness, dizziness, weakness, fatigue
Tizanidine/Zanaflex	Antispasmodic	Drowsiness, dizziness, light-headedness, weakness, dry mouth
Botulinum toxin/Botox	Antispasmodic/hypertonia	Localized muscle weakness, neck or back pain, shortness of breath
Midodrine hydrochloride/ ProAmatine	Hypotension	Supine hypertension, paresthesia, blurred vision, cardiac awareness, headache
Warfarin sodium/Coumadin	Anticoagulant	Nausea, persistent bleeding following injury, bruising
Enoxaparin sodium/Lovenox	Anticoagulant	Fatigue, persistent bleeding following injury, bruising

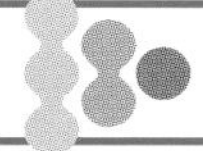

Description, Prevalence, and Etiology

The spinal cord is part of the central nervous system and is composed of longitudinally oriented spinal tracts that lie within the vertebral column. These spinal tracts consist of sensory and motor neurons that make it possible for the brain, body systems, and organs to communicate. Figure 23.2 provides an illustration of the spinal column and spinal nerves and a general description of the major muscle groups associated with each spinal cord segment.

Damage to the neural elements within the spinal canal can have a profound effect on many body systems and can lead to complete or partial loss of motor, sensory, and autonomic function below the spinal cord lesion level. SCIs can occur as a result of traumatic events or non-traumatic pathologies. Common causes of traumatic SCI include motor vehicle accidents, falls,

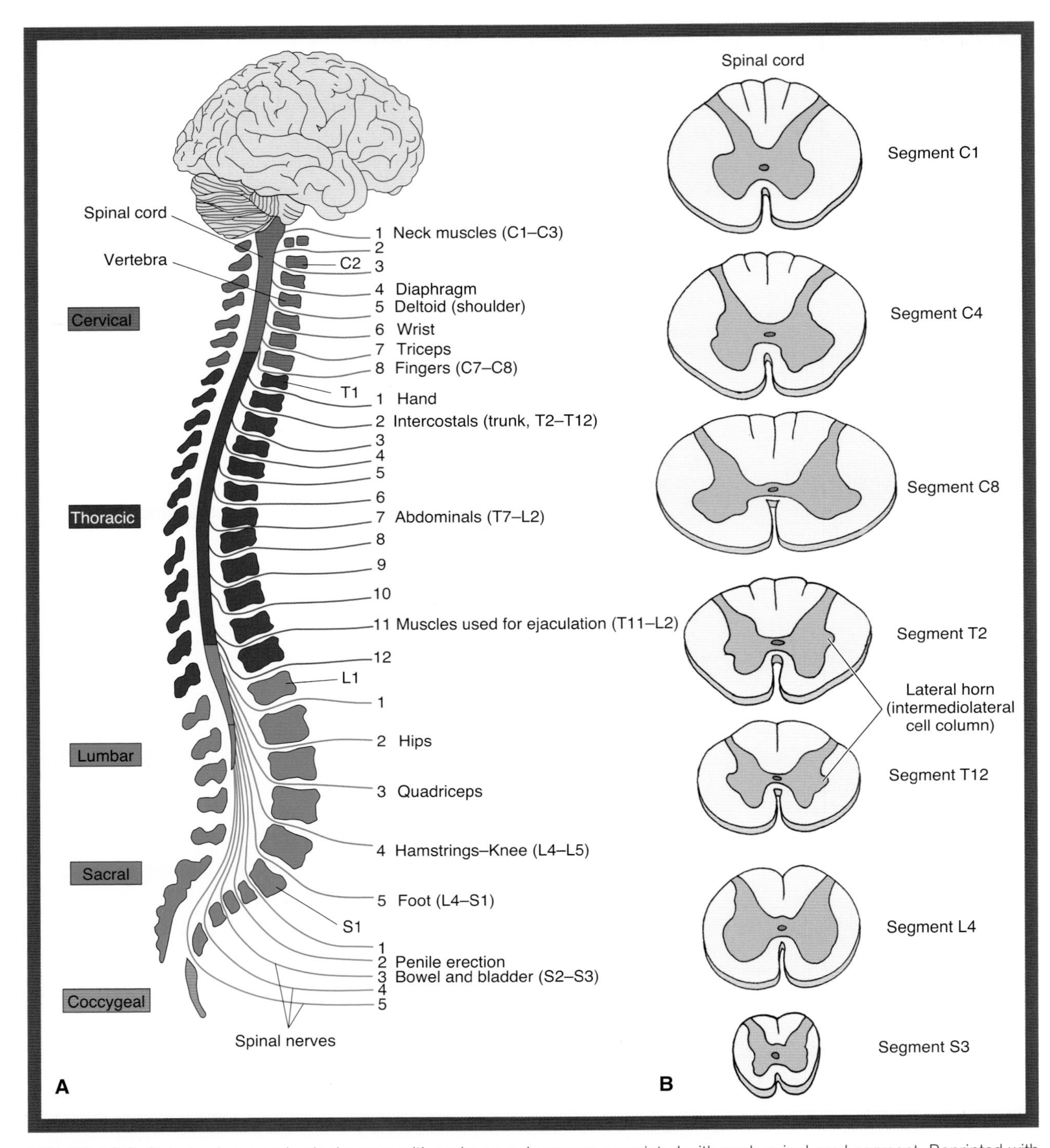

FIGURE 23.2. Spinal column and spinal nerves with major muscle groups associated with each spinal cord segment. Reprinted with permission from World Health Organization (WHO). From: Bickenbach J, et al. (2013) World Health Organization and The International Spinal Cord Society , International Perspectives on Spinal Cord Injury (ISCoS).

violence, and occupational or sports injuries (93), whereas causes of nontraumatic SCI include congenital-genetic disorders (*e.g.*, spinal dysraphism, skeletal malformations, hereditary spastic paraplegia) or acquired conditions (*e.g.*, vertebral column degeneration, infectious disease, metabolic and vascular disorders, spinal tumors, inflammatory and autoimmune diseases) (95). The nature and severity of impairments resulting from SCI are dependent on the mechanism, level, and "completeness" of the injury. Injuries to the cervical segments of the spinal cord (C1–C8) result in tetraplegia with impairment or loss of motor and/or sensory function in the arms, trunk, legs, and pelvic organs (bowels, bladder, sexual organs). Injuries to the thoracic (T1–T12), lumbar (L1–L5), or sacral (S1–S5) segments of the spinal cord result in paraplegia and result in impairment or loss of motor and/or sensory function in the trunk, legs, and pelvic organs. Neurological examinations such as the ASIA ISNCSCI are often administered to describe the neurological level and completeness of an injury and to provide a means by which standardized information regarding motor, sensory, and autonomic impairments can be communicated among health care providers. Based on examination findings, individuals with SCI are given an AIS classification based on an "A" to "E" grading system. Table 23.2 provides a description of each AIS grade based on the presence or absence of motor and sensory function below the neurological level of injury.

Globally, the annual incidence of SCI is estimated to be between 250,000 and 500,000 new cases (129). In the United States, it has been reported that SCI is the second leading cause of paralysis and that approximately 12,500 new cases occur each year (28,94). Approximately 59% of these cases involve the cervical spinal segments, and 41% involve the thoracic, lumbar, and sacral segments (94). Although differences in the average age at injury exist between traumatic SCI (15–29 yr) and nontraumatic SCI (60–70 yr), males continue to make up the majority of those who experience an SCI across injury types (28,93,130). Despite advances in emergency medical management and postacute rehabilitation, the life expectancy of persons with SCI remains lower than the general adult population, with two of the major leading causes of premature death associated with diseases of the respiratory and cardiovascular systems (26,93,130).

Owing to altered muscle morphology/physiology, impaired cardiorespiratory function, and increased sedentary time, persons with SCI are likely to experience diminished muscular strength, endurance, and aerobic capacity (70,111). It is well documented that cardiovascular control is altered

Table 23.2 American Spinal Injury Association Impairment Scale Classification

AIS Grade	Degree of Impairment
A	Complete: No motor or sensory function is preserved in the sacral segments S4–S5.
B	Sensory incomplete: Sensory function is preserved below the neurological level of injury including the sacral segments S4–S5. No motor function is preserved more than three levels below the motor level.
C	Motor incomplete: Sensory plus some motor function is preserved more than three levels below the motor level. Less than half of key muscles below the neurological level of injury have a muscle grade ≥3.
D	Motor incomplete: Sensory plus motor function is preserved more than three levels below the motor level. At least half of key muscles below the neurological level injury have a muscle grade ≥3.
E	Normal: Motor and sensory function is preserved and graded as normal.

Adapted from American Spinal Injury Association. *International Standards for Neurological Classification of Spinal Cord Injury (ISNCSCI)*. Atlanta (GA): American Spinal Injury Association; 2015.

after SCI due to disruption of descending input to the autonomic nervous system (ANS), especially for those with complete injuries at or above the level of T5 (125,126). ANS dysfunction can lead to impaired sympathetic regulation of BP, HR, and body temperature. Impaired respiratory function caused by weakness and/or stiffness of the respiratory muscles may also contribute to compromised and limited exercise capacity among persons with SCI (13,126). Further compounding the problem of physical **deconditioning** are low exercise participation and increased sedentary time among those with mobility impairments (88,105). The combination of these factors, along with pathological neuromuscular adaptations associated with SCI (*i.e.*, muscle atrophy, decrease fat-free mass, and increase fat mass) (19,53), can significantly contribute to impaired functional capacity, decreased independence with ADL, increased risk of cardiovascular and metabolic comorbidities, and decreased life expectancy (26,32,112). Consequently, physical deconditioning and its impact on health and function are major concerns for health care providers and for persons living with SCI and should be addressed using evidence-based countermeasures with measurable health and fitness outcomes.

Preparticipation Health Screening, Medical History, and Physical Examination

A detailed investigation into the medical and health history of persons with SCI will likely reveal a number of important factors that may or may not necessitate **medical clearance** but will likely be required in order to determine the most appropriate exercise testing and prescription. Compared with healthy adults and those with other chronic health conditions (i.e., known cardiovascular disease), far less evidence exists regarding the prevalence of adverse events (especially those related to cardiac episodes) during exercise participation among persons with SCI. Although current evidence within this population points to a relatively low risk of serious adverse events during exercise (123,133), it is still necessary to obtain a thorough medical and physical activity history in accordance with the American College of Sports Medicine's (ACSM) recommendations for preparticipation screening with additional consideration given to the injury-specific conditions associated with SCI (24). Self-guided questionnaires, such as the American Heart Association (AHA)/ACSM Health/Fitness Facility Pre-Participation Screening Questionnaire (11) or the revised **Physical Activity Readiness Questionnaire for Everyone (PAR-Q+)** (122), may be useful prescreening tools with the latter containing specific questions concerning SCI. Figure 23.3 provides a general decision tree for preparticipation screening for SCI. Additional considerations unique to exercise participation among persons with SCI have been provided in Table 23.3.

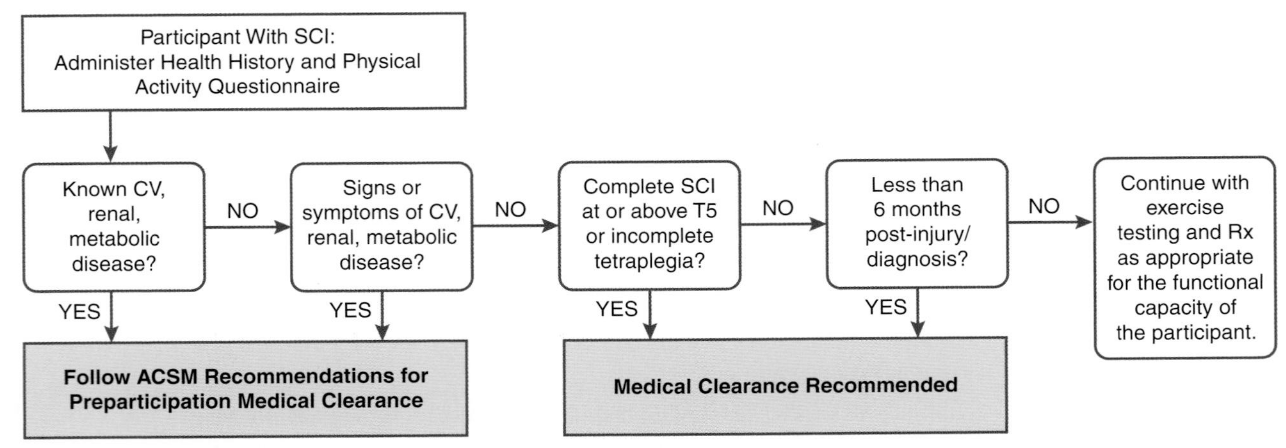

FIGURE 23.3. General preparticipation screening considerations for persons with SCI. CV, cardiovascular; Rx, prescription. (Adapted from Zehr E. Evidence-based risk assessment and recommendations for physical activity clearance: stroke and spinal cord injury. *Appl Physiol Nutr Metab.* 2011;36:S214–31.)

Table 23.3 Spinal Cord Injury Considerations for Exercise Participation

Consideration	Significance
Pharmacological	Persons with SCI will likely be subject to a specific drug regimen. Medications should be assessed and side effects considered prior to exercise testing and prescription. Table 23.1 provides a list of commonly prescribed medications associated with SCI management and their potential side effects. Common conditions for which medications might be prescribed in this population include spasticity, neuropathic pain, orthostatic hypotension, deep vein thrombosis, and neurogenic bladder.
Autonomic dysreflexia	AD is a potentially life-threatening condition often observed in persons with SCI at or above the spinal level of T5 and is most often triggered by noxious stimuli present below the lesion level (78). Impaired ANS function is the primary cause of AD, which leads to unbalanced sympathetic and parasympathetic activity resulting in peripheral and splanchnic vasoconstriction and uncontrolled elevation of BP (*i.e.*, increase in systolic BP ≥ 20–30 mm Hg) (78,89). If left untreated, AD could lead to seizures, stroke, myocardial infarction, pulmonary edema, and death (78). Immediate steps should be taken to address the signs and symptoms of AD (*i.e.*, stopping exercise, sitting upright, and identifying and removing irritating stimuli such as an obstructed catheter/urinary collection device, tight clothing, or braces) (5). If symptoms persist following appropriate countermeasures, emergency medical attention should be sought immediately. Exercise professionals working with persons with SCI, especially those with complete injuries, should be aware of the signs and symptoms of AD, which include paroxysmal hypertension, severe headaches, profuse sweating or flushing of the skin above the injury level, blurred vision, and acute anxiety. Bowel impaction and bladder distention are the most common causes of AD. Persons with SCI should be encouraged to empty their bowel and bladder or urinary bag prior to commencing exercise.
Orthostatic hypotension	OH is a common condition among persons with SCI (especially those with neurologically complete tetraplegia) and typically occurs when an individual changes body position from supine to sitting or sitting to standing. This change can lead to excessive venous pooling in the lower extremities and concomitant decrease in systolic BP of ≥20 mm Hg or decrease in diastolic BP of ≥10 mm Hg (116). The high prevalence of OH observed among persons with SCI has been attributed to impaired sympathetic control, loss of reflex vasoconstriction, impaired skeletal muscle pump, altered baroreceptor sensitivity, cardiovascular deconditioning, and altered sodium and water balance (77). Both pharmacological and nonpharmacological interventions have been suggested as countermeasures to OH. Midodrine hydrochloride is a commonly prescribed hypotensive medication that has demonstrated efficacy for increasing peripheral vasoconstriction and systolic BP during exercise (96). Nonpharmacological management of OH has included the use of abdominal binders, lower extremity stockings or wraps, FES of the lower limb muscles, and passive and active movement of the lower extremities during exercise (90). A history of frequent dizzy/fainting spells, low BP, or shortness of breath during ADL could indicate the presence of uncontrolled OH. Exercise professionals should refer participants to their physician if there are concerns of uncontrolled OH.
Spasticity	Although a consensus definition of spasticity has not been established, it has recently been described as "disordered sensorimotor control, resulting from an upper motor neuron lesion, presenting as intermittent or sustained involuntary activation of muscles including clinical presentations of hypertonia, hyperreflexia, flexor and extensor spasms, and clonus" (88,97). For some, the presence of spasticity can significantly impair functional activities such that walking, transferring, performing ADL, or operating equipment

(continued)

Table 23.3 Spinal Cord Injury Considerations for Exercise Participation *(continued)*

Consideration	Significance
	and devices can become very difficult or unsafe. For others, spasticity may create a more favorable environment in which some lower extremity muscle mass can be preserved or standing and transferring can be facilitated through enhanced activation of muscles in the lower extremities. Questions concerning the presence of spasticity and its impact on function and mobility may be valuable in the preparticipation screening process. Pharmacological treatments for spasticity and its various clinical presentations have included the use of antispasmodic medications (such as baclofen) and direct injection of botulinum toxin (Botox) into hypertonic muscles. Nonpharmacological interventions have included passive and active stretching, limb casting, and whole-body vibration. The presence and severity of spasticity should be considered when determining the most appropriate exercise test and prescription for persons with SCI.
Fracture risk	The rate of bone loss after SCI is substantially greater than that observed in other susceptible populations (14,87). As a result, persons with SCI who wish to participate in weight-bearing activities but present with limited or no recent standing history, complete injuries, longer durations postinjury, and low lesion levels may be at an increased risk for fracture (40,46). Full weight-bearing activities should be restricted to those with a recent uncomplicated history of standing or for whom prior medical clearance for weight bearing has been obtained (5).
Skin breakdown/ pressure ulcers	Pressure ulcers are soft tissue injuries resulting from unrelieved pressure over bony prominences (20). Persons with SCI are vulnerable to skin breakdown due to impaired sensation, prolonged sitting time, and contributing comorbidities such as diabetes and anemia (80). Health and fitness programs may include activities that require frequent transfers to and from the wheelchair as well as access to aquatic exercise facilities. Every attempt should be made to avoid skin damage during exercise activities. Extra foam padding, foldable floor mats, or an individual's personal wheelchair cushion can be placed over hard surfaces to help mitigate any skin pressure, shearing, or friction that might occur during exercise. Although positive fitness benefits can be derived from aquatic-based exercise for persons with SCI (74,113), individuals should be screened for the presence of skin breakdown or pressure ulcers as aquatic exercise may further exacerbate the injury and lead to further skin breakdown and possible infection.
Musculoskeletal	Paralysis and prolonged periods of immobilization can lead to musculoskeletal complications such as joint immobility, stiffness, and instability. Individuals may develop contractures following SCI due to neural and mechanical changes in the soft tissues across joints (59,131). In addition, HO is a complication in SCI characterized by the abnormal formation of bone in the soft tissues surrounding joints such as the hip, knee, or elbow (120). The presence of contractures and HO can adversely affect ROM, personal mobility, and function beyond that which might occur as a result of muscle weakness or paralysis. Muscle test scores from a neurological examination as well as general questions concerning muscle function and preexisting musculoskeletal conditions may reveal the need for adaptive or modified equipment during exercise testing and training (*i.e.*, grasping cuffs, leg/trunk stabilization straps, orthoses, splints, braces). Consideration of musculoskeletal limitations can help ensure that the most appropriate exercise tests and activities are selected based on the level of assistance and adaptive equipment needed to safely perform the desired exercises.

Case Study 23-1 Quiz:

Preparticipation Health Screening, Medical History, and Physical Examination

1. What would be the suggested guidelines regarding preparticipation screening for this patient?
2. Describe the criteria used to justify the final recommendations for exercise participation.

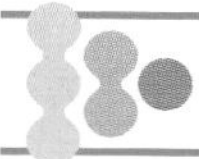

Exercise Testing Considerations

Information obtained during preparticipation screening will be needed to facilitate selection of exercise tests, equipment, protocols, and individual accommodations. Not dissimilar to exercise testing considerations for other populations, test selection for persons with SCI should be based on the individual health and fitness goals and functional limitations of the participant. A general overview of exercise testing considerations in SCI follows. Table 23.4 provides supplementary content relevant to each of the exercise testing domains described in this section.

Cardiorespiratory Fitness Testing

Cardiorespiratory exercise test selection should be determined based on consideration of neurological level of injury, motor completeness, and the extent to which the test allows the participant to utilize the largest muscle mass possible. Upon consideration of these factors, exercise professionals may choose from a variety of cardiorespiratory testing protocols and modalities including continuous, discontinuous, **submaximal**, and **maximal** assessments; however, exercise professionals should keep in mind that formulas used to estimate maximal aerobic capacity from submaximal testing in noninjured populations may not be valid for persons with SCI. Incremental multistage test protocols can be implemented for arm, leg, or combined cycle ergometry as well as recumbent stepping where workloads are increased every 1–3 minutes by increments of 5–10 W per stage for persons with tetraplegia or 10–25 W per stage for persons with paraplegia (5,56). When available, task-specific manual wheelchair tests can be performed using a stationary wheelchair roller system or a **motor-driven treadmill**. For wheelchair athletes, sport-specific **field tests** such as the 12-minute wheelchair propulsion test can be used to estimate peak cardiorespiratory capacity (41,51). Individuals who are ambulatory and present with significant preservation of trunk and lower limb function may be able to perform standardized overground or treadmill-based walking tests (119). It is important to note that individuals with motor-complete SCI above T5–T6 may exhibit lower cardiovascular performance compared to those with lower level paraplegia and motor-incomplete injuries (67,87), and it may be necessary to treat postexercise hypotension and exhaustion with rest, recumbency, and leg elevation following maximal-effort exercise testing (5). In addition to the ACSM's guidelines for healthy adults, exercise test termination criteria for persons with SCI should include any signs or symptoms of autonomic dysreflexia (AD) or orthostatic hypotension (OH).

Body Composition Testing

Field measures of **body composition** (*e.g.*, BMI, skinfold measures, bioelectrical impedance, circumference measures) can be performed relatively quickly and require minimal equipment

Table 23.4 Additional Considerations and Significance of Exercise Testing Among Persons with Spinal Cord Injury

Exercise Testing Domain	Considerations/Significance
Body composition	Spinal cord injury often results in physical, metabolic, and lifestyle changes that can lead to decreased total daily energy expenditure, reduced resting metabolic rate, and reduced thermic effect of activity (30,92,112). Consequently, there is a high prevalence of obesity among persons with SCI, and the risk of developing comorbidities is greater compared to the general population (54,86). Monitoring changes in body composition, although difficult in SCI, could provide exercise professionals with valuable information related to the effectiveness of exercise interventions aimed at combatting overweight and obesity.
Cardiorespiratory fitness	Cardiorespiratory fitness has significant health implications for those with SCI and can be affected by a number of factors including level of injury, severity of injury, degree of physical deconditioning, and extent of ANS impairment (112). Consistent with its use among other populations, results obtained from cardiorespiratory exercise testing in SCI can be used to determine **relative risk** for the development of secondary health conditions, to assist in the development and implementation of the **exercise prescription**, and to establish baseline criteria for the effectiveness of exercise interventions. Specific cardiorespiratory assessment methods, fitness profiles, and norm-referenced data have been reported for persons with SCI (50,56,111); however, clinicians and exercise professionals should use caution when comparing cardiorespiratory fitness outcomes as existing data is limited to specific modes of testing and SCI characteristics (*i.e.*, level and completeness of injury).
Muscular strength and endurance	Muscular strength and endurance testing can provide valuable information regarding changes in physical conditioning and maintenance of strength over time. Because of the heterogeneity within the SCI population, norm-referenced outcomes for **muscular strength** and endurance across all levels of injury and completeness have not been established; however, preliminary reference data has been reported for a small subset of the population (70,111). In the absence of comprehensive norm-referenced data, pre-/posttraining comparisons can be made between the maximum number of completed repetitions or the maximum weight lifted before and after training.
Flexibility	Whether propelling a manual wheelchair or using an assistive device while walking, persons with SCI are likely to rely heavily on the chest, shoulders, and arms for mobility. Assessing and maintaining range of motion across these joints should be a priority for the exercise professional.
Neuromotor	Neuromuscular function and movement quality are significantly and negatively affected as a result of SCI. Similar to aging and frail populations, persons with SCI who ambulate at home or in the community may be at an increased risk of falls due to impaired motor control, balance, coordination, and proprioception (107). Neuromotor training may be an effective strategy for improving skill-related components of fitness and may positively affect the structure and function of key brain and spinal centers involved in cognition and motor task performance, such as walking (2,22,127).

but are often based on specific assumptions regarding fat-free composition that may not be valid in SCI (15,23,112). Laboratory measures may provide greater reliability and validity but often require specialized equipment, are likely to incur greater cost, and may not be easily accessible to exercise professionals and persons with SCI. Recent evidence suggests that predictive equations developed for noninjured populations are a poor fit for those with SCI, and body fat percentage is often significantly underestimated in this population when using field techniques (15,115,132). Dual-energy x-ray absorptiometry may not be the most accessible for all persons with SCI, but the method appears to meet reliability and validity standards, can be less invasive than other measures, and may be obtained in conjunction with routine clinical assessments of bone mineral density.

Muscular Strength and Endurance Testing

Assessment options for muscular strength and endurance among persons with SCI are similar to those found in the general population and include **one repetition maximum (1-RM)**, 10-RM, isokinetic, and **isometric** testing. Special consideration should be given to the level and severity of SCI, the desired muscle(s) to be tested relative to the personal fitness goals, the extent of preserved motor function, the need for adaptive or accessible equipment, and the presence of **range-of-motion (ROM)** limitations due to contracture or HO. Traditional assessments, such as the 1-RM and 10-RM, can typically be performed using equipment found in most fitness centers and can be used to assess muscular strength across single or multiple joints. Functional exercise tests, including the modified push-up, modified pull-up, supine-to-sit, seated depression, and prone-on-elbows press-up, can also be used in conjunction with or as a supplement to traditional muscular strength tests such as the horizontal row, lateral pull-down, and bench press (111,112). For individuals with sufficient sparing of trunk and/or lower extremity muscles, it may be possible to incorporate some specific lower extremity and core **strength** assessments into the test battery (*i.e.*, seated leg press, timed modified prone plank).

Flexibility Testing

For persons with SCI, **flexibility** and adequate joint ROM are essential to maintaining mobility and decreasing the risk of injury. Upper extremity, trunk, and lower extremity ROM can be assessed using a **goniometer** and can be used to identify joint ROM deficiencies that might exist or that may begin to develop over time.

Neuromotor Testing

A number of functional assessments have been used to monitor changes in neuromotor function over time. For individuals with SCI who are ambulatory, standing balance, dynamic reach, and modified agility tests may be valuable tools for tracking functional overground performance. Specific assessments with potential utility for persons with SCI include the four-stage balance test (25), standing reach test (39,125), Timed "Up and Go" (102), the 30-second chair stand test (72), Edgren side-step test (40), and the agility T-test (100). Alternatively, the Thoracic-Lumbar Control Scale (9) may provide a means of assessing functional trunk control and seated balance for persons with limited or no lower extremity muscle activation and who require a wheelchair as their primary means of mobility. Exercise professionals who wish to incorporate tests of balance, agility, coordination, and proprioception will need to thoroughly assess each participant to determine the most appropriate and safest neuromotor assessments.

Case Study 23-1 Quiz:

Exercise Testing Considerations

3. What are the intended actions and their potential impact on exercise testing of the medications prescribed for Mrs. Case Study-SCI?
4. What exercise test protocols would you select for this participant? Justify your answer. Were the exercise tests appropriate for this participant? Why or why not?
5. What safety precaution(s) need to be taken into account for a participant with SCI performing a 1-RM test?

Exercise Prescription and Progression Considerations

Existing evidence supports the notion that participation in regular structured exercise can improve individual components of health- and skill-related fitness in the SCI population (21,38,64,71,76,83,101). Compiling evidence from available systematic reviews, randomized controlled trials, and a recent position statement, frequency, intensity, time, and type (FITT) principles for exercise recommendations in SCI have been provided in FITT table (Table 23.5) (5). The health and fitness goals of persons with SCI are likely to be similar to those in noninjured populations including improved physical conditioning, health outcomes (*i.e.*, weight management, glucose homeostasis, lower cardiovascular risk), muscular strength and endurance, and flexibility (5). Additional benefits might also be derived from exercise participation and include improved mobility, enhanced independence with ADL, prevention of falls and chronic overuse injuries, and improved performance in sports and recreational activities.

In the development of the exercise prescription, it is important to recognize that SCI is a complex condition affecting more than sensory, motor, and autonomic function. Because of the heterogeneity and unique challenges that often exist within this population, it is important to design an exercise program based on the individual intrinsic and extrinsic factors that might affect one's participation and adherence to a recommended exercise program. Individuals with SCI are often faced with a number of unique physical, environmental, and psychosocial challenges that could affect one's ability or desire to engage in exercise or leisure time **physical activity** (33,34,97,99,110). In light of this, the exercise professional is encouraged to take into consideration the World Health Organization's (WHO) framework for the International Classification of Functioning, Disability, and Health (ICF) (129). In using the ICF to support the exercise prescription process, the exercise professional can gain a better understanding of the complex interaction between the individual, their environment, and existing barriers and create a more effective strategy for overcoming obstacles and promoting long-term exercise participation and healthy lifestyle choices (111,112). Figure 23.4 provides a representation of the interactive constructs of the ICF as they might apply to Mrs. Case Study-SCI, including changes in body functions and structures, participation restrictions, activity limitations, and environmental and personal factors.

Numerous exercise strategies have been investigated for their efficacy in improving **cardiorespiratory fitness** among persons with SCI. These interventions have included functional electrical stimulation (FES) cycling, volitional arm and leg cycle ergometry, circuit training, hybrid upper and lower extremity exercise, robotic-assisted training, wheelchair propulsion, and overground ambulation for individuals with sufficient walking function (32,36,43,64,66,68). Cardiorespiratory training recommendations for individuals with SCI include selecting an exercise mode that allows the person to engage the largest muscle mass possible, performing aerobic exercise at an intensity

FITT

TABLE 23.5 FITT RECOMMENDATIONS FOR INDIVIDUALS WITH SPINAL CORD INJURY AND FOR INDIVIDUALS WITH INTELLECTUAL DISABILITY AND DOWN SYNDROME

ACSM FITT Principle of the ExR_x

Chronic Medical Condition	Frequency (How often?)	Intensity (How hard?)	Time	Type (What kind?) Primary	Resistance	Flexibility	Special Considerations
Healthy Adult	≥5 d · wk^{-1} of moderate exercise, or ≥3 d · wk^{-1} of vigorous exercise, or a combination of moderate and vigorous exercise on ≥3–5 d · wk^{-1} is recommended.	Moderate to vigorous. Light-to-moderate intensity exercise may be beneficial in deconditioned individuals.	If moderate intensity: ≥30 min · d^{-1} to total 150 min · wk^{-1}. If vigorous intensity: ≥20 min · d^{-1} to total 75 min · wk^{-1}.	Regular, purposeful exercise that involves major muscle groups and is continuous and rhythmic in nature is recommended.	Muscle strengthening 2–3 d · wk^{-1} (nonconsecutive) Moderate-to-vigorous intensity; 2–4 sets of 8–12 repetitions	2–3 d · wk^{-1}; static stretch 10–30 s; 2–4 repetitions of each exercise	Sedentary behaviors can have adverse health effects, even among those who regularly exercise. Adding short physical activity breaks throughout the day may be considered as a part of the exercise.
SCI	Minimum of 2 d · wk^{-1}; progress to 3 d · wk^{-1} Athletes can increase to 3–5 d · wk^{-1}.	Beginners: moderate intensity (40%–59% HRR) Athletes: 75%–90% HRR	Initially, bouts of 5–10 min alternating with 5-min active recovery periods Gradually increase to at least 20 min per session and decrease or eliminate rest periods.	Engage the largest possible muscle mass: voluntary arm + leg ergometry or FES-LCE and voluntary arm ergometry or rowing, recumbent stepping, arm ergometry, wheelchair ergometry/rollers, or wheeling.	Minimum of 2 d · wk^{-1} Initially, use 20-RM for each exercise. Initially, 1–2 sets of each exercise per session. Gradually progress to 3 sets of 8–10 repetitions. Accessible resistance exercise machines are convenient and safe. If not available, use dumbbells, cuff weights, or elastic bands/tubing.	Daily, especially in presence of joint contracture, spasticity or frequent wheelchair propulsion and manual transfers. Do not allow stretching discomfort >2 on the 0–10 pain scale. Stretch each muscle group repeatedly for 3–4 min · d^{-1}, preferably after warm-up or following training/competition. Active stretching is preferred, but if this is not possible, low-intensity passive stretching may be used by the individual or assistant.	Neuromotor training for this group may be appropriate. Minimum of 2 d · wk^{-1}; progress to 3 d · wk^{-1}. Minimum 20 min per session; progress to 30 min per session. Exercises involving motor skills (*e.g.*, balance, agility, coordination, and gait). Multidimensional activities such as tai chi and yoga may be appropriate when accommodations can be made for functional limitations.

(continued)

FITT

TABLE 23.5 FITT RECOMMENDATIONS FOR INDIVIDUALS WITH SPINAL CORD INJURY AND FOR INDIVIDUALS WITH INTELLECTUAL DISABILITY AND DOWN SYNDROME (*continued*)

Chronic Medical Condition	Frequency (How often?)	Intensity (How hard?)	Time	Type (What kind?) Primary	Resistance	Flexibility	Special Considerations
ID and Down Syndrome	3–7 d · wk^{-1} to maximize caloric expenditure Include 3–4 d · wk^{-1} of moderate- to vigorous-intensity exercise and light-intensity PA on remaining days.	40%–80% $\dot{V}O_2R$ or HRR; RPE may not be an appropriate indicator of intensity in this population.	30–60 min · d^{-1} Intermittent exercise bouts of 10–15 min may be used.	Primary activity is walking. Progression to running using intermittent runs is recommended. Swimming and combined. arm/leg ergometry are also effective.	2–3 d · wk^{-1} Begin with 12 repetitions using 60%–70% 1-RM for 1–2 wk. Progress to 75%–80% of 1-RM; 2–3 sets for major muscle groups. For safety purposes, machines are preferable to free weights.	At least 2–3 d · wk^{-1} but preferably daily with consideration for atlantoaxial instability in the neck. Stretch to the point of tightness or slight discomfort. Hold static stretch for 10–30 s; 2–4 repetitions of static stretch.	Additional encouragement and attention to communication in simple one-step instructions and demonstrations may be particularly important. Medications may affect exercise response. Fall risk may be increased because of motor control, gait, and balance issues.

ExR_x, exercise prescription; FES-LCE, functional electrical stimulation-leg cycle exercise; PA, physical activity; $\dot{V}O_2R$, oxygen uptake reserve.

Based on the FITT Recommendations present in *ACSM's Guidelines for Exercise Testing and Prescription*. 10th ed. Philadelphia (PA): Wolters Kluwer; 2018. 480 p.

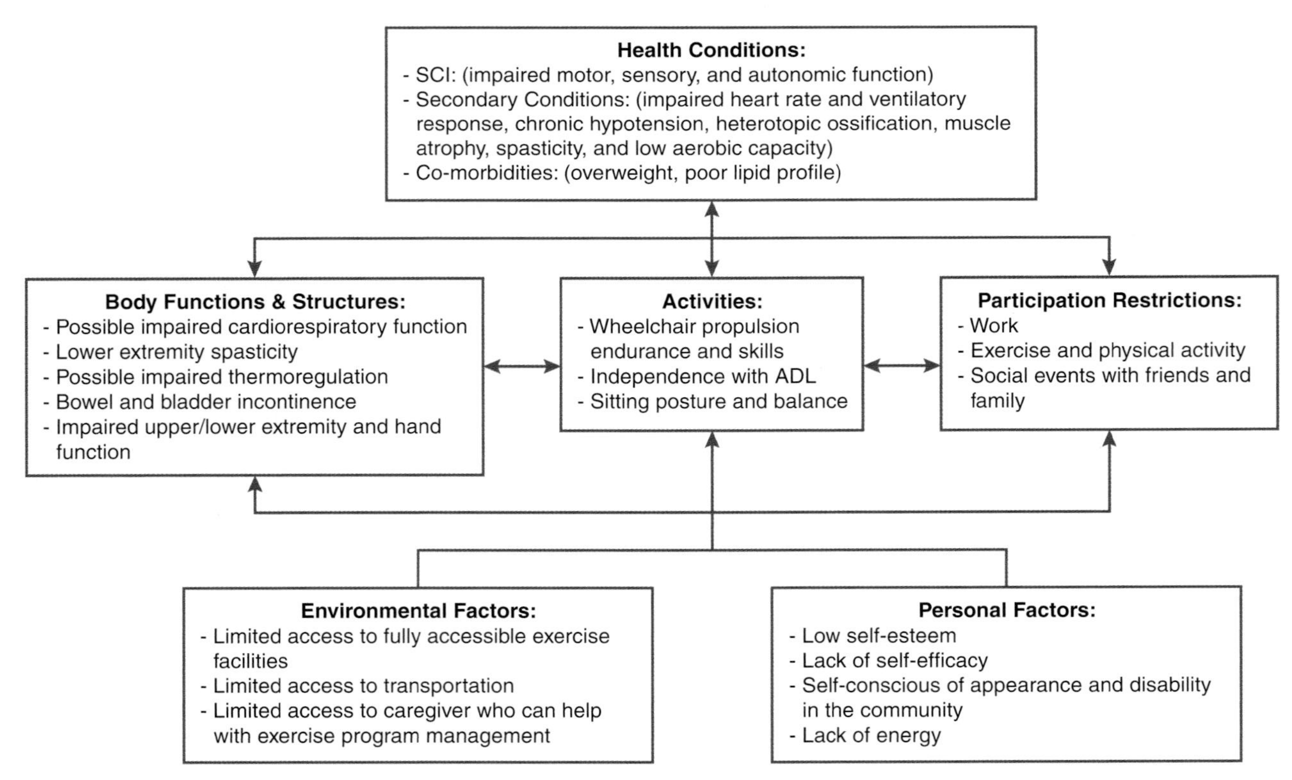

FIGURE 23.4. World Health Organization ICF framework for Mrs. Case Study-SCI. (From World Health Organization. *International Classification of Functioning, Disability and Health: ICF*. Geneva [Switzerland]: World Health Organization; 2001.)

of 40%–59% volume of oxygen consumed per unit time ($\dot{V}O_2$) or heart rate reserve (HRR) for beginners or 75%–90% $\dot{V}O_2$ or HRR for experienced exercisers, and accumulating 20–60 minutes of activity per day, 2–5 days per week. It may be possible to use rating of perceived exertion (RPE) as a basis for exercise intensity in this population; however, caution should be taken as conflicting evidence exists regarding the validity of using subjective measures of exercise intensity to prescribe exercise for persons with higher level motor-complete injuries and for those with greater physical conditioning (52,79,85). In considering exercise mode, it will be necessary to take into account the neurological level and completeness of injury along with other exercise considerations identified in the preparticipation screening process. For persons with motor-incomplete SCI with sufficient residual lower extremity function (*e.g.*, combined ISNCSCI lower extremity motor scores ≥25), consider combined voluntary arm and leg cycle ergometry or recumbent stepping. For motor-complete or individuals with combined ISNCSCI lower extremity motor scores <25, consider voluntary arm ergometry, wheelchair propulsion, or FES-augmented exercise (when available). Hybrid exercise may provide greater cardiovascular benefit compared with voluntary arm exercise or FES-leg cycle ergometry alone due to its ability to activate a larger muscle mass and elicit higher peak and submaximal training values of $\dot{V}O_2$, stroke volume, and cardiac output (10,62,121). For unfit novice exercisers and persons with injuries at or above T5, performing upper extremity exercise may result in peripheral muscular fatigue before exhausting central cardiovascular capacity. In this case, short discontinuous exercise bouts, as opposed to continuous exercise, may be required in order to reach the recommended duration and intensity of cardiorespiratory training.

During exercise, intermittent monitoring of signs or symptoms of OH and AD should take place to ensure patient safety. Individuals with a history of OH may benefit from the use of trunk and/or lower body positive pressure by applying compressive stockings, wraps, or electrical stimulation to the lower extremities; using an abdominal binder; and/or performing exercise in a recumbent position. In addition, individuals with SCI, especially those with higher level injuries, may experience thermoregulatory impairment resulting in reduced heat tolerance, the loss of sweating capacity, and dysfunctional vasomotor control below the lesion level (103). If exercising outdoors in hot and/or humid conditions, individuals with SCI should be encouraged to take time to acclimate to the environmental conditions, wear light sun-protective clothing, use ice vests, maintain hydration, and use mist spray in order to prevent heat illness (8,49,55,108).

Muscular Strength and Endurance Training

Strategies for improving muscle strength and endurance in the SCI population may include the use of free weights, elastic bands, plate-loaded machines, FES, circuit training, and body weight resistance (58,64,101,106,118). When selecting exercise mode, consideration should be given to exercises that target functionally relevant and volitionally activated muscles or muscle groups. For wheelchair users, special attention should be given to shoulder muscle imbalances and to the prevention of musculoskeletal and soft tissue injuries. For example, an emphasis should be placed on strengthening the muscles of the posterior shoulder, scapula, and upper back and stretching the muscles of the anterior shoulder, chest, and elbow flexors (35). Although muscular strength and endurance of the "pushing" muscles should be maintained, exercise professionals should resist overemphasizing exercises that target the anterior shoulder/pectoral muscles, scapular protractors, and internal rotators such as the bench press, chest fly, and rickshaw dips and emphasize "pulling" exercises that target the posterior deltoids, scapular retractors, external rotators of the shoulder, and latissimus dorsi (5).

Resistance training programs for persons with SCI should begin with one to two sets per exercise at a resistance of 15- to 20-RM. As muscle strength and exercise tolerance improves, volume can be increased to three to four sets per exercise and resistance to 5- to 10-RM. Table 23.6 provides a sample resistance training exercise progression for new or returning exercisers. Advanced exercisers and athletes may tolerate more dynamic and sport-specific activities such as ballistic medicine ball exercises, battling ropes training, weighted sled pulls, and wheelchair drills incorporating

Table 23.6 Sample Resistance Training Progression for Persons with Spinal Cord Injury

Week	Tuesday (% RM, Sets × Repetitions)	Thursday (% RM, Sets × Repetitions)
1	Baseline strength testing	50, 2 × 20
2–3	50, 2 × 20	50, 2 × 20
4–5	60–70, 2 × 12–15	60–70, 2 × 12–15
6–7	75–80, 2 × 8–10	75–80, 2 × 8–10
8–9	70, 3 × 12–15	70, 3 × 12–15
10–11	75–80, 3 × 8–10	75–80, 3 × 8–10
12	80, 1 × 8	Follow-up strength testing

power and speed. Exercises performed out of the wheelchair in a seated upright position or while sitting at the edge of a mat with legs extended can introduce an added challenge to seated balance and trunk stabilizing muscles.

Individuals should be properly oriented to the exercise program, and accommodations should be incorporated as per the functional needs of the individual. Both ANS function and medications may affect the physiological response to positional changes. Care should be taken during lifting exercises that involve postural changes, and signs and symptoms of OH and AD should be monitored to ensure participant safety. Indications of OH or AD would require cessation of exercise and additional evaluation and treatment as needed. In addition, caution should be used when transferring to and from the wheelchair to exercise equipment as impaired shoulder function and loss of sublesional sensation may place individuals with SCI at increased risk for repetitive strain injuries and skin damage (61). A well-conceived and successfully implemented resistance training program taking into account the unique considerations within this population can lead to improved functional independence and quality of life for the individual with SCI.

Flexibility Training

Flexibility and the maintenance of adequate joint ROM may be important for mobility, independence with ADL, and the prevention of muscle imbalance and musculoskeletal injury. Although conflicting evidence exists concerning the benefits of stretching in this population, the goals of flexibility training should be aimed at the prevention of contractures, the maintenance of joint ROM in the presence of spasticity, and the promotion or restoration of muscle balance around joints (1,16,57,60). Stretching should be performed daily and should target muscle groups based on the ROM and mobility needs of the individual. For persons who are confined to a seated position, flexibility training should emphasize ROM for the chest, anterior shoulders, shoulder internal rotators, elbow flexors, and trunk flexors. Lower body stretching should also be included for the hip/knee flexors, hip adductors, and ankle plantar flexors, but caution should be taken not to overstretch limbs where impaired sensation exists because this may lead to overstretching and excessive stress on soft tissues and joint structures. During stretching, stabilization of adjacent joints may be needed in order to effectively target the intended soft tissues. ROM progression should be slow and based on pain tolerance (where sensation is present), especially for persons with advanced age, arthritis, contractures, HO, existing repetitive strain injuries, or who have recently returned from a period of bed rest or hospitalization (5).

Special Note: Tenodesis is a normal anatomical action whereby, as the wrist extends, the fingers flex and naturally fall against the thumb in a position of lateral pinch. The tenodesis grip allows individuals to create a functional grasp position in spite of limited activation of hand muscles. It is important to retain the tenodesis effect, so the finger flexor muscles should not be stretched.

Neuromotor Training

Although consensus recommendations for neuromotor training have not yet been established (44), there is mounting evidence supporting the potential benefits of including neuromotor exercise as part of a comprehensive long-term training strategy for improving motor skills, function, and mobility among persons with SCI (12,42,43,73,82,109,114,117). Based on available evidence, neuromotor training may be most beneficial for persons with the capacity to ambulate where targeted interventions may be indicated for impaired standing balance, coordination, proprioception, movement speed, and agility. It has been suggested that neuromotor training performed 2–3 days per week for 20–30 minutes per session may be sufficient to improve balance, muscle strength, and agility and reduce the risk of falls and some lower limb injuries (27,44,48,63,69). A number of underlying mechanisms have been attributed to neuromotor training including increased motor unit recruitment and firing rate, improved reaction time, increased body awareness, and enhanced motor skill acquisition and retention (2,3,29,45,128). Examples of neuromotor exercises for persons with SCI are listed in Table 23.7.

Table 23.7 Sample Neuromotor Training Exercises for Persons with Spinal Cord Injury

Category	Exercise
Mobility Category (Ambulatory)	
Standing agility	Lateral side step
	Braided side step
	Backward walking
	Four-square agility
Stationary standing balance	Single-leg standing balance
	Single-leg forward reach
	Semitandem standing
	Tandem standing balance
Dynamic standing balance	Step-over hurdle
	Lunge with forward reach
	Squat with diagonal reach
Mobility Category (Wheelchair-Dependent)	
Seated balance	Propped sitting dips
	Side push-ups
	Scapular protraction/retraction
	Lateral arm raise
	Forward reach
	Side lean
Mat mobility	Prone on elbows scapular protraction
	Prone on elbows single-arm reach
	Supine on elbows scapular retraction
	Prone-to-supine/supine-to-prone roll

Exercise professionals choosing to incorporate neuromotor training in the exercise prescription should consider the personal goals and functional limitations of the individual along with a thorough risk-to-benefit analysis of each neuromotor exercise being prescribed. Given the pervasive functional limitations and subsequent compensatory strategies often observed in persons with SCI, it is important that participants performing neuromotor exercises be supervised by a trained, qualified exercise professional with experience in monitoring and appropriately correcting for improper body mechanics and joint misalignments that might occur during exercise.

Case Study 23-1 Quiz:

Exercise Prescription and Progression Considerations

6. Compare and contrast the application of the FITT principle in the preceding case study with the recommendations as presented in the FITT table (see Table 23.5). Identify any significant differences and discuss whether you agree or disagree with these different applications of the FITT recommendations. Justify your answer.
7. Can you suggest any other recommendations that would be beneficial for this participant given her goals of improving function, independence, and body composition?

COGNITIVE IMPAIRMENTS

This section provides background information and special considerations for exercise testing, prescription, and progression for individuals with a variety of cognitive impairments such as ID, autism spectrum disorder (ASD), and traumatic brain injury (TBI).

The case study that follows describes the personal health history of a young adult with Down syndrome. The case study provides a guide for exercise testing and development of a progressive aerobic and resistance training program with the primary purpose of ADL, functional skills, and the ability to successfully participate in recreational activities.

Case Study 23-2

Mr. Case Study-ID

Mr. Case Study-ID is a 22-year-old male diagnosed with Down syndrome who is brought to seek personal fitness programming and training at your clinic. His mother has expressed concern for his declining health after a recent checkup with his primary care physician. The checkup showed that the patient is currently at a BMI of 31 kg $\cdot$ m^{-2} (height: 5 ft 6 in, weight: 87 kg). Additionally, his resting BP measured at 142/73 mm Hg and his resting HR measured at 70 bpm. Baseline blood work revealed the following:

- Total cholesterol: 220 mg $\cdot$ dL^{-1} (5.70 mmol $\cdot$ L^{-1})
- LDL-C: 145 mg $\cdot$ dL^{-1} (3.76 mmol $\cdot$ L^{-1})
- HDL-C: 37 mg $\cdot$ dL^{-1} (0.96 mmol $\cdot$ L^{-1})
- Triglycerides: 190 mg $\cdot$ dL^{-1} (2.15 mmol $\cdot$ L^{-1})
- Fasting blood glucose: 123 mg $\cdot$ dL^{-1} (6.83 mmol $\cdot$ L^{-1})
- Glycolated hemoglobin (HbA1C): 6.1% (140 mg $\cdot$ dL^{-1})

Case Study 23-2 (continued)

When asked about the patient's physical activity levels, his mother explains that he participates in a seasonal Special Olympics sports program that meets once a week for several weeks in a season and 1 hour at a time. Otherwise, Mr. Case Study-ID stays at home with hired caretakers while his mother works most days of the week. In terms of other leisure activities, his mother, when she can, takes him for walks around the neighborhood. Recently, however, his mother has been increasingly busy at work, leaving less time to go on these walks. Mr. Case Study-ID typically participates in being sedentary for long periods of time. It is with this complex concern that Mr. Case Study-ID's mother asks for your help in developing an exercise program for him, with goals of weight loss and an increase of muscular fitness. She explains that Mr. Case Study-ID has previous experience and enthusiasm for resistance training through his high school physical education program. She thinks this is a great avenue to take in achieving these fitness goals.

After observing some basic movement patterns performed by Mr. Case Study-ID, such as squat patterns, walking gait, hip hinge, as well as posture, you determine that muscle imbalances are present in the form of a kyphotic posture and pelvic tilt. You later find out that Mr. Case Study-ID also has abnormally lax cervical spinal musculature, inhibiting his neck strength.

Next, 10-RM tests were performed on the seated chest press, seated row, leg press, and leg curl machines. As previously implied, Mr. Case Study-ID chest and leg pressing strength is significantly higher than either his row or leg curl strength, further emphasizing his muscle imbalance. Cardiorespiratory/muscular fitness program notes are as follows:

- Limitations
  - Activities that jar or utilize the head
    - Diving, soccer, contact sports, etc.
  - Exercise experience
  - ROM
- Target areas
  - Exercises to strengthen cephalic musculature
  - Exercises to promote scapular retraction and posture improvement
  - Exercises that balance lumbopelvic hip complex
  - Flexibility/ROM training
  - Work toward achieving the ACSM guidelines for total minutes of moderate-intensity aerobic activity per week
- Cardiorespiratory considerations
  - Frequency: four to five times per week
  - Intensity: moderate intensity (Where cognitive and motor capacity is sufficient for task comprehension and verbal communication, intensity can be estimated using the Talk Test or RPE scale; alternatively, HRR can be determined following the ACSM guidelines for aerobic intensity estimation.)
  - Type: strength training (nautilus machines), aerobic training (high-intensity interval), flexibility training, games: no-impact activities (badminton, etc.)
  - Time: 1 hour per session; 30 minutes weight training, 20 minutes aerobic, 10 minutes flexibility
  - Volume: nautilus and resistance training: (three to five sets of 5–12 repetitions periodized from hypertrophy followed by strength schemes)

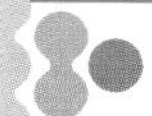

Description, Prevalence, and Etiology

There are a number of different conditions that can affect a person's cognitive functioning, including ID, ASD, and TBI. A person diagnosed with an ID possesses significant limitations in both intellectual functioning and adaptive behaviors in the areas of conceptual, social, and functional skills (4). Some of the common types of ID include Down syndrome, fragile X syndrome, Prader-Willi syndrome, and fetal alcohol syndrome. According to the *Diagnostic and Statistical Manual of Mental Disorders, 5th edition* (*DSM-5*) published by the American Psychiatric Association (6), autism is classified as one of the five pervasive developmental disorders. Based on the *DSM-5*, individuals with autism are characterized by severe and pervasive impairment in reciprocal social interaction; communication; and stereotypical behaviors, activities, and interests. Individuals diagnosed with autism often have sensory issues and may or may not have some degree of ID.

TBI is described as damage to the brain as the result of an injury or blow to the head. Individuals diagnosed with a TBI may possess different cognitive problems inducing arousal, attention, concentration, memory, problem solving, and decision making (75,93). In addition to these cognitive symptoms, individuals with TBI may possess a variety of motor impairments including, but not limited to, paralysis, paresis, ataxia, and dysarthria (motor speech disorder caused by impairment of the motor speech system).

Preparticipation Health Screening, Medical History, and Physical Examination

As with all patients, a detailed investigation into the health history of individuals diagnosed with ID, ASD, and TBI should be conducted prior to participation in a physical activity program. The ACSM recommendations for exercise **preparticipation health screening** can be used for individuals diagnosed with a cognitive impairment (104). Along with a medical history that includes current medications be used, documentation of secondary conditions needs to be addressed. Individuals with cognitive impairments, as described in this chapter, may possess a number of different comorbidities conditions such as seizure disorder, short-term and/or long-term memory issues, sensory issues, and a variety of motor issues. Self-guided questionnaires, such as the AHA/ACSM Health/Fitness Facility Pre-Participation Screening Questionnaire (11) or the revised PAR-Q+ (122), may be useful prescreening tools. Due to the nature of the specific type and severity of cognitive impairment, the patient may need assistance from a parent, guardian, and/or caregiver to accurately complete the questionnaire.

Case Study 23-2 Quiz:

Preparticipation Health Screening, Medical History, and Physical Examination

1. What are the recommendations for preparticipation screening for this individual based upon the ACSM algorithm for moderate-intensity physical activity?
2. What specific comorbid conditions should be considered for their impact on exercise tolerance for this patient?

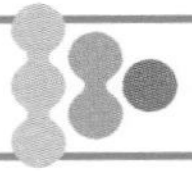

Exercise Testing Considerations

Exercise testing guidelines for individuals with cognitive impairments should follow those recommended for healthy adults wishing to begin a program of moderate-intensity aerobic activity and resistance training (104). For patients with a documented comorbid condition, appropriate modifications should be implemented. For example, some individuals diagnosed with Down syndrome may also have a congenital heart defect present as part of the syndrome. In this case, medical clearance should be obtained, and BP and HR should be monitored during exercise testing.

Table 23.8 Fitness Tests Recommendations for Individuals with Intellectual Disability

Area for Testing	Recommended	Not Recommended
Cardiorespiratory fitness	■ Walking treadmill protocols with individualized walking speeds ■ Schwinn Airdyne using both arms and legs with 25-W stages ■ 20-m shuttle run ■ Rockport One-Mile Fitness Walking Test	■ Treadmill running protocols ■ Cycle ergometry ■ Arm ergometry ■ 1–1.5-mile runs
Muscular strength and endurance	■ 1-RM using weight machines ■ Isokinetic testing ■ Isometric maximal voluntary contraction	■ 1-RM using free weights ■ Push-ups ■ Flexed arm hang
Anthropometrics and body composition	■ BMI ■ Waist circumference ■ Skinfolds ■ Air plethysmography ■ DEXA	
Flexibility	■ Sit and reach ■ Joint-specific goniometry	

DEXA, dual energy x-ray absorptiometry.

From Fernhall B. The young athlete with a mental disability. In: Hebestreit H, Bar-Or O, editors. *The Young Athlete*. Malden (MA): Blackwell; 2008. p. 403–14.

Additionally, some individuals with Down syndrome will be diagnosed with atlantoaxial instability, which is described as a greater-than-normal mobility of the upper two cervical vertebrae (C1 and C2) at the top of the neck. Atlantoaxial instability puts a patient at risk for a potential serious injury if the neck is forcibly flexed (31,84). For individuals diagnosed with TBI, the presence of paresis, paralysis, or spasticity may be presented that can challenge movement and affect balance and flexibility/ROM. Additionally, behavioral and emotional problems may be present in individuals with TBI. For individuals with ASD, sensory issues can interfere with testing and motor delays may or may not be present (81).

For all of the cognitive impairments described, simple and clear verbal directions should be provided along with demonstrations of the exercises that the patients are being asked to perform. The use of visual aids, especially for patients diagnosed with ASD, is going to be helpful, along with precise verbal cues. Additional modifications for a variety of fitness tests can be found in Table 23.8 (5).

Case Study 23-2 Quiz:

Exercise Testing Considerations

3. Was exercise testing necessary for Mr. Case Study-ID? Why or why not?
4. If a congenital heart defect is present, what precautions should be taken during exercise testing?
5. If atlantoaxial instability is present, what precautions should be taken during exercise nesting?

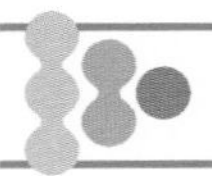

Exercise Prescription and Progression Consideration

When prescribing and monitoring exercise programs for individuals with cognitive impairments, guidelines for healthy individuals can generally be applied. There are, however, a number of factors that should be additionally considered. Obesity is a common comorbidity in individuals with cognitive impairment, in particular, Down syndrome. Low levels of daily physical activity and higher body weights suggest an exercise prescription that emphasizes caloric expenditure, 250–300 minutes per week (5). Exercise intensity can be prescribed and monitored using various self-report exertion scales such as the Borg RPE; however, evidence suggests that, in the presence of moderate-to-severe cognitive deficits, modified and condensed versions of a verbal anchor scale may be needed to accurately reflect changes in exercise intensity among persons with brain injury (37). In addition, the exercise professional should ensure that extra time is given to thoroughly explain the scale and images reflecting the various intensity categories at each level of exertion. Additional explanation and verbal cueing may be needed to ensure that the participant understands exactly what it is that is being asked.

Monitoring cardiovascular biometrics such as BP and HR during exercise would likely yield more accurate reflections of the physiological demands and intensity of the activity being performed by the participant (47). Consequently, an examination of the patient's current medications will be warranted in order to identify any pharmacological effects that may exist with respect to the cardiorespiratory response to exercise. For example, some medications such as β-blockers can have an effect on BP and HR (39). When working with patients with cognitive impairments in an exercise setting, it is important to remember that some patients, depending on the nature and severity of their cognitive impairments, may have difficulties with communication (either verbal or nonverbal), may have impaired short- or long-term memory, and may have limited ability to attend to specific cognitive or motor tasks. Exercise programs should be developed with thorough consideration of these factors.

Determining the best way to communicate, keeping instructions simple, and planning for a variety of activities prior to the training session will afford the patient with the greatest opportunity for success, enjoyment, and improvement of health-related **physical fitness**. Complete FITT guidelines can be found in FITT table (see Table 23.5).

Case Study 23-2 Quiz:

Exercise Prescription and Progression Considerations

6. What weight/resistance exercise should Mr. Case Study-ID begin for upper body?
7. What additional exercises would you recommend that would facilitate Mr. Case Study-ID's participation in Special Olympics or recreational activities?
8. How would you recommend progressing Mr. Case Study-ID's aerobic routine?

SUMMARY

This chapter presents relevant information regarding exercise testing, prescription, and progression recommendations for individuals with SCI and cognitive impairments (ID, ASD, and TBI). Two case studies provided help to clarify the concepts presented.

Spinal Cord Injury

When prescribing exercise and monitoring training sessions for persons with SCI, exercise professionals should remember these key points:

- Knowledge of and access to prior neurological examinations such as the ISNCSCI may be extremely valuable in identifying strengths and impairments that might inform the exercise prescription. Note that not all persons with SCI will have completed a neurological examination in the course of their rehabilitation. Preparticipation screening and participant inquiry will reveal whether examination results are available and can be obtained.
- It is essential that the exercise prescription be based on the personal goals and functional abilities of the individual with additional consideration given to the unique environmental and psychosocial barriers that might limit participation and long-term adherence to the exercise program.
- During exercise, participants should be monitored for signs and symptoms of AD. If present, exercise should be discontinued immediately and countermeasures should be taken to identify and remove any irritating stimuli that might be causing the dysreflexic response.
- Individuals with complete injuries at or above the level of T5 or with incomplete tetraplegia may have impaired ANS function and, as a result, may demonstrate a diminished cardiorespiratory response to exercise. Care should be taken and extra time given to participants when transitioning between exercises and exercise positions to allow the individual the opportunity to accommodate to changes in body position and venous pooling and to minimize the effects of OH.
- Neuromotor training may be a valuable tool for improving functional ability and skill-related components of fitness, and exercise selection should be based on the functional needs of the individual. Performing neuromotor exercises will likely require direct, hands-on supervision in order to ensure safety and maximize effectiveness.

It should be noted that SCI often exists alongside other comorbidities such as diabetes (see Chapter 14), pulmonary disease (see Chapter 17), and aging (see Chapter 9), so the clinician or exercise professional working with this population should be familiar with the exercise testing, prescription, and progressions for a variety of clinical populations.

Cognitive Impairments

When prescribing exercise and monitoring training sessions for individuals with cognitive impairments, exercise professionals should remember these key points:

- Be aware of any secondary conditions that may affect the individual's participation in an exercise program and make appropriate modifications.
- Determine the extent of the cognitive impairment and how it affects the individual's ability to communicate. If needed, work with a parent, guardian, or caregiver to determine the best method for communication.
- Provide simple and precise verbal instructions and verbal cues accompanied by good physical demonstrations as methods to convey important information.
- Plan for a variety of exercises during a training session in order to account for any attentional problems that may be present.

RECOMMENDED RESOURCES

American Spinal Injury Association (ASIA) Learning Center: http://www.asia-spinalinjury.org/elearning/elearning.php
National Center on Health, Physical Activity and Disability: http://www.nchpad.org/Articles/9/Exercise~and~Fitness
Peter Harrison Centre for Disability Sport: http://www.lboro.ac.uk/research/phc/educational-toolkit/
SCI Action Canada: http://sciactioncanada.ca/guidelines/toolkit
Spinal Cord Injury Rehabilitation Evidence (SCIRE): http://www.scireproject.com/rehabilitation-evidence/cardiovascular-health/exercise-rehabilitation-and-cardiovascular-fitness/fun

REFERENCES

1. Adams M, Hicks A. Spasticity after spinal cord injury. *Spinal Cord*. 2005;43:577–86.
2. Adkins D, Boychuk J, Remple M, Kleim JA. Motor training induces experience-specific patterns of plasticity across motor cortex and spinal cord. *J Appl Physiol (1985)*. 2006;101:1776–82.
3. Aman JE, Elangovan N, Yeh IL, Konczak J. The effectiveness of proprioceptive training for improving motor function: a systematic review. *Front Hum Neurosci*. 2015;8:1075.
4. American Association on Intellectual and Developmental Disabilities Web site [Internet]. Washington (DC): American Association on Intellectual and Developmental Disabilities; [cited 2017]. Available from: http://www.aaidd.org
5. American College of Sports Medicine. *ACSM's Guidelines for Exercise Testing and Prescription*. 10th ed. Philadelphia (PA): Wolters Kluwer; 2018. 480 p.
6. American Psychiatric Association. *Diagnostic and Statistical Manual of Mental Disorders*. 5th ed. Arlington (VA): American Psychiatric Association; 2013. 991 p.
7. American Spinal Injury Association. *International Standards for Neurological Classification of Spinal Cord Injury (ISNCSCI)*. Atlanta (GA): American Spinal Injury Association; 2015.
8. Armstrong L, Casa D, Millard-Stafford M, Moran DS, Pyne SW, Roberts WO. American College of Sports Medicine position stand. Exertional heat illness during training and competition. *Med Sci Sports Exerc*. 2007;39(3):556–72.
9. Atkinson D, Atkinson K, Kern M, Hale J, Feltz M, Graves D. Poster 38: reliability of a thoracic-lumbar control scale for use in spinal cord injury research. *Arch Phys Med Rehabil*. 2008;89(10):e18.
10. Bakkum A, Paulson T, Bishop N, et al. Effects of hybrid cycle and handcycle exercise on cardiovascular disease risk factors in people with spinal cord injury: a randomized controlled trial. *J Rehabil Med*. 2015;47:523–30.
11. Balady G, Chaitman B, Driscoll D, et al. ACSM/AHA joint position statement: recommendations for cardiovascular screening, staffing, and emergency policies at health/fitness facilities. *Med Sci Sports Exerc*. 1998;30(6):1009–18.
12. Basso D, Hansen C. Biological basis of exercise-based treatments: spinal cord injury. *PM R*. 2011;3:S73–7.
13. Battikha M, Sà L, Porter A, Taylor JA. Relationship between pulmonary function and exercise capacity in individuals with spinal cord injury. *Am J Phys Med Rehabil*. 2014;93(5):413–21.
14. Bauman W, Cardozo C. Osteoporosis in individuals with spinal cord injury. *PM R*. 2015;7:188–201.
15. Beck L, Lamb J, Atkinson E, Wuermser LA, Amin S. Body composition of women and men with complete motor paraplegia. *J Spinal Cord Med*. 2014;37(4):359–65.
16. Ben M, Harvey L, Denis S, et al. Does 12 weeks of regular standing prevent loss of ankle mobility and bone mineral density in people with recent spinal cord injuries? *Aust J Physiother*. 2005;51:251–6.
17. Beres-Jones J, Johnson T, Harkema S. Clonus after human spinal cord injury cannot be attributed solely to recurrent muscle-tendon stretch. *Exp Brain Res*. 2003;149(2):222–36.
18. Betz R, Murray H, Patel N, et al. Musculoskeletal complications. In: Chhabra H, editor. *ISCoS Textbook on Comprehensive Management of Spinal Cord Injuries*. Philadelphia (PA): Wolters Kluwer; 2015. p. 761–75.
19. Biering-Sørenson B, Kristensen I, Kjaer M, Biering-Sørenson F. Muscle after spinal cord injury. *Muscle Nerve*. 2009;40:499–519.
20. Black J, Edsberg L, Baharestani M, et al. Pressure ulcers: avoidable or unavoidable? Results of the National Pressure Ulcer Advisory Panel Consensus Conference. *Ostomy Wound Manage*. 2011;57(2):24–37.
21. Bochkezanian V, Raymond J, de Oliveira C, Davis GM. Can combined aerobic and muscle strength training improve aerobic fitness, muscle strength, function and quality of life in people with spinal cord injury? A systematic review. *Spinal Cord*. 2015;53(6):418–31.
22. Brach J, Lowry K, Perera S, et al. Improving motor control in walking: a randomized clinical trial in older adults with subclinical walking difficulty. *Arch Phys Med Rehabil*. 2015;96(3):388–94.
23. Buchholz AC, Bugaresti J. A review of body mass index and waist circumference as markers of obesity and coronary heart disease risk in persons with chronic spinal cord injury. *Spinal Cord*. 2005;43(9):513–8.
24. Burr J, Shephard R, Zehr E. Physical activity after stroke and spinal cord injury: evidence-based recommendations on clearance for physical activity and exercise. *Can Fam Physician*. 2012;58:1236–9.
25. Centers for Disease Control and Prevention. STEADI (Stopping Elderly Accidents, Deaths & Injuries) materials for health care providers [Internet]. Atlanta (GA): Centers for Disease Control and Prevention; [cited 2015]. Available from: www.cdc.gov/injury/steadi/materials.html

26. Chamberlain J, Meier S, Mader L, von Groote PM, Brinkhof MW. Mortality and longevity after a spinal cord injury: systematic review and meta-analysis. *Neuroepidemiology*. 2015;44:182–98.
27. Chin Paw A MJ, van Uffelen J, Riphagen I, van Mechelen W. The functional effects of physical exercise training in frail older people: a systematic review. *Sports Med*. 2008;38(9):781–93.
28. Christopher & Dana Reeve Foundation. *One Degree of Separation: Paralysis and Spinal Cord Injury in the United States*. Short Hills (NJ): The Reeve Foundation Paralysis Resource Center; 2009. 28 p.
29. Chung P, Ng G. Taekwondo training improves the neuromuscular excitability and reaction of large and small muscles. *Phys Ther Sport*. 2012;13:163–9.
30. Collins E, Gater D, Kiratli J, Butler J, Hanson K, Langbein WE. Energy cost of physical activities in persons with spinal cord injury. *Med Sci Sports Exerc*. 2010;42(4):691–700.
31. Cooke RE. Atlantoaxial instability in individuals with Down syndrome. *Phys Activity Q*. 1984;1:194–6.
32. Cowan R, Nash M. Cardiovascular disease, SCI and exercise: unique risks and focused countermeasures. *Disabil Rehabil*. 2010;32(26):2228–36.
33. Cowan R, Nash M, Anderson K. Exercise participation barrier prevalence and association with exercise participation status in individuals with spinal cord injury. *Spinal Cord*. 2013;51:27–32.
34. Cowan R, Nash M, Anderson-Erisman K. Perceived exercise barriers and odds of exercise participation among persons with SCI living in high-income households. *Top Spinal Cord Inj Rehabil*. 2012;18(2):126–7.
35. Cratsenberg K, Deitrick C, Harrington T, et al. Effectiveness of exercise programs for management of shoulder pain in manual wheelchair users with spinal cord injury. *J Neurol Phys Ther*. 2015;39:197–203.
36. Davis G, Hamzaid N, Fornusek C. Cardiorespiratory, metabolic, and biomechanical responses during functional electrical stimulation leg exercise: health and fitness benefits. *Artif Organs*. 2008;32(8):625–9.
37. Dawes HN, Barker KL, Cockburn J, Roach N, Scott O, Wade D. Borg's rating of perceived exertion scales: do the verbal anchors mean the same for different clinical groups? *Arch Phys Med Rehabil*. 2005;86:912–6.
38. Duncan PW, Weiner DK, Chandler J, Studenski S. Functional reach: a new clinical measure of balance. *J Gerontol*. 1990;45(6):M192–7.
39. Durstine L, Moore G. *ACSM's Exercise Management for Person's With Chronic Diseases and Disabilities*. 2nd ed. Champaign (IL): Human Kinetics; 2003. 374 p.
40. Fattal C, Mariano-Goulart D, Thomas E, Rouays-Mabit H, Verollet C, Maimoun L. Osteoporosis in persons with spinal cord injury: the need for a targeted therapeutic education. *Arch Phys Med Rehabil*. 2011;92:59–67.
41. Franklin B, Swantek K, Grais S, Johnstone KS, Gordon S, Timmis GC. Field test estimation of maximal oxygen consumption in wheelchair users. *Arch Phys Med Rehabil*. 1990;71(8):574–8.
42. Fritz S, Merlo-Rains A, Rivers E, et al. An intensive intervention for improving gait, balance, and mobility in individuals with chronic incomplete spinal cord injury: a pilot study of activity tolerance and benefits. *Arch Phys Med Rehabil*. 2011;92:1776–84.
43. Galea M. Physical modalities in the treatment of neurological dysfunction. *Clin Neurol Neurosurg*. 2012;114:483–8.
44. Garber C, Blissmer B, Deschenes M, et al. American College of Sports Medicine position stand. Quantity and quality of exercise for developing and maintaining cardiorespiratory, musculoskeletal, and neuromotor fitness in apparently healthy adults: guidance for prescribing exercise. *Med Sci Sports Exerc*. 2011;43(7):1334–59.
45. Gatts S. Neural mechanics underlying balance control in Tai Chi. *Med Sports Sci*. 2008;52:87–103.
46. Giangregorio L, McCartney N. Bone loss and muscle atrophy in spinal cord injury: epidemiology, fracture prediction, and rehabilitation strategies. *J Spinal Cord Med*. 2006;29:489–500.
47. Gigure H, Kelly L. Non-progressive brain injuries. In: Wing C, editor. *ACSM/NCHPAD Resources for Inclusive Fitness Trainer*. Indianapolis (IN): American College of Sports Medicine; 2012. p. 128–39.
48. Gillespie L, Robertson M, Gillespie W. Interventions for preventing falls in older people living in the community. *Cochrane Database Syst Rev*. 2009;(2):CD007146.
49. Girard O. Thermoregulation in wheelchair tennis — how to manage heat stress? *Front Physiol*. 2015;6:175. doi:10.3389/fphys.2015.00175.
50. Goosey-Tolfrey V, Castle P, Webborn N, Abel T. Aerobic capacity and peak power output of elite quadriplegic games players. *Br J Sports Med*. 2006;40:684–7.
51. Goosey-Tolfrey V, Leicht C. Field-based physiological testing of wheelchair athletes. *Sports Med*. 2013;43(2):77–91.
52. Goosey-Tolfrey V, Lenton J, Goddard J, Oldfield V, Tolfrey K, Eston R. Regulating intensity using perceived exertion in spinal cord-injured participants. *Med Sci Sports Exerc*. 2010;42(3):608–13.
53. Gorgey A, Dudley G. Skeletal muscle atrophy and increased intramuscular fat after incomplete spinal cord injury. *Spinal Cord*. 2007;45:304–9.
54. Gorgey A, Gater D. Prevalence of obesity after spinal cord injury. *Top Spinal Cord Inj Rehabil*. 2007;12(4):1–7.
55. Griggs K, Price M, Goosey-Tolfrey V. Cooling athletes with a spinal cord injury. *Sports Med*. 2015;45(1):9–21.
56. Haisma J, van der Woude L, Stam H, Bergen MP, Sluis TA, Bussman JB. Physical capacity in wheelchair-dependent persons with a spinal cord injury: a critical review of the literature. *Spinal Cord*. 2006;44:642–52.
57. Harvey L, Byak A, Ostrovskaya M, Glinsky J, Katte L, Herbert RD. Randomised trial of the effects of four weeks of daily stretch on extensibility of hamstring muscles in people with spinal cord injuries. *Aust J Physiother*. 2003;49:176–81.

58. Harvey L, Fornusek C, Bowden J, et al. Electrical stimulation plus progressive resistance training for leg strength in spinal cord injury: a randomized controlled trial. *Spinal Cord*. 2010;48(7):570–5.
59. Harvey L, Glinsky J, Katalinic O, Ben M. Contracture management for people with spinal cord injuries. *NeuroRehabilitation*. 2011;28:17–20.
60. Harvey L, Herbert R. Muscle stretching for treatment and prevention of contracture in people with spinal cord injury. *Spinal Cord*. 2002;40:1–9.
61. Hasnan N, Engkasan J, Ramakrishnan K, et al. Follow-up after spinal cord injury. In: Chhabra H, editor. *ISCoS Textbook on Comprehensive Management of Spinal Cord Injuries*. Philadelphia (PA): Wolters Kluwer; 2015. p. 897–901.
62. Hettinga D, Andrews B. Oxygen consumption during functional electrical stimulation-assisted exercise in persons with spinal cord injury: implications for fitness and health. *Sports Med*. 2008;38(10):825–38.
63. Hewett T, Myer G, Ford K. Reducing knee and anterior cruciate ligament injuries among female athletes: a systematic review of neuromuscular training interventions. *J Knee Surg*. 2005;18(1):82–8.
64. Hicks A, Martin Ginis K, Pelletier C, Ditor DS, Foulon B, Wolfe DL. The effects of exercise training on physical capacity, strength, body composition and functional performance among adults with spinal cord injury: a systematic review. *Spinal Cord*. 2011;49:1103–27.
65. Hidler J, Rymer W. A simulation study of reflex instability in spasticity: origins of clonus. *IEEE Trans Rehabil Eng*. 1999;7(3):327–340.
66. Hoekstra F, van Nunen M, Gerrits K, Stolwijk-Swüste JM, Crins MH, Janssen TW. Effect of robotic gait training on cardiorespiratory system in incomplete spinal cord injury. *J Rehabil Res Dev*. 2013;50(10):1411–22.
67. Hopman M. Circulatory responses during arm exercise in individuals with paraplegia. *Int J Sports Med*. 1994;15(3):126–31.
68. Hornby T, Kinnaird C, Holleran C, Rafferty MR, Rodriguez KS, Cain JB. Kinematic, muscular, and metabolic responses during exoskeletal-, elliptical-, or therapist-assisted stepping in people with incomplete spinal cord injury. *Phys Ther*. 2012;92(10):1278–91.
69. Hübscher M, Refshauge K. Neuromuscular training strategies for preventing lower limb injuries: what's new and what are the practical implications of what we already know? *Br J Sports Med*. 2013;47(15):939–40.
70. Janssen T, Dallmeijer A, Veeger D, van der Woude LH. Normative values and determinants of physical capacity in individuals with spinal cord injury. *J Rehabil Res Dev*. 2002;39(1):29–39.
71. Jayaraman A, Thompson C, Rymer W, Hornby TG. Short-term maximal-intensity resistance training increases volitional function and strength in chronic incomplete spinal cord injury: a pilot study. *J Neurol Phys Ther*. 2013;37:112–7.
72. Jones C, Rikli R, Beam W. A 30-s chair-stand test as a measure of lower body strength in community-residing older adults. *Res Q Exerc Sport*. 1999;70(2):113–9.
73. Jones M, Evans N, Tefertiller C, et al. Activity-based therapy for recovery of walking in individuals with chronic spinal cord injury: results from a randomized clinical trial. *Arch Phys Med Rehabil*. 2014;95:2239–46.
74. Jung J, Chung E, Kim K, Lee BH, Lee J. The effects of aquatic exercise on pulmonary function in patients with spinal cord injury. *J Phys Ther Sci*. 2014;26:707–9.
75. Katz DI, Ashley MJ, O'Shanick GI, Connors SH. *Cognitive Rehabilitation: the Evidence, Funding, and Case for Advocacy in Brain Injury*. McLean (VA): Brain Injury Association of America; 2006. 28 p.
76. Kim D, Lee H, Lee B, Kim J, Jeon JY. Effects of a 6-week indoor hand-bike exercise program on health and fitness levels in people with spinal cord injury: a randomized controlled trial study. *Arch Phys Med Rehabil*. 2015;96:2033–40.
77. Krassioukov A, Eng J, Warburton D, Teasell R. A systematic review of the management of orthostatic hypotension following spinal cord injury. *Arch Phys Med Rehabil*. 2009;90(5):876–85.
78. Krassioukov A, Rapidi C, Wecht J, et al. Autonomic dysreflexia. In: Chhabra H, editor. *ISCoS Textbook on Comprehensive Management of Spinal Cord Injuries*. Philadelphia (PA): Wolters Kluwer; 2015. p. 814–24.
79. Kressler J, Cowan R, Ginnity K, Nash MS. Subjective measures of exercise intensity to gauge substrate partitioning in persons with paraplegia. *Top Spinal Cord Inj Rehabil*. 2012;18(3):205–11.
80. Kruger E, Pires M, Ngann Y, Sterling M, Rubayi S. Comprehensive management of pressure ulcers in spinal cord injury: current concepts and future trends. *J Spinal Cord Med*. 2013;36(6):572–85.
81. Kutik C, Malone LA. General exercise program design considerations. In: Wing C, editor. *ACSM/NCHPAD Resources for Inclusive Fitness Trainer*. Indianapolis (IN): American College of Sports Medicine; 2012. p. 84–95.
82. Lee G, Bae H, Yoon T, Kim JS, Yi TI, Park JS. Factors that influence quiet standing balance of patients with incomplete cervical spinal cord injuries. *Ann Rehabil Med*. 2012;36:530–7.
83. Lee Y, Oh K, Kong I, et al. Effect of regular exercise on cardiopulmonary fitness in males with spinal cord injury. *Ann Rehabil Med*. 2015;39(1):91–9.
84. Leshin L. Atlantoaxial instability in Down syndrome: controversy and commentary [Internet]. [cited 2003]. Available from: http://www.ds-health.com/aai.htm
85. Lewis J, Nash M, Hamm L, Martin SC, Groah SL. The relationship between perceived exertion and physiologic indicators of stress during graded arm exercise in persons with spinal cord injuries. *Arch Phys Med Rehabil*. 2007;88:1205–11.
86. Libin A, Tinsley E, Nash M, et al. Cardiometabolic risk clustering in spinal cord injury: results of exploratory factor analysis. *Top Spinal Cord Inj Rehabil*. 2013;19(3):183–94.

87. Machač S, Radvanský J, Kolář P, Kříž J. Cardiovascular response to peak voluntary exercise in males with cervical spinal cord injury. *J Spinal Cord Med.* 2016;39(4):412–20.
88. Martin Ginis K, Latimer A, Arbour-Nicitopoulos K, et al. Leisure time physical activity in a population-based sample of people with spinal cord injury part I: demographic and injury-related correlates. *Arch Phys Med Rehabil.* 2010;91:722–8.
89. McKay WB, Ovechkin AV, Vitaz TW, Terson de Paleville DG, Harkema SJ. Long-lasting involuntary motor activity after spinal cord injury. *Spinal Cord.* 2011;49(1):87–93.
90. Mills P, Fung C, Travlos A, Krassioukov A. Nonpharmacologic management of orthostatic hypotension: a systematic review. *Arch Phys Med Rehabil.* 2015;96:366–75.
91. Mirbagheri M, Kindig M, Niu X. Effects of robotic-locomotor training on stretch reflex function and muscular properties in individuals with spinal cord injury. *Clin Neurophysiol.* 2015;126:997–1006.
92. Monroe MB, Tataranni PA, Pratley R, Manore MM, Skinner JS, Ravussin E. Lower daily energy expenditure as measured by a respiratory chamber in subjects with spinal cord injury compared with control subjects. *Am J Clin Nutr.* 1998;68(6):1223–7.
93. National Institute of Neurological Disorders and Stroke. *Traumatic Brain Injury. Hope Through Research.* Bethesda (MD): National Institutes of Health; 2002. 158 p.
94. National Spinal Cord Injury Statistical Center. *Spinal Cord Injury (SCI): Facts and Figures at a Glance.* Birmingham (AL): University of Alabama at Birmingham; 2015. 2 p.
95. New P, Marshall R. International spinal cord injury data sets for non-traumatic spinal cord injury. *Spinal Cord.* 2014;52:123–32.
96. Nieshoff EC, Birk TJ, Birk CA, Hinderer SR, Yavuzer G. Double-blinded, placebo-controlled trial of midodrine for exercise performance enhancement in tetraplegia: a pilot study. *J Spinal Cord Med.* 2004;27:219–25.
97. Nooijen C, Post M, Spooren A, et al. Exercise self-efficacy and the relation with physical behavior and physical capacity in wheelchair-dependent persons with subacute spinal cord injury. *J Neuroeng Rehabil.* 2015;12:103.
98. Pandyan A, Gregoric M, Barnes M, et al. Spasticity: clinical perceptions, neurological realities and meaningful measurement. *Disabil Rehabil.* 2005;27(1–2):2–6.
99. Papathomas A, Williams T, Smith B. Understanding physical activity participation in spinal cord injured populations: three narrative types for consideration. *Int J Qual Stud Health Well-being.* 2015;10:27295.
100. Pauole K, Madole K, Garhammer J, Lacourse M, Rozenek R. Reliability and validity of the T-test as a measure of agility, leg power, and leg speed in college-aged men and women. *J Strength Cond Res.* 2000;14(4):443–50.
101. Pelletier C, Totosy de Zepetnek J, MacDonald MJ, Hicks AL. A 16-week randomized controlled trial evaluating the physical activity guidelines for adults with spinal cord injury. *Spinal Cord.* 2015;53:363–7.
102. Podsiadlo D, Richardson S. The timed "Up & Go": a test of basic functional mobility for frail elderly persons. *J Am Geriatr Soc.* 1991;39(2):142–8.
103. Price M. Thermoregulation during exercise in individuals with spinal cord injuries. *Sports Med.* 2006;36(10):863–79.
104. Reibe D, Franklin BA, Thompson PD, et al. Updating ACSM's recommendations for exercise preparticipation health screening. *Med Sci Sports Exerc.* 2015;47(11):2473–9.
105. Rimmer JH, Riley B, Wang E, Rauworth A, Jurkowski J. Physical activity participation among persons with disabilities: barriers and facilitators. *Am J Prev Med.* 2004;26(5):419–25.
106. Sasso E, Backus D. Home-based circuit resistance training to overcome barriers to exercise for people with spinal cord injury: a case study. *J Neurol Phys Ther.* 2013;37(2):65–71.
107. Saunders LL, Dipiro ND, Krause JS, Brotherton S, Kraft S. Risk of fall-related injuries among ambulatory participants with spinal cord injury. *Top Spinal Cord Inj Rehabil.* 2013;19(4):259–66.
108. Sawka M, Burke L, Eichner ER, Maughan RJ, Montain SJ, Stachenfeld NS. American College of Sports Medicine position stand. *Exercise and fluid replacement. Med Sci Sports Exerc.* 2007;39(2):377–90.
109. Sayenko D, Alekhina M, Masani K, et al. Positive effect of balance training with visual feedback on standing balance abilities in people with incomplete spinal cord injury. *Spinal Cord.* 2010;48:886–93.
110. Scelza W, Kalpakjian CZ, Zemper E, Tate G. Perceived barriers to exercise in people with spinal cord injury. *Am J Phys Med Rehabil.* 2005;84(8):576–83.
111. Simmons O, Kressler J, Nash M. Reference fitness values in the untrained spinal cord injury population. *Arch Phys Med Rehabil.* 2014;95:2272–8.
112. Sisto S, Evans N. Activity and fitness in spinal cord injury: review and update. *Curr Phys Med Rehabil Rep.* 2014;2:147–57.
113. Stevens S, Caputo J, Fuller D, Morgan DW. Effects of underwater treadmill training on leg strength, balance, and walking performance in adults with incomplete spinal cord injury. *J Spinal Cord Med.* 2015;38(1):91–101.
114. Tamburella F, Scivoletto G, Molinari M. Balance training improves static stability and gait in chronic incomplete spinal cord injury: a pilot study. *Eur J Phys Rehabil Med.* 2013;49(3):353–64.
115. Terson de Paleville D, Lorenz D, McCulloch J, et al. Development of protocols to estimate maximal oxygen consumption and body composition in individuals with spinal cord injury. *FASEB J.* 2014;28(1 suppl):884.827.
116. The Consensus Committee of the American Autonomic Society and the American Academy of Neurology. Consensus statement on the definition of orthostatic hypotension, pure autonomic failure, and multiple system atrophy. *Neurology.* 1996;46:1470.

117. Tsang WW, Gao KL, Chan KM, Purves S, Macfarlane DJ, Fong SS. Sitting Tai Chi improves the balance control and muscle strength of community-dwelling persons with spinal cord injuries: a pilot study. *Evid Based Complement Alternat Med.* 2015;2015:523852.
118. Turbanski S, Schmidtbleicher D. Effects of heavy resistance training on strength and power in upper extremities in wheelchair athletes. *J Strength Cond Res.* 2010;24(1):8–16.
119. van Hedel H, Wirz M, Dietz V. Assessing walking ability in subjects with spinal cord injury: validity and reliability of 3 walking tests. *Arch Phys Med Rehabil.* 2005;86:190–6.
120. van Kuijk A, Geurts A, van Kuppevelt H. Neurogenic heterotopic ossification in spinal cord injury. *Spinal Cord.* 2002;40:313–26.
121. Verellen J, Vanlandewijck Y, Andrews B, Wheeler GD. Cardiorespiratory responses during arm ergometry, functional electrical stimulation cycling, and two hybrid exercise conditions in spinal cord injured. *Disabil Rehabil Assist Technol.* 2007;2(2):127–32.
122. Warburton D, Jamnik V, Bredin S, Gledhill N. The 2014 Physical Activity Readiness Questionnaire for Everyone (PAR-Q+) and Electronic Physical Activity Readiness Medical Examination (EPARMED-X+). *Health & Fitness Journal of Canada.* 2014;7(1):80–3.
123. Warms CA, Backus D, Rajan S, Bombardier CH, Schomer KG, Burns SP. Adverse events in cardiovascular-related training programs in people with spinal cord injury: a systematic review. *J Spinal Cord Med.* 2014;37(6):672–92.
124. Waters R, Adkins R, Yakura J. Definition of complete spinal cord injury. *Paraplegia.* 1991;29:573–81.
125. Weiner DK, Duncan PW, Chandler J, Studenski SA. Functional reach: a marker of physical frailty. *J Am Geriatr Soc.* 1992;40(3):203–7.
126. West C, Campbell I, Shave R, Romer LM. Resting cardiopulmonary function in Paralympic athletes with cervical spinal cord injury. *Med Sci Sports Exerc.* 2012;44(2):323–9.
127. Wolpaw J. Spinal cord plasticity in acquisition and maintenance motor skills. *Acta Physiol.* 2007;189:155–69.
129. Wong J, Kistemaker D, Chin A, Gribble PL. Can proprioceptive training improve motor learning? *J Neurophysiol.* 2012;108:3313–21.
129. World Health Organization. *International Classification of Functioning, Disability and Health: ICF.* Geneva (Switzerland): World Health Organization; 2001. 207 p.
130. World Health Organization. *WHO-ISCoS International Perspectives on Spinal Cord Injury.* Geneva (Switzerland): World Health Organization; 2013. 247 p.
131. Yaeshima K, Negishi D, Yamamoto S, Ogata T, Nakazawa K, Kawashima N. Mechanical and neural changes in plantar-flexor muscles after spinal cord injury in humans. *Spinal Cord.* 2015;53:526–33.
132. Yarar-Fisher C, Chen Y, Jackson A, Hunter GR. Body mass index underestimates adiposity in women with spinal cord injury. *Obesity.* 2013;21(6):1223–5.
133. Zehr E. Evidence-based risk assessment and recommendations for physical activity clearance: stroke and spinal cord injury. *Appl Physiol Nutr Metab.* 2011;36:S214–31.

Glossary

2C model Partitions body mass into fat mass (FM) and fat-free mass (FFM) and has the widest application to body composition analysis. This model is limited by the assumptions that water and mineral contents of the body remain constant throughout life and between all individuals and that the density of FFM is constant among all individuals.

Activities of daily living (ADL) Activities such as lifting and carrying groceries, housework, toileting, and care of pets and children as well as grandchildren.

Adolescent A person who has begun puberty but has not yet reached maturation; age ranges from 13 to 18 years.

Aerobic Refers to a physical activity or exercise that requires sufficient oxygen to maintain.

Anthropometry The measurement of the human body using simple physical techniques. Height should be assessed with a stadiometer (a vertical ruler mounted on a wall with a wide horizontal headboard).

Body composition Describes the amount and relative proportions of FM and FFM in the human body.

Body mass index (BMI) Used to assess an individual's mass relative to height (BMI = body mass / height squared; $kg \cdot m^{-2}$). The primary advantages of BMI are that it is a relatively easy measure to obtain and it is useful for categorizing the extent of overweight and obesity in large populations.

Cardiorespiratory fitness The ability to perform large-muscle, dynamic, moderate- to vigorous-intensity exercise for prolonged periods of time.

Child A person in the age range from the first birthday until the beginning of adolescence.

Concentric Movement in which the muscle ends are drawn closer together.

Deconditioning A partial or complete reversal of physiological adaptions to exercise resulting from a significant reduction or cessation of exercise.

Detraining The process that occurs after the cessation of training in which adaptions to exercise are gradually reduced or lost.

Eccentric Movement in which a force external to the muscle overcomes the muscle force and the ends of the muscle are drawn further apart.

Exercise A subset of physical activity performed for the purpose of improving or maintaining physical fitness.

Exercise prescription Individualizing a program for the patient to achieve the goals of enhancing health through a sustainable physical activity program.

Field tests Non-laboratory based tests often performed in the natural setting.

FITT-VP Five components of exercise prescription are reported as Frequency, Intensity, Time, and Type (FITT) with the Volume (V) of exercise added along with the Progression (P) component.

Flexibility The ability of a joint to move through its full range of motion (ROM).

Frequency A component of exercise prescription (see *FITT-VP*).

Functional movement ability Movement through a necessary ROM without incurring pain or limiting performance.

Goniometer An instrument for the precise measurement of angles.

Graded exercise test An exercise test involving a progressive increase in work rate over time that is often used to determine a subject's $\dot{V}O_{2max}$ or lactate threshold.

Hydrostatic weighing (HW; also known as *hydrodensitometry*) Considered the criterion method for body composition.

Inclinometer A device for measuring the angle of inclination of something, especially from the horizontal plane.

Intensity Light-intensity physical activity (*e.g.*, walking) can be defined as requiring <3.0 METs, moderate-intensity physical activity (*e.g.*, jogging) as 3.0–5.9 METs, and vigorous-intensity physical activity (*e.g.*, running) as ≥6 METs.

Isometric Movement in which the ends of the muscle are prevented from drawing closer together, with no change in length.

Light-intensity activity Seated and nonseated activities with an energy expenditure between 1.5 and 3.0 METs.

Maturation The process of reaching the adult or mature state.

Maximal An exercise intensity that is preformed to the point of volitional fatigue.

Maximal oxygen consumption The greatest rate of oxygen consumption of the body measured during dynamic exercise which is determined by maximal cardiac output and maximal arteriovenous oxygen difference.

Medical clearance Approval from a health care provider for an individual to participate in exercise based on the presence of signs or symptoms and/or known cardiovascular, metabolic, or renal disease and his or her current physical activity level.

Metabolic disorder An abnormality or disorder of one of the body's physiological systems, for example: metabolic syndrome, hypertension, and dyslipidemia.

Metabolic equivalent of task (MET) Amount of nutritional energy required to complete an activity or exercise.

Moderate intensity Activities with an energy expenditure of between 3.0 and 6.0 METs.

Motor performance The ability of the neuromuscular system to perform specific motor tasks, including locomotor and object control skills.

Multicompartment models These models divide the body into more than two compartments and require fewer assumptions about the composition of the FFM. Thus, multicompartment models provide more accurate results.

Muscular endurance The time limit of a person's ability to maintain either an isometric force or a power level involving combinations of concentric and/or eccentric muscle actions (SI unit: second).

Muscular power The rate of performing work; the product of force and velocity; the rate of transformation of metabolic potential energy to work or heat (SI unit: watt).

Muscular strength The maximal force or torque a muscle or muscle group can generate at a specified or determined velocity.

Older adult Healthy individuals ≥65 years and/or individuals 50 years through 64 years with disabilities, chronic disease, and/or functional impairments.

One repetition maximum (1-RM) The highest load that can be lifted through a full ROM utilizing correct form one time.

Physical activity Any type of movement produced by the musculature that results in an increase in energy expenditure.

Physical activity domains Include recreation, transport, occupation, and household. *Active living* incorporates exercise, recreational activities, household and occupational activities, and active transportation.

Physical Activity Readiness Questionnaire for Everyone (PAR-Q+) An evidence-based physical activity questionnaire that can be used by qualified exercise professionals to determine if an individual would be placed at risk during exercise based on risk factors and/or signs and symptoms of disease.

Physical fitness A set of attributes (*e.g.*, muscular strength and endurance, cardiorespiratory fitness, flexibility, and body composition) that people have or achieve that relate to the ability to perform physical activity.

Physical inactivity Failure to perform sufficient amounts of moderate and/or vigorous physical activity, as typically determined by *2008 Physical Activity Guidelines for Americans.*

Physical literacy The application of competence, confidence, and motivation to fundamental movement skills and sport-related skills; relies on the building of a "movement vocabulary."

Preparticipation health screening The goals are to (a) identify who should receive medical clearance prior to initiating an exercise program or increasing the frequency, intensity, and/or volume of their current exercise program; (b) identify those with clinically significant disease(s) to determine if they would benefit from participating in a medically supervised exercise program; and (c) identify those with medical conditions who should be restricted from participating in an exercise program until their disease conditions are abated or better controlled.

Range of motion (ROM) Movement potential of a joint.

Rate of force development The capacity to produce maximal voluntary activation of motor units during first 0–200 milliseconds.

Relative risk The risk of an adverse health outcome among a group with a specific condition compared to a group without the condition. For physical activity, relative risk is the ratio of the risk of a disease or disorder when comparing groups of people who vary in their amount of physical activity.

Sarcopenia The degenerative loss of skeletal muscle mass and strength as a result of aging, reduced physical activity, and certain diseases can be assessed.

Sedentary behavior Any waking behavior characterized by an energy expenditure ≤1.5 METs while in a sitting or reclined posture.

Sedentary physiology A subdiscipline of biology dedicated to the study of the body's response to short- and long-term sedentary behavior with a particular focus on identifying unique mechanisms that are distinct from the biological basis of exercising.

Skeletal muscle mass The weight of skeletal muscles in the body, typically decreases with age.

Steady state Condition where the metabolic demands of the body are being met aerobically.

Strength The ability of a muscle or muscle group to continue to perform without fatigue.

Submaximal An exercise intensity that is performed below the anaerobic threshold and allows the body to reach a steady state.

Systematic review and meta-analysis Meta-analysis is a type of review that systematically analyses results from a number of studies on the same topic for the purpose of increasing the power and drawing important and relevant conclusions.

Time A component of exercise prescription (see *FITT-VP*).

Type A component of exercise prescription (see *FITT-VP*).

Vigorous intensity An exercise intensity that elicits a heart rate that is between 76% and 96% of an individual's age-predicted maximal heart rate or between 60% and <90% of heart rate reserve.

Index

Note: Page numbers followed by *b* indicate boxes, those followed by *f* indicate figures, and those followed by *t* indicate tables.

A

D

E

F

G

H

M

N

O

P

Q

R

W

Y